Teaching Atlas
of Brain Imaging

Teaching Atlas
of Brain Imaging

Nancy J. Fischbein, M.D.

Assistant Professor of Radiology
Department of Radiology
University of California, San Francisco
San Francisco, California

William P. Dillon, M.D.

Professor of Radiology, Neurology, and Neurosurgery
Department of Radiology
University of California, San Francisco
San Francisco, California

A. James Barkovich, M.D.

Professor of Radiology, Neurology, Pediatrics, and Neurosurgery
Department of Radiology
University of California, San Francisco
San Francisco, California

2000

Thieme
New York • Stuttgart

Thieme New York
333 Seventh Avenue
New York, NY 10001

Teaching Atlas of Brain Imaging
Nancy J. Fischbein, M.D.
William P. Dillon, M.D.
A. James Barkovich, M.D.

Executive Editor: Jane Pennington, Ph.D.
Editorial Director: Avé McCracken
Developmental Editor: Carol A. Bader
Developmental Manager: Kathleen P. Lyons
Director, Production and Manufacturing: Anne Vinnicombe
Senior Production Editor: Eric L. Gladstone
Marketing Director: Phyllis Gold
Sales Manager: Ross Lumpkin
Chief Financial Officer: Seth S. Fishman
President: Brian D. Scanlan
Cover Designer: Kevin Kall
Compositor: Alexander Graphics
Printer: Maple-Vail

Library of Congress Cataloging-in-Publication Data

Teaching atlas of brain imaging / editors, Nancy Fischbein, William P. Dillon,
  James Barkovich.
      p.   cm.
    Includes bibliographical references and index.
    ISBN 0-86577-862-0. — ISBN 3-13-116341-0
    1. Brain—Tomography—Atlases.   2. Brain—Magnetic resonance
imaging—Atlases.   3. Brain—Tomography—Case studies.   4. Brain—
Magnetic resonance imaging—Case studies.   I. Fischbein, Nancy.   II. Dillon,
William P., 1952-   .   III. Barkovich, A. James, 1952-   .
    [DNLM: 1. Brain Diseases—radiography atlases.   2. Brain Diseases—
radiography case studies.]
RC386.6.T64T43   1999
616.8'04754—dc21
DNLM/DLC
for Library of Congress   98-32391
                                                                                                      CIP

Important note: Medical knowledge is ever-changing. As new research and clinical experience broaden our knowledge, changes in treatment and drug therapy may be required. The authors and editors of the material herein have consulted sources believed to be reliable in their efforts to provide information that is complete and in accord with the standards accepted at the time of publication. However, in view of the possibility of human error by the authors, editors, or publisher of the work herein, or changes in medical knowledge, neither the authors, editors, publisher, nor any other party who has been involved in the preparation of this work, warrants that the information contained herein is in every respect accurate or complete, and they are not responsible for any errors or omissions or for the results obtained from use of such information. Readers are encouraged to confirm the information contained herein with other sources. For example, readers are advised to check the product information sheet included in the package of each drug they plan to administer to be certain that the information contained in this publication is accurate and that changes have not been made in the recommended dose or in the contraindications for administration. This recommendation is of particular importance in connection with new or infrequently used drugs.

Some of the product names, patents, and registered designs referred to in this book are in fact registered trademarks or proprietary names even though specific reference to this fact is not always made in the text. Therefore, the appearance of a name without designation as proprietary is not to be construed as a representation by the publisher that it is in the public domain.

Printed in the United States of America
5 4

TNY ISBN 0-86577-862-0
GTV ISBN 3-13-116341-0

We dedicate this book to T. Hans Newton, M.D. In addition to his numerous other contributions to the field of neuroradiology, Dr. Newton initiated UCSF Neuroradiology Grand Rounds at which many of these cases were presented.

CONTENTS

Preface xiii

Acknowledgments xv

Commonly Used Abbreviations xvii

I. NEOPLASM

  A. Supratentorial

    Case 1.   Grade II Astrocytoma 3

    Case 2.   Gliosarcoma 6

    Case 3.   Oligodendroglioma 10

    Case 4.   Ganglioglioma 13

    Case 5.   Gliomatosis Cerebri 16

    Case 6.   Metastatic Disease 19

    Case 7.   Ependymoma 23

    Case 8.   Dysembryoplastic Neuroepithelial Tumor 26

    Case 9.   Lymphoma (non-AIDS-related) 29

    Case 10. Lymphoma (AIDS-related) 32

    Case 11. Primitive Neuroectodermal Tumor 36

    Case 12. Hamartoma of the Tuber Cinereum 39

    Case 13. Pineoblastoma 42

    Case 14. Germ Cell Neoplasm of Pineal Region 46

    Case 15. Pituitary Microadenoma 49

    Case 16. Pituitary Macroadenoma 52

    Case 17. Rathke's Cleft Cyst 55

    Case 18. Craniopharyngioma 58

    Case 19. Germ Cell Neoplasm 62

    Case 20. Neurocytoma 65

    Case 21. Meningioma 68

    Case 22. Subependymoma 71

    Case 23. Choroid Plexus Papilloma 75

    Case 24. Arachnoid Cyst 78

    Case 25. Dermoid Cyst 82

    Case 26. Colloid Cyst 85

  B. Infratentorial

    Case 27. Juvenile Pilocytic Astrocytoma 91

    Case 28. Hemangioblastoma 95

    Case 29. Tectal Glioma 98

    Case 30. Pontine Glioma 101

    Case 31. Medulloblastoma 104

    Case 32. Ependymoma 108

    Case 33. Acoustic Neuroma 111

    Case 34. Meningioma 115

    Case 35. Epidermoid 118

    Case 36. Glioblastoma Multiforme of Cerebellopontine Angle ... 121

    Case 37. Lipoma 124

II. INFECTION

Case 38.	Congenital Cytomegalovirus	129
Case 39.	Congenital Toxoplasmosis	132
Case 40.	Herpes Simplex Virus Type 2	135
Case 41.	Neonatal Meningitis with Infarct	139
Case 42.	*H. flu* Meningitis with Subdural Effusion	143
Case 43.	Pediatric AIDS	146
Case 44.	Acute Cerebellitis	149
Case 45.	Brain Abscess	153
Case 46.	Herpes Simplex Virus Type 1	157
Case 47.	Neurocysticercosis	161
Case 48.	Tuberculosis	165
Case 49.	Lyme Disease	169
Case 50.	CNS Aspergillosis	172
Case 51.	HIV Encephalitis	176
Case 52.	Progressive Multifocal Leukoencephalopathy	179
Case 53.	CNS Toxoplasmosis	183
Case 54.	Cryptococcosis	187
Case 55.	Cytomegalovirus Ventriculitis	191
Case 56.	Meningovascular Syphilis	194
Case 57.	Subdural Empyema	198

III. DURAL/LEPTOMENINGEAL PROCESSES

Case 58.	Meningioma	205
Case 59.	Dural Metastases (Pachymeningitis Hemorrhagica)	209
Case 60.	Sarcoid	213
Case 61.	Spontaneous Intracranial Hypotension	216
Case 62.	Meningeal Carcinomatosis	220
Case 63.	Bacterial Meningitis	223
Case 64.	Coccidioides Meningitis	227
Case 65.	Superficial Siderosis	230

IV. VASCULAR/ISCHEMIC

Case 66.	Berry Aneurysm	235
Case 67.	Giant Aneurysm	239
Case 68.	Benign Perimesencephalic Hemorrhage	243
Case 69.	Middle Cerebral Artery Infarction	247
Case 70.	Watershed Injury	252
Case 71.	Basilar Artery Thrombosis	256
Case 72.	Arterial Dissection	260
Case 73.	Hypotensive Bleed	264
Case 74.	Global Anoxic Injury	268
Case 75.	Cavernous Malformation	272
Case 76.	Arteriovenous Malformation	277
Case 77.	Venous Angioma	282
Case 78.	Carotid Cavernous Fistula	286
Case 79.	Dural Arteriovenous Fistula	290
Case 80.	Primary Angiitis of CNS	294
Case 81.	Fibromuscular Dysplasia	298
Case 82.	Takayasu Arteritis	302
Case 83.	Periventricular Leukomalacia	306
Case 84.	Neonatal Hypoxic-Ischemic Encephalopathy	310

Case 85.   Moyamoya Disease 315
Case 86.   Vein of Galen Malformation 320
Case 87.   Sickle Cell Disease 325
Case 88.   Dural Sinus Thrombosis/Venous Infarction 329

V.   WHITE MATTER DISEASE/METABOLIC

Case 89.   Multiple Sclerosis 335
Case 90.   Acute Disseminated Encephalomyelitis 339
Case 91.   Central Pontine/Extrapontine Myelinolysis 343
Case 92.   Post-Seizure Changes 347
Case 93.   Carbon Monoxide Poisoning 351
Case 94.   Adrenoleukodystrophy 354
Case 95.   Leigh Disease 358
Case 96.   Krabbe's Disease 362
Case 97.   Pelizaeus-Merzbacher Disease 366
Case 98.   Organic Acidopathy 370

VI.   NON-INFECTIOUS INFLAMMATORY/IDIOPATHIC

Case 99.   Systemic Lupus Erythematosus 377
Case 100. Langerhans' Cell Histiocytosis 381
Case 101. Wernicke's Encephalopathy 386
Case 102. Mesial Temporal Sclerosis 390

VII.   NEURODEGENERATIVE/BASAL GANGLIA DISORDERS

Case 103. Amyotrophic Lateral Sclerosis 397
Case 104. Creutzfeldt-Jakob Disease 401
Case 105. Hallervorden-Spatz Disease 404
Case 106. Wilson's Disease 408
Case 107. Huntington's Disease 412
Case 108. Olivopontocerebellar Atrophy 416
Case 109. Primary Cerebral Amyloid Angiopathy 419

VIII.   TRAUMA

Case 110. Epidural Hematoma 425
Case 111. Subdural Hematoma 428
Case 112. Diffuse Axonal Injury 431
Case 113. Parenchymal Contusion 435
Case 114. Non-Accidental Trauma 438

IX.   PHAKOMATOSES

Case 115. Neurofibromatosis Type 1 445
Case 116. Neurofibromatosis Type 2 449
Case 117. Tuberous Sclerosis 453
Case 118. von Hippel-Lindau Disease 457
Case 119. Sturge-Weber Syndrome 461
Case 120. Neurocutaneous Melanosis 465

X.   CONGENITAL MALFORMATIONS/SYNDROMES

A.   Supratentorial

Case 121. Agenesis of the Corpus Callosum 471
Case 122. Holoprosencephaly 474
Case 123. Septo-optic Dysplasia 478

Case 124. Hydranencephaly 481
Case 125. Cephalocele 484

B. Infratentorial
Case 126. Chiari I 489
Case 127. Chiari II 492
Case 128. Dandy-Walker Spectrum 495
Case 129. Lhermitte-Duclos 499

XI. MALFORMATIONS OF CORTICAL DEVELOPMENT
Case 130. Hemimegalencephaly 505
Case 131. Subependymal Nodular Heterotopia 508
Case 132. Band Heterotopia 512
Case 133. Lissencephaly 515
Case 134. Polymicrogyria 518
Case 135. Schizencephaly 522
Case 136. Focal Cortical Dysplasia 525

XII. CRANIAL NERVES
Cranial Nerve I 531
Case 137. Olfactory Neuroblastoma 532
Case 138. Neurosarcoidosis 535

Cranial Nerve II 538
Case 139. Optic Neuritis 540
Case 140. Chiasmal Glioma 542
Case 141. Occipital Lobe Infarction 544

Cranial Nerve III 547
Case 142. Aneurysm of Posterior Communicating Artery 549
Case 143. Radiation Injury 552
Case 144. Brainstem Infarction 554

Cranial Nerve IV 556
Case 145. Pseudotumor of the Cavernous Sinus 557
Case 146. Traumatic CN IV Palsy 559

Cranial Nerve V 561
Case 147. Acute Disseminated Encephalomyelitis 563
Case 148. Herpetic Neuritis 565
Case 149. Schwannoma of CN V 568
Case 150. Squamous Cell Carcinoma 571

Cranial Nerve VI 574
Case 151. Brainstem Abscess and Meningitis 576
Case 152. Duane's Syndrome 579

Cranial Nerve VII 581
Case 153. Bell's Palsy 583
Case 154. Hemifacial Spasm 585
Case 155. Hemangioma of the Facial Canal 587
Case 156. Perineural Spread of Tumor Along CN VII 589

Cranial Nerve VIII 592
Case 157. Vestibular Schwannoma 593
Case 158. Intralabyrinthine Vestibular Schwannoma 595

Cranial Nerve IX 597
Case 159. Aneurysm of the Posterior Inferior Cerebellar Artery ... 598
Case 160. Meningioma of the Jugular Foramen 600
Case 161. Schwannoma of CN IX 602

Cranial Nerve X 605
Case 162. Lateral Medullary Infarction 607
Case 163. Glomus Jugulare Tumor 610

Cranial Nerve XI 613
Case 164. Iatrogenic Injury to CN XI 614
Case 165. Schwannoma of CN XI 616

Cranial Nerve XII 618
Case 166. Nasopharyngeal Adenoid Cystic Carcinoma 620
Case 167. Skull Base Osteomyelitis 623

Index 627

The publisher plans to post additional cases on its web site. Please check the following URL: http://www.thieme.com/display/663.

PREFACE

For many years, the UCSF Neuroradiology Section has presented the "Unknown Case Conference" on Thursday afternoons. Fellows and residents present unknown cases for members of the audience to discuss and to generate a differential diagnosis and a specific diagnosis.

Over time we have accumulated an extensive teaching file based on these and many other interesting cases that covers a broad spectrum of disease entities that affect the brain, its coverings and the cranial nerves. Broad categories include neoplasm, infection, dural and leptomeningeal processes, white matter disease, trauma, congenital malformations, and phakomatoses, among others. Some cases are relatively straightforward; others are a bit more challenging.

We feel this book will provide a useful review to the senior resident studying for radiology boards as well as to the neuroradiology fellow or practitioner preparing for the CAQ exam. We also hope that practicing general radiologists and neuroradiologists will enjoy testing themselves on these cases and benefiting from the "Pearls and Pitfalls" section included for each case. This book can be read cover-to-cover by those desiring a case-based review of numerous brain pathologies that can be diagnosed with CT and MR. Alternatively, the book can be used in "review-mode" by those who desire to test themselves in neuroradiology by looking at the images for each case and comparing their differential diagnosis and diagnosis with ours.

Each case is supported by a brief discussion of etiology, pathology, imaging findings, treatment and prognosis, all in concise bulleted format for easy reference. Discussions are based on up-to-date reviews of current literature, and a few suggested readings are listed for each case. In many cases, additional images ("margin cases") are provided to illustrate entities one might consider in the differential diagnosis or to illustrate additional manifestations of a given disease entity.

It should be noted that the Cranial Nerves section has a slightly different format from that of the other sections in the book. Each nerve is introduced with a review of its function and anatomy. Certain pathologies that affect the intracranial and skull base segments of each cranial nerve are then illustrated and discussed briefly. Extracranial pathologies are covered in another volume (*Teaching Atlas of Head and Neck Imaging*), to be published soon by Thieme.

In developing this book we realized that there were many more cases with excellent teaching points than we could possibly include in this atlas. To avoid creating a huge and expensive tome, we decided to make some additional cases available on the Thieme web site. This site can of course be accessed free of charge, and more information about this can be found in the table of contents.

We have tried to keep our comments to the point and hope that our readers will benefit from what we consider to be the major teaching points concerning a broad spectrum of disorders of brain parenchyma, meninges, and cranial nerves in both adults and children.

Nancy J. Fischbein, M.D.
William P. Dillon, M.D.
A. James Barkovich, M.D.

ACKNOWLEDGMENTS

We gratefully acknowledge the contribution of Paul Cazier, M.D., one of our excellent neuroradiology fellows (1996–1998), to the Congenital Malformations: Infratentorial and Phakomatoses sections, as well as the many UCSF Neuroradiology Fellows, past and present, for their ongoing contributions to the UCSF neuroradiology teaching file.

COMMONLY USED ABBREVIATIONS

MR/CT Terminology

CECT	contrast-enhanced CT scan
FLAIR	fluid-attenuated inversion recovery
FSE	fast spin-echo
MPGR	multiplanar gradient-echo
NECT	non-enhanced CT scan
PD-WI	proton density-weighted image
SPGR	spoiled gradient-recalled acquisition in the steady state
T1-W1	T1-weighted image
T2-W1	T2-weighted image

Anatomic Terminology

ACA	anterior cerebral artery
acomm	anterior communicating artery
AICA	anterior inferior cerebellar artery
CPA	cerebellopontine angle
ECA	external carotid artery
IAC	internal auditory canal
ICA	internal carotid artery
MCA	middle cerebral artery
PCA	posterior cerebral artery
pcomm	posterior communicating artery
PICA	posterior inferior cerebellar artery
SCA	superior cerebellar artery

Other Abbreviations

ADEM	acute disseminated encephalomyelitis
AIDS	acquired immunodeficiency syndrome
AVM	arteriovenous malformation
CMV	cytomegalovirus
GBM	glioblastoma multiforme
HIV	human immunodeficiency virus
HSV	herpes simplex virus
MS	multiple sclerosis
PML	progressive multifocal leukoencephalopathy
TB	tuberculosis

Section I

Neoplasm

A. Supratentorial

Case 1

Clinical Presentation

A 25-year-old man presents with a generalized tonic-clonic seizure. He reports having had an increasing number of headaches over the past 6 months.

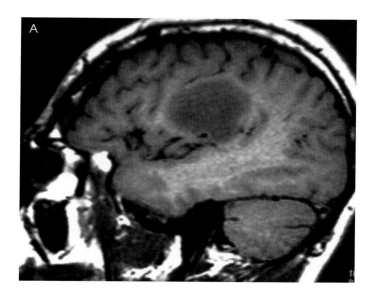

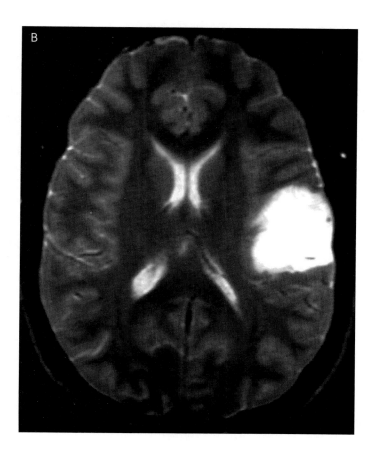

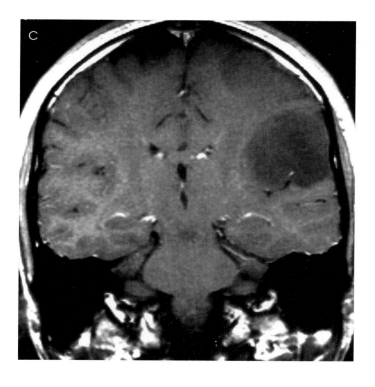

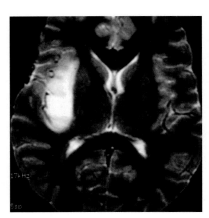

Fig. D. An axial T2-WI in a patient with a low-grade glioma mimics a right MCA infarct. However, this patient's symptoms were chronic and progressive.

Radiologic Findings

A sagittal T1-WI (Fig. A) demonstrates a well-demarcated intraaxial mass that is hypointense compared with brain parenchyma, centered in the left inferior frontal lobe just above the sylvian fissure. An axial T2-WI (Fig. B) demonstrates that the mass is hyperintense to brain parenchyma. No surrounding edema is noted. No enhancement is present on a post-gadolinium coronal T1-WI (Fig. C). Note the mild mass effect associated with this process, with depression of the left sylvian fissure as compared with the right side.

Diagnosis

Grade II astrocytoma

Differential Diagnosis

• Grade III astrocytoma (typically more infiltrative, and more likely to be associated with surrounding edema, but generally indistinguishable on imaging)
• Oligodendroglioma (often calcified)
• Ganglioglioma (often contains cysts or calcification, has a predilection for the temporal lobe)
• Arachnoid cyst (extra-axial, follows CSF intensity on all sequences)

Discussion

Background

Astrocytoma is a primary brain tumor of astrocytic origin. Most primary brain tumors in adults arise supratentorially: approximately 50% of these are gliomas, and approximately 90% of gliomas are astrocytomas. Ten to 15% of these tumors are "low grade" (see below). These lesions are most commonly located in the frontal lobes.

Clinical Findings

Low-grade astrocytomas usually present in young adults, and the symptoms vary with tumor location. Headache, seizures, and focal neurologic deficits are common.

Pathology

Astrocytomas are divided into grades I to IV according to the World Health Organization (WHO) classification:

• Grade I: juvenile pilocytic astrocytoma, benign
• Grade II: fibrillary/diffuse astrocytoma
• Grade III: anaplastic astrocytoma
• Grade IV: glioblastoma multiforme

Grades II-IV constitute the malignant gliomas, with increasing malignancy corresponding to higher grades. Grading is useful to assess prognosis and guide management. The ultimate tumor grade is determined by the most malignant-appearing tissue submitted for evaluation.

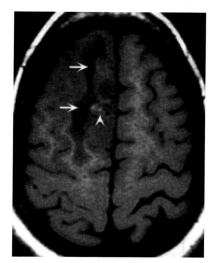

Fig. E. An axial T1-WI in a patient with a right frontal grade II astrocytoma shows areas of cystic change (*arrows*) and hemorrhage (*arrowhead*).

Imaging Findings

Typical imaging findings of low-grade astrocytomas include:

CT

- Low density mass on noncontrast scan
- Little or no contrast enhancement

MR

- Mass lesion with low-signal intensity on T1-WI, and high-signal intensity on T2-WI
- Generally a lack of contrast enhancement
- Little or no surrounding edema
- Occasional cystic degeneration and/or hemorrhage (Fig. E)

Treatment

- Initial: surgical excision, if accessible, often followed by radiation therapy
- Recurrent disease: often of a higher grade histologically ("dedifferentiation")
    - Re-resection
    - Stereotactic radiosurgery
    - Chemotherapy

Prognosis

- The major cause of mortality from a low-grade astrocytoma is differentiation into a high-grade astrocytoma
- Younger age, gross total resection, and long course of preoperative symptoms are associated with longer survival. Most series report median survivals of 7 to 10 years.

Suggested Readings

Kondziolka D, Lunsford LD, Martinez AJ. Unreliability of contemporary neurodiagnostic imaging in evaluating suspected adult supratentorial (low-grade) astrocytoma. *J Neurosurg* 79:533–536, 1993.

Madison MT, Hall WA, Latchaw RE, Loes DJ. Radiologic diagnosis, staging, and follow-up of adult central nervous system primary malignant glioma. *Radiolog Clin North Am* 32:183–196, 1994.

Piepmeier J, Christopher S, Spencer D, et al. Variations in the natural history and survival of patients with supratentorial low-grade astrocytomas. *Neurosurgery* 38:872–879, 1996.

Case 2

Clinical Presentation

A 58-year-old previously healthy professor presents with confusion and a generalized seizure.

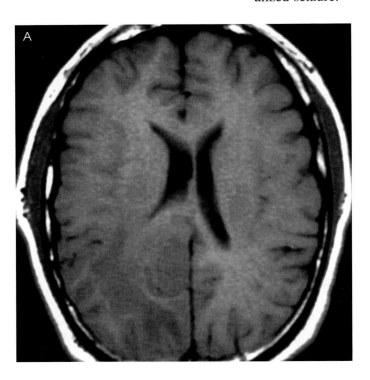

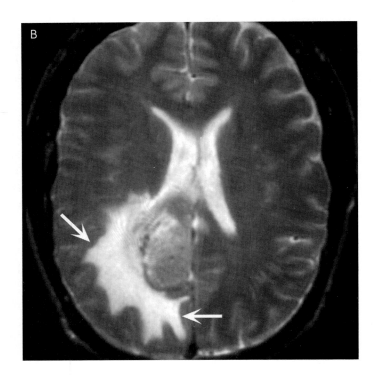

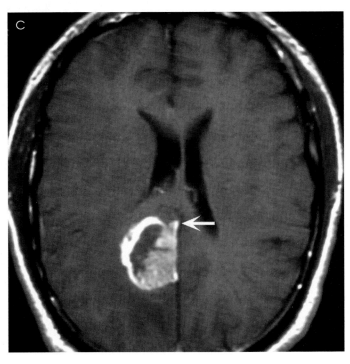

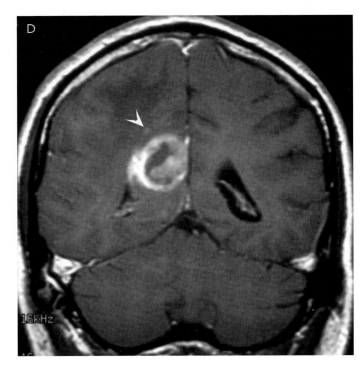

Pearls

- There is a large overlap in appearance between low-grade and high-grade malignancies.

- It is difficult to accurately determine tumor margins. Microscopic tumor is frequently seen beyond the radiologic tumor boundary.

- A favored location for high-grade gliomas is the corpus callosum, which gives rise to the so-called "butterfly" glioma (Figs. E and F).

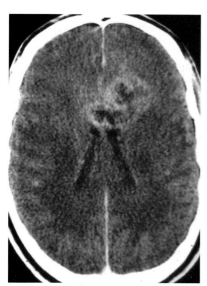

Fig. E. A non-contrast CT scan demonstrates an intrinsically dense irregular mass lesion with central cyst formation or necrosis involving the genu of the corpus callosum and the left frontal lobe in a young man.

Radiologic Findings

An axial T-WI (Fig. A) demonstrates a mildly hypointense ovoid mass in the right parietal lobe adjacent to the falx, with significant surrounding edema and mass effect. On an axial T2-WI (Fig. B), the mass is moderately heterogeneous and mostly isointense to gray matter. Surrounding vasogenic edema (*arrows*) is well demonstrated. Post-gadolinium, a T1-WI (Fig. C) shows thick and nodular peripheral enhancement with central necrosis. A broad dural base is seen, with enhancing tissue extending linearly along the falx ("dural tail," *arrow*). On a coronal post-gadolinium T1-WI (Fig. D), an enhancing satellite nodule is seen in the adjacent parenchyma (*arrowhead*). This is a helpful finding as the presence of a satellite nodule suggests that this lesion is intraaxial in origin, despite its broad dural base.

Diagnosis

Gliosarcoma

Differential Diagnosis

- Glioblastoma multiforme (indistinguishable from gliosarcoma)
- Metastasis (often multiple; typically centered at gray-white junction; rarely invades overlying meninges)
- Malignant meningioma (often invades brain parenchyma and incites a large amount of vasogenic edema; does not typically have satellite nodules)
- Lymphoma (non-AIDS-related CNS lymphoma typically enhances intensely and homogeneously and does not show areas of necrosis)

Discussion

Background

Primary malignancies of the CNS account for ~1.5% of all malignant disease, and primary malignant gliomas represent 45 to 50% of all intracranial tumors. In adults, the majority of gliomas are supratentorial; in childhood, 70 to 80% are infratentorial. Glioblastoma multiforme is the most common primary supratentorial neoplasm in an adult; most of these patients are 45 to 55 years of age, and there is a 3:2 male predominance. Gliosarcoma is a rare primary brain tumor that is composed of neoplastic glial cells mixed with a spindle-cell sarcomatous element. The sarcomatous element is thought to arise from neoplastically transformed vascular elements within the glioblastoma itself. Gliosarcomas are usually solitary, but may be multicentric. The distinction between glioblastoma and gliosarcoma is usually made at histopathological examination.

Clinical Findings

Findings vary with tumor size and location: focal neurological deficits; seizures; symptoms related to an overall elevation of intracranial pressure (headache, altered mental status).

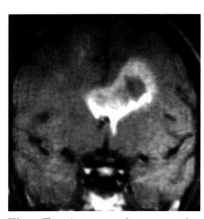

Fig. F. A coronal post-gadolinium T1-WI in the patient in Fig. E demonstrates the involvement of the corpus callosum and left frontal lobe in this patient with glioblastoma multiforme.

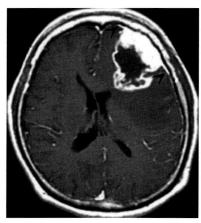

Fig. G. An axial post-gadolinium T1-WI demonstrates a left frontal intraaxial lesion with thick, nodular, irregular peripheral enhancement and central necrosis. The lesion has extended to the brain surface and is growing along the dura (*arrowheads*). Surrounding vasogenic edema is present. At surgery glioblastoma multiforme was confirmed.

Pathology

Gross

- Firm, lobulated masses with central areas of necrosis

Microscopic

- Malignant glial and mesenchymal elements
- The glial element resembles glioblastoma multiforme

Imaging Findings

High-grade gliomas are usually large, irregular lesions with indistinct margins that show severe surrounding edema and mass effect. The description below applies to glioblastoma multiforme as well as to gliosarcoma.

CT

- Non-contrast CT: irregular, hypo- or isodense mass
    - Calcification is rare
    - Foci of hemorrhage may be seen
- Post-contrast CT: usually heterogeneous, often ringlike enhancement with thick, irregular, nodular walls
- Nonenhancing high-grade gliomas are uncommon

MR

- T1-WI: mass is usually hypointense, with a large amount of surrounding edema and mass effect
- T2-WI: mass is often very heterogeneous, reflecting hemorrhage, necrosis, cyst formation, and varying degrees of cellularity. Adjacent white matter tracts usually demonstrate extensive high signal, reflecting a combination of infiltrating tumor and peritumoral edema.
- Post-gadolinium images: enhancement is often very heterogeneous but is commonly ringlike, with thick, nodular, irregular walls around an area of central necrosis (Fig. G)

Treatment

- Surgery
- Radiation therapy
- Treatment of recurrence may include: chemotherapy, stereotactic radiosurgery, and Iodine-125 interstitial radiotherapy (brachytherapy)

Prognosis

Poor, with a median survival of 6 months (similar to glioblastoma multiforme)

Pitfalls

- In this case, the broad dural base and the "dural tail" might suggest an extraaxial lesion. However, peripherally located intraaxial lesions may invade the dura or incite an inflammatory reaction.

- The dural tail sign is most commonly associated with meningioma. However, it has also been described with other extraaxial lesions including acoustic neuroma, metastases, chloroma, and sarcoidosis, and with peripherally located intraaxial lesions such as glioma.

Selected Readings

Gupta S, Gupta RK, Banerjee D, Gujral RB. Problems with the "dural tail" sign. *Neuroradiology* 35:541–542, 1993.

Madison MT, Hall WA, Latchaw RE, Loes DJ. Radiologic diagnosis, staging, and follow-up of adult central nervous system primary malignant glioma. *Radiol Clin North Am* 32:183–196, 1994.

Meis JM, Ho KL, Nelson JS. Gliosarcoma: a histologic and immunohistochemical reaffirmation. *Mod Pathol* 3:19–23, 1990.

Case 3

Clinical Presentation

A 42-year-old man complains of increasing headache and blurred vision. He reports two recent accidents at the same freeway off-ramp.

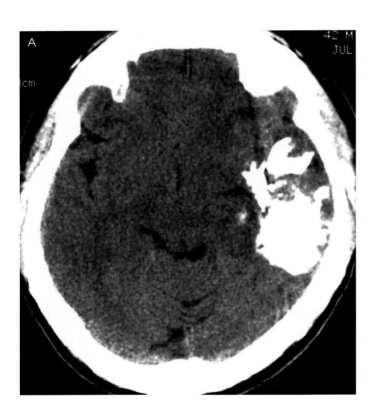
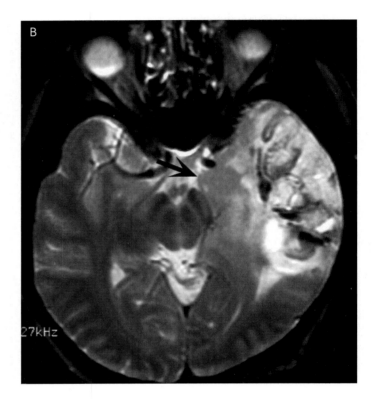

Radiologic Findings

A non-contrast CT scan (Fig. A) demonstrates extensive calcification in the left temporal lobe. There is mild mass effect on the midbrain, with obliteration of the left ambient cistern. An axial T2-WI (Fig. B) at the level of the midbrain demonstrates a heterogenous mass extensively involving the left temporal lobe. There is mild uncal herniation (*arrow*) with compression of the left cerebral peduncle. Without the correlative CT scan, it could be difficult to determine whether the linear areas of low signal intensity on this image represent hemosiderin or possibly even flow voids versus calcification.

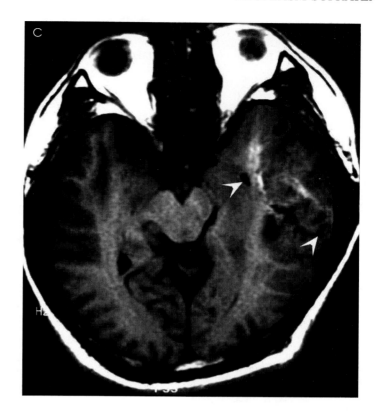

An axial T1-WI (Fig. C) demonstrates that the left temporal lobe mass is also heterogenous on T1-weighted images, with areas of cyst formation (*arrowheads*) as well as linear areas of T1 shortening presumably related to the parenchymal calcification.

Diagnosis

Oligodendroglioma

Differential Diagnosis

• Astrocytoma (may be indistinguishable)
• Ganglioglioma (typically presents at a younger age, often cortical location)
• Thrombosed and calcified vascular malformation (should not usually cause mass effect)

Discussion

Background

Oligodendrogliomas account for 4 to 7% of primary intracranial gliomas. They are most frequently discovered in young adults 35 to 45 years of age and are usually located peripherally in the cerebrum, with a tendency to involve the frontal lobes. They typically begin in the hemispheric white matter and grow toward the cortex. Rarely they may arise in the ventricular system (1 to 10%). Oligodendrogliomas are classified as low-, intermediate-, or high-grade (least common), and the grades cannot be reliably differentiated with imaging.

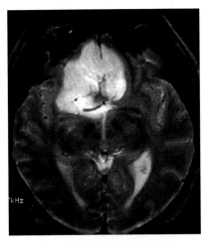

Fig. D. Axial T2-WI from a patient presenting with insidious onset of personality change. A hyperintense slightly heterogeneous mass involving the frontal lobes bilaterally is identified.

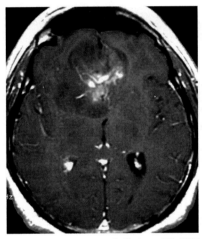

Fig. E. A post-gadolinium T1-WI in the patient in Figure D shows heterogenous linear and nodular enhancement of a portion of this mass. The histologic diagnosis was oligodendroglioma.

Clinical Findings

The interval between the onset of symptoms and the diagnosis of tumor is quite variable, ranging in one series from a few days to 15 years. Symptoms include seizure, headache, and focal neurologic deficits that depend on the location of the lesion.

Pathology

Gross

- Typically unencapsulated but relatively well-circumscribed

Microscopic

- Approximately 50% are classified as "mixed," containing glial elements other than oligodendrocytes
- High cellularity and high nuclear to cytoplasmic ratio are typical
- Often calcified and often contain areas of cystic degeneration
- Hemorrhage and necrosis are relatively infrequent

Imaging Findings

CT

- Isodense or hypodense pre-contrast
- Hyperdense in regions of hemorrhage or calcification (75 to 90%)
- Cysts in ~20%
- Large peripherally located tumors may erode and remodel the calvarium

MR

- Usually hypointense on T1-WI (unless areas of hemorrhage or calcification)
- Typically hyperintense on T2-WI (Fig. D)
- Calcification is often not seen well on MR
- Heterogeneous enhancement is common (Fig. E)

Treatment

- Total or subtotal excision, depending on size and location
- External beam radiotherapy for subtotally resected tumors
- Consideration of gamma knife radiosurgery and/or chemotherapy for recurrent disease

Prognosis

- Variable depending on grade of tumor and extent of resection
- Five-year survival is ~75% for low-grade tumors, 40% for high-grade tumors

Suggested Readings

Lee Y-Y, Van Tassel P. Intracranial oligodendrogliomas: imaging findings in 35 untreated cases. *AJR* 152:361–369, 1989.

Shaw EG, Scheithauer BW, O'Fallon JR, et al. Oligodendrogliomas: the Mayo Clinic experience. *J Neurosurg* 76:428–434, 1992.

Case 4

Clinical Presentation

An 8-year-old boy presents with medically refractory seizures.

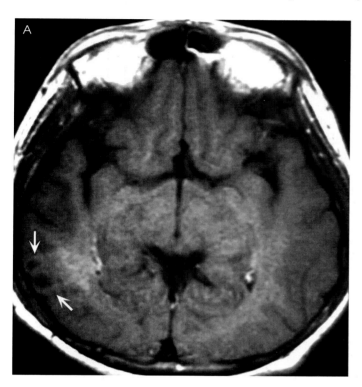

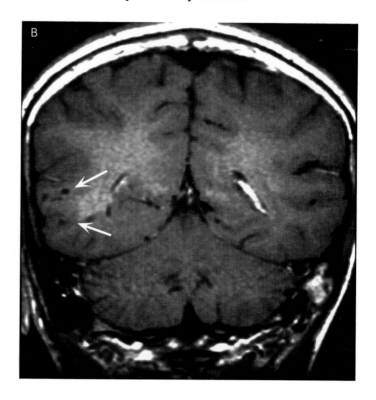

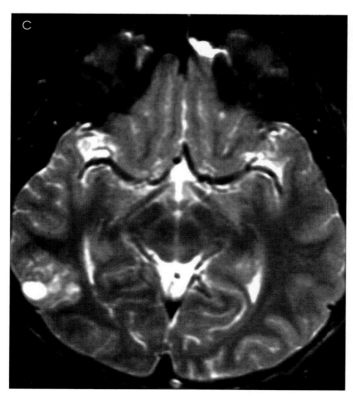

Radiologic Findings

Axial (Fig. A) and coronal (Fig. B) post-gadolinium T1-WIs demonstrate a non-enhancing mass in the right posterior temporal lobe (*arrows*). The mass has a predominantly cortical location and contains two small cysts. A T2-WI (Fig. C) demonstrates that the mass is mildly hyperintense, and the cyst more focally hyperintense, compared with brain parenchyma.

Diagnosis

Ganglioglioma

Differential Diagnosis

• Low-grade astrocytoma (often indistinguishable)
• Oligodendroglioma (tend to be larger and more heterogeneous)
• Dysembryoplastic neuroepithelial tumor (favors frontal and anterior temporal lobes, but may be indistinguishable)
• Gangliocytoma (contains only neuronal elements, differentiated pathologically)

Discussion

Background

Ganglioglioma is a slow-growing primary brain tumor that contains both neuronal and glial elements. It occurs most commonly in children and young adults and constitutes 0.4 to 0.9% of primary brain neoplasms. Gangliogliomas are most commonly located in the cerebral hemispheres, especially the temporal lobes. Other locations include the posterior fossa, thalamus, and pineal gland. They are usually solitary, though multiple tumors within the same patient have been reported.

Clinical Findings

Patients usually have a long-standing history of seizures and headache. Focal neurologic signs, symptoms of elevated intracranial pressure, and intellectual impairment are less common presentations. Malignant transformation of a ganglioglioma is unusual.

Pathology

Gross

• Usually a firm, well-circumscribed mass

Microscopic

• Neoplastic ganglion cells are interspersed within a glial stroma. The degree of malignancy is based upon the extent of differentiation of these cells and is graded from I to III, with ~85% being low-grade (Grade I) lesions
• May be cystic or contain foci of calcification

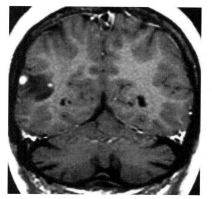

Fig. D. A coronal post-gadolinium T1-WI demonstrates two nodular foci of enhancement in this right temporal ganglioglioma.

Imaging Findings

CT

- Usually low density or cystic mass
- Focal enhancement in 50%
- Calcification in 35%

MR

- Hemispheric lesions generally have a cortical location
- Small cysts are common
- Usually hypointense or isointense on T1-WI, hyperintense on T2-WI
- Gadolinium enhancement is variable; if present, it is often focal or nodular (Fig. D). Enhancement may also be peripheral around a cystic component

Treatment

- Surgical excision
- If resection is partial, radiotherapy is generally reserved for progressive lesions

Prognosis

- Generally excellent, with ~80% seizure-free after surgery
- An increased risk of recurrence is seen in patients over the age of 30, tumors with a high degree of anaplasia, and patients with symptoms for less than 1 year

Suggested Readings

Castillo M, Davis PC, Takei Y, Hoffman JC. Intracranial ganglioglioma: MR, CT, and clinical findings in 18 patients. *AJNR* 11:109–114, 1990.

Dorne HL, O'Gorman AM, Melanson D. Computed tomography of intracranial gangliogliomas. *AJNR* 7:281–285, 1986.

Wacker MR, Cogen PH, Etzell JE, et al. Diffuse leptomeningeal involvement by a ganglioglioma in a child. *J Neurosurg* 77:302–306, 1992.

Case 5

Clinical Presentation

A 48-year-old patient has become increasingly confused and disoriented over the past few months. A lumbar puncture is unremarkable.

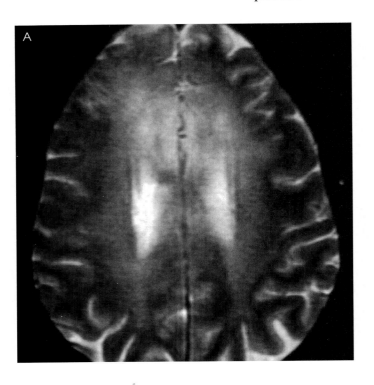

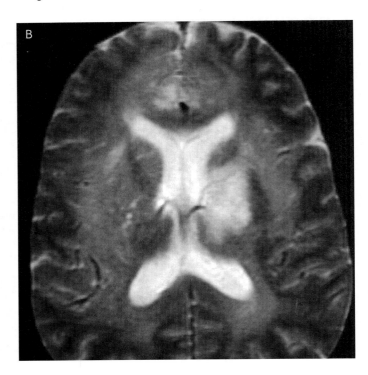

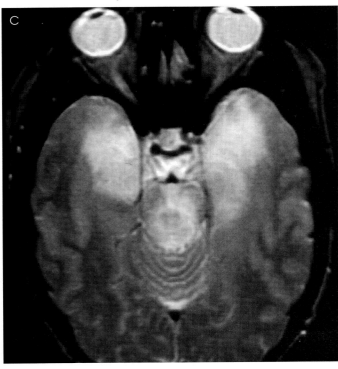

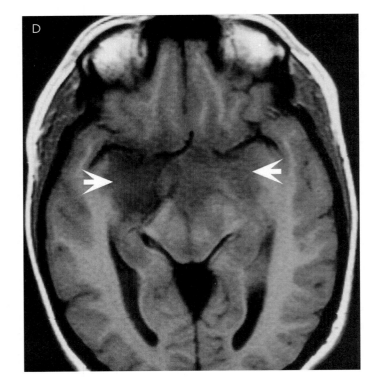

Radiologic Findings

Axial T2-WIs (Figs. A, B, and C) demonstrate extensive T2 prolongation throughout the white matter of the cerebral hemispheres bilaterally, extending into the corpus callosum. Abnormal T2 prolongation also involves the deep gray nuclei bilaterally (left greater than right), as well as the midbrain and the anteromedial temporal lobes bilaterally. Note the relative lack of mass effect on an axial T1-WI (Fig. D). The hypointense tumor infiltrates the medial temporal lobes (*arrows*) and hypothalamic region. No abnormal parenchymal enhancement was noted following administration of gadolinium (not shown).

Diagnosis

Gliomatosis cerebri

Differential Diagnosis

- Lymphomatosis cerebri (usually shows multifocal enhancement, but may be indistinguishable from gliomatosis cerebri)
- Multicentric glioma (often patchy enhancement, but may be indistinguishable)
- Viral encephalitis (often a more acute presentation; cerebrospinal fluid usually abnormal with cells and elevated protein)
- Vasculitis (usually causes multifocal areas of infarction; often patchy, multifocal areas of enhancement)
- Extensive active demyelinating disease such as ADEM (acute disseminated encephalomyelitis) or acute multiple sclerosis (typically lack mass effect, usually shows focal areas of enhancement)

Discussion

Background

Gliomatosis cerebri is an uncommon primary brain tumor characterized by diffuse neoplastic proliferation of astrocytes, with preservation of underlying brain architecture and relative sparing of neurons. The process shows a relentless progression over time and typically presents with a slow decline in cognitive function. The peak incidence is in the second to fourth decades.

Clinical Findings

Clinical findings are often relatively minor compared to the extent of parenchymal involvement. Patients most commonly manifest personality changes and mental status disturbances. Other symptoms and signs include ataxia, headache, hemiparesis, cranial nerve palsies, and seizures.

Pathology

Gross

- Tumor infiltrates at least two, usually three, lobes of the brain and is often bihemispheric
- Tumor typically crosses midline via the corpus callosum or the interthalamic adhesion

Microscopic

- Neoplastic astrocytes infiltrate both gray and white matter, but white matter involvement is usually more extensive than gray
- Little or no damage to nerve cells or axons
- Underlying brain architecture is relatively preserved

Imaging Findings

CT

- Evidence for subtle mass effect or apparent expansion of normal structures
- May observe mild hypodensity in the white matter
- No or minimal contrast enhancement

MR

- Extensive T2 prolongation throughout involved white matter
- Iso- or hypointense on T1-WI
- Does not form a defined mass
- Subtle to marked sulcal/ventricular effacement
- Variable contrast enhancement which is patchy and subtle if present. It may be parenchymal or leptomeningeal, and may increase if there is focal transformation to higher grade malignancy.

Treatment

- Too extensive for surgery–usually only a biopsy is obtained
- Radiation therapy and chemotherapy are relatively ineffective

Prognosis

Poor, with a relentlessly progressive course lasting weeks to years

Suggested Readings

del Carpio-O'Donovan R, Korah I, Salazar A, Melancon D. Gliomatosis cerebri. *Radiology* 198:831–835, 1996.

Shin YM, Chang KH, Han MH, et al. Gliomatosis cerebri: comparison of MR and CT features. *AJR* 161:859–862, 1993.

Spagnoli MV, Grossman RI, Packer RJ, et al. Magnetic resonance determination of gliomatosis cerebri. *Neuroradiology* 34:331–333, 1987.

Case 6

Clinical Presentation

A 67-year-old woman with a history of breast cancer presents with headaches and visual changes.

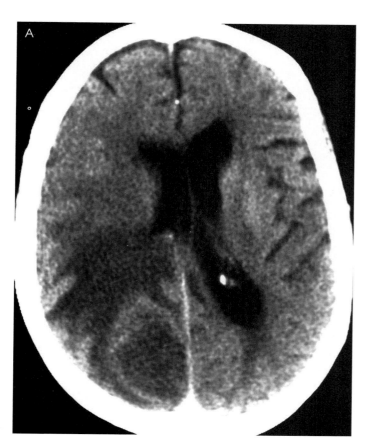
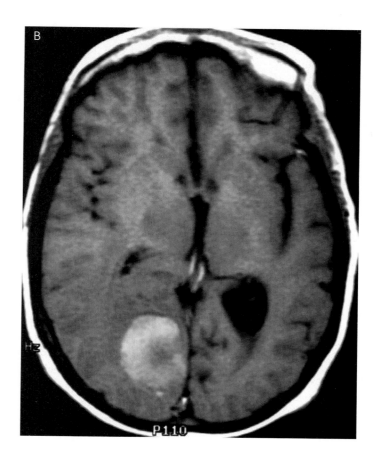

Radiologic Findings

An axial non-contrast CT scan demonstrates a mass in the right occipital lobe (Fig. A). The mass shows central hypodensity, an irregular rim of isodensity, and a surrounding zone of vasogenic edema. There is mass effect on the right ventricular atrium. An MR was recommended for further evaluation. An axial T1-WI (Fig. B) demonstrates T1 shortening in the center of the mass, consistent with proteinaceous or hemorrhagic contents. Surrounding vasogenic edema and mass effect are again noted.

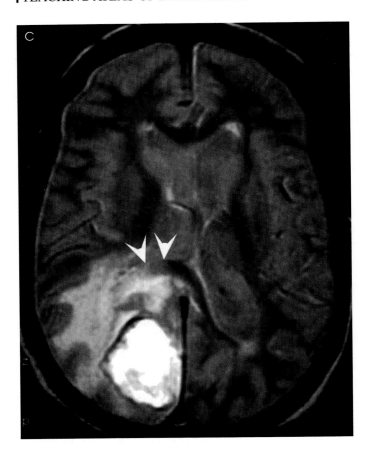

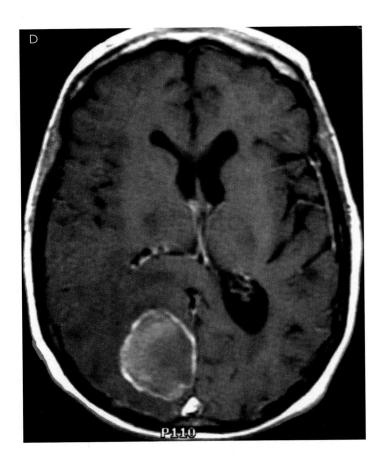

An axial PD-WI (Fig. C) demonstrates hyperintensity within the center of the mass, and peripheral hypointensity. These findings are most consistent with subacute hemorrhage. Note again the extensive vasogenic edema, with extension into the splenium of the corpus callosum (*arrowheads*). A post-gadolinium T1-WI (Fig. D) demonstrates irregular linear enhancement around the periphery of this lesion. At surgery, a mostly cystic lesion containing hemorrhagic fluid was encountered.

Diagnosis

Metastatic breast cancer

Differential Diagnosis

- Single lesion: abscess, glioma, subacute hematoma
- Multiple lesions: multiple abscesses, multifocal glioma

Discussion

Background

Parenchymal metastases are the most common CNS complication of extracranial primary neoplasms. The most common primary sites to metastasize to the CNS include lung, breast, and skin (melanoma). Parenchymal metastases represent 25 to 33% of all brain tumors in adults and are present in 10 to 25% of patients with extracranial neoplasms at autopsy. They are multiple in 60 to 85% of cases.

Pearls

- Contrast-enhanced MR is more sensitive than CT in detecting metastases.

- Triple-dose contrast allows a 20 to 30% increase in the number of detected metastases. If a "solitary" metastatic lesion is seen, it is wise to consider a triple-dose study before proceeding with surgery or stereotactic radiosurgery to look for small additional lesions (Fig. F, *arrowhead*).

- Magnetization transfer plus single-dose contrast is comparable to triple-dose contrast in improving lesion detection.

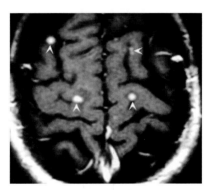

Fig. E. Post-gadolinium T1-WI in a patient with a history of breast cancer demonstrates multiple nodular foci of enhancement located peripherally in the cortex and at the gray-white matter junction (*arrowheads*).

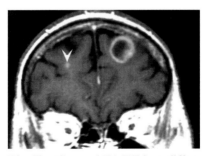

Fig. F. Coronal T1-WI in a different patient with a history of breast cancer. On a triple-dose gadolinium study, an unsuspected small lesion in the right frontal lobe (*arrowhead*) is identified.

Clinical Findings

CNS metastases may be asymptomatic and discovered incidentally on staging neuroimaging studies. Symptoms, when present, vary with the location of lesion(s).

Complications

Metastases are typically accompanied by surrounding brain edema, which may be severe. Hemorrhage may complicate vascular metastases. The incidence of hemorrhage is highest with choriocarcinoma, thyroid carcinoma, melanoma, and renal cell carcinoma (mnemonic "CT/MR"), but lung and breast carcinomas account for the greatest number by virtue of their prevalence.

Pathology

Gross

- Usually well-circumscribed rounded nodules of variable size
- Any area may be affected, but the gray-white junction is a favored location (Fig. E)
- May be solid, cystic or mixed
- Calcification or hemorrhage may be present

Microscopic

- Varies with histology of primary tumor

Imaging Findings

CT

- Usually iso- or hypodense pre-contrast
- May be hyperdense if hemorrhagic or calcified, or if there is a high nuclear to cytoplasmic ratio
- Homogeneous or peripheral enhancement post-contrast

MR

- T1-WI: usually hypointense, although T1 shortening may be related to hemorrhage or melanin; if small, the lesion(s) may not be visible on pre-contrast images
- T2-WI: typically hyperintense; iso- or hypointensity on T2-WI may be related to hemorrhage, mucin secretion (adenocarcinomas), or a high nuclear to cytoplasmic ratio; surrounding vasogenic edema is usually seen
- Post-gadolinium: enhancement may be solid, peripheral, or mixed

Treatment

- Depends on whether solitary or multiple. Solitary lesion can be treated by surgical resection, if feasible, or stereotactic radiosurgery. Multiple lesions require whole-brain radiation or stereotactic radiosurgery (depending on number and location).
- Chemotherapy may have a role

Pitfalls

- Vessels are prominent on triple-dose studies – do not mistake a vessel for a lesion.

- Small metastases may be missed if too wide an interslice gap is used.

- Intracortical metastases may not elicit surrounding edema and will be missed if gadolinium is not given. Also, there may be essentially no edema with "miliary metastases."

- Enhancing lesions may be less conspicuous on spoiled gradient-echo images compared with spin-echo T1-WI.

Prognosis

Variable: multiple metastases treated with whole-brain radiation generally have median survival time on the order of 3 to 6 months. Patients with solitary metastases treated with surgery and/or stereotactic radiosurgery have median survival on the order of 1.3 years.

Suggested Readings

Davis PC, Hudgins PA, Peterman SB, Hoffman JC Jr. Diagnosis of cerebral metastases: double-dose delayed CT vs. contrast-enhanced MR imaging. *AJNR* 12:293–300, 1991.

Matthews VP, Caldemeyer KS, Ulmer JL, et al. Effects of contrast dose, delayed imaging, and magnetization transfer saturation on gadolinium-enhanced MR imaging of brain lesions. *JMRI* 1997; 7:14–22.

Case 7

Clinical Presentation

An 18-year-old male presents with several months of progressive headache and mild right sided weakness.

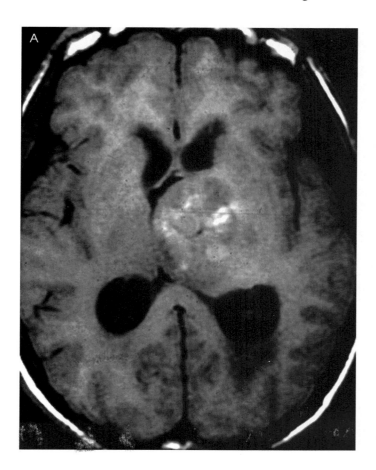 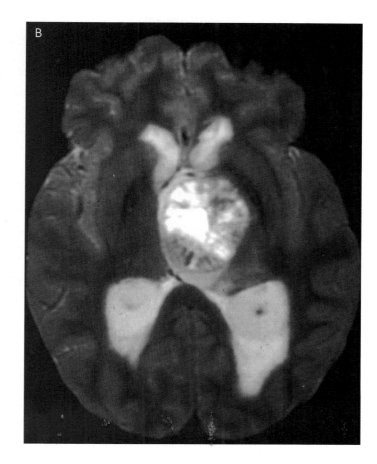

Radiologic Findings

An axial T1-WI (Fig. A) demonstrates a heterogeneous mass centered in the left thalamus, exerting mass effect on the displaced and compressed third ventricle. The lateral ventricles are enlarged, and there is evidence of transependymal flow of CSF, seen as left periatrial hypointensity. Areas of heterogenous high signal are noted within the mass, consistent with focal areas of hemorrhage or calcification. An axial T2-WI (Fig. B) demonstrates foci of probable necrosis within the mass and only minimal edema in adjacent brain parenchyma.

Pearls

- Proximity to a ventricular surface can be a helpful clue to the diagnosis of supratentorial ependymoma.

- Remember to include ependymoma in the differential diagnosis of a supratentorial parenchymal mass lesion, particularly in a child.

- If the lesion extends into the ventricle, it is best to screen the spine preoperatively with contrast-enhanced MR to detect CSF spread of disease.

Pitfall

- Ependymomas may have large hemorrhagic cysts and significant surrounding edema, similar to supratentorial PNETs (Figs. D and E).

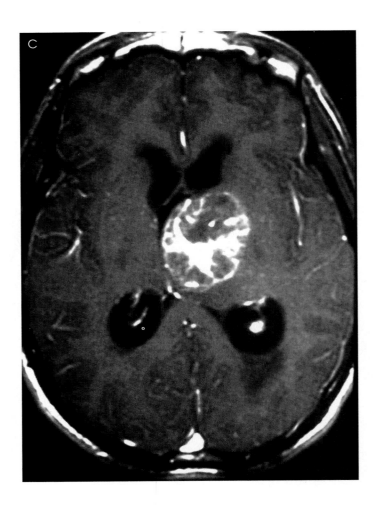

A post-contrast T1-WI (Fig. C) demonstrates irregular enhancement.

Diagnosis

Supratentorial ependymoma

Differential Diagnosis

- Primitive neuroectodermal tumor (PNET) (often more peripheral, more edema)
- Malignant rhabdoid tumor (generally seen in infants and young children)
- Glioblastoma multiforme (typically significant surrounding edema)
- Anaplastic astrocytoma (may be indistinguishable, but less likely to be in proximity to a ventricular surface)
- Metastatic disease (often multifocal, with significant surrounding edema)

Discussion

Background

Ependymomas are four to six times more common in children than adults. Approximately 60% of ependymomas are infratentorial, and 40% are supratentorial. When ependymomas occur supratentorially, approximately 70% are extraventricular in location, though they often arise close to the ventricular surface and may extend into the ventricle.

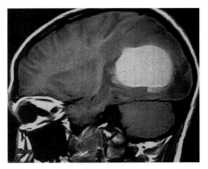

Fig. D. Sagittal T1-WI in a 21-year-old male with supratentorial ependymoma shows a large hemorrhagic cyst.

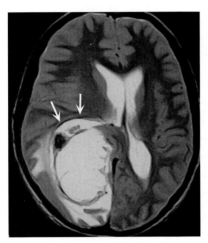

Fig. E. An axial T2-WI in the patient in Fig. D shows the tumor's close relationship to and displacement of the right ventricular atrium (*arrows*). This lesion was thought to be a primitive neuroectodermal tumor (PNET) preoperatively.

Clinical Findings

Nonspecific symptoms related to mass effect and/or hydrocephalus

Etiology

Supratentorial ependymomas are thought to arise from periventricular ependymal cell rests. The majority are benign, but malignant ependymomas occur as well.

Pathology

Gross

- Lobulated, often partly cystic mass
- Calcification and hemorrhage may be seen

Microscopic

- Cellular ependymomas, the most frequent subtype, demonstrate "perivascular pseudorosettes," a characteristic finding

Imaging Findings

The supratentorial ependymoma is generally a heterogeneous mass often lying deep within the cerebral hemisphere, close to a ventricular surface. Moderate inhomogeneous enhancement is present on both CT and MR.

CT

- Calcification in 50%

MR

- Variable signal intensity on T1- and T2-WIs
- Often very heterogeneous secondary to necrosis, hemorrhage, and calcification

Treatment

- Total resection if possible
- Postoperative radiation therapy if resection is incomplete, histology is malignant, or there is an apparent total resection but the lesion is located near eloquent brain areas. XRT must be used with caution in the growing brain of a child.
- Spinal irradiation is not usually administered unless CSF metastases are detected

Prognosis

- Varies with histology
- Overall 45 to 60% 5-year survival

Suggested Readings

Armington WG, Osborn AG, Cubberley DA, et al. Supratentorial ependymoma: CT appearance. *Radiology* 157:367–372, 1985.

Centeno LS, Lee AA, Winter J, Barba D. Supratentorial ependymomas: neuroimaging and pathological correlation. *J Neurosurg* 64:209–215, 1986.

Palma L, Celli P, Cantore G. Supratentorial ependymomas of the first two decades of life. *Neurosurgery* 32:169–175, 1993.

Case 8

Clinical Presentation

A 24-year-old man with complex partial seizures presents for evaluation.

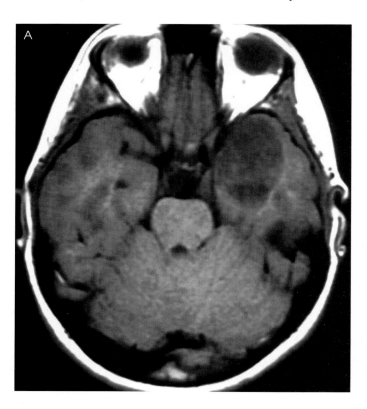

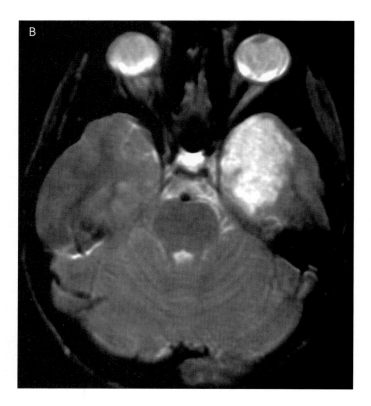

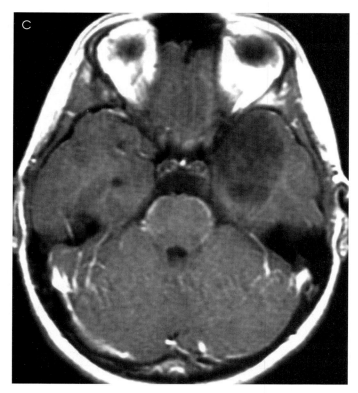

Radiologic Findings

An axial T1-WI (Fig. A) demonstrates an ovoid intraaxial mass in the left antero-medial temporal lobe which is hypointense to brain parenchyma. On a T2-WI, the mass is hyperintense to brain parenchyma (Fig. B). No surrounding edema is seen. No enhancement is detected on an axial post-gadolinium T1-WI (Fig. C).

Diagnosis

Dysembryoplastic neuroepithelial tumor (DNET)

Differential Diagnosis

• Ganglioglioma (may be indistinguishable)
• Oligodendroglioma (often heterogeneous, calcified)
• Low-grade astrocytoma (often more infiltrative)

Note: The above tumors do not have the propensity for cortical involvement that is seen with DNETs, but preoperative distinction can be difficult.

Discussion

Background

DNET, first reported as a new entity in 1988, is an uncommon benign intracortical lesion that is usually diagnosed in adolescence or young adulthood. Histologically DNETs resemble gliomas but behave as stable lesions. The classification of these lesions is controversial, and they may not represent true neoplasms as their stable course and histology suggest a cortical dysplastic process. A temporal lobe location is most common (>60%), and the lesion often involves or lies close to mesial temporal structures. Other locations include the frontal lobes (30%), followed by parietal and/or occipital lobes, and rarely the basal ganglia. Infratentorial DNET has been reported but is rare.

Clinical Findings

Patients commonly present with partial complex seizures that are often long-standing and intractable.

Etiology

DNETs are thought to originate from secondary germinal layers of the developing CNS. The presence of associated foci of cortical dysplasia suggests that these lesions arise during formation of the cortex. It remains somewhat uncertain if the DNET is a true brain neoplasm or a form of cerebral dysgenesis.

Pathology

At present, DNET is classified by the World Health Organization (WHO) as a "neuronal and mixed neuronoglial tumor." Important pathologic features include an intracortical location, multinodular architecture, and heterogeneity of cellular composition with astrocytes, oligodendrocytes, and neurons.

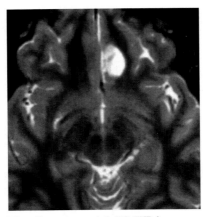

Fig. D. An axial T2-WI in a patient with seizures demonstrates an ovoid hyperintense lesion centered in the frontal cortex.

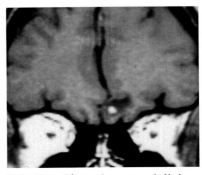

Fig. E. Coronal post-gadolinium T1-WI in the patient in Fig. D demonstrates a nodular focus of enhancement at the medial aspect of a dysembryoplastic neuroepithelial tumor (DNET).

Imaging Findings

CT

- Well-demarcated low-density lesion that may contain cysts
- Focal contrast enhancement may be present
- Calcification is present in <25% of cases
- Calvarial deformity may be present adjacent to the lesion, indicative of a long-standing process

MR

- Low signal on T1-WI, high signal on T2-WI
- Cortical location more easily appreciated than on CT (Fig. D)
- The lesion often has a "thick gyriform" or "nodular" configuration
- Little mass effect, no surrounding edema
- May see focal marginal or nodular contrast enhancement (Fig. E)
- Hemorrhage is uncommon but has been observed
- Small "daughter cysts" are typical

Treatment

- Surgical resection, if accessible
- Radiotherapy is not of definite benefit, even with subtotal resection

Prognosis

- Excellent, with long survival even with incomplete tumor resection
- The majority of patients are seizure-free after surgery, or have a significant reduction in seizure frequency

Suggested Readings

Daumas-Duport C, Scheithauer BW, Chodkiewicz JP, et al. Dysembryoplastic neuroepithelial tumor: a surgically curable tumor of young patients with intractable partial seizures: report of 39 cases. *Neurosurgery* 23:545–556, 1988.

Koeller KK, Dillon WP. Dysembryoplastic neuroepithelial tumors: MR appearance. *AJNR* 13:1319–1325, 1992.

Ostertun B, Wolf HK, Campos MG, et al. Dysembryoplastic neuroepithelial tumors: MR and CT evaluation. *AJNR* 17:419–430, 1996.

Case 9

Clinical Presentation

A 66-year-old man presents with headache and confusion.

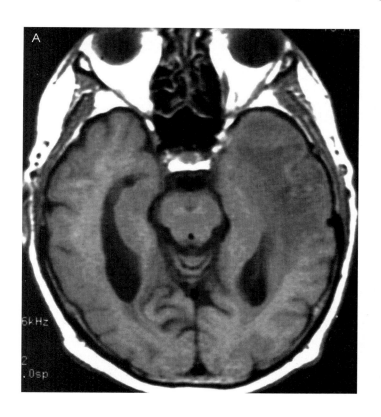

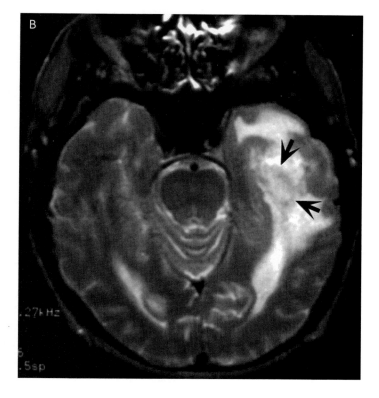

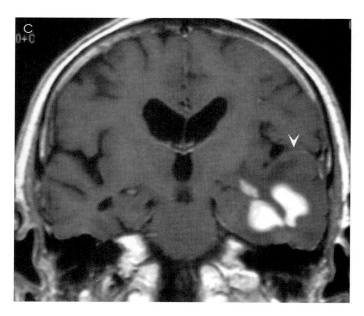

Radiologic Findings

An axial T1-WI (Fig. A) demonstrates abnormal hypointensity involving an expanded left temporal lobe. An axial T2-WI (Fig. B) shows subcortical T2 prolongation consistent with vasogenic edema within the left temporal lobe. A more focal area of intermediate signal intensity (*arrows*) is noted. Post-gadolinium, a T1-WI (Fig. C) shows intense, lobulated, homogenous enhancement within the white matter of the temporal lobe. Note the overall expansion of the left temporal lobe and the mass effect on the left sylvian fissure (*arrowhead*).

Diagnosis

Primary CNS lymphoma (PCNSL), non-AIDS-related

Differential Diagnosis

- Metastatic disease (often multiple lesions, significant vasogenic edema)
- High-grade glioma (often areas of necrosis, hemorrhage, or cyst formation)
- Pyogenic abcess (usually peripheral enhancement)

Discussion

Background

PCNSL represents about 1% of intracranial neoplasms in the nonimmunocompromised population and about 1% of all lymphomas. The incidence of PCNSL has been increasing in recent years. It usually affects older adults, with a median age of 60 years. It may present as a solitary mass or multiple lesions (40%), or be diffusely infiltrative. The diffusely infiltrative form may be radiologically indistinguishable from gliomatosis cerebri. Supratentorial disease is more common than infratentorial. Intracranial spread of systemic lymphoma (secondary CNS lymphoma) usually manifests as either leptomeningeal or dural-based disease, and only rarely presents as an isolated parenchymal mass.

Clinical Findings

The most common presenting symptoms are headache, confusion, and seizures.

Pathology

Gross

- Well-circumscribed or infiltrative mass
- Calcification and hemorrhage are rare in untreated lymphoma
- Necrosis is uncommon in the absence of AIDS

Microscopic

- Usually non-Hodgkin's B-cell lymphoma
- Lesions frequently abut the ventricular system and may show a diffuse periventricular pattern

Imaging Findings

PCNSL often involves the deep gray matter, periventricular regions, and corpus callosum.

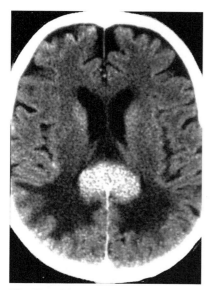

Fig. D. Non-contrast CT scan in a patient with PCNSL demonstrates an intrinsically dense and homogenous mass with surrounding edema involving the splenium of the corpus callosum.

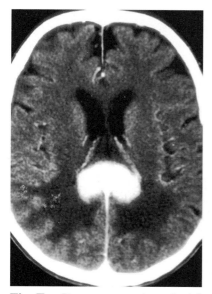

Fig. E. Post-contrast, the splenial lesion shown in Fig. D demonstrates intense and homogenous enhancement.

CT

- Often intrinsically dense prior to contrast administration (Fig. D)
- Enhances homogeneously in most cases (Fig. E)

MR

- T1-WI: iso- or hypointense to gray matter
- T2-WI: usually iso- or hypointense to gray matter. This is thought to be related to high cellularity and scant cytoplasm in these lesions
- Post-gadolinium: typically enhances with a homogeneous pattern. Less commonly a peripheral pattern of enhancement is seen

Treatment

- Radiation therapy and/or chemotherapy
- Steroids

Prognosis

- Poor, with a median survival of 13.5 months
- The tumor is exquisitely radiosensitive, but has a high rate of relapse

Suggested Readings

Michalski JM, Garcia DM, Kase E, et al. Primary central nervous system lymphoma: analysis of prognostic variables and patterns of treatment failure. *Radiology* 176:855–860, 1990.

Roman-Goldstein SM, Goldman DL, Howieson J, et al. MR of primary CNS lymphoma in immunologically normal patients. *AJNR* 13:1207–1213, 1992.

Schwaighofer BW, Hesselink JR, Press GA, et al. Primary intracranial CNS lymphoma: MR manifestations. *AJNR* 10:725–729, 1989.

Case 10

Clinical Presentation

A 28-year-old HIV-positive male was brought to the emergency room following a seizure. Confusion and a right hemiparesis prompted an imaging evaluation.

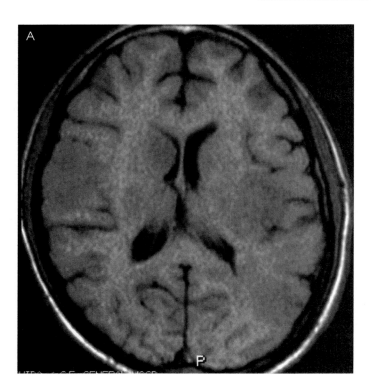

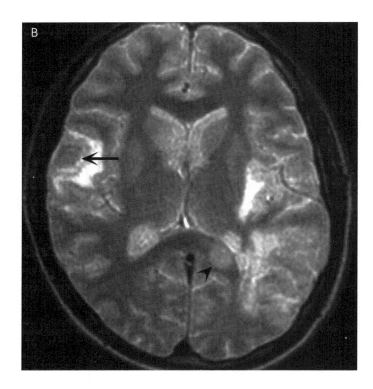

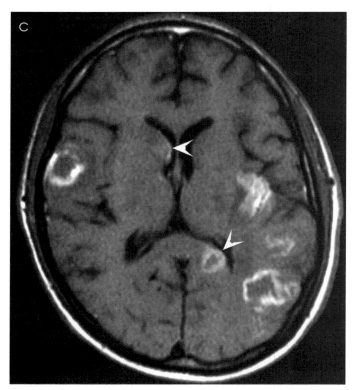

Radiologic Findings

An axial T1-WI (Fig. A) demonstrates multiple areas of parenchymal hypodensity involving the sylvian regions bilaterally, the left temporal lobe, and the right caudate head. On an axial T2-WI (Fig. B), multifocal areas of high signal intensity are seen. Note that a right frontal lesion is centrally isointense to brain parenchyma (*arrow*). In addition, a lesion in the splenium is appreciated far more easily on the T2-WI (*arrowhead*) than on the T1-WI. Post-gadolinium (Fig. C), all lesions demonstrate enhancement. Note that the enhancement pattern is generally peripheral. The left sylvian lesion shows gyral and subcortical enhancement, while the caudate and splenial lesions show enhancement of the adjacent ependymal surfaces (*arrowheads*).

Diagnosis

AIDS-related primary CNS lymphoma

Differential Diagnosis

• Toxoplasmosis (in some cases may be indistinguishable from lymphoma, but lacks subarachnoid and ependymal spread)
• Other brain abscess (usually hyperintense on T2-WI, not hyperdense on noncontrast CT scan)
• Cytomegalovirus (CMV) (may mimic lymphoma that involves only the ependymal surfaces)
• Glioblastoma multiforme (may be indistinguishable though typically a large, solitary lesion)
• Metastatic disease (typically does not show the ependymal and subarachnoid enhancement that is common with lymphoma)

Discussion

Background

Primary CNS lymphoma (PCNSL) has an incidence of 2 to 6% among AIDS patients. The risk of developing PCNSL is 1000 times greater in AIDS patients than in the non-AIDS population. In an HIV-positive individual, PCNSL is an AIDS-defining condition. Because of the epidemiology of AIDS, affected patients are usually in their 20s and 30s. Lesions are usually supratentorial (75%) and may be single or multiple. A solitary mass lesion in an AIDS patient is more often due to lymphoma than to infection (71%), but is still nonspecific. Lesions may be located superficially or in deep structures. Furthermore, they may coexist with other pathologic processes, which may make the imaging diagnosis confusing.

Clinical Findings

Symptoms reflect the location of the lesion(s): focal neurological deficits (hemiparesis, ataxia), signs of increased intracranial pressure, seizures, mental status changes.

Etiology

The brain is devoid of lymphatics and lymphocytes. AIDS-related PCNSL is considered to be the result of activation of a population of B-cells by an opportunis-

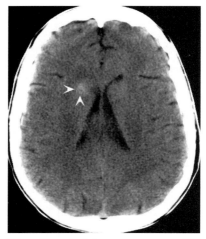

Fig. D. Axial non-contrast CT scan in an HIV-positive woman with confusion demonstrates mild hyperdensity in the right caudate head (*arrowheads*).

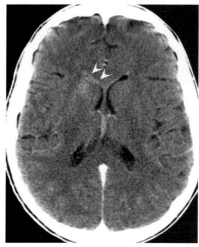

Fig. E. Following administration of contrast to the patient in Fig. D, mild enhancement of the right caudate lesion and the ependymal surface of the adjacent right frontal horn (*arrowheads*) occurs. Lymphoma was confirmed by stereotactic biopsy.

Table 1. Features of Lymphoma and Toxoplasmosis

	Lymphoma	Toxoplasmosis
Single lesion	+	+/−
Deep gray nuclear involvement	+	+
Dense on noncontrast CT	++	+/−
Eccentric target sign	−	++
Callosal involvement	++	very rare
Ependymal spread	++	−
Subarachnoid spread	++	−
201-thallium scanning	++	−

Symbols: ++, strongly favors; +, favors; +/−, not helpful; −, not associated

tic oncogenic virus (HIV, Epstein-Barr Virus, CMV). These cells subsequently undergo numerous cell divisions in an environment lacking immune surveillance secondary to a deficient T-cell system.

Pathology

Gross

- Lesions commonly affect diencephalic structures and basal ganglia
- Peripheral portions of the cerebral hemispheres are also involved
- Lesions are often necrotic, occasionally hemorrhagic
- Calcification is rare prior to therapy

Microscopic

- Immunoblastic histology (a high-grade malignancy) predominates
- Tumor cells are often found in a perivascular distribution

Imaging Findings

CT

- Isodense or hyperdense on noncontrast scan (Figs. D and E)
- May enhance homogeneously or peripherally (non-AIDS-related PCNSL rarely shows a peripheral enhancement pattern)

MR

- Isointense to gray matter on T1-WI and T2-WI
- Peripheral enhancement is typical
- Ependymal extension is frequent
- Hemorrhage is rare in the absence of treatment
- ^{1}H MR spectroscopy shows elevated choline
- MR perfusion shows elevated RCBV (regional cerebral blood volume)

Treatment

- Patients are often treated initially with empiric antitoxoplasmosis therapy
- When lesions fail to respond, brain biopsy is generally performed
- Once PCNSL is diagnosed, treatment may include steroids (significant decrease in size, but not a durable response), radiation therapy, and chemotherapy in selected cases (CD4 count > 200)

Prognosis

Poor, with a median survival of 5 months

Suggested Readings

Ioachim HL, Dorsett B, Cronn W, et al. Acquired immunodeficiency syndrome associated lymphomas: clinical, pathologic, immunologic and viral characteristics of 111 cases. *Hum Pathol* 22:659–673, 1991.

Lee YY, Bruner JM, Van Tassell P, Libshitz HI. Primary central nervous system lymphoma: CT and pathologic correlation. *AJR* 147:747–752, 1986.

Ruiz A, Donovan Post MJ, Bundschu C, et al. Primary central nervous system lymphoma in patients with AIDS. *Neuroim Clin North Am* 7:281–296, 1997.

Case 11

Clinical Presentation

A 16-year-old male presents with gradually progressive left-sided weakness. He has also noted headaches for several months.

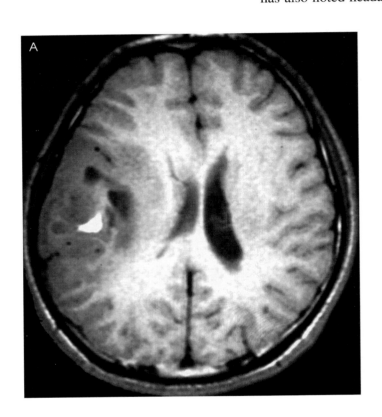

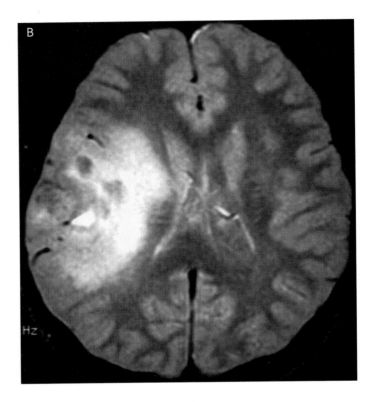

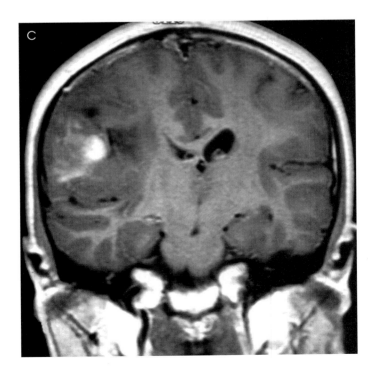

Radiologic Findings

An axial T1-WI (Fig. A) demonstrates a heterogeneous intraaxial lesion in the right frontal lobe. Areas of cyst formation and hemorrhage are present. A PD-WI (Fig. B) demonstrates a heterogeneous, infiltrative lesion. There is relatively little surrounding edema. A coronal post-gadolinium T1-WI (Fig. C) demonstrates only mild enhancement lateral to the area of hemorrhage. This lesion exerts mass effect, with inferior displacement of the right sylvian fissure and compression of the right lateral ventricle.

Diagnosis

Supratentorial primitive neuroectodermal tumor (PNET)

Differential Diagnosis

• Ependymoma (may be indistinguishable)
• Ependymoblastoma (rare, usually in neonates, very large and heterogeneous)
• Malignant rhabdoid tumor (may be indistinguishable)
• Glioblastoma multiforme (typically more surrounding edema)
• Teratoma/teratocarcinoma (usually midline; may contain fat)

Discussion

Background

PNET, also known as cerebral neuroblastoma, is a rare neoplasm typically described in children as a large, heterogeneous parenchymal supratentorial mass. These tumors usually displace the adjacent ventricle but may extend into the ventricle. Infants and young children are most commonly affected, with 80% of cases occurring in the first decade of life. This tumor may be congenital. Overall supratentorial PNET accounts for <1% of primary brain tumors but 18% of brain neoplasms that are diagnosed within the first 2 months of life. Parietal and occipital locations are most common, but multiple lobes of the brain are frequently involved.

Clinical Findings

Clinical findings are nonspecific: headache, seizures, signs of elevated intracranial pressure, and/or focal neurologic findings may be present. Infants may demonstrate macrocephaly.

Pathology

Gross

• Usually large hemispheric masses that appear sharply circumscribed
• Frequently contains cysts, necrosis, calcification, hemorrhage

Microscopic

• Highly cellular tumors composed of 90 to 95% undifferentiated cells
• Electron microscopy is useful in demonstrating neuronal differentiation

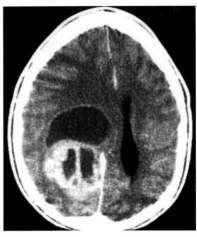

Fig. D. Contrast-enhanced scan in a different patient with PNET demonstrates a large heterogeneously enhancing parenchymal mass that has both cystic and solid components.

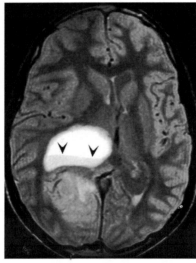

Fig. E. Axial PD-WI from the patient in Fig. D shows a cystic and solid lesion with no surrounding edema. The cyst is hyperintense compared with CSF, and also contains a fluid level (*arrowheads*) consistent with hemorrhage.

Imaging Findings

CT

- Large heterogeneous parenchymal mass (Fig. D)
- Solid portions tend to be dense on pre-contrast images
- Inhomogeneous enhancement post-contrast
- Cysts, calcification, and hemorrhage are common
- Frequently little edema relative to the size of lesion

MR

- Inhomogeneous on both T1- and T2-WIs
- Variable enhancement characteristics
- Hemorrhage is frequent and often occurs into tumor cysts (Fig. E)
- Calcification and hemosiderin may mimic flow voids

Treatment

- Surgical excision (usually subtotal because of the large size of these lesions)
- Postoperative radiation therapy depending on the age of the patient
- Chemotherapy

Prognosis

- Poor: this is a malignant lesion with a high rate of recurrence after therapy and frequent subarachnoid metastases
- 5-year survival is on the order of 30%

Suggested Readings

Davis PC, Wichman RD, Takei Y, Hoffman JC Jr. Primary cerebral neuroblastoma: CT and MR findings in 12 cases. *AJNR* 11:115–120, 1990.

Robles HA, Smirniotopoulos JG, Figueroa RE. Understanding the radiology of intracranial primitive neuroectodermal tumors from a pathological perspective: a review. *Semin US, CT, MR* 13:170–181, 1992.

Case 12

Clinical Presentation

An 11-year-old boy has a history of unusual laughing (gelastic) seizures.

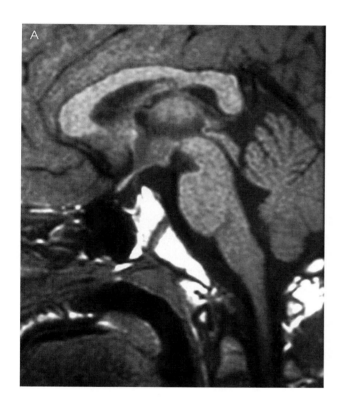

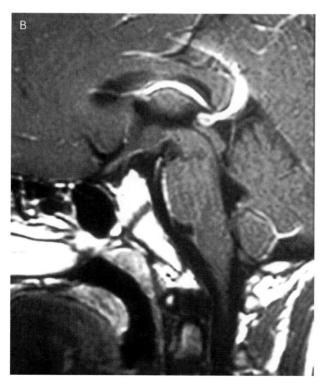

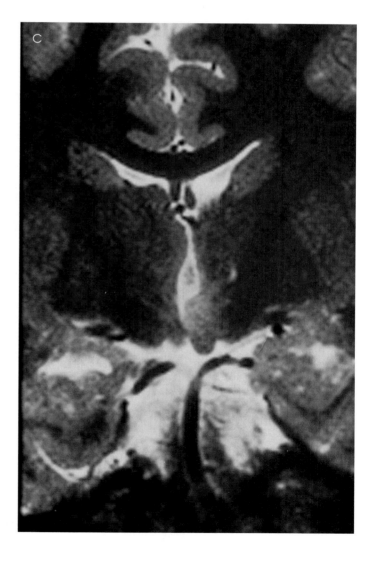

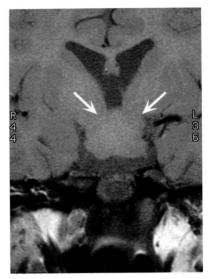

Fig. D. Coronal T1-WI demonstrates a large lesion isointense to gray matter arising from the inferior hypothalamus and extending into the suprasellar cistern (*arrows*). This lesion was initially noted on a neonatal sonogram performed in a patient with the characteristic phenotypic features of Pallister-Hall syndrome.

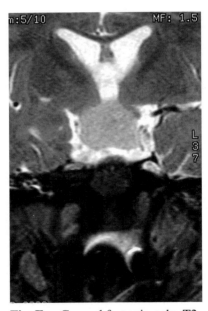

Fig. E. Coronal fast spin-echo T2-WI of the patient in Fig. D shows the mass to be mildly hyperintense to gray matter.

Radiologic Findings

A sagittal T1-WI (Fig. A) demonstrates a sessile mass isointense to gray matter arising in the region of the tuber cinereum. Incidentally noted is a small sella turcica and hypoplastic pituitary gland. On a post-gadolinium sagittal T1-WI (Fig. B), the mass does not enhance. A coronal fast spin-echo T2-WI (Fig. C) shows that the mass is slightly hyperintense compared with gray matter.

Diagnosis

Hamartoma of the tuber cinereum

Differential Diagnosis

- Astrocytoma (infiltrative, enhancing)
- Other glial neoplasm (unusual location, usually brighter on T2-WI)

Discussion

Background

The "tuber cinereum" is located between the infundibular stalk anteriorly and the mamillary bodies posteriorly, and includes the middle hypothalamic nuclei. Hamartomas of this region are congenital, nonneoplastic heterotopia composed of normal neuronal tissue. These rare lesions are more commonly seen in males than in females. The hamartoma is typically pedunculated and is attached to the tuber cinereum or mammillary body by a thin stalk, but the lesion may be completely contained in the hypothalamus and have a "sessile" appearance. Large lesions may be associated with syndromes such as Pallister-Hall, which includes specific facial anomalies, polydactyly, imperforate anus, and hypothalamic hamartoma (Figs. D and E).

Clinical Findings

Two distinct clinical presentations have been noted. (1) Precocious puberty (symptom onset usually prior to 2 years of age) and (2) seizures (often of a characteristic "gelastic" type [spasmodic laughter], associated with a sessile morphology). Neurodevelopmental delay and hyperactivity are associated with lesions over 1 cm in diameter.

Pathology

Gross

- Pedunculated or sessile mass

Microscopic

- Closely resembles gray matter
- Neurons may be similar to those in the adjacent hypothalamus
- Variable amounts of fibrillary gliosis

Imaging Findings

The lesions range in size from a few millimeters to 3 to 4 centimeters and are nonenhancing on both CT and MR.

Pearls

- MR is much more sensitive and specific for this diagnosis than CT, and coronal and sagittal imaging should be performed with both T1- and T2-WIs.

- Thin sections are essential to look for small lesions: consider a T1-weighted volumetric acquisition such as 3D-SPGR (spoiled grass) with 1.5-mm partitions and a coronal high-resolution fast spin-echo T2-weighted acquisition with 2- to 3-mm slice thickness.

- The floor of the third ventricle should be smooth from infundibulum to mammillary bodies. Any nodularity should raise suspicion for a hamartoma in the appropriate clinical setting.

Pitfall

- Small lesions are easy to miss with conventional imaging. Thin-section coronal and sagittal imaging should be performed as described above in any child with precocious puberty or gelastic seizures in whom standard sequences are unrevealing.

CT

- Rounded mass that is isodense with brain tissue
- Cystic component may rarely be seen
- In axial plane, appears to lie within suprasellar/interpeduncular cisterns
- No hemorrhage, rare calcification

MR

- Isointense to gray matter on T1-WI
- Iso- or hyperintense to gray matter on T2-WI
- Posterior pituitary bright spot is usually preserved
- No enhancement

Treatment

Treatment is controversial as these lesions are nonneoplastic: Surgical treatment is recommended for pedunculated lesions with refractory symptoms, while medical therapy is recommended for sessile lesions.

Prognosis

- Surgical resection of pedunculated lesion is generally curative
- Sessile lesions are more difficult to resect without damaging adjacent structures
- Medical therapy with gonadotropin-releasing hormone is an option, but it is very expensive as many years of treatment may be required

Suggested Readings

Albright AL, Lee PA. Neurosurgical treatment of hypothalamic hamartomas causing precocious puberty. *J Neurosurg* 78:77–82, 1993.

Boyko OB, Curnes JT, Oakes WJ, Burger PC. Hamartomas of the tuber cinereum: CT, MR, and pathologic findings. *AJNR* 12:309–314, 1991.

Diebler C, Ponsot G. Hamartomas of the tuber cinereum. *Neuroradiology* 25:93–101, 1983.

Case 13

Clinical Presentation

A teenage boy presents with increasingly severe headaches over the past several months.

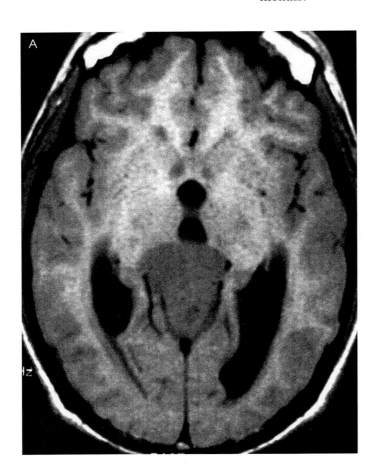

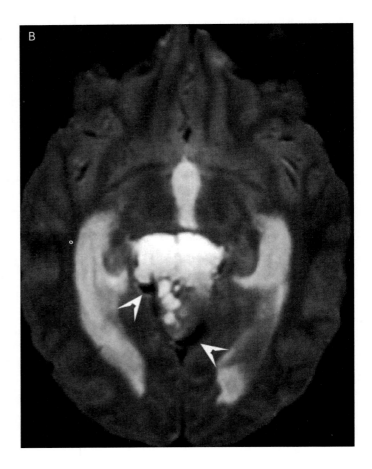

Radiologic Findings

An axial T1-WI (Fig. A) demonstrates a well-circumscribed pineal region mass that is slightly hypointense compared with cortex. Mild obstructive hydrocephalus is present. An axial T2-WI (Fig. B) shows heterogeneous signal intensity within the mass. Areas of low signal (*arrowheads*) are consistent with hemorrhage.

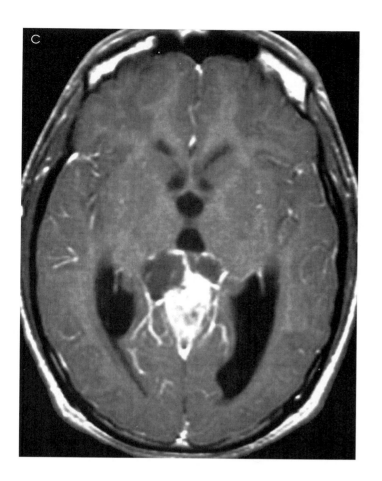

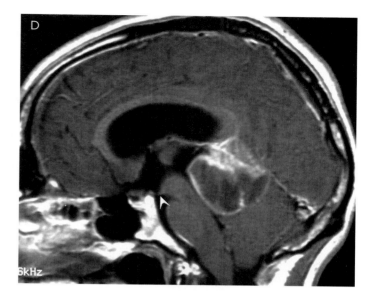

An axial post-gadolinium T1-WI (Fig. C) shows heterogeneous enhancement, with nonenhancement of the anterior cystic portions and intense and homogeneous enhancement of solid regions. A sagittal post-gadolinium T1-WI (Fig. D) again demonstrates the heterogeneously enhancing mass centered in the pineal region. There is mass effect on the cerebellar vermis. In addition, there is obstructive hydrocephalus with enlargement of the lateral and third ventricles. The floor of the third ventricle is depressed (*arrowhead*).

Diagnosis

Pineoblastoma

Differential Diagnosis

- Pineocytoma (more likely to be calcified, but often indistinguishable)
- Germ-cell neoplasm (typically more homogeneous)
- Astrocytoma (often more infiltrative)

Discussion

Background

Pineal region tumors constitute 0.4 to 1% of brain tumors in adults and 3 to 8% of brain tumors in children. Germinomas and astrocytomas account for the ma-

Pearls

- Imaging findings are generally nonspecific among pineal region tumors, so tissue confirmation of histology is required.
- Pineocytomas tend to be smaller and better circumscribed (Fig. E) and are more often calcified.

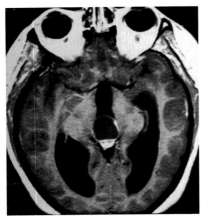

Fig. E. Axial post-gadolinium T1-WI demonstrates nodular enhancement around the periphery of a cystic mass. Pineocytoma was confirmed histologically.

Pitfalls

- Benign pineal cysts should not be confused with a pineal-region tumor.
- Follow-up scans done in patients with familial and/or bilateral retinoblastoma should always include the pineal region.

jority of pineal region masses. Pineal parenchymal cell tumors include pineoblastomas and pineocytomas, and together these account for <15% of pineal region neoplasms. In the so-called "trilateral retinoblastoma," pineoblastomas may develop in patients with familial and/or bilateral retinoblastoma (RB). There is a 3 to 10% incidence of pineoblastoma in patients with familial and/or bilateral RB, with these lesions usually occurring later than RBs (age at diagnosis of pineoblastoma is typically 2 to 3 years, whereas RBs usually occur at 3 to 6 months of age).

Clinical Findings

Nonspecific signs are related to local mass effect and hydrocephalus secondary to aqueductal obstruction: patients may demonstrate symptoms and signs of elevated intracranial pressure, ataxia, and/or Parinaud's sign (paresis of upward gaze).

Etiology

Both pineoblastoma and pineocytoma arise from pineal parenchymal cells. Pineoblastoma cells are undifferentiated and immature and are considered a type of primitive neuroectodermal tumor.

Pathology

Gross

- Unencapsulated masses that invade adjacent brain when large

Microscopic

- Densely cellular small round cell tumors
- Mixed histologies with elements of both pineoblastoma and pineocytoma may occur

Imaging Findings

CT

- Usually noncalcified, often hyperdense, may be hemorrhagic
- Solid portions enhance homogeneously or mildly heterogeneously

MR

- Usually large, lobulated masses that may invade adjacent parenchyma
- Hypo- to isointense on T1-WI
- Iso- to slightly hyperintense on T2-WI, like other small round cell tumors
- May contain areas of cyst formation, necrosis, and/or hemorrhage

Treatment

- Surgical resection
- Radiation therapy
- Chemotherapy

Prognosis

- Varies with the extent of disease at time of diagnosis. Initial staging should include examination of CSF and MR of the spine to look for subarachnoid spread of tumor.
- Patients with pineoblastoma and a history of bilateral RB ("trilateral retinoblastoma") have a uniformly poor prognosis

Suggested Readings

Chang SM, Lillis-Hearne PK, Larson DA, et al. Pineoblastoma in adults. *Neurosurgery* 37:383–390, 1995.

Chiechi MV, Smirniotopoulos JG, Mena H. Pineal parenchymal tumors: CT and MR features. *J Comput Assist Tomogr* 19:509–517, 1995.

Edwards MSB, Hudgins RJ, Wilson CB, et al. Pineal region tumors in children. *J Neurosurg* 68:689–697, 1988.

Case 14

Clinical Presentation

A 23-year-old man presents with headache and paresis of upward gaze.

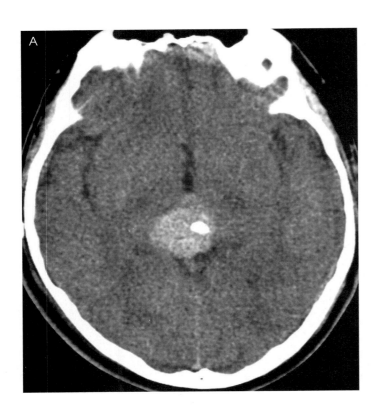

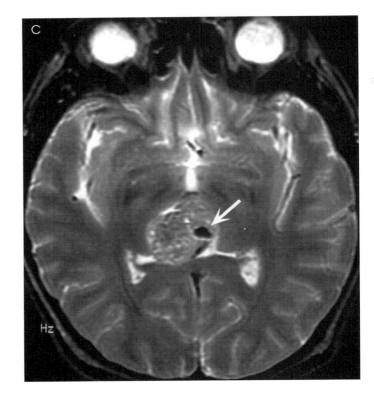

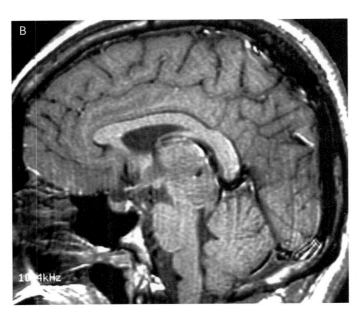

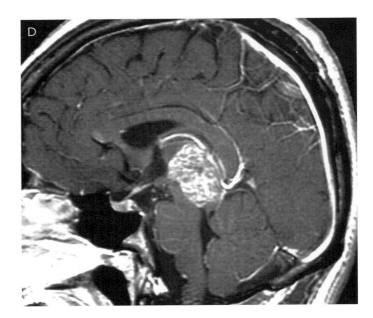

Radiologic Findings

A non-contrast CT scan (Fig. A) demonstrates a lobulated intrinsically dense mass centered at the level of the pineal gland. A focal calcification is noted within the mass. A sagittal T1-WI (Fig. B) demonstrates an isointense mass with a punctate focus of hypointensity representing the known calcification. Surprisingly, there is no significant hydrocephalus. An axial T2-WI (Fig. C) again demonstrates the apparently well-circumscribed mass, which is largely isointense to brain parenchyma. The calcification appears as a focal hypointensity (*arrows*). No edema is noted in the adjacent brain parenchyma. A sagittal post-gadolinium T1-WI (Fig. D) demonstrates moderate enhancement of the lesion.

Diagnosis

Germinoma

Differential Diagnosis

- Other germ cell tumors (generally need tissue to distinguish among these)
- Lymphoma (typically an older patient, not usually calcified)
- Pineocytoma (more heterogeneous, often cyst formation)
- Pineoblastoma (more heterogeneous, may be hemorrhagic)
- Astrocytoma (large, irregular, heterogeneous)

Discussion

Background

The most common neoplasm of the pineal region is the germ cell tumor, accounting for 3 to 8% of pediatric brain tumors. Germ cell tumors include germinomas, nongerminomas (teratoma, endodermal sinus tumor, choriocarcinoma), and mixed lesions. Germinomas account for over 50% of pineal region neoplasms, and most of these lesions occur in the second and third decades. Thirty-five percent of intracranial germinomas occur in the suprasellar region. Pineal region germinomas have a 10:1 male predominance, while suprasellar germinomas have an equal gender incidence. Fewer than 10% of germ cell tumors originate in the basal ganglia or thalamus, though these locations are more commonly involved in the Japanese.

Clinical Findings

Patients typically present with hydrocephalus and Parinaud's syndrome (paresis of upward gaze).

Etiology

Germinomas are considered to arise embryologically from a midline streaming of totipotential cells that occurs early in the development of the rostral part of the neural tube.

Pathology

Gross

- Usually a well-defined round or lobulated mass

Microscopic

• Intracranial germinomas are histologically identical to testicular seminomas
• Unencapsulated mass with large polygonal cells and clusters of lymphocytes in a dense connective tissue stroma
• Mixed histologies (germinoma with foci of embryonal carcinoma, choriocarcinoma, yolk sac tumor, and/or teratoma/teratocarcinoma) are common

Imaging Findings

Imaging findings are similar to other highly cellular tumors:

CT

• Iso- to hyperdense on non-contrast study
• Homogeneous enhancement
• Usually noncalcified (except for engulfed pineal gland), and noncystic

MR

• Well-marginated, lobulated mass
• Usually isointense on both T1- and T2-WIs
• Homogeneous intense enhancement post-gadolinium

Treatment

• Germinoma is exquisitely sensitive to radiation therapy
• Chemotherapy is used for recurrent disease or more aggressive histologies

Prognosis

Varies with histology:

• Germinoma = 92.7% 10-year survival
• Malignant teratoma = 70.7% 10-year survival
• Embryonal carcinoma, yolk sac tumor, choriocarcinoma = 27.3% 3-year survival

Table 1. Hormone Production by Germ Cell Neoplasms

Histology	AFP	Beta-HCG	PLAP
Germinoma	–	–	+
Embryonal carcinoma	+	+	
Choriocarcinoma	–	+	
Yolk sac tumor	+	–	
Teratoma	+/–	+/–	

PLAP: placental alkaline phosphatase

AFP: alpha-fetoprotein

Beta-HCG: beta subunit of human chorionic gonadotropin

Suggested Readings

Matsutani M, Sano K, Takakura K, et al. Primary intracranial germ cell tumors: a clinical analysis of 153 histologically verified cases. *J Neurosurg* 86:446–455, 1997.

Moon WK, Chang KH, Kim IO, et al. Germinomas of the basal ganglia and thalamus: MR findings and a comparison between MR and CT. *AJR* 162:1413–1417, 1994.

Tien RD, Barkovich AJ, Edwards MSB. MR imaging of pineal tumors. *AJNR* 11:557–565, 1990.

Case 15

Clinical Presentation

Three different women in their 20s with a history of secondary amenorrhea and galactorrhea are referred for MR imaging.

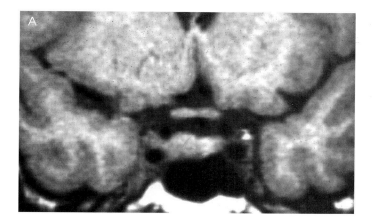

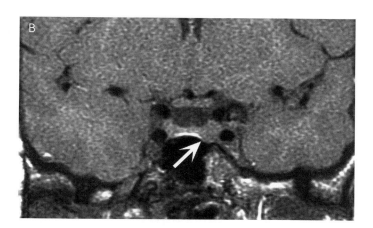

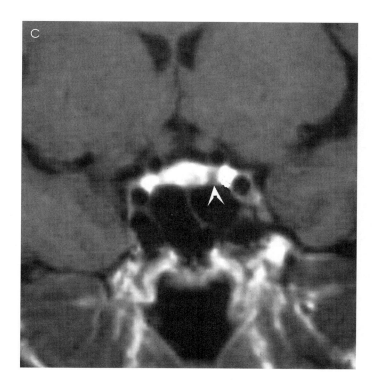

Radiologic Findings

A coronal T1-WI (Fig. A) demonstrates asymmetry of the pituitary gland, with a low signal intensity mass in the right side of the gland. The floor of the sella is depressed on the right as compared with the left. A coronal T1-WI in a second patient (Fig. B) demonstrates a rounded lesion in the left pituitary gland that is isointense to the remainder of the gland (*arrow*). Note also the downsloping of the left sellar floor. A post-gadolinium coronal T1-WI in a third patient (Fig. C) demonstrates a small nonenhancing focus in the left side of the gland (*arrowhead*).

Diagnosis

Pituitary microadenomas, prolactin-secreting

Differential Diagnosis

• Pituitary cyst (does not enhance, usually lower in signal intensity on T1-WI)
• Intrasellar craniopharyngioma (very rare)
• Pituitary metastasis (also very rare, usually in older patient)

Discussion

Background

Pituitary adenomas account for ~10% of primary intracranial neoplasms. Microadenomas are 400 times more common than macroadenomas, and both occur most frequently in adults. A pituitary microadenoma is defined as an adenoma ≤10 mm in diameter. Hormonally active tumors are more likely to present when small because symptoms of hormone overproduction cause the patient to seek medical attention. Prolactin-secreting and adrenocorticotropic hormone (ACTH)-secreting tumors are more common in females but do occur in males as well. Growth hormone-secreting tumors are more common in males. Overall, prolactin-secreting adenomas account for 30% of all pituitary adenomas.

Clinical Findings

In females, hyperprolactinemia results in amenorrhea and galactorrhea. In males, hyperprolactinemia results in decreased libido.

Complications

• Vary with type of hormone produced: ACTH-producing adenoma causes complications of Cushing's disease (obesity, hypertension, elevated blood sugar) and growth-hormone-secreting adenoma causes complications of acromegaly (coarsened facial features, growth of hands and feet, etc.)
• Cavernous sinus and/or clivus invasion may occur with microadenomas as well as macroadenomas and generally prevents surgical cure
• Pituitary apoplexy (typically seen with macroadenomas, see Case 16)

Pathology

Gross
• Well-defined, encapsulated, benign, slow-growing lesion

Microscopic
• Generally monotonous sheets of uniform cells
• Subclassified by immunohistochemical criteria

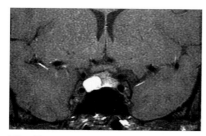

Fig. D. A coronal pre-gadolinium T1-WI demonstrates a well-circumscribed intrinsically bright mass in the right pituitary gland. Hemorrhagic adenoma was proved surgically.

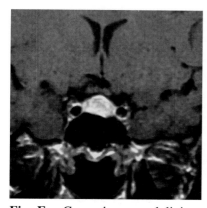

Fig. E. Coronal post-gadolinium T1-WI in a 27-year-old woman with acromegaly. The pituitary gland is prominent, which is common in menstruating females, but no focal low–intensity lesion is detected.

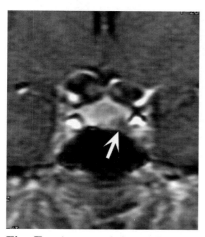

Fig. F. A coronal fast spin-echo T1-WI obtained 40 seconds after dynamic gadolinium infusion in the patient in Figure D demonstrates a focal hypointensity within the left inferior aspect of the pituitary gland (*arrow*) not visible on routine post-gadolinium images. At surgery, this was confirmed to represent a growth-hormone-secreting microadenoma.

Imaging Findings

CT

- Less sensitive than MR because of bone artifact, and poor soft tissue contrast
- If a lesion is visible, it is typically isodense to normal gland pre-contrast and shows delayed enhancement post-contrast

MR

- Usually isointense on T1- and T2-WIs
- Rarely demonstrate cyst formation or hemorrhage (Fig. D)
- Usually appear hypointense compared with normal enhancing pituitary parenchyma (pituitary lacks a blood-brain barrier) on post-contrast images, but may occasionally be iso- or hyperintense post-contrast
- In general, microadenomas are difficult to detect because of their small size. Dynamic scanning during bolus infusion of gadolinium may increase sensitivity (Figs. E and F) because of the relatively delayed enhancement of an adenoma as compared with normal pituitary gland, and therefore greater conspicuity of the adenoma on early enhanced images (under 2 minutes).

Treatment

- Surgical excision
- Medical therapy is an option which varies with the type of hormone produced

Prognosis

Excellent

Suggested Readings

Davis WL, Lee JN, King BD, Harnsberger HR. Dynamic contrast-enhanced MR imaging of the pituitary gland with fast spin-echo technique. *JMRI* 4:509–511, 1994.

Teramoto A, Hirakawa K, Sanno N, Osamura Y. Incidental pituitary lesions in 1,000 unselected autopsy specimens. *Radiology* 193:161–164, 1994.

Case 16

Clinical Presentation

A 27-year-old female presents with abrupt onset of bitemporal hemianopia.

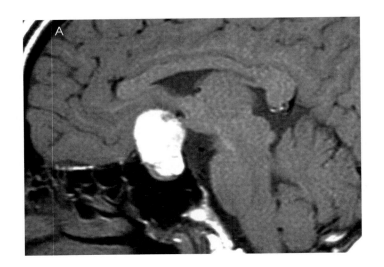

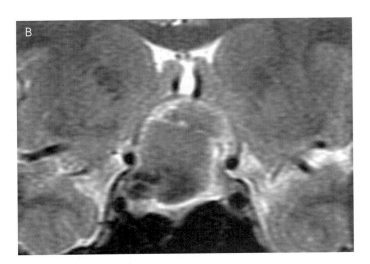

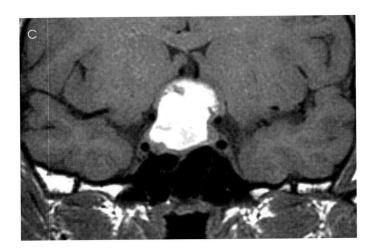

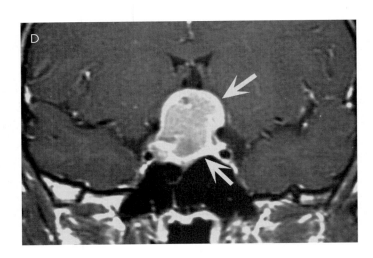

Radiologic Findings

A sagittal T1-WI (Fig. A) demonstrates a well-circumscribed sellar and suprasellar mass of intrinsic high signal intensity. The sella turcica is enlarged. A coronal fast spin-echo T2-WI (Fig. B) demonstrates areas of low and intermediate signal intensity within the mass. The signal characteristics are consistent with subacute blood products (intracellular methemoglobin). A coronal T1-WI (Fig. C) again demonstrates the sellar and suprasellar mass. The optic chiasm is superiorly displaced by the mass. A post-gadolinium T1-WI (Fig. D) demonstrates moderate homogeneous enhancement of the solid peripheral components of the mass (arrows).

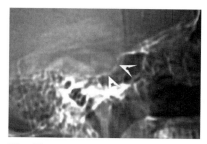

Fig. E. A lateral digital scout view from a CT scan demonstrates enlargement of the sella turcica (*arrowheads*).

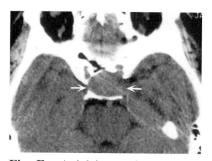

Fig. F. Axial image from a noncontrast CT scan (same patient as Fig. E) demonstrates enlargement of the sella secondary to a homogeneous soft tissue mass (*arrows*).

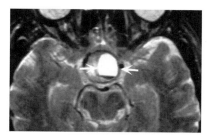

Fig. G. Axial T2-WI shows a hemorrhagic cyst with a fluid-fluid level within the left aspect of a pituitary macroadenoma (*arrows*) in a different patient without any acute change in symptoms.

Pearls

• For most pituitary MR imaging studies, pre- and postcontrast T1-WIs are adequate, but T2-WIs are indicated in cases of apoplexy to assess acute hemorrhage. *(continued)*

Diagnosis

Pituitary macroadenoma complicated by hemorrhage ("pituitary apoplexy")

Differential Diagnosis

• Craniopharyngioma (usually does not enlarge sella; dominant component of mass usually suprasellar even if mass extends into sella, does not enhance)
• Rathke's cleft cyst (usually does not enlarge sella)
• Pituitary carcinoma (rare, more invasive)
• Pituitary metastasis (more irregular, usually does not enlarge sella, also rare)
• Pituitary abscess (usually not hemorrhagic, often associated with sphenoid sinus disease)

Discussion

Background

A pituitary macroadenoma is defined as a pituitary adenoma >10 mm. Non-hormone-secreting adenomas are more likely to present at a large size because hormone production generally brings secreting lesions to early attention when patients complain of symptoms related to excess hormone production. Pituitary macroadenomas often grow superiorly through the diaphragma sella, accounting for half of all suprasellar masses.

Clinical Findings

Common complaints include visual changes (often bitemporal hemianopia) secondary to mass effect on the optic chiasm, cranial nerve palsies secondary to cavernous sinus compression/invasion, and symptoms of hypopituitarism (i.e., decreased libido).

Complications

"Pituitary apoplexy" is due to sudden infarction, either bland or hemorrhagic, within a normal or neoplastic pituitary gland and occurs in ~7% of patients with pituitary adenomas. The gland suddenly enlarges and may acutely compress adjacent structures such as the optic chiasm. Patients complain of sudden loss of visual acuity, oculomotor palsies, decreased sensorium, and/or severe headache. Subarachnoid hemorrhage may occur and mimic the presentation of a ruptured aneurysm.

Pathology

Gross

• Lobulated well-demarcated mass that usually bulges superiorly through the diaphragma sella into the suprasellar cistern
• Characteristic "figure-of-eight" appearance, with waist at level of the diaphragma sella

Microscopic

• Sheets, cords, or nests of uniform cells
• May be "invasive" or "aggressive" in behavior, but in these cases the histology remains indistinguishable from benign counterpart

- Fat packing is generally placed in the sphenoid sinus at the time of surgery, so use fat-saturation on post-operative post-contrast scans. Note that over time the fat will necrose and scar down and may appear similar to residual or recurrent tumor.

- Macroadenoma encasing the cavernous carotid artery usually does not cause narrowing (Fig. H), unlike meningiomas which typically narrow the vessels they surround.

Pitfalls

- Pituitary apoplexy is a clinical diagnosis, because pituitary hemorrhage may occur without apoplectic symptoms.

- Within the first 12 hours, coronal thin-section CT may be better for visualizing intratumoral hemorrhage. However, MR is more sensitive in detecting and following hemorrhage in the subacute stage.

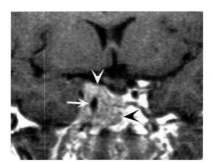

Fig. H. Coronal T1-WI in a patient with an invasive pituitary macroadenoma (*arrowheads*) demonstrates extension into the clivus and the right cavernous sinus. The cavernous carotid artery (*arrow*) is surrounded by the soft tissue mass but not narrowed.

Imaging Findings

Typically both a sellar and suprasellar component to the mass.

CT

- Sellar expansion, with bone erosion and remodeling (Figs. E and F)
- Intermediate-density soft tissue mass; hyperdense mass if hemorrhagic

MR

- "Figure-of-eight"-shaped sellar and suprasellar mass
- Usually homogeneously isointense on T1- and T2-WI
- May show areas of cyst formation, necrosis, and/or hemorrhage (Fig. G)
- Enhances moderately and homogeneously if solid
- May see cavernous sinus compression or invasion

Treatment

- Pituitary apoplexy is a surgical emergency usually treated with steroids and prompt surgical decompression
- Macroadenoma in general is treated by surgical resection, medical therapy if the lesion is hormonally active (i.e., bromocriptine for prolactinoma), or radiation therapy if there is subtotal resection and/or aggressive disease

Prognosis

- The outcome of pituitary apoplexy is good with rapid diagnosis and treatment
- However, in some cases, visual deficits and ocular palsies may persist

Suggested Readings

Donovan JL, Nesbit GM. Distinction of masses involving the sella and suprasellar space: specificity of imaging features. *AJR* 167:597–603, 1996.

Ostrov SG, Quencer RM, Hoffman JC, et al. Hemorrhage within pituitary adenomas: how often associated with pituitary apoplexy syndrome? *AJNR* 10:503–510, 1989.

Wakai S, Fukushima T, Teramoto A, Sano K. Pituitary apoplexy: its incidence and clinical significance. *J Neurosurg* 55:187–193, 1981.

Case 17

Clinical Presentation

A 45-year-old female underwent MR scanning for evaluation of headaches.

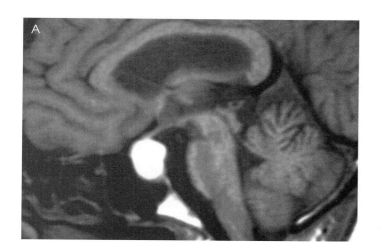

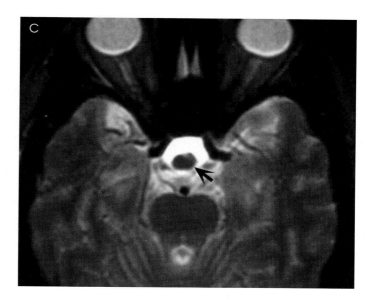

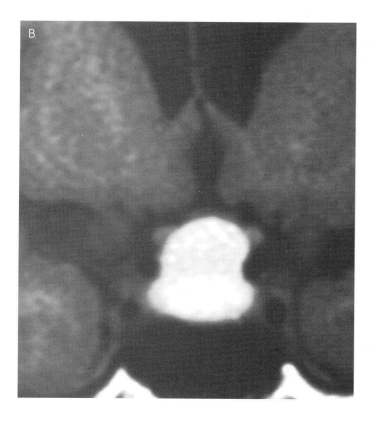

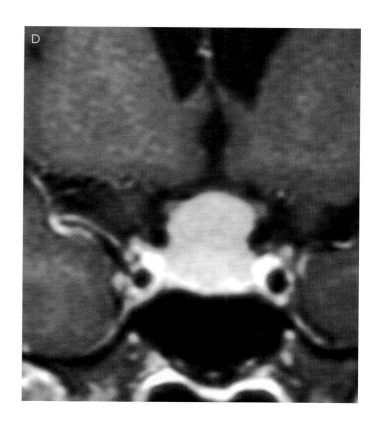

Radiologic Findings

Sagittal (Fig. A) and coronal (Fig. B) T1-WIs demonstrate a well-circumscribed sellar and suprasellar mass that shows intrinsic high-signal intensity. An axial T2-WI (Fig. C) shows that the mass is heterogeneous, containing a focal area of T2 shortening likely representing focal aggregation of particulate material (*arrow*). Following administration of gadolinium (Fig. D), a coronal T1-WI shows no evidence of enhancement around the periphery of or within this lesion.

Diagnosis

Rathke's cleft cyst

Differential Diagnosis

- Craniopharyngioma (frequently mixed cystic and solid, often calcified)
- Pituitary micro- or macroadenoma (usually solid, but may have cystic or hemorrhagic areas)
- Arachnoid cyst (contains fluid identical to CSF in density/intensity)
- Epidermoid cyst (often slightly hyperintense to CSF, irregular margin)
- Abscess (often a shaggy or irregular margin, thick enhancing rim)

Discussion

Background

Rathke's cleft cysts are found incidentally in up to 25% of autopsies. These lesions may be purely intrasellar (~25%), purely suprasellar (rare), or combined (most common, ~70%). Their size is variable, usually ranging from 3 mm to 3 cm. These lesions are rarely symptomatic and are usually undetected in life or are detected incidentally. If symptomatic, they usually present in middle-aged adults and are more commonly seen in females.

Clinical Findings

Symptoms are the result of local mass effect and include headache, amenorrhea/galactorrhea, or visual field cuts, and less commonly hypopituitarism, diabetes insipidus, diplopia, or ptosis.

Etiology

Rathke's pouch develops as a rostral outpouching of the primitive oral cavity during the third or fourth week of gestation. If the lumen of the pouch does not obliterate, then a cyst may arise between the anterior and intermediate lobes of the pituitary. Competing theories state that this lesion may originate directly from neuroepithelial tissue or represent reverse metaplasia of anterior lobe cells.

Pathology

Gross

- Smoothly marginated lobulated lesion
- Cyst contents range from serous fluid to gray mucoid material
- Clumps of calcification may occasionally be present

Pearl

• Rathke's cleft cysts have a much more variable appearance on MR than is generally appreciated due to the variable protein content of cyst fluid.

Pitfall

• This lesion may mimic pituitary adenoma or craniopharyngioma both clinically and on imaging.

Microscopic

• Cyst wall consists of a single layer of pseudostratified epithelium with an underlying layer of connective tissue

Imaging Findings

These lesions are discrete and well-defined on both CT and MR. Most Rathke's cleft cysts do not enlarge the sella.

CT

• Cysts are usually low density, but may be mixed high and low density
• High density is presumed secondary to inspissated contents

MR

• Variable signal intensity on both T1- and T2-WIs.
• This variability is related to protein content, cholesterol crystals, and blood products
• Post-gadolinium images may show a thin rim of enhancement, which reflects residual pituitary gland displaced around the cyst

Treatment

• Symptomatic lesions: transsphenoidal cyst drainage with biopsy of the cyst wall. Purely suprasellar lesions require craniotomy or stereotactic aspiraiton
• Asymptomatic lesions: follow-up imaging to evaluate growth

Prognosis

Excellent, but may recur in 5 to 10% of cases

Suggested Readings

El-Mahdy W, Powell M. Transsphenoidal management of 28 symptomatic Rathkes cleft cysts, with special reference to visual and hormonal recovery. *Neurosurgery* 42:7–17, 1998.

Ross DA, Norman D, Wilson CB. Radiologic characteristics and results of surgical management of Rathke's cysts in 43 patients. *Neurosurgery* 30:173–179, 1992.

Voelker JL, Campbell RL, Muller J. Clinical, radiographic, and pathologic features of symptomatic Rathke's cleft cysts. *J Neurosurg* 74:535–544, 1991.

Case 18

Clinical Presentation

A 4-year-old male with increasing irritability and developmental delay compared with his twin brother.

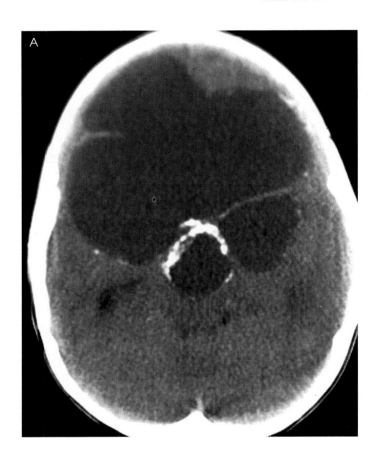

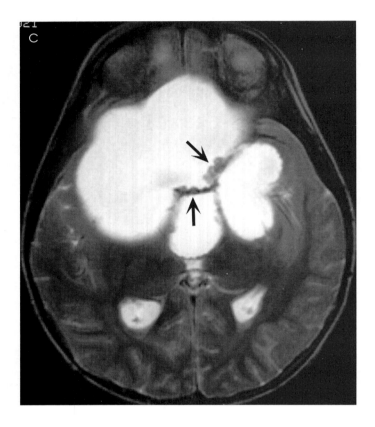

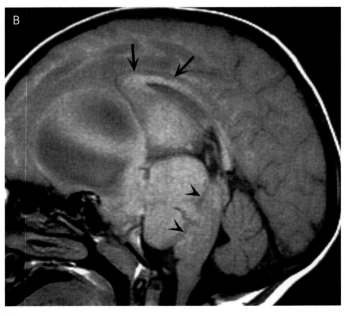

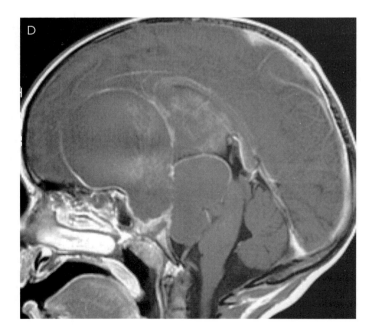

Radiologic Findings.

A non-contrast CT scan (Fig. A) demonstrates a large well-circumscribed multicystic lesion with calcification around the periphery of one of the cysts. Its site of origin is unclear on this image. A sagittal T1-WI (Fig. B) demonstrates a heterogeneous, extraaxial, mixed cystic and solid lesion involving the sellar and suprasellar regions, as well as the interpeduncular and prepontine cisterns. The signal intensity of the cysts is greater than that of CSF. Note the marked displacement and elevation of the corpus callosum (*arrows*) and the mass effect on the brainstem (*arrowheads*). On an axial T2-WI (Fig. C), the extraaxial cystic masses have high-signal intensity and incite no edema in the adjacent brain parenchyma. Areas of irregular hypointensity around the periphery of portions of the cyst (*arrows*) correspond to calcifications noted on CT scan. A sagittal post-gadolinium T1-WI (Fig. D) demonstrates a slightly irregular rim of linear enhancement around the cystic components of the lesion.

Diagnosis

Craniopharyngioma

Differential Diagnosis

- Essentially none in this case
- General differential of "cystic" suprasellar masses includes (1) Rathke's cyst (smaller, less heterogeneous, nonenhancing, no solid component), (2) pituitary adenoma (more homogeneous, enlarges sella), (3) glioma (not typically calcified), (4) metastasis (uncommon location), and (5) aneurysm (lamellated thrombus, phase artifact)

Discussion

Background

Craniopharyngiomas account for about 3% of primary intracranial tumors. Over 50% of these tumors occur in children and young adults. These tumors are usually suprasellar, though they may be purely intrasellar. Intrasellar extension is relatively frequent, with enlargement of the sella and erosion of the dorsum sella. Two types of craniopharyngioma are classically described, though recently there has been some controversy over the correlation of age with histologic subtype:

1. Childhood form: peaks at 10 to 14 years and has frequent cyst formation and calcification, an adamantinomatous microscopic pattern, and a generally poor prognosis
2. Adult form: peaks in the sixth decade, has less frequent cysts and calcification, and demonstrates papillary squamous epithelium.

Clinical Findings

Symptoms are typically related to mass effect: headache and visual disturbances due to pressure on chiasm, cognitive/behavioral changes due to mass effect on the frontal lobes, hydrocephalus, and endocrine dysfunction.

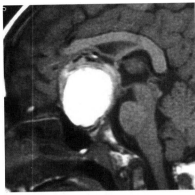

Fig. E. A sagittal T1-WI demonstrates a large sellar and suprasellar mass with a rim of soft tissue around a markedly hyperintense central cyst. Craniopharyngioma.

Pearls

- The "90%" rule: it is generally quoted that childhood craniopharyngiomas are cystic in 90% and calcified in 90%.

- High-signal intensity within a suprasellar mass on T1-WI should raise suspicion of a craniopharyngioma.

- Plain film (Fig. F) or CT demonstration of calcification may add specificity to the diagnosis but is usually unnecessary.

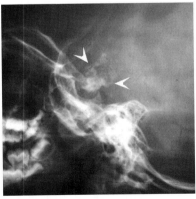

Fig. F. A lateral plain film of the skull demonstrates amorphous sellar and supersellar calcification (*arrowheads*). Note also the enlargement of the sella turcica in this patient with a craniopharyngioma.

Etiology

The two major hypotheses are that craniopharygiomas arise from remnants of the craniopharyngeal duct, which connects the stomodeal ectoderm with the evaginated Rathke's pouch, or they arise from squamous epithelial cells in the pars tuberalis of the adenohypophysis.

Pathology

Gross

- Lobulated, well-defined mass
- Cyst fluid contents varies from highly proteinaceous yellowish fluid to "crankcase oil" containing cholesterol and blood products

Microscopic

- Very heterogeneous: cysts, cholesterol clefts, inflammation, giant cell reaction, and calcification
- The cell type is often mixed or transitional: squamous epithelium in continuation with adamantinomatous epithelium

Imaging Findings

CT

- Large, lobulated, heterogeneous suprasellar mass
- Frequent calcification that may be linear and peripheral or irregular and nodular
- Cysts vary in density depending on contents
- Mass may enlarge sella, erode dorsum sella

MR

- Cysts may vary greatly in signal intensity depending on contents (Fig. E)
- Calcification is more difficult to detect on MR than on CT
- A solid enhancing portion is almost always present
- The cyst rim usually enhances
- Infiltration of adjacent structures (i.e., hypothalamus, optic chiasm and tracts) is frequent

Treatment

- Surgical resection–usually subtotal due to adherence to adjacent structures
- For residual/recurrent disease options include: radiation therapy, cyst aspiration if symptoms are due to an enlarging cyst, or instillation of phosphorous-32 or other sclerosing agents into the cyst

Prognosis

- Varies with age, size of tumor, and extent of resection
- Fewer recurrences are seen if radiation is given after subtotal resection

Pitfall

- In some cases craniopharyngioma can be difficult to distinguish from a cystic and/or hemorrhagic pituitary macroadenoma.

Suggested Readings

Eldevik OP, Blaivas M, Gabrielsen TO, et al. Craniopharyngioma: radiologic and histologic findings and recurrence. *AJNR* 17:1427–1439, 1996.

Sartoretti-Schefer S, Wichmann W, Aguzzi A, Valavanis A. MR differentiation of adamantinomatous and squamous-papillary craniopharyngiomas. *AJNR* 18:77–87, 1997.

Yasargil MG, Curcic M, Kis M, et al. Total removal of craniopharyngiomas. Approaches and long-term results in 144 patients. *J Neurosurg* 73:3–11, 1990.

Case 19

Clinical Presentation

A 12-year-old boy presents with frequent urination and is dignosed with diabetes insipidus.

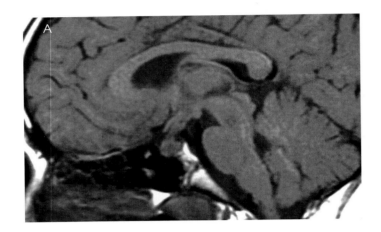

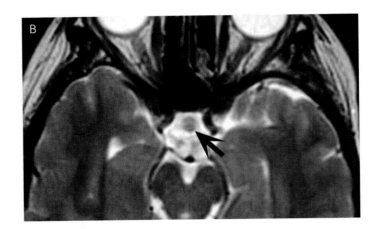

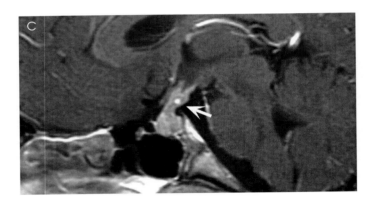

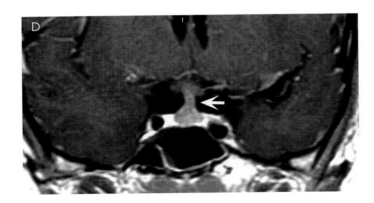

Radiologic Findings

A sagittal T1-WI (Fig. A) shows thickening of the pituitary infundibular stalk and slight prominence of the pituitary gland. The normal posterior pituitary bright spot is not observed. An axial T2-WI (Fig. B) demonstrates that the thickened infundibulum (*arrow*) is isointense to gray matter. Sagittal (Fig. C) and coronal (Fig. D) post-gadolinium T1-WIs demonstrate moderately intense and homogeneous enhancement of abnormal soft tissue which involves the infundibulum (*arrows*) and floor of the third ventricle.

Diagnosis

Germinoma

Differential Diagnosis

• Sarcoid (look for associated systemic findings such as hilar adenopathy)
• Langerhans' cell histiocytosis (typically occurs in children, look for associated destructive skull and temporal bone lesions)
• Lymphoma (look for evidence of systemic disease)
• Glioma (more irregular, heterogeneous)
• Tuberculosis (look for evidence of remote or active disease on chest x-ray)
• Metastatic disease (often parenchymal lesions as well, older patient)

Discussion

Background

Germ cell neoplasms make up 0.3 to 3% of pediatric brain tumors in Western countries and 4.8 to 15% of those in Japan. Forty-five percent of germ cell neoplasms are germinomas. These lesions generally occur in the midline. The suprasellar region is the second most common location for intracranial germinomas after the pineal region and these lesions tend to involve the hypothalamic stalk. Suprasellar germinomas occur in both sexes with equal frequency, and 70% of them occur in adolescents. Spread through subarachnoid spaces and along ependymal surfaces is a common feature of this neoplasm.

Clinical Findings

These tumors usually present in adolescence with visual or pituitary axis dysfunction: diabetes insipidus (DI), panhypopituitarism, and precocious puberty. DI may be present prior to any definite imaging findings. DI frequently persists even after a response to therapy is shown by MR imaging.

Pathology

Gross

• Unencapsulated, may invade adjacent structures

Microscopic

• Histologically identical to testicular seminoma
• Loosely cohesive aggregates of germ cells associated with scattered small lymphocytes

Imaging Findings

CT

• Homogeneous mass which is intrinsically dense prior to contrast
• Typically noncalcified

MR

• May be an infiltrative process rather than masslike
• Isointense on T1-WI, mildly hyperintense on T2-WI
• Enhances homogeneously post-gadolinium

Treatment

- Biopsy to establish accurate diagnosis
- Definitive radiation therapy

Prognosis

Good, with survival as high as 90% at 10 years

Suggested Readings

Hoffman HJ, Otsubo H, Hendrick EB, et al. Intracranial germ-cell tumors in children. *J Neurosurg* 74:545–551, 1991.

Simmons GE, Suchnicki JE, Rak KM, Damiano TR. MR imaging of the pituitary stalk: size, shape, and enhancement pattern. *AJR* 159:375–377, 1992.

Sumida M, Uozumi T, Kiya K, et al. MRI of intracranial germ cell tumors. *Neuroradiology* 37:32–37, 1995.

Case 20

Clinical Presentation

A 20-year-old female presents with progressive headaches.

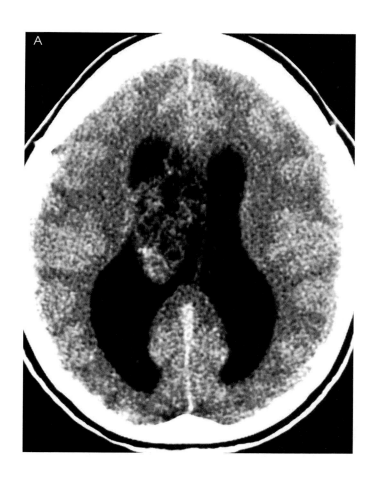

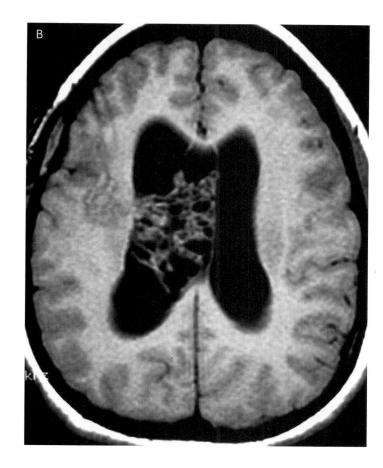

Radiologic Findings

An axial non-contrast CT scan (Fig. A) demonstrates an intraventricular mass with a "feathery" appearance. This mass is attached along its medial margin to the septum pellucidum. Moderate enlargement of the lateral ventricles secondary to hydrocephalus is present. An axial T1-WI demonstrates that the solid component is isointense to brain parenchyma (Fig. B).

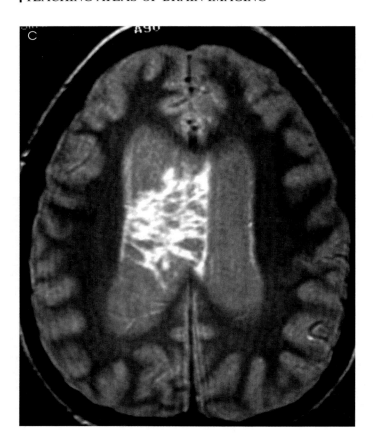

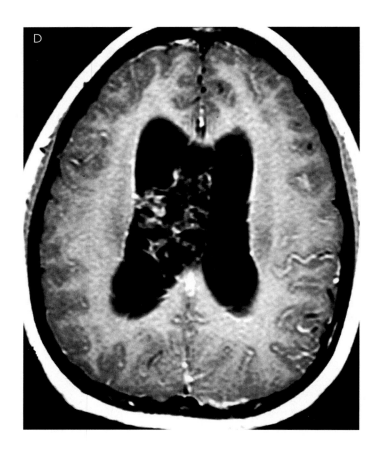

An axial PD-WI demonstrates that the solid component is hyperintense to brain parenchyma (Fig. C). An axial post-gadolinium T1-WI shows mild enhancement of the solid portions of the mass (Fig. D).

Pearls

- The tumor often has a "feathery" appearance on CT and MR due to multiple cysts

- When central neurocytoma arises within the lateral ventricle it is usually attached to the septum pellucidum.

Pitfalls

- In the past, these tumors were often misdiagnosed as oligodendrogliomas.

- Neurocytomas are generally localized lesions, but cases of craniospinal dissemination of histologically typical central neurocytoma lacking malignant change have been reported.

Diagnosis

Central neurocytoma

Differential Diagnosis

- Oligodendroglioma (may be indistinguishable)
- Astrocytoma (may be indistinguishable, though generally lacks feathery appearance)
- Ependymoma (often centered in periventricular parenchyma when supratentorial)
- Choroid plexus tumor (more commonly located within the fourth ventricle in an adult)
- Intraventricular metastasis (often invades brain, incites edema)

Discussion

Background

The entity of central neurocytoma was first described in 1982. It is a benign tumor of neuronal origin that is usually located within the ventricular system, typically the lateral ventricle, and is often attached to the septum pellucidum. Central neurocytoma is relatively uncommon, accounting for ~0.5% of primary brain

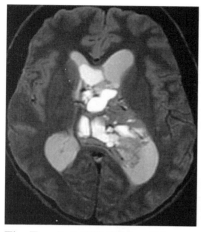

Fig. E. Axial T2-WI in a 28-year-old female demonstrates a mixed cystic and solid intraventricular mass. Areas of low-signal intensity are consistent with hemorrhage or calcification.

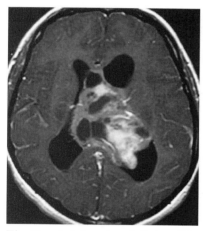

Fig. F. Axial post-gadolinium T1-WI in the same patient demonstrates a lobulated intraventricular mass with the solid portions showing variable enhancement. Neurocytoma was diagnosed at surgery.

tumors. It usually affects young adults, with an average age at presentation of 31 years. Extraventricular neoplasms with neurocytoma-like features have been reported, but controversy exists over their classification.

Clinical Findings

Nonspecific: headache and other signs of elevated intracranial pressure

Etiology

Central neurocytoma is a tumor of neuronal (as opposed to glial) lineage.

Pathology

Gross

- Well-defined and sharply circumscribed intraventricular mass, though the tumor may infiltrate into adjacent brain parenchyma, precluding total resection
- Neurocytomas are primarily solid but contain cysts in ~85% of cases

Microscopic

- Resembles oligodendroglioma on light microscopy. Immunoreactivity stains show neuronal markers (synaptophysin) and electron microscopy shows neurosecretory granules

Imaging Findings

CT

- Often calcified (70%)
- May have a "feathery" appearance due to multiple cysts and thin intervening septa
- Calcification is variable

MR

- Hypo- or isointense to gray matter on T1-WI
- Heterogeneously hyperintense on T2-WI
- Intratumoral hemorrhage may occur
- Cyst formation is common
- Solid portions tend to enhance moderately and homogeneously or heterogeneously (Figs. E and F)

Treatment

Combination of surgery, radiation therapy, and/or chemotherapy

Prognosis

Generally excellent with overall 5-year survival of 81%

Suggested Readings

Chang KH, Han MH, Kim DG, et al. MR appearance of central neurocytoma. *Acta Radiologica* 34:520–526, 1993.

Goergen SK, Gonzales MF, McLean CA. Intraventricular neurocytoma: radiologic features and review of the literature. *Radiology* 182:787–792, 1992.

Schild SE, Scheithauer BW, Haddock MG, et al. Central neurocytomas. *Cancer* 79:790–795, 1996.

Case 21

Clinical Presentation

An elderly male was referred for a head CT after a series of falls.

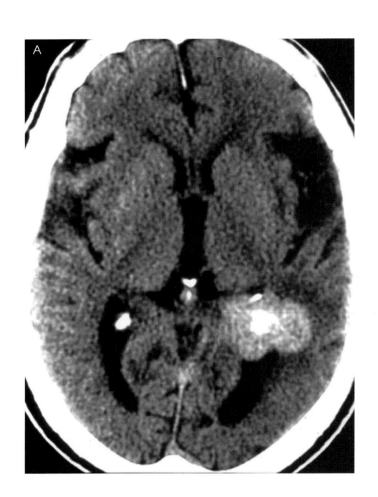
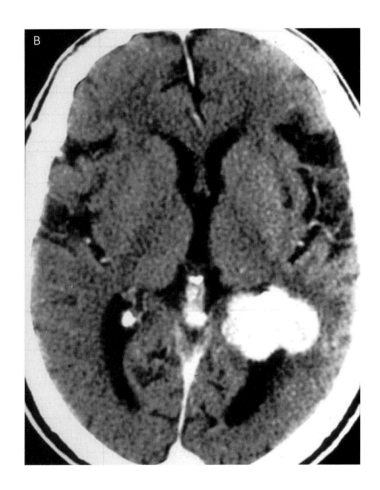

Radiologic Findings

A non-contrast CT scan (Fig. A) demonstrates a lobulated mass centered in the atrium of the left lateral ventricle. The mass is mildly hyperdense compared with brain parenchyma, and an area of central calfication is present. Following the administration of intravenous contrast (Fig. B), the mass intensely and homogeneously enhances. An axial T2-WI obtained the following day (Fig. C) demonstrates the well-circumscribed intraventricular mass within a mildly enlarged ventricular atrium. The mass is minimally hyperintense compared with brain parenchyma, while the central calcification is hypointense. Post-gadolinium (Fig. D), a T1-WI shows intense and homogenous enhancement of the intraventricular mass. Note the focus of central hypointensity corresponding to the known calcification.

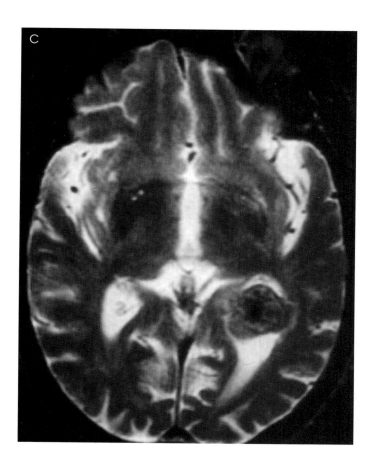

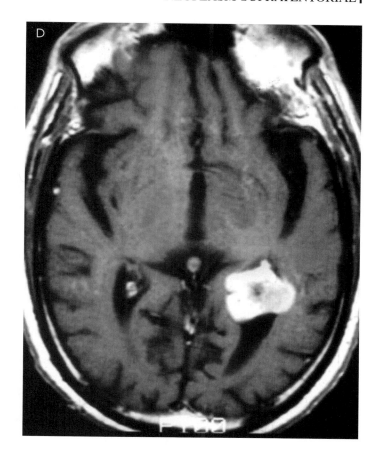

Diagnosis

Intraventricular meningioma

Differential Diagnosis

- Adult patient with a mass within the *atrium* of the lateral ventricle
  - –Meningioma or metastasis
- Adult patient with a mass within the *body* of the lateral ventricle
  - –Astrocytoma, oligodendroglioma, central neurocytoma, and/or subependymoma
- Choroid plexus cyst: should follow CSF in signal intensity; nonenhancing
- Choroid plexus papilloma (usually in fourth ventricle in the adult)
- Xanthogranuloma of choroid plexus: typically contains fat

Discussion

Background

Meningioma is the most common tumor of the ventricular atrium in people over the age of 30. Of all intracranial meningiomas, only 0.5 to 2% are intraventricular. As with most meningiomas, there is a female predominance of 2:1. In an older patient with a mass arising in the atrium of the lateral ventricle, the differential diagnosis usually lies between meningioma and metastasis.

Clinical Findings

Patients usually present with signs and symptoms of hydrocephalus.

Complications

Meningiomas may be associated with intraventricular hemorrhage.

Etiology

Intraventricular meningiomas arise from the stroma of the choroid plexus or from rests of arachnoid tissue within the choroid.

Pathology

Cross

• Intraventricular meningiomas are usually spherical, lobulated, and benign

Microscopic

• Exhibit a wide range of histologic patterns, though meningothelial and fibrous variants predominate
• Usually benign

Imaging Findings

Well-circumscribed mass within ventricular atrium

CT

• Often contain dense calcification (50%)
• Intrinsically dense even if noncalcified

MR

• May be hypointense on T1- and T2-WI if heavily calcified
• Isointense on T1- and T2-WI if noncalcified
• Intense, usually homogeneous enhancement in noncalcified portions of the mass

Treatment

• Surgical resection
• Radiation therapy for subtotal resection or if malignant

Prognosis

Good

Suggested Readings

Guidetti B, Delfini R, Gagliardi FM, Vagnozzi R. Meningiomas of the lateral ventricles: clinical, neuroradiologic, and surgical considerations in 19 cases. *Surg Neurol* 24:364–370, 1985.

Jelinek J, Smirniotopoulos JG, Parisi JE, Kanzer M. Lateral ventricular neoplasms of the brain: differential diagnosis based on clinical, CT, and MR findings. *AJNR* 11:567–574, 1990.

Rohringer M, Sutherland G, Louw DF, Sima AAF. Incidence and clinicopathological features of meningioma. *J Neurosurg* 71:665–672, 1989.

Case 22

Clinical Presentation

A 44-year-old male is evaluated for progressive headache.

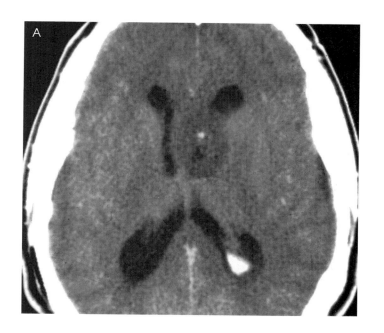

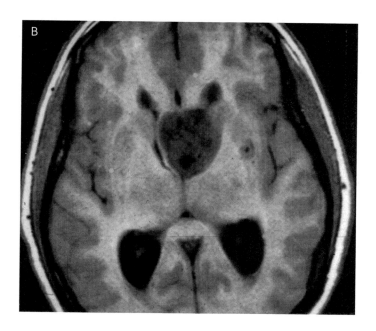

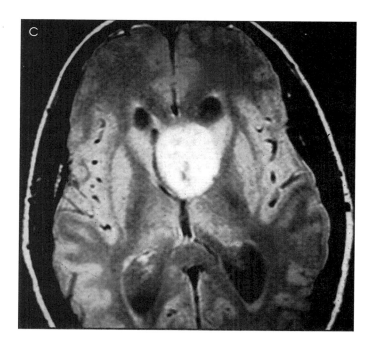

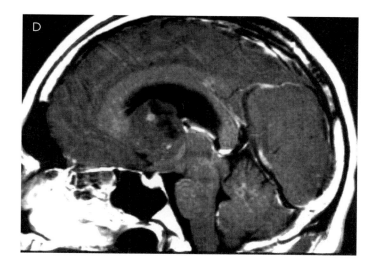

Radiologic Findings

An axial non-contrast CT scan (Fig. A) demonstrates a mass centered in the frontal horn of the left lateral ventricle. It contains a small cyst, as well as a punctate focus of calcification. There is mild dilatation of the lateral ventricles. An axial T1-WI (Fig. B) demonstrates a hypointense mass centered at the level of the left frontal horn. Again note mild heterogeneity secondary to cyst formation within the mass. An axial PD-WI (Fig. C) demonstrates marked hyperintensity of the mass lesion. A sagittal post-gadolinium T1-WI (Fig. D) demonstrates that the mass is largely nonenhancing, with the exception of a few punctate foci of enhancement.

Diagnosis

Subependymoma of the lateral ventricle

Differential Diagnosis

- Subependymal giant cell astrocytoma (occurs at level of foramen of Monro and is typically seen in patients with tuberous sclerosis)
- Oligodendroglioma (often more irregular in appearance)
- Central neurocytoma (often a feathery appearance, associated with septum pellucidum)
- Meningioma (enhances, usually arises in the trigone in older patients)
- Ependymoma (younger patients, usually centered in parenchyma when supratentorial)

Discussion

Background

Subependymoma is classically described as an asymptomatic fourth ventricular tumor found incidentally at autopsy in elderly males. The incidence of this relatively uncommon tumor was 0.4% in 1000 serial autopsies. Overall approximately 66% of these tumors arise in the fourth ventricle and 33% arise in the lateral ventricles, though in some individual series a lateral ventricular location is more common. Tumors that are symptomatic are usually large, measuring 5 cm or more.

Clinical Findings

Patients usually present with symptoms and signs related to elevated intracranial pressure such as headache.

Complications

Complications include hydrocephalus and intratumoral or subarachnoid hemorrhage.

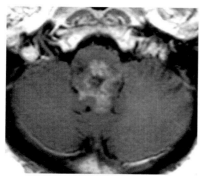

Fig. E. Axial post-gadolinium T1-WI in an older male demonstrates a heterogenously enhancing mass at the level of the inferior fourth ventricle. Subependymoma.

Pearl

- Unlike ependymomas, subependymomas tend not to seed the subarachnoid space.

Pitfalls

- Lesions may be multiple, so postoperative imaging is important to evaluate for additional lesions after mass effect from the dominant lesion has been relieved.

- A subependymoma located in the midline at the junction of the septum pellucidum with the roof of the third ventricle may be mistaken for a colloid cyst (Fig. F).

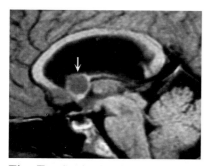

Fig F. Sagittal T1-WI demonstrates a rounded mass at the level of the anterosuperior third ventricle (*arrow*). Surgery confirmed a subependymoma.

Etiology

The histogenesis and exact nature of subependymoma are controversial, as ultrastructural assessment shows both ependymal and astrocytic features.

Pathology

Gross

- Benign lesion that is usually well-circumscribed and sometimes multiple

Microscopic

- Approximately 20% are mixed histologically and have a component of ependymoma
- Microcysts are common, mitoses are absent

Imaging Findings

- Some variations in imaging appearance are noted depending on location. In general, on MR, subependymomas are hypo- or isointense on T1-WI and iso- or hyperintense on PD- and T2-WI
- In the lateral ventricular location (Table 1):
  usually noncalcified; minimal or no enhancement; small cysts frequently seen
- In the fourth ventricular location:
  frequently calcified; moderate heterogeneous enhancement (Fig. E)
- In both locations, there is only rare transependymal extension and generally little or no associated parenchymal edema

Table 1. Lateral Ventricular Masses

Location	Adult	Child
Atrium	Meningioma	CP papilloma
	Metastasis	CP carcinoma
	CP xanthogranuloma	Ependymoma
Body	Subependymoma	Astrocytoma
	Oligodendroglioma	PNET
	Central neurocytoma	Teratoma
	Astrocytoma	CP papilloma
Foramen of Monro	Giant cell astrocytoma	Giant cell astrocytoma

Legend: CP = choroid plexus; PNET = primitive neuroectodermal tumor

Treatment

- Surgical excision if possible
- Radiation therapy may be indicated for residual or recurrent disease

Prognosis

- Depends on degree of resection
- Perioperative mortality may be as high as 10% because of extensive attachment to adjacent structures

Suggested Readings

Chiechi MV, Smirniotopoulos JG, Jones RV. Intracranial subependymomas: CT and MR imaging features in 24 cases. *AJR* 165:1245–1250, 1995.

Hoeffel C, Boukobza M, Polivka M, et al. MR manifestations of subependymomas. *AJNR* 16:2121–2129, 1995.

Jelinek J, Smirniotopoulos JG, Parisi JE, Kanzer M. Lateral ventricular neoplasms of the brain. *AJNR* 11:567–574, 1990.

Case 23

Clinical Presentation

A 3-month-old male presents with increasing head size and irritability.

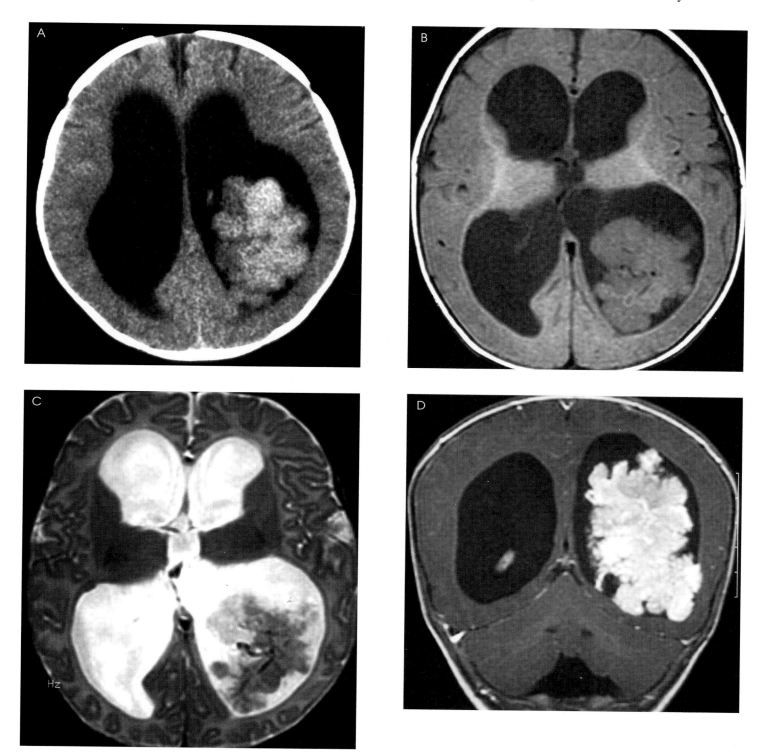

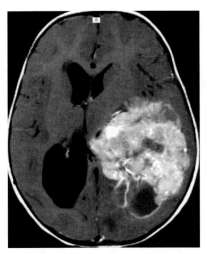

Fig. E. Post-gadolinium T1-WI from a 12-month-old male shows a heterogenous enhancing mass which infiltrates adjacent brain parenchyma. At surgery, this choroid plexus carcinoma was found to invade adjacent brain parenchyma.

Radiologic Findings

An axial non-contrast CT scan (Fig. A) demonstrates a lobulated mass in the left lateral ventricle which is mildly hyperdense compared with brain parenchyma. The lateral ventricles are markedly enlarged. An axial T1-WI (Fig. B) demonstrates a lobulated intraventricular mass that is isointense to gray matter. Note the linear flow voids within the mass, consistent with prominent vascularity. The mass is isointense to gray matter on an axial T2-WI (Fig. C). Post-gadolinium (Fig. D), a T1-WI shows intense, relatively homogenous enhancement of the cauliflowerlike mass.

Diagnosis

Choroid plexus papilloma

Differential Diagnosis

• Choroid plexus carcinoma (no clearly distinguishing features, but tends to be more invasive, Fig. E)
• Intraventricular metastasis (very rare in a child)
• Malignant rhabdoid tumor (may be intraventricular, tends to invade adjacent brain and incite significant edema)
• Primitive neuroectodermal tumor (invades adjacent brain parenchyma, may be indistinguishable from choroid plexus carcinoma)
• Ependymoma (typically centered in parenchyma, often more irregular and heterogeneous, often hemorrhagic)

Discussion

Background

Choroid plexus papillomas are relatively uncommon, accounting for only 2 to 4% of intracranial neoplasms of childhood. Seventy percent of patients diagnosed with choroid plexus papilloma are less than 2 years old, and ~90% of these tumors occur during the first 5 years of life. Choroid plexus papillomas may rarely present in the newborn period or be diagnosed on prenatal sonograms. In children, choroid plexus papillomas usually occur in the lateral ventricles, while in adults they usually occur in the fourth ventricle. Choroid plexus papillomas are usually benign, but carcinoma is seen in ~25% of choroid plexus tumors of childhood.

Clinical Findings

Patients present with symptoms and signs of elevated intracranial pressure/hydrocephalus.

Complications

Hydrocephalus is common and is probably multifactorial, related to CSF overproduction, obstruction of CSF pathways by mass effect, and obstruction of arachnoid granulations secondary to proteinaceous or hemorrhagic CSF.

Etiology

Choroid plexus papillomas arise from the epithelium of the choroid plexus.

Pathology

Gross

- Usually globular with an irregular papillary surface. These tumors are very vascular and often appear dark pink or red. They frequently contain areas of hemorrhage or calcification, and they range in size from <1 cm to >8 cm

Microscopic

- Choroid plexus papillomas most commonly have papillary architecture and simple columnar epithelium

Imaging Findings

CT

- Isodense or hyperdense on non-contrast CT
- Punctate foci of calcification are common
- Intense, homogeneous enhancement postcontrast

MR

- Homogeneous, lobulated, intensely enhancing intraventricular mass
- Isointense on T1-WI, iso- or mildly hypointense on T2-WI
- Foci of hemorrhage or calcification may be seen

Note that choroid plexus *carcinoma* tends to be irregular and of mixed density/intensity, and may invade into the brain, inciting vasogenic edema

Treatment

- Total excision if possible
- Adjuvant therapy (radiation, chemotherapy) reserved for specific cases

Prognosis

- Favorable for papillomas (88% 5-year survival)
- Less favorable for carcinomas (25 to 80% 5-year survival depending on the extent of surgical resection)

Suggested Readings

Boyd MC, Steinbok P. Choroid plexus tumors: problems in diagnosis and management. *J Neurosurg* 66:800–805, 1987.

Ellenbogen RG, Winston KR, Kupsky WJ. Tumors of the choroid plexus in children. *Neurosurgery* 25:327–335, 1989.

Tacconi L, Delfini R, Cantore G. Choroid plexus papillomas: consideration of a surgical series of 33 cases. *Acta Neurochirurgica* 138:802–810, 1996.

Case 24

Clinical Presentation

A 12-day-old male infant with irritability and enlarging head size is referred for MR imaging.

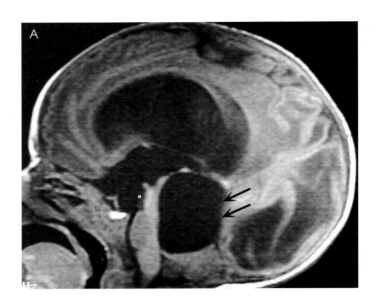

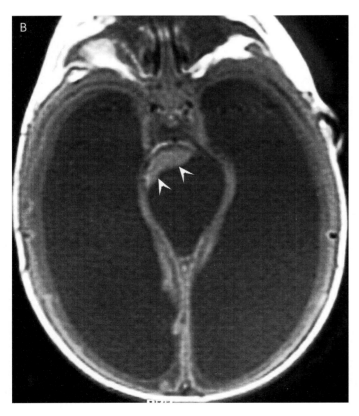

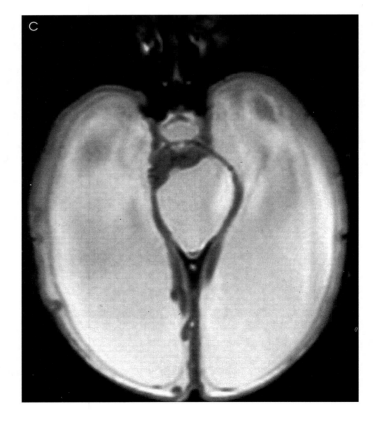

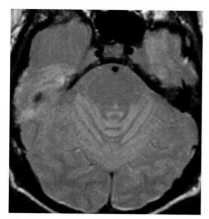

Fig D. An axial PD-WI shows an extra-axial mass located at the anterior aspect of the middle cranial fossa that is isointense to CSF.

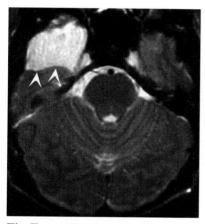

Fig E. A T2-WI in the same patient shows that the mass remains isointense to CSF and exerts mass effect on the tip of the temporal lobe (*arrowheads*). Arachnoid cyst.

Radiologic Findings

A sagittal T1-WI (Fig. A) demonstrates a well-circumscribed fluid intensity mass in the supravermian cistern (*arrows*). There is marked obstructive hydrocephalus with enlargement of the third ventricle and lateral ventricles. Note the marked hyperintensity of the normal neonatal pituitary gland. An axial T1-WI (Fig. B) demonstrates compression of the brainstem (*arrowheads*) by the cyst. In addition, there is marked enlargement of the lateral ventricles secondary to noncommunicating (obstructive) hydrocephalus. The overlying parenchymal mantle is severely compressed. An axial T2-WI (Fig. C) demonstrates that the cyst follows CSF in signal intensity. Mild heterogeneity of signal is related to CSF flow within the large cyst and the grossly enlarged lateral ventricles. Contrast was not administered in this case.

Diagnosis

Arachnoid cyst of supravermian cistern

Differential Diagnosis

- Cystic neoplasm (usually not a perfectly thin, smooth wall; rim usually enhances)
- Epidermoid cyst (often does not follow CSF exactly, rare in children)
- Parasitic cyst (wall usually enhances)

Discussion

Background

Arachnoid cysts are benign congenital intra-arachnoid collections of CSF. They occur in characteristic locations including the middle cranial fossa (50 to 66% of arachnoid cysts, Figs. D and E), over the convexities, in the retrocerebellar region, and in the perimesencephalic cisterns. Arachnoid cysts represent 1% of all atraumatic intracranial masses. Arachnoid cysts may gradually enlarge over time, and theories of growth include diffusion of fluid into the cyst due to osmotic gradients, a "ball-valve" mechanism (fluid gets in but cannot get out), and active cyst wall secretion.

Clinical Findings

Arachnoid cysts are usually asymptomatic and discovered incidentally on imaging exams. Symptoms may be produced by compression of adjacent neural tissue or obstruction of CSF flow: symptoms include intracranial hypertension, seizures, and focal neurological deficits.

Complications

Hemorrhage into a cyst may result in sudden expansion or subdural hematoma. Arachnoid cysts may rarely become secondarily infected.

Etiology

Congenital arachnoid cysts are thought to form by variations in the condensation of the meninx primitiva and/or slight variations in the flow of CSF into the

Table 1. Arachnoid Cyst versus Epidermoid

	Arachnoid Cyst	Epidermoid
SI relative to CSF on T1-WI	isointense	mildly hyperintense
SI relative to CSF on PD-WI	isointense	usually hyperintense
SI relative to CSF on T2-WI	isointense	isointense
Enhancement	no	no
Margin of lesion	smooth	irregular
Effect on adjacent structures	displaces	engulfs, insinuates
Pulsation artifact	often present	absent
Appearance on DW-MRI	follows CSF	hyperintense to CSF
Appearance on FLAIR	suppresses like CSF	usually hyperintense to CSF

Legend: SI = signal intensity; DW-MRI = diffusion-weighted MRI

forming pia-arachnoid. "Acquired" arachnoid cysts (better termed "arachnoid loculations") are caused by arachnoid adhesions, scarring, and trapping of CSF. These may occur in association with extra-axial neoplasms such as meningioma or vestibular schwannoma.

Pathology

Gross

• Thin but distinct transparent wall. Cyst fluid is usually clear and colorless, but may be hemorrhagic or proteinaceous

Microscopic

• The cyst wall consists of a vascular collagenous membrane lined by flattened arachnoid cells

Imaging Findings

CT

• Smoothly demarcated extra-axial mass
• Noncalcified, nonenhancing
• Contents similar to CSF unless hemorrhage has occurred

MR

• Well-defined extra-axial nonenhancing mass lesion that should follow CSF on all sequences. May be hyperintense to CSF if proteinaceous or hemorrhagic.
• Specialized sequences such as diffusion-weighted MR imaging may help distinguish from epidermoid, as arachnoid cysts will be similar to CSF on diffusion-weighted images while epidermoids are typically higher in signal

Treatment

• Most arachnoid cysts are discovered incidentally and need no therapy
• When cysts are symptomatic, the various treatment options depend on symptoms and location. Options include needle aspiration, cyst-peritoneal shunting, ventriculocystostomy, and craniotomy for partial or complete resection or for marsupialization into the subarachnoid space, basilar cisterns, or ventricle.
• Shunting of arachnoid cysts is generally more successful than fenestration. However, craniotomy and cyst fenestration rate is generally preferred for treatment of quadrigeminal cistern cysts.

Prognosis

Excellent

Suggested Readings

Ciricillo SF, Cogen PH, Harsh GR, Edwards MSB. Intracranial arachnoid cysts in children. *J Neurosurg* 74:230–235, 1991.

Maeda M, Kawamura Y, Tamagawa Y, et al. Intravoxel incoherent motion (IVIM) MRI in intracranial, extra-axial tumors and cysts. *JCAT* 16:514–518, 1992.

Tien RD, Felsberg GJ, Lirng JF. Variable bandwidth steady-state free-precession MR imaging: a technique for improving characterization of epidermoid tumor and arachnoid cyst. *AJR* 164:689–692, 1995.

Case 25

Clinical Presentation

A young male patient presents with acute onset of severe headache. An MR is performed as the CT scanner is being repaired.

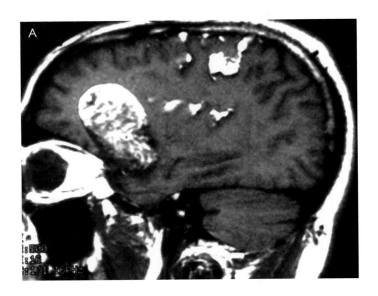

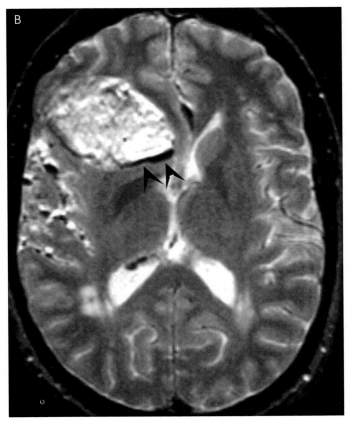

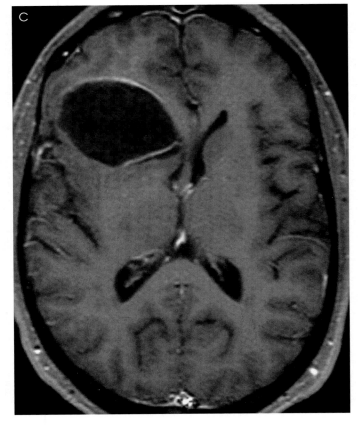

Radiologic Findings

A sagittal T1-WI (Fig. A) demonstrates a heterogenously hyperintense right frontotemporal extra-axial mass. In addition, multiple focal areas of T1 shortening are present within the subarachnoid space, associated with linear hypointensity representing chemical shift artifact. On an axial T2-WI (Fig. B), foci of mixed-signal intensity are present in the right frontal mass, as well as the subarachnoid space. Note the prominent linear low signal along the posterior margin of the mass consistent with chemical shift artifact (*arrowheads*). An axial post-gadolinium T1-WI with fat saturation (Fig. C) demonstrates loss of signal from the right-sided mass lesion.

Diagnosis

Dermoid cyst with rupture into the subarachnoid space

Differential Diagnosis

- Lipoma (more homogeneously fatty, does not spread via subarachnoid space)
- Subarachnoid hemorrhage (should not see chemical shift artifact)
- Lipoblastic meningioma (solid enhancing elements usually seen)

Discussion

Background

Dermoid cysts are included in the category of congenital ectodermal inclusion cysts. They are rare, accounting for only 0.04 to 0.6% of primary intracranial tumors. They are 5-10 times less common than epidermoids (Table 1), they are typically found in or just off midline, and usually present in young adults.

Clinical Findings

Patients often have long-standing headaches and/or seizures. Rupture of a dermoid into the subarachnoid space or ventricle presents acutely with worsening headache, visual symptoms, new seizures, confusion, and/or hemiparesis due to chemical meningitis.

Table 1. Differentiating Epidermoid from Dermoid

	Dermoid	Epidermoid
Age at presentation	2nd to 3rd decade	4th to 6th decade
Incidence	0.04-0.6% of primary intracranial mass lesions	0.2-1% of primary intracranial mass lesions
Location	Midline, supra >infratentorial	Paramedian, usually infratentorial
Path: dermal appendages	Present	Absent
CT appearance	Hypodense, follows fat	Isodense to CSF (usually)
MR appearance: T1-WI	Mixed iso- and hyperintense	Slightly hyperintense to CSF
MR appearance: T2-WI	Mixed iso- and hypointense	Slightly hyperintense to CSF
MR appearance: chemical shift	Present	Absent
MR appearance: fat saturation	Saturates	Does not saturate
Subarachnoid space rupture	Common	Rare

Note: This table lists the typical appearance of these lesions; atypical presentations of both do occur.

Pearls

- A ruptured dermoid cyst has characteristic features on CT and MR: cyst rupture leads to droplets of fat scattered throughout the subarachnoid space.
- In the posterior fossa or subfrontal region, look for a dermal sinus in association with an intracranial dermoid.

Pitfall

- Fat can mimic air if a CT is viewed only with soft tissue windows–check appearance with widened window.

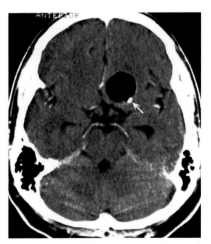

Fig. D. Axial contrast-enhanced CT scan shows a hypointense, well circumscribed, left frontal dermoid. A focus of calcification is noted posterolaterally (*arrow*).

Complications

Rupture into the subarachnoid space with acute chemical meningitis may be fatal.

Etiology

A dermoid is a congenital inclusion cyst containing epithelial elements and dermal appendages. As with epidermoids, these slowly expand over time.

Pathology

Gross

- Well-defined lobulated mass containing viscous, oily fluid

Microscopic

- Dense fibrous capsule lined with squamous epithelium and containing dermal appendages (hair follicles, sebaceous glands, sweat glands)
- Cyst contents include desquamated debris containing keratin and cholesterol
- Areas of hemorrhage, calcification, and/or ossification may be present

Imaging Findings

CT

- Mixed-density regions that are iso- and hypodense relative to brain parenchyma
- Calcification may occur, typically in the rim (Fig. D)

MR

- Isointense soft tissue mixed with hyperintense fatty material
- Usually nonenhancing, though the fibrous capsule may enhance
- Fatty areas will saturate out with fat-saturation sequences and also produce chemical shift artifact

Treatment

- Surgical excision of primary mass
- Steroids are helpful to treat the chemical meningitis

Prognosis

- Generally good
- May require ventricular shunting for communicating hydrocephalus due to chronic arachnoiditis caused by chemical meningitis

Suggested Readings

Hahn FJ, Ong E, McComb RD, et al. MR imaging of ruptured intracranial dermoid. *J Comput Assist Tomogr* 10:888–892, 1986.

Lunardi P, Missori P. Supratentorial dermoid cysts. *J Neurosurg* 75:262–266, 1991.

Smith AS, Benson JE, Blaser SI, et al. Diagnosis of ruptured intracranial dermoid cyst: value of MR over CT. *AJNR* 12:175–180, 1991.

Case 26

Clinical Presentation

A young man presents for evaluation of chronic progressive headache.

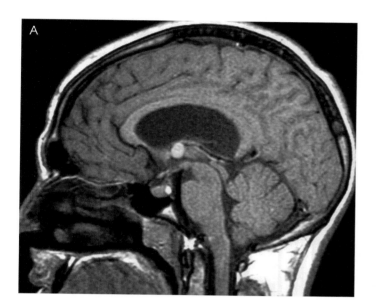

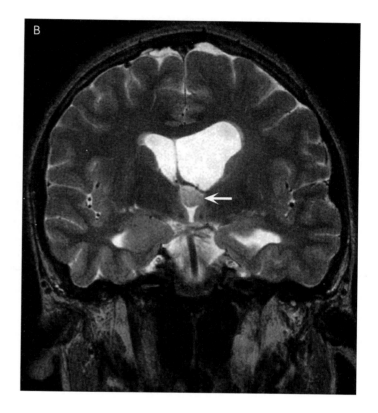

Radiologic Findings

A sagittal T1-WI (Fig. A) demonstrates a rounded mass in the anterosuperior aspect of the third ventricle that shows mild intrinsic hyperintensity. A coronal fast-spin echo T2-WI (Fig. B) demonstrates that the mass (*arrow*) is mildly hyperintense compared with brain parenchyma. Note the enlargement of the left lateral ventricle due to obstruction at the level of the foramen of Monro.

Diagnosis

Colloid cyst

Differential Diagnosis

- Subependymoma (less dense on non-enhanced CT, more heterogeneous)
- Astrocytoma (usually iso- or hypointense on T1-WI)
- Lymphoma (more infiltrative, usually enhances homogeneously)
- Meningioma (usually located in atrium in an older patient)
- Choroid plexus papilloma (usually located in fourth ventricle in an adult)
- Tumefactive intraventricular hemorrhage (usually more irregular, often dependent)
- Cysticercal cyst (not typically dense on CT or hyperintense on a T1-WI)

Discussion

Background

Colloid cysts represent 0.5 to 1% of intracranial tumors. They occupy a strategic position in the anterosuperior aspect of the third ventricle and typically range in size from 5 to 33 mm in diameter. They are generally detected in adults and are rare in children. If they are detected incidentally and followed over time, they will usually demonstrate slow growth.

Clinical Findings

Patients typically present with chronic headache as obstruction of one or both foramina of Monro leads to hydrocephalus.

Complications

Colloid cysts may present with acute hydrocephalus leading to coma and death.

Etiology

The probable origin is the primitive neuroepithelium of the tela choroidea.

Pathology

Gross

- The content of the cyst is usually a homogeneous, amorphous eosinophilic substance containing cholesterol, blood breakdown products, and macrophages

Microscopic

- Nonneural intracranial epithelial cyst with a thin wall consisting of an inner layer of cuboidal or cylindrical cells and an outer layer of connective tissue including vessels

Imaging Findings

CT

- Located in anterior third ventricle near foramen of Monro

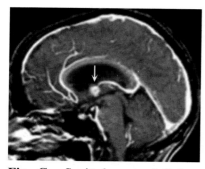

Fig. C. Sagittal postgadolinium T1-WI in a 32-year-old woman with headaches shows a high-signal intensity mass (*arrow*) in the anterosuperior third ventricle as well as hydrocephalus.

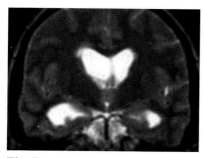

Fig. D. Coronal T2-WI (same patient as Fig. C) demonstrates that the mass is isointense to gray matter. The patient was informed preoperatively that she had a benign colloid cyst. Intraoperatively, this mass was found to represent lymphoma.

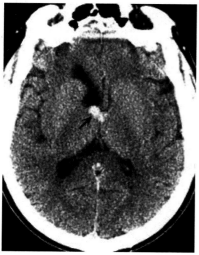

Fig. E. Non-contrast CT scan demonstrates a rounded hyperdense lesion dumbbelling through the right foramen of Monro (*arrow*). The right lateral ventricle is enlarged due to obstructive hydrocephalus. Colloid cyst.

- Most commonly hyperdense to brain parenchyma (Fig. E), but may be hypo- or isodense
- Increased density is probably due to highly proteinaceous fluid because hemorrhage or gross calcification are rarely found

MR

- Very variable signal patterns: often hyperintense on T1-WI, iso- or hypointense on T2-WI
- May contain a nonenhancing, often dependent nodule representing inspissated debris that is usually hyperdense on CT and hypointense on T2-WI
- A very thin rim of enhancement representing the cyst capsule may be seen on post-gadolinium imaging

Treatment

- Transcallosal microsurgical removal is favored
- Aspiration of the cyst alone has an 80% recurrence rate

Prognosis

- Microsurgical removal is curative
- Major complication is transient or permanent memory deficit due to damage to the fornix

Suggested Readings

Maeder PP, Holtas SL, Basibuyuk LN, et al. Colloid cysts of the third ventricle: correlation of MR and CT findings with histology and chemical analysis. *AJR* 155:135–141, 1990.

Mathiesen T, Grane P, Lindgren L, Lindquist C. Third ventricle colloid cysts: a consecutive 12-year series. *J Neurosurg* 86:5–12, 1997.

Waggenspack GA, Guinto FC Jr. MR and CT of masses of the anterosuperior third ventricle. *AJNR* 10:105–110, 1989.

Section I

Neoplasm

B.   Infratentorial

Case 27

Clinical Presentation

A 9-year-old male presents with headache and vomiting.

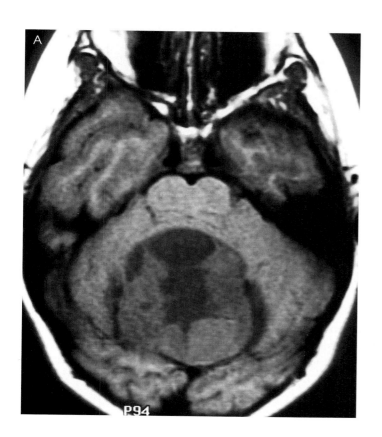 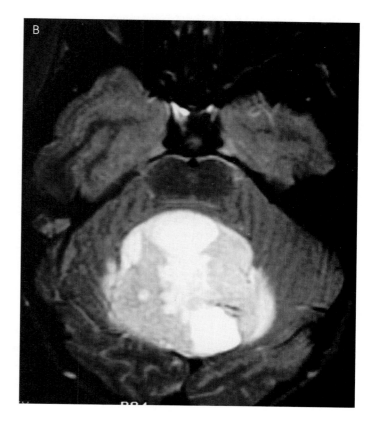

Radiologic Findings

An axial T1-WI (Fig. A) shows a mixed cystic and solid mass centered in the middle of the cerebellum. A T2-WI (Fig. B) demonstrates that the solid portions of the mass are hyperintense compared with brain parenchyma, while the fluid-filled areas are isointense with CSF.

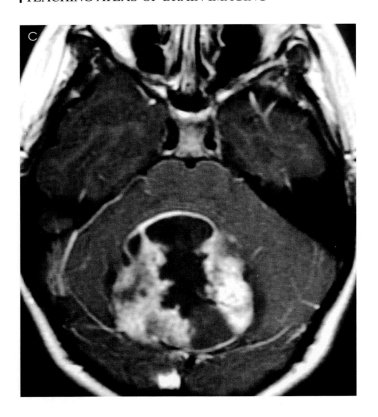

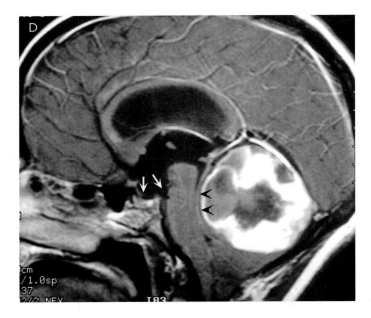

Following administration of gadolinium (Fig. C), the solid portions of the mass enhance somewhat heterogenously. There is also enhancement along the rim of the cystic area anteriorly. On a sagittal post-gadolinium T1-WI (Fig. D), cerebellar tonsillar herniation is present. It is clear that the mass arises in cerebellar parenchyma rather than the fourth ventricle, as a strip of compressed brain tissue can be identified between the mass and the distorted fourth ventricle (*black arrowheads*). In addition, there is evidence of non-communicating obstructive hydrocephalus, and the floor of the third ventricle is severely depressed (*white arrows*).

Diagnosis

Juvenile pilocytic astrocytoma (JPA) of the cerebellum

Differential Diagnosis

- Higher grade astrocytoma (more infiltrative, often incites edema)
- Hemangioblastoma (young adult, may see enlarged feeding vessels)
- Medulloblastoma (usually arises in midline, large cysts uncommon, solid portions usually iso- or hypointense to gray matter)
- Ependymoma (arises in inferior fourth ventricle, often extends through basal foramina)

Discussion

Background

Astrocytomas account for ~50% of primary CNS neoplasms in children. Sixty percent of them arise in the posterior fossa, 40% in the cerebellum and 20% in

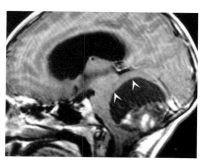

Fig. E. A sagittal post-gadolinium T1-WI demonstrates a mixed cystic and solid midline cerebellar mass consistent with JPA. The cyst wall is nonenhancing (*arrowheads*).

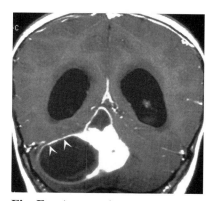

Fig. F. A coronal post-gadolinium T1-WI demonstrates a mixed cystic and solid cerebellar mass consistent with JPA. Note the thin, linear enhancement of the cyst wall (*arrowheads*).

the brainstem. Eighty to 85% of cerebellar astrocytomas in children are World Health Organization II (WHO II)-classified grade I tumors, so-called JPAs. The remainder are higher grade malignant astrocytomas. JPAs usually occur before age 10 and have an equal sex incidence. Other common locations for JPAs include the hypothalamus, optic nerves, brainstem, and cerebral hemispheres. Cerebellar JPAs most often originate in the midline and extend into the cerebellar hemispheres, but they may involve only the cerebellar hemispheres.

Clinical Findings

Symptoms are related to mass effect in the posterior fossa and obstructive hydrocephalus and include headache, irritability, vomiting, and ataxia.

Etiology

JPAs arise from a unique class of astrocytes that are inconspicuous in normal brain.

Pathology

Gross

- Well-circumscribed masses that most commonly demonstrate a large cyst and a focal mural nodule. May be mostly solid or have cystic degeneration within their solid portion, as in this case

Microscopic

- Patterns include compact regions of elongated cells with pilocytic processes and more loosely organized spongiform foci.
- Typically prominent Rosenthal fibers, low or absent mitotic activity, and no necrosis

Imaging Findings

JPAs may be cystic with a mural nodule, solid, or solid with cystic degeneration.

CT

- Sharply demarcated mass with minimal if any surrounding edema
- The solid portion of the tumor usually enhances intensely and homogeneously
- The cyst wall often does not enhance, though areas of cystic degeneration within solid tumor will show peripheral enhancement related to the tumor mass itself
- Calcification is present in ~10% of cases

MR

- The tumor cyst usually has an intensity similar to CSF, though this may vary with protein content
- The mural nodule and other solid portions of the tumor enhance intensely and are usually iso- or hypointense on T1-WI and hyperintense on T2-WI. Enhancement of the cyst wall is variable (Figs. E and F), though the cyst wall is most commonly nonenhancing.
- Significant flow voids in or near the solid tumor are not generally seen

Treatment

- Surgical resection is generally curative

- Radiation therapy or chemotherapy may be given if the resection is subtotal. In general, residual disease is followed closely with serial MR examinations, and chemotherapy and/or radiation therapy are reserved until there is evidence of disease progression.

Prognosis

Postoperative survival rate is 85 to 100% at 5 years and 70% at 20 years

Suggested Readings

Davis CH, Joglekar VM. Cerebellar astrocytomas in children and young adults. *J Neurol Neurosurg Psych* 44:820–828, 1981.

Lee YY, Van Tassel P, Bruner JM, et al. Juvenile pilocytic astrocytomas: CT and MR characteristics. *AJNR* 10:363–370, 1989.

Obana WG, Cogen PH, Davis RL, Edwards MSB. Metastatic juvenile pilocytic astrocytoma: case report. *J Neurosurg* 75:972–975, 1991.

Case 28

Clinical Presentation

A 25-year-old man presents with progressive headache and ataxia.

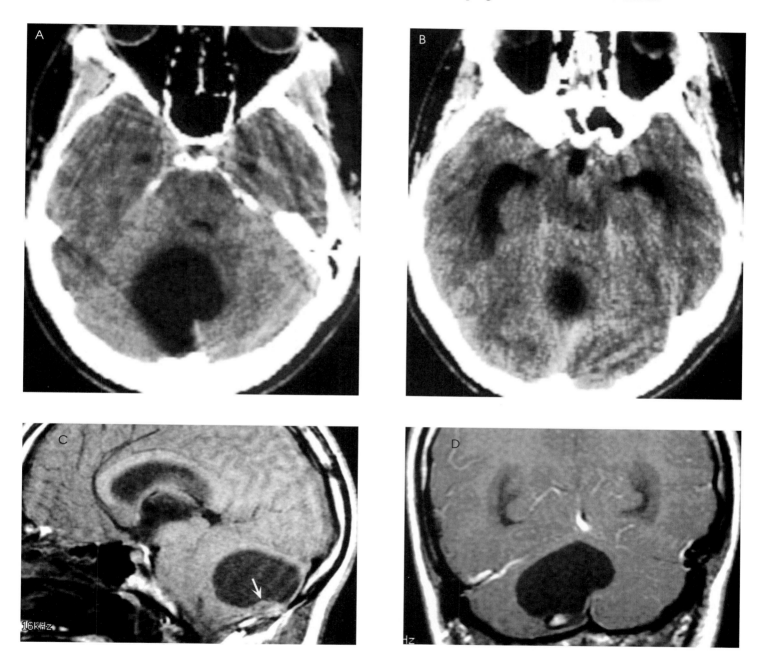

Radiologic Findings

A non-contrast CT scan (Fig. A) demonstrates a well-circumscribed mass of CSF density centered in the right cerebellar hemisphere. A more cephalad image

Fig. B) from the CT scan demonstrates upward herniation of the cerebellar vermis through the tentorial incisura, as well as evidence for obstructive hydrocephalus with dilatation of the temporal horns bilaterally. A sagittal T1-WI (Fig. C) demonstrates that the mass is isointense to CSF and appears cystic. There is a suggestion of a solid isointense nodule along the inferior aspect of the cyst (*arrow*). A coronal post-gadolinium T1-WI (Fig. D) demonstrates intense enhancement of the solid nodule but no enhancement of the cyst wall.

Diagnosis

Hemangioblastoma

Differential Diagnosis

- Metastatic disease (usually in an older age group, often multiple lesions)
- Juvenile pilocytic astrocytoma (unlikely at this age, not generally associated with enlarged feeding vessels)
- Cysticercosis (usually smaller cyst, multiple lesions, calcifications on CT scan)

Discussion

Background

Hemangioblastoma is a benign tumor that accounts for 1 to 2.5% of intracranial neoplasms. It is the most common posterior fossa tumor in adults after metastases. Eighty-five percent of hemangioblastomas occur in the cerebellum, but they also occur in the spinal cord (10%), the medulla (3%), and the cerebrum (2%). They typically present in young adults, and there is a slight male predominance. Solitary hemangioblastomas are associated with von Hippel-Lindau disease (VHL) in 10 to 20% of cases (see discussion of VHL in Case 118).

Clinical Findings

A long history of mild symptoms including headache, disequilibrium, nausea/vomiting, and vertigo usually precedes an acute exacerbation of symptoms. Polycythemia secondary to erythropoietin production occurs in up to 40% of cases and is more common with solitary than with multiple hemangioblastomas.

Complications

Acute hemorrhage or acute obstructive hydrocephalus may occur.

Pathology

Gross

- Typically a well-circumscribed solid mural nodule which abuts a pial surface and is associated with an adjacent cyst containing CSF-like fluid
- May be predominantly solid (40%) or both cystic and solid (60%). If both cystic and solid, the cyst may be within the solid portion or a large cyst may be associated with a mural nodule.

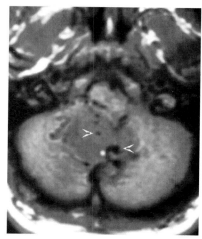

Fig. E. An axial T1-WI demonstrates a hypointense mass in the right cerebellum, distorting the dorsal medulla and obliterating the inferior fourth ventricle. Multiple punctate hypointensities are consistent with flow voids (*arrowheads*).

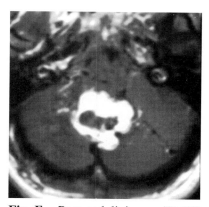

Fig. F. Post-gadolinium, a T1-WI in the patient from Fig. E shows intense enhancement of the solid portions of the mass, with a central area of cystic degeneration or necrosis.

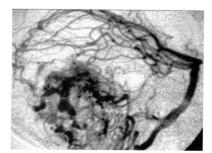

Fig. G. A lateral view from a cerebral angiogram (same patient as in Figs. E and F) after injection of the vertebral artery demonstrates marked hypervascularity of the posterior fossa mass.

Microscopic

- The nodule consists of thin-walled, tightly packed blood vessels on a connective tissue background. The cyst wall is composed of compressed brain parenchyma and reactive glia and does not represent tumor. A cyst found within the nodule itself may represent focal necrosis.

Imaging Findings

CT

- Isodense nodule within thin-walled hypodense cyst
- Mural nodule enhances homogeneously
- Cyst wall does not enhance unless there is neoplastic extension (rare)

MR

- Nodule usually hypo- or isointense on T1-WI, hyperintense on T2-WI
- Cyst fluid is usually mildly hyperintense to CSF on all sequences
- Intense enhancement of solid tumor post-contrast, while the cyst wall rarely enhances
- Flow voids representing feeding and draining vessels are often identified adjacent to or within the nodule

Angiography

- Solid portions are hypervascular (Figs. E through G)

Treatment

- Surgical excision of nodule and drainage of cyst
- Preoperative endovascular embolization may be useful in aiding surgical resection

Prognosis

- Generally good, with ~85% 10-year survival
- Recurrence rate ranges from 8 to 16%

Suggested Readings

Eskridge JM, McAuliffe W, Harris B, et al. Preoperative endovascular embolization of craniospinal hemangioblastomas. *AJNR* 17:525–531, 1996.

Ho VB, Smirniotopoulos JG, Murphy FM, Rushing EJ. Radiologic-pathologic correlation: hemangioblastoma. *AJNR* 13:1343–1352, 1992.

Lee SR, Sanches J, Mark AS, Dillon WP, Norman D, Newton TH. Posterior fossa hemangioblastomas: MR imaging. *Radiology* 171:463–468, 1989.

Case 29

Clinical Presentation

An 18-year-old girl previously shunted for hydrocephalus of uncertain cause presents for MR evaluation.

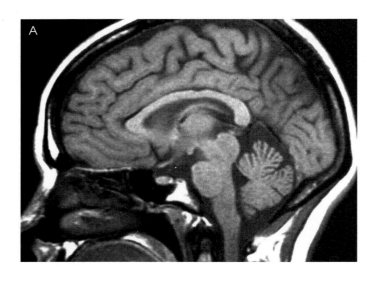

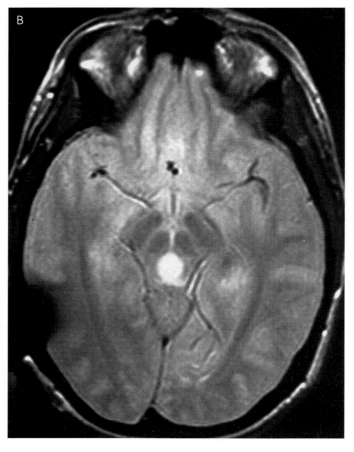

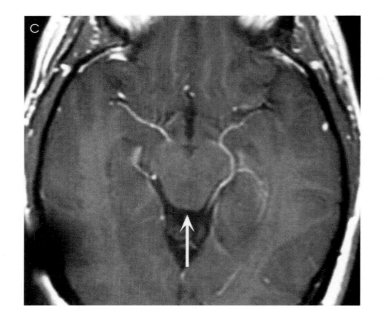

Pearls

- Consider this diagnosis in unexplained "aqueductal stenosis."

- Enhancement is atypical and may indicate a need for biopsy and treatment.

- If a lesion extends beyond the tectum but is still confined to the midbrain, it is referred to as a "peritectal" tumor (Figs. D and E); these tumors have a worse prognosis than purely tectal lesions.

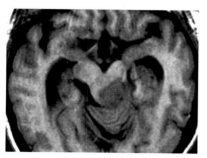

Fig. D. Axial T1-WI in a 56-year-old woman with headaches demonstrates a mildly hypointense exophytic mass that is not confined to the tectum, as well as obstructive hydrocephalus with dilatation of the temporal horns.

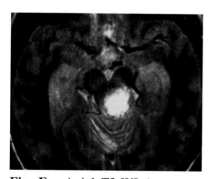

Fig. E. Axial T2-WI (same patient as Fig. D) demonstrates that the mass is hyperintense and has an ill-defined margin with the adjacent brain parenchyma. Peritectal brain stem tumor.

Radiologic Findings

A sagittal T1-WI (Fig. A) demonstrates bulbous enlargement of the tectum. The aqueduct of Sylvius is obliterated. An axial PD-WI (Fig. B) demonstrates focal hyperintensity confined to the tectum. A focal area of susceptibility artifact over the right temporal region is related to a prior shunt catheter. A post-gadolinium T1-WI (Fig. C) shows subtle hypointensity in the tectum, but no abnormal enhancement. Note the loss of the normal intercollicular depression (*arrow*).

Diagnosis

Focal midbrain glioma (tectal glioma)

Differential Diagnosis

- Benign aqueductal stenosis (on CT a mass may not be evident)
- Pineal region cyst or tumor (sagittal MR best localizes a mass to the tectum or the pineal gland)

Discussion

Background

Brainstem tumors have increasingly been recognized as a heterogeneous group of neoplasms, and focal tumors confined to the tectal plate ("tectal gliomas") constitute a distinct subset of brainstem tumors. These tumors are usually diagnosed on the basis of MR imaging. As tectal gliomas have a good long-term prognosis and are located deep near particularly delicate regions of the brain, they are usually followed without biopsy and with serial imaging to document stability. Treatment is reserved for progressive disease.

Clinical Findings

Patients usually present with symptoms and signs of hydrocephalus and elevated intracranial pressure due to aqueductal obstruction.

Pathology

These lesions are rarely biopsied, but when they are studied histologically they are usually low-grade astrocytomas (WHO II grade I or II)

Imaging Findings

CT

- If small, one may just see aqueductal obliteration and/or subtle distortion of the posterior third ventricle
- Calcification may be present
- Usually nonenhancing

MR

- Bulbous enlargement of the tectal plate is seen on sagittal images
- Loss of the intercollicular depression of the tectal plate is seen on axial images
- Usually isointense on T1-WI, hyperintense on PD- and T2-WI
- Enhancement is usually absent or subtle

Pitfalls

- In the axial plane, it may be difficult to differentiate pineal region tumors from tectal lesions.

- A normal CT scan does not exclude the diagnosis of a tectal glioma (i.e., in a patient with unexplained hydrocephalus), and MR should be performed.

Treatment

- Shunting (internal or external) to treat hydrocephalus
- Close radiographic follow-up with serial MR scans. Evidence of progression usually mandates stereotactic or open biopsy followed by radiation therapy

Prognosis

Excellent, usually 100% 5-year survival unless there are shunt complications

Suggested Readings

May PL, Blaser SI, Hoffman HJ, et al. Benign intrinsic tectal "tumors" in children. *J Neurosurg* 74:867–871, 1991.

Pollack IF, Pang D, Albright AL. The long-term outcome in children with late-onset aqueductal stenosis resulting from benign intrinsic tectal tumors. *J Neurosurg* 80:681–688, 1994.

Vandertop WP, Hoffman HJ, Drake JM, et al. Focal midbrain tumors in children. *Neurosurgery* 31:186–194, 1992.

Case 30

Clinical Presentation

An 8-year-old boy presents with failure to thrive and multiple cranial nerve palsies.

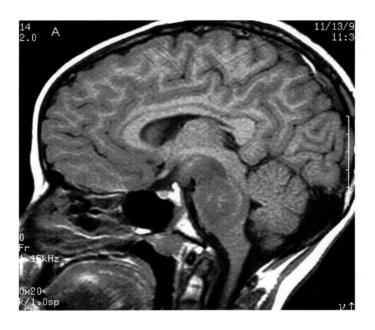

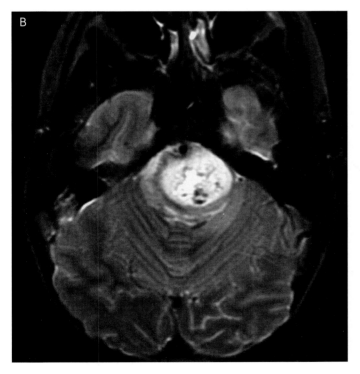

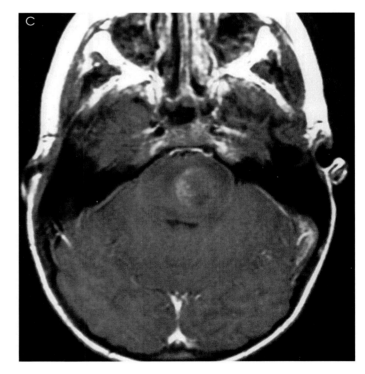

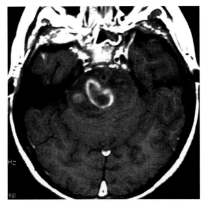

Fig. D. Axial post-gadolinium T1-WI of a 6-year-old girl demonstrates an expansile pontine mass with ring and nodular enhancement.

Pearls

- MR is the study of choice to evaluate the margins of the lesion and thus to determine whether it is diffuse or focal. Sagittal fast spin-echo T2-WIs are particularly useful for assessing infiltration of adjacent areas of the brainstem, while fluid-attenuated inversion recovery (FLAIR) sequences are also useful to fully assess the extent of tumor (Fig. E).

- Biopsy is not required prior to radiation therapy if clinical and imaging findings are typical of diffuse pontine glioma, as stereotactic biopsy is subject to sampling error and complications.

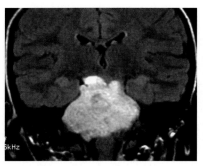

Fig. E. A coronal heavily T2-weighted FLAIR image in the patient from Figure D beautifully demonstrates invasion of the midbrain by this diffuse pontine glioma.

Radiologic Findings

A sagittal T1-WI (Fig. A) demonstrates an expansile, hypointense mass involving the pons and midbrain. Foci of central T1 shortening are consistent with focal hemorrhage. An axial T2-WI (Fig. B) demonstrates expansion and T2 prolongation within the pons. Irregular areas of T2 shortening are consistent with hemorrhage. Exophytic growth of the mass engulfs the basilar artery anteriorly. A post-gadolinium T1-WI (Fig. C) demonstrates mild enhancement of a portion of the tumor.

Diagnosis

Diffuse pontine glioma

Differential Diagnosis

- Brainstem encephalitis (more acute history, may have fever and a reactive CSF profile)
- Infiltrating neoplasm such as leukemia or lymphoma (usually patchier and more heterogeneous; patients with CNS involvement by leukemia or lymphoma usually have known systemic disease)
- Acute demyelination, such as multiple sclerosis or ADEM (typically multiple lesions that are both supra- and infratentorial)

Discussion

Background

Brainstem tumors constitute 10 to 15% of all pediatric CNS neoplasms and 25% of posterior fossa tumors in children. They have a peak incidence at 3 to 10 years of age and are equally common in males and females. They also occur in adults but are significantly less common. In recent years there has been increasing recognition of the heterogeneity of brainstem tumors. Diffuse pontine gliomas, which represent approximately 50% of brainstem tumors in children, are the most common subtype of brainstem tumor and carry the worst prognosis. Focal brain stem tumors and dorsally exophytic cervicomedullary tumors have a better prognosis than diffuse tumors.

Clinical Findings

Diffuse pontine gliomas generally present with the insidious onset of pyramidal tract signs, cranial nerve palsies (most commonly cranial nerves VI and VII), and cerebellar dysfunction. Focal gliomas generally have focal symptoms such as isolated cranial neuropathy. Hydrocephalus is usually a late finding with diffuse pontine gliomas but is the common presenting feature of a tectal glioma.

Complications

Involvement of cranial nerves and the reticular activating system may lead to aspiration and respiratory depression. Acute hemorrhage occasionally complicates gliomas.

Pitfalls

- Brainstem encephalitis may mimic a diffuse pontine glioma. Therefore accurate history is critical since diffuse gliomas usually present insidiously, while encephalitis is generally more acute.

- The use of hyperfractionated radiation therapy may lead to rapid tumor necrosis on follow-up scans which may be difficult to distinguish from tumor progression, so correlation with history and close interval follow-up scans are essential.

Pathology

Diffuse gliomas are most commonly anaplastic astrocytomas (grade III). In diffuse tumors, neoplastic cells infiltrate widely along fiber tracts.

Imaging Findings

CT

- Diffuse pontine enlargement
- The pons is hypodense pre-contrast and variably enhances

MR

- Expansion of the pons
- Abnormal pontine signal: hypointense on T1-WI and hyperintense on T2-WI
- The basilar artery may be "engulfed" by exophytic growth of tumor
- Often infiltrative extension to midbrain and medulla
- Associated edema is usually minimal
- Enhancement characteristics are variable: the tumors are usually either nonenhancing or contain areas of focal nodular or peripheral enhancement (Fig. D)
- Cyst formation, hemorrhage, or areas of focal necrosis are variably present

Treatment

- Diffuse glioma: typically hyperfractionated radiation therapy with or without chemotherapy. However, it is not clear that hyperfractionation confers an advantage over standard radiotherapy
- Focal glioma: biopsy and resection if possible. Radiation therapy for residual disease

Prognosis

Poor for diffuse gliomas, with 35 to 45% survival at 1 year and 10 to 20% at 5 years

Suggested Readings

Epstein FJ, Farmer JP. Brainstem glioma growth patterns. *J Neurosurg* 78:408–412, 1993.

Fischbein NJ, Prados MD, Wara W, et al. Radiologic classification of brain stem tumors: correlation of magnetic resonance imaging appearance with clinical outcome. *Pediatr Neurosurg* 24: 9–23, 1996.

Packer RJ, Boyett JM, Zimmerman RA, et al. Outcome of children with brain stem gliomas after treatment with 7800 cGy of hyperfractionated radiotherapy. *Cancer* 74:1827–1834, 1994.

Case 31

Clinical Presentation

A 7-year-old male presents with progressive headache and ataxia.

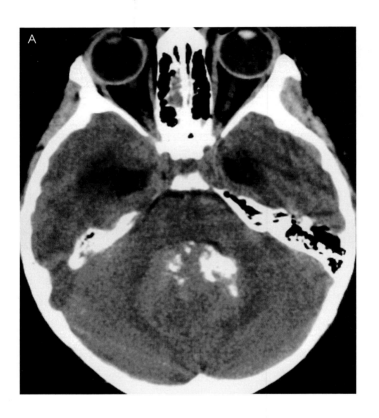

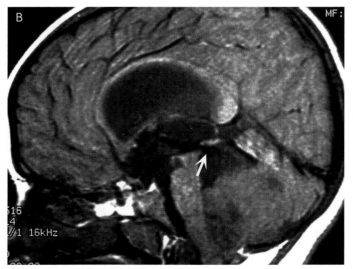

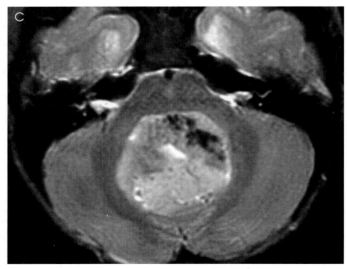

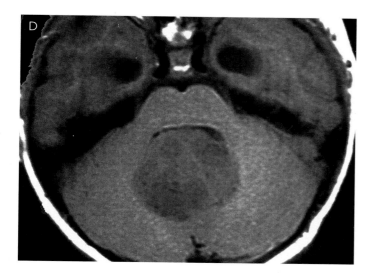
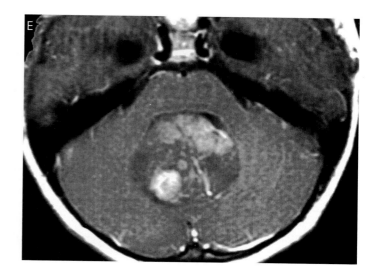

Radiologic Findings

An axial non-contrast CT scan (Fig. A) demonstrates a mass that is isodense to brain parenchyma centered in the cerebellar vermis, with areas of focal high density consistent with calcification. A sagittal T1-WI (Fig. B) demonstrates the mass growing exophytically into the inferior aspect of the fourth ventricle. Obstructive hydrocephalus is present, with dilatation of the superior fourth ventricle, third ventricle, and lateral ventricle; the corpus callosum is thinned and elevated, and a prominent aqueductal flow void is noted (*arrow*). An axial T2-WI (Fig. C) shows that the mass is mildly hyperintense to brain parenchyma, with areas of low-signal intensity corresponding to the calcification seen on CT. Axial pre- (Fig. D) and post-gadolinium (Fig. E) T1-WIs demonstrate moderate patchy enhancement of the mass.

Diagnosis

Medulloblastoma

Differential Diagnosis

- Ependymoma (typically off midline, often more heterogeneous, often extends through foramina of Luschka or Magendie)
- Choroid plexus papilloma (typically located in lateral ventricle in a child, more lobulated and more intensely enhancing)
- Astrocytoma (usually a cystic component but may be solid, usually more intensely enhancing)
- Metastasis (uncommon in a child unless there is a known primary tumor)
- Hemangioblastoma (often a cyst and large vessels, more intensely enhancing)
- Atypical teratoid/rhabdoid tumor (typically affects patients <2 years old, usually more irregular and heterogeneous)
- Oligodendroglioma (rare in posterior fossa)

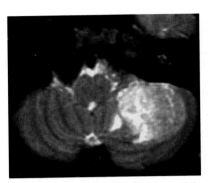

Fig F. An axial T2-WI in a 14-year-old boy with ataxia demonstrates a relatively homogenous mass of intermediate-signal intensity in the left cerebellar hemisphere.

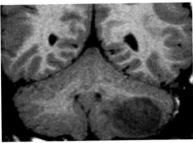

Fig G. A coronal T1-WI (same patient as Fig. F) demonstrates a relatively homogenous rounded mass in the left cerebellar hemisphere, hypointense to brain parenchyma. Medulloblastoma.

Pearls

• Systemic metastases are rare but do occur (bone, lymph nodes, lung). Metastatic medulloblastoma may cause sclerotic lesions in bone, while metastases to the abdominal cavity may occur via a ventriculoperitoneal shunt catheter.

• Medulloblastomas may occur in association with certain syndromes such as Gorlin's syndrome (basal cell nevi, odontogenic keratocysts, falx calcification) or Turcot's syndrome (colonic polyps and CNS malignancy, usually either medulloblastoma or glioblastoma multiforme).

Discussion

Background

Cerebellar medulloblastoma accounts for 15% of childhood brain tumors and 0.4 to 1% of adult brain tumors. Medulloblastoma represents 30 to 40% of posterior fossa neoplasms in children. Childhood medulloblastoma generally arises from the vermis and is located in the midline. In adolescents and adults, medulloblastomas more commonly arise laterally in the cerebellar hemispheres (Figs. F and G). Unfortunately, metastases to the spinal subarachnoid space and cauda equina occur in ~40% of medulloblastoma cases, so a screening post-gadolinium MR of the total spine is essential prior to posterior fossa craniotomy.

Clinical Findings

The duration of symptoms is generally shorter than for patients with astrocytoma. Symptoms of hydrocephalus (headache, nausea/vomiting) predominate with midline lesions while cerebellar dysfunction (dysequilibrium, ataxia) predominates with hemispheric lesions. In young children (<1 year), increasing head size is often the presenting problem.

Etiology

Medulloblastomas are thought to originate from a group of neuroepithelial cells located in roof of fourth ventricle that migrate outward and laterally to form the cerebellar external granular layer, thus explaining the occurrence in the cerebellar hemispheres in older patients.

Pathology

Gross

• Medulloblastomas are usually rounded, well-circumscribed masses that demonstrate mild to moderate surrounding edema
• Cysts, hemorrhage, and calcification may occur but are less common than with ependymoma and more often seen with large lesions
• Heterogeneity is more common in adults than in children

Microscopic

• Medulloblastoma is part of the group of primitive neuroectodermal tumors, a family of highly malignant tumors composed of undifferentiated small round cells
• The lateral hemispheric lesions often have a desmoplastic histopathology, which is considered to have a somewhat more favorable prognosis than midline tumors

Imaging Findings

CT

• Hyperdense prior to contrast
• Typically enhance, with a diffuse or patchy pattern
• Calcification in <20%, hemorrhage rare
• Cystic degeneration and focal necrosis may be seen

Pitfalls

- Medulloblastomas may occur off the midline in children, but this is more common in older patients.

- Medulloblastomas may occasionally grow in an exophytic fashion into the cerebellopontine angle, mimicking ependymoma (Figs. H and I)

MR

- Iso- or mildly hyperintense on T1-WI
- Usually iso- or hypointense on T2-WI, like other highly cellular small round cell neoplasms
- Enhancement is often mild to moderate and relatively homogeneous

Treatment

- Surgical resection
- Radiation therapy, usually craniospinal
- Chemotherapy

Prognosis

Overall 5-year survival is on the order of 50%, but children who undergo gross total resection and have no evidence of spinal metastases have 5-year survival rates of ~73%

Suggested Readings

Bourgouin PM, Tampieri D, Grahovac SZ, et al. CT and MR imaging findings in adults with cerebellar medulloblastoma: comparison with findings in children. *AJR* 159:609–612, 1992.

Meyers SP, Kemp SS, Tarr RW. MR imaging features of medulloblastomas. *AJR* 158:859–865, 1992.

Robles HA, Smirniotopoulos JG, Figueroa RE. Understanding the radiology of intracranial primitive neuroectodermal tumors from a pathological perspective: a review. *Semin US, CT, MR* 13:170–181, 1992.

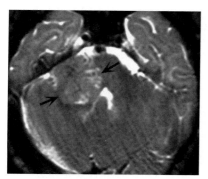

Fig. H. A T2-WI in a 9-month-old female demonstrates a lobulated mass isointense to cortex growing exophytically into the right cerebellopontine angle (*arrows*).

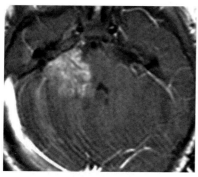

Fig. I. Post-gadolinium, a T1-WI (same patient as Fig. H) shows moderate heterogenous enhancement of the slightly lobulated, exophytic mass extending into the right cerebellopontine angle. Medulloblastoma was diagnosed at surgery.

Case 32

Clinical Presentation

A 19-month-old female presents with irritability and vomiting.

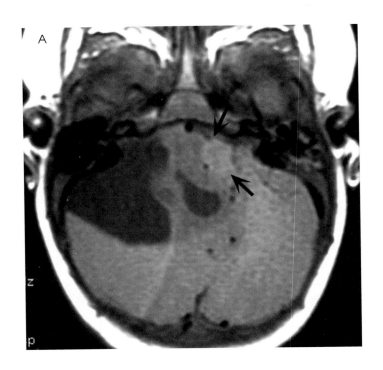

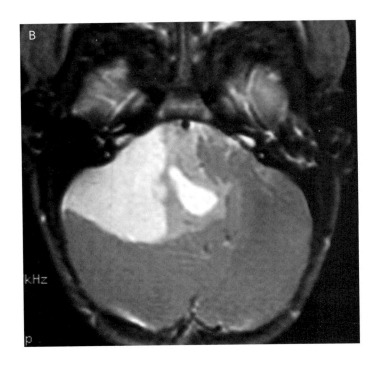

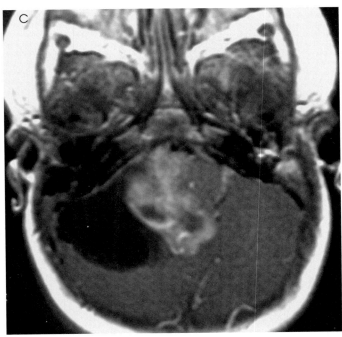

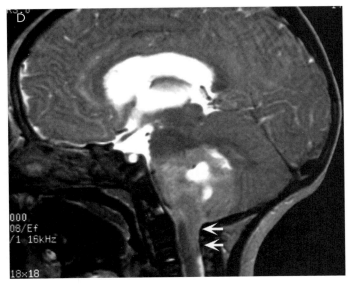

Radiologic Findings

An axial T1-WI (Fig. A) demonstrates a heterogenous, mixed cystic and solid mass which appears extra-axial and displaces the medulla to the left (*arrows*). The solid component is slightly hypointense to brain parenchyma. A T2-WI (Fig. B) demonstrates that the solid component of the mass is mildly hyperintense to brain parenchyma. The cystic components are isointense with CSF. A post-gadolinium T1-WI (Fig. C) demonstrates moderate enhancement of the solid component of the lesion. A sagittal fast-spin echo T2-WI (Fig. D) again demonstrates the heterogenous cystic and solid mass. Note that the solid component is extruding down through the foramen magnum into the upper cervical canal (*arrows*).

Diagnosis

Ependymoma

Differential Diagnosis

- Medulloblastoma (usually involves vermis, more homogeneous)
- Cerebellar astrocytoma (arises in cerebellar hemisphere)
- Brain stem glioma (may be exophytic, but arises from brainstem rather than just displacing it)
- Choroid plexus papilloma (usually a lateral ventricular mass in a child)
- Subependymoma (typically seen in adults)
- Intraventricular metastasis (rare, and particularly uncommon in children)

Discussion

Background

Ependymomas constitute 9% of primary CNS neoplasms in children, and 15% of childhood posterior fossa tumors. They are much less frequent supratentorially (see Case 7). Children are usually 5 years or younger at the time of diagnosis, but there is a bimodal age distribution with peaks at 3 and 34 years.

Clinical Findings

Symptoms of hydrocephalus and brainstem/cerebellar compression are prominent, including headache, nausea/vomiting, and disequilibrium.

Etiology

Ependymomas arise from ependymal cell rests that line the fourth ventricle and the foramina of Luschka.

Pathology

Gross

- Lobulated heterogeneous intraventricular masses that may be cystic, hemorrhagic, or partly calcified
- Ependymomas often appear soft and pliable or "plastic," and they have a characteristic tendency to extend out the foramina of Luschka into the cerebellopontine and cerebellomedullary angles and out the foramen of Magendie into the upper cervical canal

Microscopic

- Infiltrative tumor composed of uniform cells which invades the ventricular walls and the cerebellar parenchyma. Ependymomas demonstrate a spectrum of anaplasia and are graded by the presence of mitotic figures, endothelial proliferation, and necrosis
- "Pseudorosettes" are a hallmark of ependymoma

Imaging Findings

CT

- Large, apparently well-circumscribed mass isodense to brain parenchyma which fills or displaces the fourth ventricle
- Multifocal calcification in 50%, small cysts in 15%, occasional hemorrhage
- Heterogeneous enhancement post-contrast

MR

- Multilobulated mass filling and extending out of the fourth ventricle
- Isointense on T1-WI, iso- or hyperintense on T2-WI
- Often heterogeneous due to calcification, cysts, or hemorrhage
- Moderate, usually heterogeneous enhancement post-gadolinium
- Invasion of adjacent brain parenchyma and peritumoral edema may be seen

Treatment

- Surgical resection, the extent of which is determined by adherence of tumor to the fourth ventricular floor and local invasion of surrounding brain
- Postoperative radiation therapy
- Chemotherapy for recurrent or high-grade disease

Prognosis

- Better prognosis for adults (60 to 70% 5-year survival in adults vs. 15 to 20% for children)
- Better survival if gross total resection is performed

Suggested Readings

Lyons MK, Kelly PJ. Posterior fossa ependymomas: report of 30 cases and review of the literature. *Neurosurgery* 28:659–665, 1991.

Steinbok P, Hentschel S, Cochrane DD, Kestle JR. Value of post-operative surveillance imaging in the management of children with some common brain tumors. *J Neurosurg* 84:726–732, 1996.

Tortori-Donati P, Fondelli MP, Cama A, et al. Ependymomas of the posterior cranial fossa: CT and MRI findings. *Neuroradiology* 37:238–243, 1995.

Case 33

Clinical Presentation

A young woman presents with progressive right-sided hearing loss.

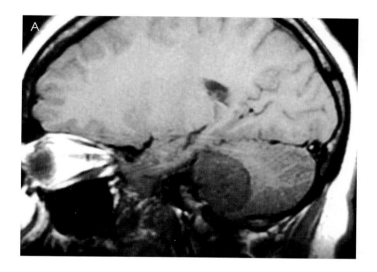

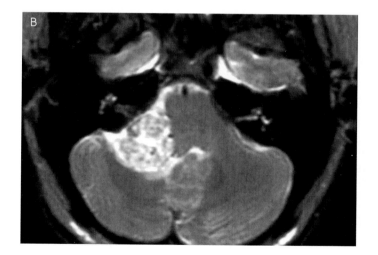

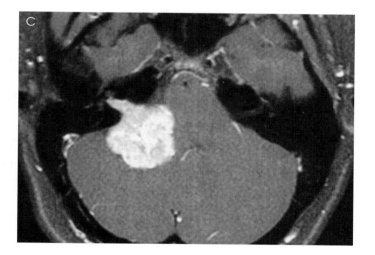

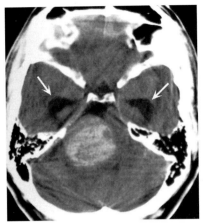

Fig. D. Non-contrast CT scan in a patient with right-sided hearing loss and progressive headache shows a large mass with intrinsic hyperdensity in the right CPA, markedly compressing the pons and cerebellar peduncle. Expansion of the CPA cistern suggests an extra-axial mass. Dilatation of the temporal horns (*arrows*) is consistent with obstructive hydrocephalus.

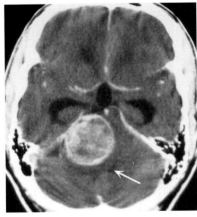

Fig. E. Post-contrast, the mass shown in Fig. D enhances moderately and heterogeneously. The fourth ventricle is severely compressed and distorted (*arrow*).

Radiologic Findings

A sagittal T1-WI (Fig. A) demonstrates a mass that is mildly hypointense compared with brain parenchyma in the cerebellopontine angle (CPA). The mass is sharply demarcated from adjacent brain parenchyma and appears extra-axial. A T2-WI (Fig. B) demonstrates that the right CPA mass is heterogenously hyperintense. In addition, the right internal auditory canal appears midly expanded. The adjacent pons and cerebellar peduncle are distorted, but there is no evidence for parenchymal edema. A post-gadolinium T1-WI with fat saturation (Fig. C) demonstrates intense homogenous enhancement of the right CPA mass. Enhancing tissue extends to the fundus of the expanded right internal auditory canal.

Diagnosis

Vestibular schwannoma (acoustic neuroma)

Differential Diagnosis

- Meningioma (dural-based, dural tail, low- or intermediate-signal on T2-WI, uncommonly cystic or hemorrhagic)
- Giant aneurysm (phase artifact if any flow within the lesion, does not expand internal auditory canal)
- Epidermoid (nonenhancing, similar to CSF on T1- and T2-WI)
- Cavernous malformation (very rare, intrinsic T1 shortening, hemosiderin ring)
- Choroid plexus papilloma (typically centered in the fourth ventricle or foramen of Luschka, no erosion of porus acousticus)

Discussion

Background

Vestibular schwannomas account for 75-80% of CPA masses. These tumors are seen most commonly in older patients, usually presenting in the fifth to sixth decades. While usually unilateral, vestibular schwannomas are bilateral in ~5% of cases, which is characteristic of neurofibromatosis type II (NF2). In patients with NF2, vestibular schwannomas are bilateral in >90% of cases. Vestibular schwannomas are rare in children in the absence of NF2.

Clinical Findings

Patients commonly present with sensorineural hearing loss and/or tinnitus. If the lesion is large, symptoms of hydrocephalus and brainstem compression may occur (Figs. D through F).

Complications

Patients may present acutely following intratumoral hemorrhage and rapid expansion of the tumor, or with subarachnoid hemorrhage. Fifth and seventh cranial nerve palsies may occur in this setting.

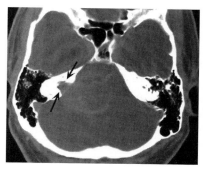

Fig. F. An image photographed in bone windows at the level of the IAC of the same patient as Figures D and E shows irregular enlargement and erosion of the right IAC (*arrows*). Vestibular schwannoma.

Pearls

- To exclude a small tumor of the IAC or labyrinth, post-gadolinium thin-section (≤3 mm) T1-WI with fat saturation in the axial and coronal planes are most useful.

- High-resolution fast spin-echo T2-WI of the IAC detects many small and all large tumors and does not require gadolinium administration, but meticulous attention to technique is necessary and small tumors of the labyrinth in particular may be overlooked.

- The seventh cranial nerve is rarely affected by vestibular schwannomas. If an acute seventh nerve palsy occurs in association with a vestibular schwannomas, consider intratumoral hemorrhage.

Pitfalls

- A large hemorrhagic vestibular schwannoma (Figs. G and H) may mimic a giant aneurysm. Look for phase artifact (typical of aneurysm but may be absent with a thrombosed aneurysm), extension into or widening of the IAC (favors schwannoma), other schwannomas (unlikely to have NF2 and an aneurysm). *(continued)*

Etiology

Vestibular schwannomas usually arise from the inferior or superior division of the vestibular nerve at the glial-Schwann cell interface near Scarpa's ganglion. The cochlear nerve is rarely affected.

Pathology

Gross

- Benign slow-growing encapsulated tumors that arise eccentrically from the parent nerve. Cystic degeneration is common, hemorrhage less so.

Microscopic

- Typically composed of two types of tissue: Antoni A, highly cellular compact tissue interspersed with mature collagen; and Antoni B, widely separated cells in a looser mucoid matrix

Imaging Findings

Most vestibular schwannomas arise within the internal auditory canal (IAC), though they may be purely intravestibular or intracochlear

CT

- Enhancing extra-axial mass positioned at the CPA and/or IAC
- Widening of the IAC or undercutting of the posterior lip of the porus acusticus may occur with lesions larger than 8 to 10 mm
- The portion of the mass in the CPA cistern forms acute angles with the petrous bone (meningiomas tend to have a broad dural base and form obtuse angles)
- Small lesions are usually isodense to brain and enhance homogeneously
- Larger lesions are often heterogeneous (cysts, hemorrhage, fatty degeneration)

MR

- Lesions are usually iso- or hypointense to brain parenchyma on T1-WI
- Iso- or mildly hyperintense on T2-WI
- Small lesions enhance homogeneously, large lesions heterogeneously
- Areas of hemorrhage and cyst formation may be present

Treatment

- Depends on the size of the tumor, the age of the patient, the preferences of the patient, and the status of hearing
- Options include close observation and serial follow-up scans to assess growth pattern; surgical resection; and gamma knife radiosurgery

Prognosis

Excellent, though tumor may regrow if subtotally resected. Vestibular schwannomas are not known to undergo malignant degeneration

- Small intracanalicular enhancing foci may represent leptomeningeal metastases, meningitis, neuritis, sarcoid, or a vascular malformation.

- Labyrinthine hemorrhage in the setting of viral labyrinthitis may cause high signal in the cochlea and/or vestibule which may be mistaken for an enhancing neoplasm if pre-gadolinium T1-WIs have not been obtained.

Suggested Readings

Allen RW, Harnsberger HR, Shelton C, et al. Low-cost high-resolution fast spin-echo MR of acoustic schwannoma: an alternative to enhanced conventional spin-echo MR? *AJNR* 17:1205–1210, 1996.

Mulkens TH, Parizel PM, Martin JJ, et al. Acoustic schwannoma: MR findings in 84 tumors. *AJR* 160:395–398, 1993.

Smirniotopoulos JG, Yue NC, Rushing EJ. Cerebellopontine angle masses: radiologic-pathologic correlation. *Radiographics* 13:1131–1147, 1993.

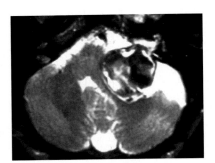

Fig. G. Axial T2-WI shows a heterogenous, mostly hypointense mass centered in the left CPA. The preoperative dignosis was thrombosed giant aneurysm of the posterior inferior cerebellar artery.

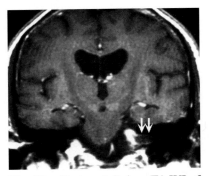

Fig. H. Post-gadolinium T1-WI of the same patient as Fig. G demonstrates widening of the left internal auditory canal (*arrows*). A hemorrhagic vestibular schwannoma was diagnosed at surgery.

Case 34

Clinical Presentation

A 55-year-old woman presents with gradually progressive left-sided hearing loss and left facial numbness.

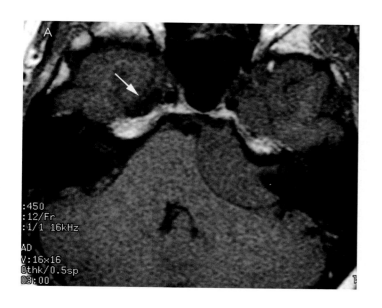

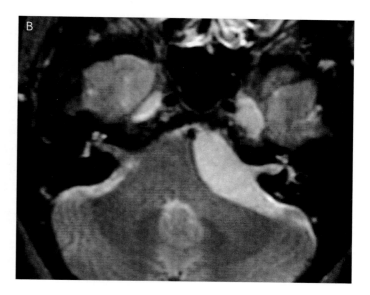

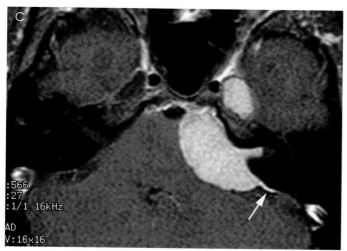

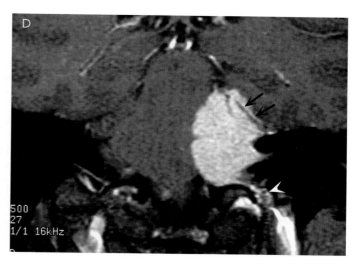

Radiologic Findings

An axial T1-WI (Fig. A) demonstrates an ovoid lesion centered in the left cerebellopontine angle (CPA), extending into the left internal auditory canal (IAC). The lesion is sharply demarcated from adjacent brain parenchyma and appears extra-axial. In addition, the mass extends to Meckel's cave on the left. Note the normal CSF in Meckel's cave on the right (*arrow*). A T2-WI (Fig. B) shows that this mass is mildly hyperintense compared with brain parenchyma. Again note the sharp demarcation from adjacent brain parenchyma and the lack of edema within the brain. Post-gadolinium (Fig. C), a T1-WI shows that the left CPA mass enhances intensely and homogenously, with extension of enhancing tissue into the left internal auditory canal and Meckel's cave. Note also the dural tail (*arrow*) extending away from this lesion posteriorly. A coronal post-gadolinium T1-WI (Fig. D) demonstrates that the mass involves both sides of the tentorium cerebelli, which appears mildly thickened (*arrows*), as well as extending into the jugular foramen (*arrowhead*).

Diagnosis

Meningioma of the CPA

Differential Diagnosis

- Vestibular schwannoma (should extend into the IAC and frequently expands the IAC, typically rounded, often areas of cyst formation or hemorrhage)
- Dural metastasis (often multiple lesions, may incite edema in adjacent brain)
- Hemangiopericytoma (cannot be distinguished without tissue)

Discussion

Background

Meningioma is the second most common CPA tumor after vestibular schwannoma (acoustic neuroma). However, less than 5% of all meningiomas arise in this location. Meningiomas usually occur in middle-aged patients and are more common in women than in men.

Clinical Findings

Meningiomas of the CPA are often asymptomatic until large. Symptoms are usually related to mass effect on nearby cranial nerves such as III, V, VII, and VIII. Hearing loss is less frequent than with vestibular schwannomas.

Etiology

Meningiomas arise from meningothelial cells of the arachnoid villi that are found in association with small veins and along the root sleeves of exiting cranial and spinal nerves

Pathology

Distinct histologic subtypes of meningioma have been defined historically, but meningiomas are now generally classified as typical, atypical, and malignant.

- Typical meningiomas are benign
- Atypical meningioma frequently demonstrates a growth pattern of syncytial sheets, has areas of micronecrosis, and contains large distinct nucleoli. Atypical meningiomas have a Ki-67 labeling index and a recurrence rate between typical and malignant meningiomas.
- Both atypical and malignant meningiomas demonstrate frequent loss of the long arm of chromosome 14, as well as abnormalities of chromosomes 1, 3, and 6
- Over time, atypical meningiomas may transform and become malignant (1 to 2% of cases)

Pearls

- Axial and coronal images through the skull base with post-gadolinium fat-saturated T1-weighted sequences best define the extent of the lesion.

- Compared with vestibular schwannoma, CPA meningiomas tend to be larger, are more hemispheric than round in shape, have a wide dural base, are rather flat, may be associated with hyperostosis, and rarely extend into or widen the IAC.

Pitfalls

- The "dural tail" sign is not specific for meningioma, as it may be seen with any tumor that invades the dura or incites a dural reaction.

- The dural tail most often represents hypervascular dural reaction rather than actual tumor involvement.

- Small meningiomas may be easily overlooked on noncontrast images.

Imaging Findings

CT

- Extra-axial mass that is typically iso- or hyperdense pre-contrast and enhances intensely post-contrast
- May see adjacent bony hyperostosis

MR

- Extra-axial mass that is usually isointense on both T1- and T2-WI
- Intense, homogeneous enhancement post-gadolinium
- May see a "dural tail" sign (nonspecific but frequent)

Treatment

- Surgical resection if possible
- External beam radiation and gamma knife radiosurgery are options for lesions in surgically inaccessible locations (95% control at 5 years for benign lesions)
- Incomplete resection is usually followed with postoperative radiation therapy

Prognosis

- Excellent for typical meningiomas
- Atypical and malignant meningioma subtypes have a higher recurrence rate and poorer survival. Survival at 10 years is 79% in atypical meningiomas and 35% in patients with malignant meningioma

Suggested Readings

Buetow MP, Buetow PC, Smirniotopoulos JG. Typical, atypical, and misleading features in meningioma. *Radiographics* 11:1087–1100, 1991.

Bydder GM, Kingsley DP, Brown J, et al. MR imaging of meningiomas including studies with and without gadolinium-DTPA. *JCAT* 9:690–697, 1985.

Smirniotopoulos JG, Yue NC, Rushing EJ. Cerebellopontine angle masses: radiologic-pathologic correlation. *Radiographics* 13:1131–1147, 1993.

Case 35

Clinical Presentation

A 14-year-old girl presents with gradually progressive right-sided hearing loss.

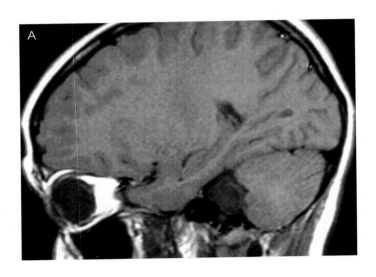

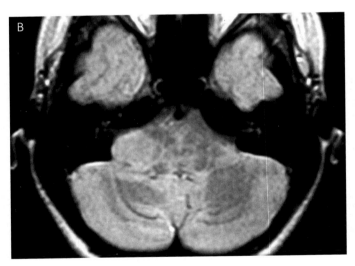

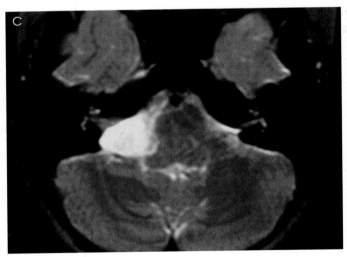

Radiologic Findings

A sagittal T1-WI (Fig. A) demonstrates a hypointense lesion in the right cerebellopontine angle (CPA). An axial PD-WI (Fig. B) demonstrates a rounded mass in the right CPA that is mildly hyperintense compared with CSF. An axial T2-WI (Fig. C) also demonstrates that the mass is hyperintense compared with CSF. Post-gadolinium (Fig. D), there is only a thin irregular margin of enhancement along the posterior aspect of this lesion. Note that fat saturation has been applied. A post-gadolinium coronal T1-WI with fat saturation (Fig. E) demonstrates extension of the mass into the right internal auditory canal (*arrows*), which is expanded as compared with the left side.

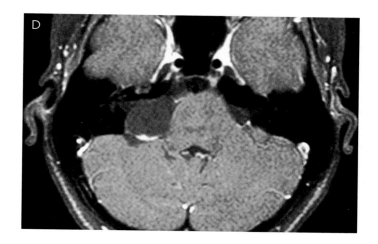
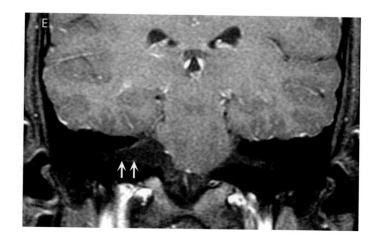

Diagnosis

Epidermoid tumor of the CPA

Differential Diagnosis (Table 1)

- Arachnoid cyst (follows CSF on all imaging sequences, nonenhancing)
- Vestibular schwannoma (usually more solid, solid portions enhance, though can be cystic)
- Dermoid (usually fatty signal intensity)
- Meningioma (usually ovoid, enhancing, older age group)
- Neurenteric cyst (usually midline in location, rare)

Discussion

Background

Epidermoids represent 0.2 to 1% of intracranial tumors and 5% of CPA tumors. Forty percent of intracranial epidermoids occur in the CPA, with other common locations being the parasellar and suprasellar regions and the middle cranial fossa. They are slow-growing benign lesions that expand gradually over many years and therefore typically present in adulthood.

Table 1. Differential Diagnosis of Cerebellopontine Angle Masses*

Tumor	Incidence	NECT	T1-WI	PD-WI	T2-WI	Post-gad	Comments
Vestibular schwannoma	75-80%	Hypo	Hypo	Hyper	Hyper	++	C, Ca, Hem
Meningioma	10%	Iso	Hypo or iso	Usually hyper	Iso or hyper	++	Dural tail common
Epidermoid	5%	Iso or mildly hyper to CSF	Hypo (can be hyper)	Hyper to CSF	Iso or hyper to CSF	- - (may have thin rim)	May have peripheral Ca
Arachnoid cyst	1%	Iso to CSF	Iso to CSF	Iso to CSF	Iso to CSF	–	no C,Ca,Hem
Astrocytoma	1%	Iso	Hypo or iso	Hyper	Hyper	+	Exophytic

Note: Densities/intensities are compared with brain parenchyma unless otherwise specified.

Hypo = hypodense for CT, hypointense for MR; Iso = isodense for CT, isointense for MR; Hyper = hyperdense for CT, hyperintense for MR; ++ = intense enhancement, + = moderate enhancement, -- = non-enhancing; C = cyst; Ca = calcification; Hem = hemorrhage; NECT = non-enhanced CT

*Other rare masses of the CPA include neuromas of other cranial nerves, metastasis, paraganglioma.

Clinical Findings

Epidermoids of the CPA generally present with cranial nerve dysfunction (facial pain or palsy, diplopia, hearing loss) or symptoms of brainstem compression.

Etiology

Epidermoids are thought to arises from incomplete cleavage of neural and cutaneous ectoderm between 3 and 5 weeks gestation. Because CPA epidermoids are laterally located, they are thought to result from inclusion of epithelial elements at a later stage of embryogenesis. These tumors grow slowly (at the rate of skin turnover), and therefore rarely present before the third or fourth decade.

Pathology

Gross

• Lobulated, "cauliflowerlike," pearly lesions

Microscopic

• Lined by simple squamous epithelium
• Contains desquamated keratin, lipids, and cholesterol crystals

Imaging Findings

CT

• Usually hypodense, nonenhancing
• Patchy peripheral calcification in ~25%

MR

• Intensity often similar to CSF: hypointense on T1-WI and hyperintense on T2-WI compared with brain parenchyma. However, epidermoids do not usually follow CSF exactly, being mildly hyperintense to CSF on T1- and PD-WI and having internal areas of mixed-signal intensity that indicate a solid mass.
• Occasionally may be very hyperintense on T1-WI (this is thought to be related to triglycerides and/or polyunsaturated fatty acids)
• May rarely show mild rim enhancement post-gadolinium, probably representing an inflammatory reaction at the periphery of the lesion

Treatment

Surgical removal (adherence of capsule to brainstem and cranial nerves may limit resection)

Prognosis

Excellent, though lesions may recur following subtotal resection

Suggested Readings

Gao P, Osborn AG, Smirniotopoulos JG, Harris CP. Radiologic-pathologic correlation: epidermoid tumor of the cerebellopontine angle. *AJNR* 13:863–872, 1992.

Mohanty A, Venkatrama SK, Rao BR, et al. Experience with cerebellopontine angle epidermoids. *Neurosurgery* 40:24–30, 1997.

Tampieri D, Melanson D, Ethier R. MR imaging of epidermoid cysts. *AJNR* 10:351–356, 1989.

Case 36

Clinical Presentation

A 70-year-old male presents with 1 month of rapidly progressing left-sided hearing loss.

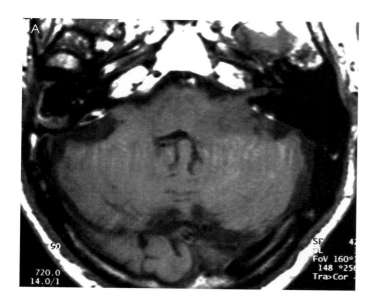

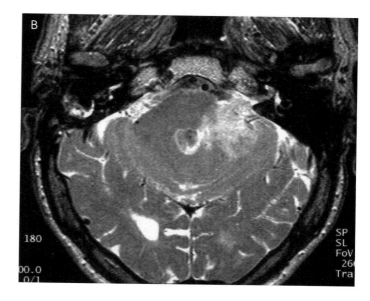

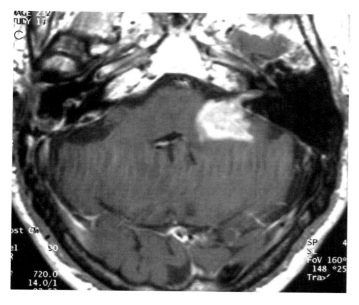

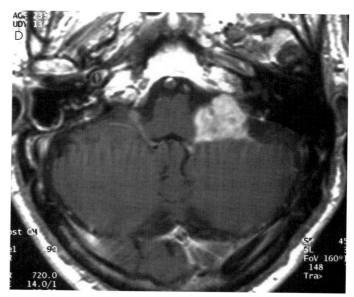

Radiologic Findings

An axial T1-WI (Fig. A) shows a soft tissue mass in the left cerebellopontine angle, with extension into the left internal auditory canal. On this image, it is somewhat difficult to determine whether this mass is intra- or extra-axial. The mass is heterogeneously hyperintense on an axial T2-WI (Fig. B), and the mar-

Pearls

- MR is generally preferred over CT for evaluation of brain tumors, especially in the posterior fossa, because MR better assesses extent of tumor and helps plan surgical resection, allows a more accurate preoperative differential diagnosis to be formulated, is more sensitive to CSF spread of disease, and avoids bone artifacts that compromise CT.

- A screening examination of the spine is generally indicated in the setting of posterior fossa disease to rule out drop metastases.

Pitfalls

- An exophytic lesion arising from the cerebellar hemisphere or middle cerebellar peduncle may mimic an extra-axial mass. In this setting, MR's multiplanar capabilities and excellent soft tissue contrast are very helpful in establishing the origin of the mass.

- An exophytic parenchymal lesion may extend into the internal auditory canal (IAC), so IAC involvement does not rule out a parenchymal lesion.

- An irregular interface between the mass and adjacent brain favors an intra-axial origin of the tumor.

- GBMs usually incite significant edema and exert mass effect, but this may be limited when a lesion is predominantly exophytic.

gins are ill-defined with respect to adjacent brain parenchyma. Post-gadolinium (Fig. C), there is intense and relatively homogenous enhancement of the soft tissue mass, with enhancement extending into the left internal auditory canal. A more inferior post-gadolinium T1-WI (Fig. D) demonstrates enhancement of the exophytic component of the mass in the cerebellomedullary angle.

Diagnosis

Glioblastoma multiforme (GBM)

Differential Diagnosis

- Metastasis (often multiple)
- Choroid plexus neoplasm (extra-axial, intensely enhancing)
- Ependymoma (may have an irregular interface with parenchyma, usually occurs in children)
- Acoustic neuroma (extra-axial, cerebellopontine angle component is usually rounded and smooth rather than irregular)

Discussion

Background

GBM is the most malignant of all glial neoplasms (grade IV) and represents 15 to 20% of primary CNS neoplasms in adults. It is usually located supratentorially, involving the cerebral hemispheres or the corpus callosum. Posterior fossa involvement is rare and is seen in <1% of GBMs. In the posterior fossa, GBMs may involve the cerebellar hemisphere, the vermis, or the brain stem. They often grow in an exophytic fashion into the fourth ventricle or basal cisterns. Posterior fossa GBMs tend to generate less edema than metastases and less often calcify. Overall, metastatic disease is the most common posterior fossa neoplasm in an adult.

Clinical Findings

In the posterior fossa, typical symptoms include headache, nausea/vomiting, dizziness, and hearing loss.

Complications

Complications include obstructive hydrocephalus and parenchymal or subarachnoid hemorrhage.

Etiology

An abnormal p53 tumor-suppressor gene has been implicated in some cases of GBM.

Pathology

Gross

- Irregular, heterogeneous, vascular neoplasm

Microscopic

- Marked neovascularity, increased mitoses, cellular pleomorphism, necrosis, and pseudopalisading are observed
- Less malignant gliomas (grades II, III) have less mitotic activity and pleomorphism and lack necrosis and pseudopalisading

Imaging Findings

CT

- Irregular mass lesion, often hyperdense on nonenhanced scan
- Post-contrast: heterogeneous enhancement, areas of necrosis

MR

- Intra-axial mass that is typically heterogeneous due to cysts, hemorrhage, and/or necrosis
- Solid portions of the mass are usually iso- or hypointense to parenchyma on T1-WI and iso- or hyperintense to parenchyma on T2-WI
- Enhancement is heterogeneous in most cases, and is rarely absent (<5% of cases)

Treatment

- Surgical resection
- Radiation therapy
- Adjuvant chemotherapy

Prognosis

Poorly differentiated gliomas of the cerebellum (grade III and IV lesions) shows a median survival of 31 months

Suggested Readings

Ahn MS, Jackler RK. Exophytic brain tumors mimicking primary lesions of the cerebellopontine angle. *Laryngoscope* 107:466–471, 1997.

Kuroiwa T, Numaguchi Y, Rothman MI, et al. Posterior fossa glioblastoma multiforme: MR findings. *AJNR* 16:583–589, 1995.

Rees JH, Smirniotopoulos JG, Jones RV, Wong K. Glioblastoma multiforme: radiologic-pathologic correlation. *Radiographics* 16:1413–1438, 1996.

Case 37

Clinical Presentation

A 32-year-old woman with long-standing hearing loss presents for evaluation.

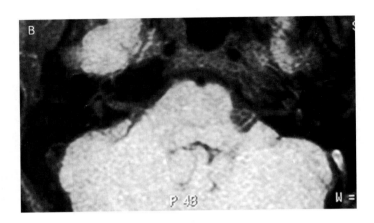

Radiologic Findings

An axial pre-contrast T1-WI (Fig. A) demonstrates a hyperintense lesion in the left cerebellopontine angle (CPA). A linear low-signal intensity structure runs through this mass. In addition, a second lesion with intrinsic T1 shortening is identified in the expected location of the left vestibule (*arrow*). With a fat-saturation pulse applied to a T1-WI (Fig. B), the previously identified hyperintense lesions are now barely visualizable.

Diagnosis

Lipoma of CPA and vestibule

Differential Diagnosis

- Dermoid (displaces neurovascular structures)
- Epidermoid (usually isointense to CSF but may show T1 shortening, does not show chemical shift artifact, and does not lose signal on fat-saturated sequence)
- Vestibular schwannoma (not homogeneously hyperintense even when hemorrhagic)
- Fat within petrous bone (located within bone rather than within a CSF space)

Discussion

Background

Intracranial lipomas most commonly occur in the midline and involve the subarachnoid space adjacent to the corpus callosum (Fig. C) and dorsal midbrain. In

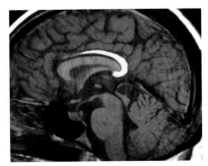

Fig. C. Sagittal T1-WI shows a lipoma in the pericallosal subarachnoid space, associated with hypogenesis of the corpus callosum and deficiency of the splenium. An incidental pineal cyst is also seen.

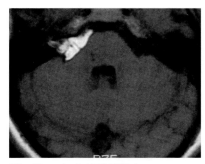

Fig. D. Axial T1-WI demonstrates a hyperintense lesion in the right CPA, extending into the right internal auditory canal.

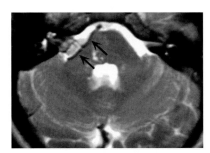

Fig. E. Axial T2-WI (same patient as Fig. D) demonstrates linear hypointensity along the margin of the lesion (*arrows*) representing chemical shift artifact. Irregular T2 prolongation in the right pons was thought to represent ischemic change. Diagnosis: lipoma.

Pearls

• The fatty nature of the lesion can be confirmed with fat-saturation techniques or by demonstration of chemical shift artifact, which is generally best seen on PD-WIs.

• CNS lipomas are malformations, not neoplasms.

• Nerves (i.e., cranial nerve VIII) and blood vessels traverse these lesions and may be damaged in attempted resections.

these locations, they are often associated with other congenital malformations. Approximately 9% of intracranial lipomas occur in the CPA, and they are usually isolated malformations. Lipoma of the internal auditory canal is less common than the lipoma of the CPA, but more common than the lipoma of the vestibule.

Clinical Findings

Lipomas of the CPA generally present with cranial nerve symptoms including sensorineural hearing loss, trigeminal neuralgia, and hemifacial spasm.

Etiology

Intracranial lipomas are congenital malformations rather than true neoplasms. They result from abnormal persistence and maldifferentiation of the *meninx primitiva*, which is the precursor of the leptomeninges. Thus lipomas actually occur within the subarachnoid space and are often traversed by normal neurovascular structures.

Pathology

Composed of mature adipose tissue, but may be traversed by nerves and vessels

Imaging Findings

Intracranial lipomas follow fat on all imaging sequences:

CT

• Hypodense, and may mimic air on soft tissue windows

MR

• Characteristic T1 shortening
• Signal loss on fat-saturated images
• Evidence of chemical shift artifact (Figs. D and E)
• Neurovascular structures traversing the lesion are often identified

Treatment

• In evolution: observation with periodic follow-up imaging is recommended for relatively small lesions in difficult locations because normal vessels and nerves traverse these lesions and resection can injure these delicate structures
• For particularly large lesions with significant symptoms, a conservative surgical approach may be taken: accomplish decompression without risking damage to traversing or adjacent structures by attempting total removal
• In certain cases, weight loss may decrease the size of a lipoma

Prognosis

Excellent for isolated lesions

Suggested Readings

Bohrer PS, Chole RA. Unusual lesions of the internal auditory canal. *Am J Otol* 17:143–149, 1996.

Pitfalls

- Chemical shift will be less pronounced as the bandwidth is increased

- Fat within the marrow cavity of the petrous bone may be confused with a lipoma of the internal auditory canal.

- If T1-WI is performed only post-gadolinium, a lipoma may be mistaken for an enhancing lesion such as an acoustic neuroma.

Huang TS. Primary intravestibular lipoma. *Ann Otol Rhinol Laryngol* 98:393–395, 1989.

Truwit CL, Barkovich AJ. Pathogenesis of intracranial lipoma: an MR study in 42 patients. *AJR* 155:855–864, 1990.

Section II

Infection

Case 38

Clinical Presentation

A 10-month-old female with developmental delay, microcephaly, and seizures presents for evaluation.

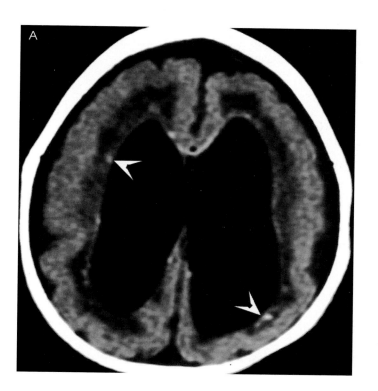

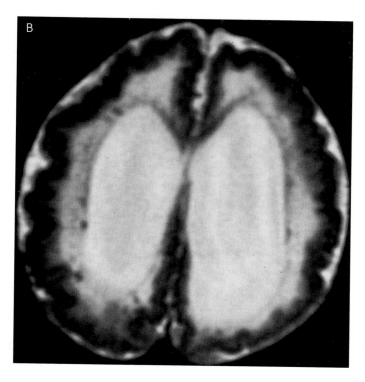

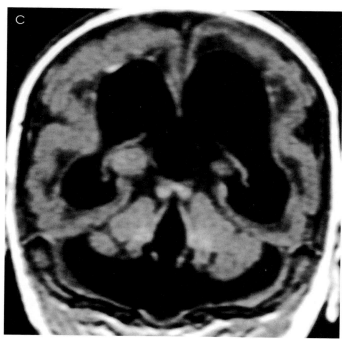

Radiologic Findings

An axial T1-WI (Fig. A) demonstrates marked enlargement of the lateral ventricles, as well as prominence of the subarachnoid spaces. The cortex is diffusely abnormal, without normal formation of sulci and gyri. In addition, multiple puncate hyperintensities (*arrowheads*) are noted around the ventricular margins, and the white matter is abnormally hypointense. An axial T2-WI (Fig. B) demonstrates the diffuse cortical abnormality to better advantage and shows a pattern of multiple small sulci and gyri suggesting polymicrogyria. The white matter is diffusely abnormally hyperintense. Multiple punctate hypointensities are noted along the ventricular surface, correlating with the T1 hyperintensities, consistent with calcifications. On a coronal T1-WI (Fig. C), the above-described findings are again observed, as is striking cerebellar hypoplasia.

Diagnosis

Congenital cytomegalovirus (CMV) infection

Differential Diagnosis

- Toxoplasmosis (lacks cerebral cortical abnormality, more irregular and scattered pattern of Ca^{2+})
- Rubella (microcephaly, congenital cataracts, congenital heart disease)
- Herpes encephalitis (usually presents at a few weeks of age)
- Neonatal bacterial meningitis (acute clinical presentation)

Discussion

Background

CMV is one of the "TORCH" infections, an acronym that is applied to describe common infections of the fetus and neonate: toxoplasmosis, other (e.g., syphilis), rubella, CMV, and herpes simplex virus type 2. Congenital CMV infection affects ~1% of newborns in the United States. When a woman is infected with CMV for the first time during pregnancy or has reactivation of a prior infection, the virus is transmitted to the fetus in utero via the placenta and then disseminates hematogenously. Preexisting maternal antibodies do seem to lessen the incidence and severity of the manifestations of congenital CMV infection. In most cases, the infection is subclinical at birth, with symptoms developing later in childhood.

Etiology

CMV is a linear double-stranded DNA virus that is a member of the herpesvirus group. It replicates in the cell nucleus, causing either a lytic and productive or latent infection. The diagnosis is made by polymerase chain reaction (PCR) identification of viral DNA and/or by viral culture.

Clinical Findings

Five to 10% of infants with congenital CMV are symptomatic at birth, while an additional 10 to 15% become symptomatic during the first year of life. CNS symptoms include sensorineural deafness, seizures, mental retardation, chorioretinitis, optic neuritis, microcephaly, anophthalmia, and microphthalmia. Non-CNS symptoms include intrauterine growth retardation, jaundice, hepatosplenomegaly, hemolytic anemia, thrombocytopenic purpura, and pneumonitis.

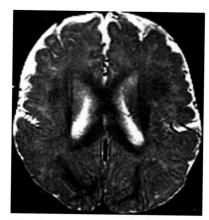

Fig. D. An axial T2-WI appears relatively normal except for prominence of the subarachnoid spaces and a questionably abnormal cortical folding pattern in the left frontal lobe.

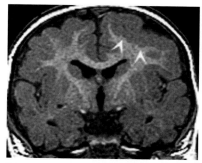

Fig. E. A coronal T1-WI in the same patient as Fig. D confirms localized left frontal polymicrogyria (*arrowheads*) in this patient with congenital CMV.

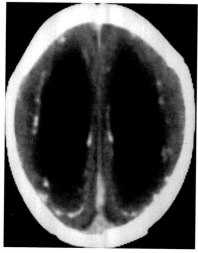

Fig. F. A non-enhanced CT scan in a patient with a congenital CMV demonstrates ventriculomegaly and a pattern of multiple periventricular calcifications.

Complications

Hydrocephalus may be obstructive secondary to ventriculitis and obstruction of CSF flow by inflammatory exudate, or *ex vacuo* related to brain atrophy. Hydrocephalus is more common in congenital toxoplasmosis than in congenital CMV.

Pathology

- CMV causes a necrotizing inflammation with a predilection for the subependymal germinal matrix of the lateral ventricles. This results in: paraventricular subependymal cystic lesions, postinflammatory calcifications (usually periventricular in distribution), disturbed neuronal migration (lissencephaly, cortical dysplasia), and cerebellar hypoplasia/dysplasia.
- Mineralizing vasculopathy with thickening of the walls of the lenticulostriate vessels is also commonly observed.
- The severity of the findings is directly related to the gestational age of the fetus at the time of infection. Earlier infection leads to more severe migrational and developmental anomalies. Early second trimester infection often leads to complete lissencephaly, while later second trimester infection causes polymicrogyria. With infection in the third trimester, the gyral pattern may be normal or show focal areas of polymicrogyria (Figs. D and E).

Imaging Findings

Both CT and MR demonstrate ventricular enlargement due to hydrocephalus and/or brain atrophy.

CT

- Predominantly periventricular pattern of calcification (Fig. F)
- May show subependymal cysts and lenticulostriate calcifications

MR

- Much more sensitive to areas of polymicrogyria
- Allows evaluation of cerebellar hypogenesis/dysgenesis
- Delayed or abnormal myelination is common

Treatment

Ganciclovir (an antiviral agent) reduces viremia/viruria and may stabilize or even improve hearing

Prognosis

Variable: depends on extent of brain injury and visceral organ injury

Suggested Readings

Barkovich AJ, Lindan CE. Congenital cytomegalovirus infection of the brain: imaging analysis and embryological considerations. *AJNR* 15:703–715, 1994.

Boesch C, Issakainen J, Kewitz G, et al. Magnetic resonance imaging of the brain in congenital cytomegalovirus infection. *Pediatr Radiol* 19:91–93, 1989.

Whitley RJ, Cloud G, Gruber W, et al. Ganciclovir treatment of symptomatic congenital cytomegalovirus infection: results of a phase II study. *J Infect Dis* 175:1080–1086, 1997.

Case 39

Clinical Presentation

A neonate was noted to be microcephalic and hypotonic. Clinical examination showed evidence of bilateral chorioretinitis. Following a seizure, a CT scan was obtained.

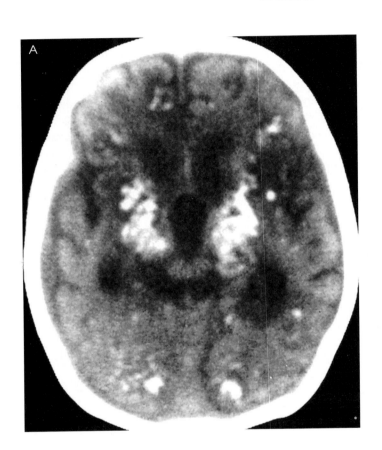 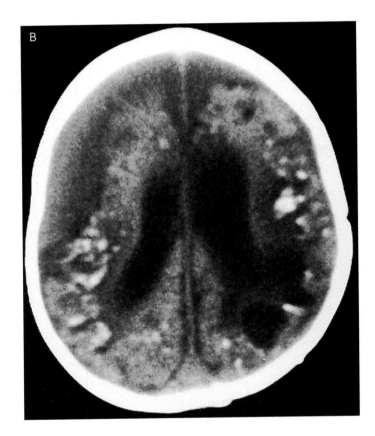

Radiologic Findings

An axial non-contrast CT (Fig. A) shows prominence of the lateral ventricles and third ventricle out of proportion to the sulci, consistent with hydrocephalus. In addition, multiple irregular calcifications are present within the basal ganglia bilaterally and also scattered throughout the brain parenchyma. A more cephalad image (Fig. B) shows bifrontal extra-axial collections consistent with subdural hygromas or chronic hematomas. Areas of cystic encephalomalacia are present, and mutlifocal irregular parenchymal calcifications are again identified.

Diagnosis

Congenital toxoplasmosis

Differential Diagnosis

- Congenital cytomegalovirus (periventricular Ca^{2+}, often polymicrogyria)
- Congenital rubella (severe microcephaly, more subtle pattern of Ca^{2+})

Discussion

Background

Congenital toxoplasmosis develops after the parasite *Toxoplasma gondii* is passed to the fetus transplacentally. This usually occurs when an immunocompetent mother is infected for the first time during gestation, but congenital transmission may also occur from a mother who is immunocompromised and chronically infected. Congenital toxoplasmosis is second in frequency to cytomegalovirus infection among the TORCH infections. The incidence of congenital toxoplasmosis is about 1 to 2 cases per 1000 births per year.

Etiology

Toxoplasmosis is caused by the obligate intracellular protozoan parasite *Toxoplasma gondii*. This usually infects human beings via inadequately cooked meat that harbors oocysts (cattle, sheep, and pigs are intermediate hosts), but may also be acquired from contact with cats (the definitive hosts) and from unwashed fruits and vegetables via a fecal-oral route. CSF adds pleocytosis and elevated protein.

Clinical Findings

Most infants are asymptomatic at birth, with onset of symptoms in the first days to weeks of postnatal life. Infection may be generalized or concentrated primarily in the CNS. CNS findings include chorioretinitis (bilateral in 85%), hydrocephalus, and seizures. Severely affected patients have microcephaly, tetraplegia, mental retardation, and/or blindness.

Complications

The earlier the in utero infection, the more severe the above-mentioned findings.

Pathology

Gross

- Ventricular dilatation, scattered calcifications

Microscopic

- Multifocal necrotizing granulomatous infection that is often accompanied by a granular ependymitis

Imaging Findings

Both CT and MR may show ventricular dilatation and areas of encephalomalacia

CT

- Scattered multifocal cerebral calcifications with less of a periventricular predilection than CMV

MR

- Delayed myelination
- Focal areas of parenchymal destruction

Treatment

- Usually long-term treatment with the antimicrobials pyrimethamine and sulfadiazine
- If infection is diagnosed in utero, maternal treatment with spiramycin can reduce the incidence and severity of congenital infection

Prognosis

Variable, depending on early identification and prompt institution of therapy. This has been greatly aided by neonatal screening programs. In children treated for 1 year, signs of active CNS infection (CSF pleocytosis, elevated CSF protein) resolved, and this group had significantly better neurologic and developmental outcomes than a group that was untreated or treated for less than 1 month.

Suggested Readings

Becker LE. Infections of the developing brain. *AJNR* 13:537–549, 1992.

Patel DV, Holfels EM, Vogel NP, et al. Resolution of intracranial calcifications in infants with treated congenital toxoplasmosis. *Radiology* 199:433–440, 1996.

Roizen N, Swisher CN, Stein NA, et al. Neurologic and developmental outcome in treated congenital toxoplasmosis. *Pediatrics* 95:11–20, 1995.

Case 40

Clinical Presentation

A 4-week-old infant who had been been febrile and irritable for several days presented to the emergency room in status epilepticus. She progressed to a chronic vegetative state, and serial studies were obtained.

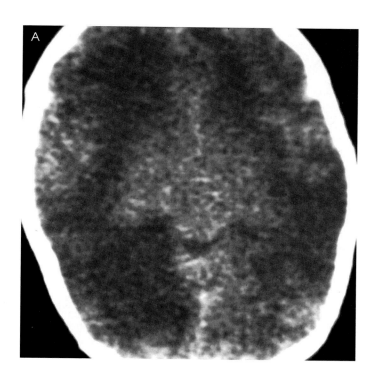

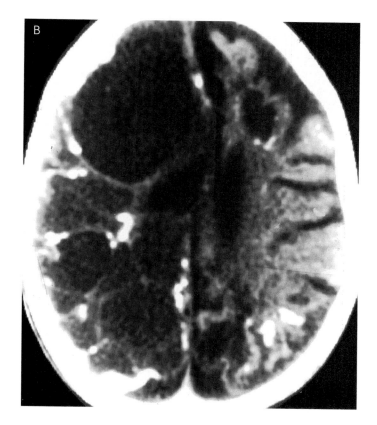

Radiologic Findings

A non-contrast CT scan (Fig. A) obtained at the time of presentation demonstrates bifrontal and biparietal areas of low density involving cortex and underlying white matter. A follow-up CT scan obtained several months later (Fig. B) shows extensive macrocystic encephalomalacia and multiple areas of irregular parenchymal calcification.

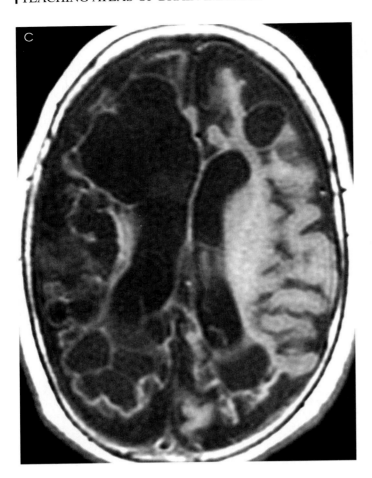

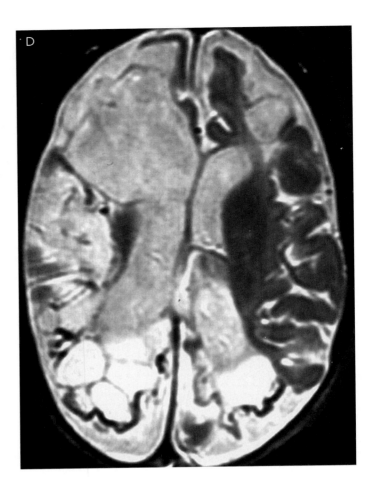

An axial T1-WI (Fig. C) from an MR scan obtained shortly thereafter also demonstrates the extensive cystic encephalomalacia involving both hemispheres, right greater than left. A T2-WI (Fig. D) confirms the extensive parenchymal volume loss. Linear low signal in the posterior cortex is related to calcification.

Diagnosis

Neonatal herpes meningoencephalitis (herpes simplex virus type 2)

Differential Diagnosis

- Neonatal bacterial meningitis (organisms may be isolated from blood or CSF)
- Congenital cytolomegalovirus (cerebral cortical malformations, periventricular calcifications)
- Congenital toxoplasmosis (chorioretinitis, irregular calcifications)
- Congenital rubella (rare, cataracts, microcephaly)

Discussion

Background

The neonate typically becomes infected with herpes simplex virus type 2 (HSV2) via contact with active herpetic lesions in the maternal birth canal during delivery. Rarely, hematogenous transplacental infection in utero may occur. The CNS

Pearls

- Both CT and MR clearly demonstrate the late sequelae of the infection, but MR is more sensitive in the acute stage of the disease.
- Consider this diagnosis in a neonate who presents in the second or third week of life with diffuse brain edema and leptomeningeal enhancement.

Pitfalls

- Neonatal herpes encephalitis does not demonstrate the temporal and inferior frontal lobe predominance associated with herpes infections in older patients.
- This diagnosis must not be missed as early treatment is imperative.

is involved in 30 to 60% of cases. Primary HSV2 infection in neonates causes a diffuse brain infection that is distinct from the predominantly inferior frontal and temporal lobe involvement that is typical of reactivated latent HSV1 or HSV2 infection in older children and adults.

Etiology

HSV2 is a DNA virus of the herpesvirus group.

Clinical Findings

Fever, irritability, and lethargy usually develop within the first 2 to 4 weeks of life.

Complications

There may be a rapid progression to seizures, coma, and death. Disseminated intravascular coagulopathy and hepatic failure are often present.

Pathology/Laboratory

- HSV2 causes a necrotizing meningoencephalitis with areas of focal hemorrhagic necrosis. Findings include inflammatory cells in the meninges, perivascular inflammatory infiltrates, severe multifocal necrosis of all cellular elements of brain parenchyma, and reactive microglial and astroglial proliferation. CSF analysis shows elevated protein and pleocytosis, sometimes with red blood cells. Isolation of the virus is the definitive means for establishing the diagnosis. Virus may be isolated from vesicular skin lesions (if present), throat, stool, urine, or CSF. The polymerase chain reaction is often used to amplify small quantities of viral DNA. Brain biopsy is generally not necessary to make the diagnosis.
- In the chronic phase, there is parenchymal calcification, macrocystic encephalomalacia, and failure of brain growth

Imaging Findings

Early disease

CT

- Subtle hypodensity in periventricular white matter and cortex

MR

- Brain edema with T1 and T2 prolongation that may be difficult to detect in the unmyelinated brain. A clue to cortical edema is isointensity of cortex to white matter.
- Gyral swelling
- Postcontrast: mild leptomeningeal enhancement

Late disease

CT

- High density in the cortex secondary to petechial hemorrhage
- Progression to atrophy and multicystic encephalomalacia
- Punctate parenchymal and/or gyral calcifications may develop

MR

- Focal hemorrhagic necrosis and extensive cyst formation
- Parenchymal volume loss, "Swiss cheese brain"

Treatment

Acyclovir, a drug of limited toxicity and high specificity, is a deoxyguanosine analogue that is activated by a herpes-specific thymidine kinase. It inhibits viral DNA polymerase and therefore viral replication.

Prognosis

- CNS disease carries a 15% mortality and a 60 to 70% risk of neurologic compromise
- Disseminated disease (multiple organ systems) is associated with a 50 to 65% mortality

Suggested Readings

Noorbehesht B, Enzmann DR, Sullinder W, et al. Neonatal herpes simplex encephalitis: correlation of clinical and CT findings. *Radiology* 162:813–819, 1987.

Shaw DWW, Cohen WA. Viral infections of the CNS in children: imaging features. *AJR* 160:125–133, 1993.

Tien RD, Felsberg GJ, Osumi AK. Herpesvirus infections of the CNS: MR findings. *AJR* 161:167–176, 1993.

Case 41

Clinical Presentation

A 5-week-old male infant was admitted to an outside hospital with fever and lethargy. Because of progressive obtundation, he was transferred to a tertiary care hospital.

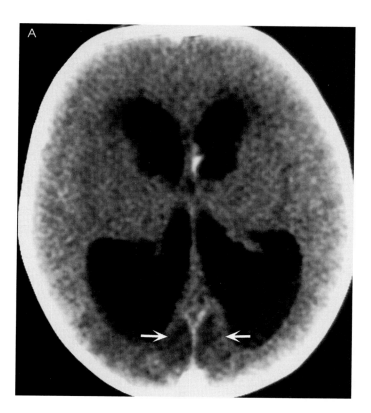

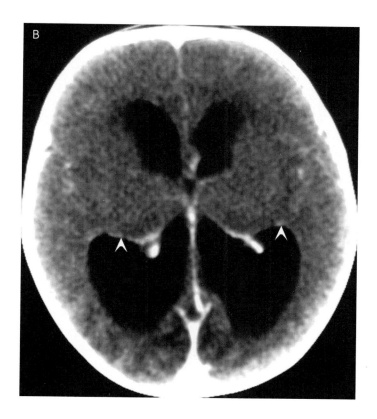

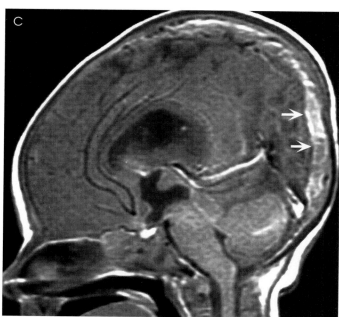

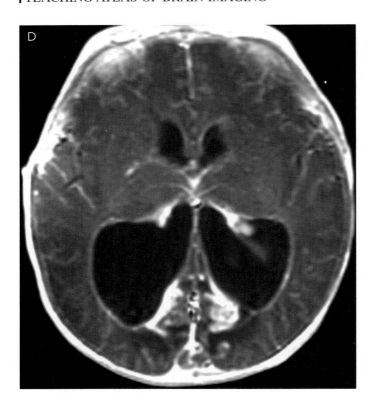

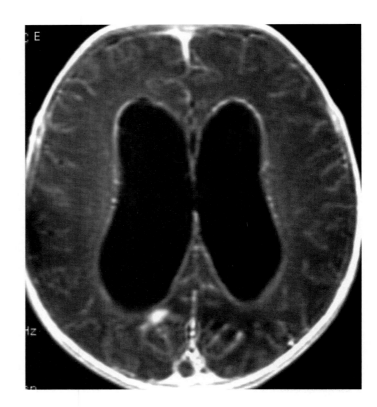

Radiologic Findings

A non-contrast CT scan (Fig. A) demonstrates marked enlargement of the lateral ventricles and effacement of cerebral sulci, consistent with obstructive hydrocephalus. Low density is present in the occipital lobes bilaterally (*arrows*). Mild low density around the frontal horns is likely due to transependymal flow of CSF. In addition, the sagittal sinus is abnormally dense for a non-contrast CT, suggesting sagittal sinus thrombosis. Post-contrast (Fig. B), there is subtle linear enhancement of the ependymal surfaces of the ventricular atria bilaterally (*arrowheads*). Because of concern for sagittal sinus thrombosis, an MR scan was obtained. A sagittal T1-WI (Fig. C) demonstrates high-signal-intensity material filling and expanding the sagittal sinus (*arrows*) and straight sinus. Subcortical hypointensity is present in the occipital lobe. Dilatation of the anterior recesses of the third ventricle is consistent with known hydrocephalus. There is also evidence for downward herniation, with obliteration of the quadrigeminal plate cisterns. An axial post-gadolinium T1-WI (Fig. D) demonstrates ependymal and leptomeningeal enhancement significantly better than the CT scan. Hypointensity and gyral enhancement involving the occipital lobes is noted. A post-gadolinium T1-WI at a somewhat higher level (Fig. E) also demonstrates diffuse ependymal and leptomeningeal enhancement. In addition, note the filling defect within the sagittal sinus, consistent with venous sinus thrombosis.

Diagnosis

Neonatal bacterial meningitis (group B streptococci) complicated by dural sinus thrombosis and brain infarction

Differential Diagnosis

- Arterial infarction of noninfectious etiology (affects an arterial distribution)
- Viral meningitis (usually more benign except herpes simplex virus type 2, typically less enhancement)

Discussion

Background

Meningitis is the most common form of CNS infection in children. Neonatal meningitis can be divided into early-onset and late-onset disease. Early-onset disease usually occurs in setting of premature birth or obstetric complications (i.e., prolonged internal monitoring) and is dominated by nonneurologic signs such as hypotension, apnea, and jaundice. Late-onset disease has its onset after the first week of life and is characterized by lethargy, seizures, bulging fontanelle, and focal neurologic signs. Group B streptococcus is a common cause of neonatal meningitis. It is usually acquired during passage through an infected birth canal, but it may also be caused by ascending infection in the setting of premature rupture of the membranes. The incidence of group B streptococcal neonatal meningitis is ~1.8 cases per 1000 live births.

Etiology

Group B streptococcal species and *Escherichia coli* are the most common causes of neonatal meningitis (~60% of cases), but many pathogens have been implicated.

Clinical Findings

Neonatal infection with group B streptococci may cause pneumonia, sepsis, and/or meningitis. Group B streptococcal meningitis is characterized by severe obtundation and seizures.

Complications

CNS complications include cranial nerve palsies, hydrocephalus, cerebral infarction, parenchymal abscess, and intracranial empyema. Systemic complications include disseminated intravascular coagulation, shock, and respiratory failure.

Pathology

- Acute inflammation in the subarachnoid space
- Ventriculitis and a necrotizing infectious vasculopathy with secondary infarction may occur in advanced cases

Imaging Findings

The CT and MR findings in meningitis are similar, though MR is more sensitive to leptomeningeal or ependymal enhancement and early infarction. The spectrum of CT and MR findings includes:

- Uncomplicated meningitis: normal study (this does not exclude the diagnosis of meningitis), communicating or noncommunicating hydrocephalus, leptomeningeal and/or ependymal enhancement

- Complicated of meningitis: arterial infarction secondary to infectious vasculopathy, venous infarction secondary to sepsis and dehydration with venous thrombosis, brain abscess, subdural and/or epidural empyema

Treatment

- Antistreptococcal agent with good CSF penetration (e.g., penicillin)
- Corticosteroids
- Vaccines against group B streptococci are currently under trial

Prognosis

Case-fatality ratio of 10 to 20%

Suggested Readings

Boyer KM. Neonatal group B streptococcal infections. *Curr Opin Pediatr* 7:13–18, 1995.

Platt MW, Gilson GJ. Group B streptococcal disease in the perinatal period. *Am Fam Physician* 49:434–442, 1994.

Yancey MK, Duff P, Kubilis P, et al. Risk factors for neonatal sepsis. *Obstet Gynecol* 87:188–194, 1996.

Case 42

Clinical Presentation

A 6-month-old infant with fever and irritability is admitted to the hospital to rule out meningitis. An admission CT scan (not shown) suggested an extra-axial fluid collection. An MR scan was obtained for further evaluation.

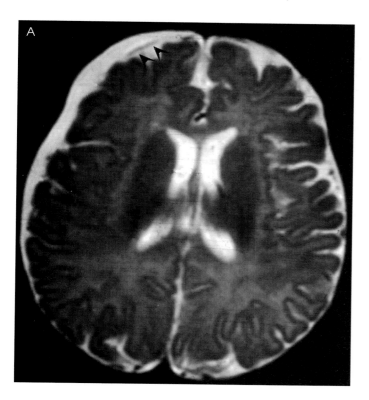

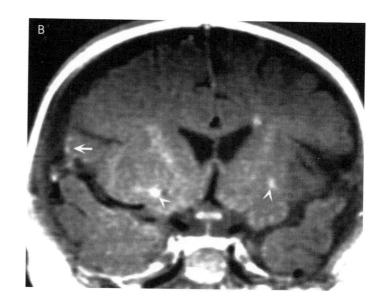

Radiologic Findings

An axial T2-WI (Fig. A) demonstrates prominence of the extra-axial spaces bilaterally, right greater than left. On the right, a displaced vessel (*arrowheads*) clearly demonstrates that the holohemispheric lentiform collection is subdural in location. A coronal post-gadolinium T1-WI (Fig. B) demonstrates bilateral lentiform, holohemispheric collections consistent with subdural effusions, right larger than left. Note that there is also mild enhancement of the pial surface beneath the collection on the right (*arrow*). A few punctate foci of enhancement are noted in the deep gray nuclei bilaterally (*arrowheads*).

Diagnosis

Haemophilus influenzae meningitis complicated by subdural effusion

Pearls

- Imaging studies are useful to assess the complications of meningitis and are usually ordered in the setting of persistent or secondary fever. Seizures and focal neurologic deficits are also indications for scanning.

- MR is more sensitive than CT to extensive enhancement that would favor subdural empyema over subdural effusion.

Pitfalls

- It can be difficult to differentiate subdural effusion from subdural empyema. Helpful features include: (1) Subdural effusion should follow CSF exactly on all sequences, while empyema may be more heterogeneous and proteinaceous. In particular, increased signal of the collection relative to CSF on a PD-WI is concerning for empyema. (2) Empyema usually results in marked dural/pial enhancement. (3) Subdural effusions are usually bilateral while subdural empyema is usually unilateral. (4) Note that superinfection of an effusion may occur, and a collection may need to be aspirated and cultured if a child fails to improve or worsens.

Differential Diagnosis

- Other bacterial meningitides (need CSF for gram stain, culture)
- Viral meningitis (rare to have subdural effusion)
- Non-infectious cause of subdural collections
    - Benign enlargement of the subarachnoid space
    - Prior trauma, accidental or nonaccidental

Discussion

Background

Haemophilus influenzae is the most common organism to cause meningitis in older infants (beyond the neonatal period) and children. Other common organisms in this age group include pneumococcus and meningococcus. Overall, however, viral meningitides are more common than bacterial meningitides. Subdural effusion is a not uncommon complication of meningitis that is frequently associated with *H. influenzae* meningitis, but may be seen with any bacterial meningitis. Overall, subdural effusion occurs in 15 to 39% of children with bacterial meningitis.

Etiology

Subdural effusion is presumably related to irritation of the meninges with transudation of fluid.

Clinical Findings

Meningitis may cause fever, irritability, nuchal rigidity, headache, nausea/vomiting, and/or diplopia. It may progress to seizures, coma, and death without appropriate therapy.

Complications

Complications of meningitis are outlined in Case 41. Superinfection of subdural effusion may lead to subdural empyema.

Pathology

Sterile fluid collections within subdural the space.

Imaging Findings

CT and MR

- Subdural effusions are usually located over the frontal and temporal regions and follow the density or intensity of CSF on all imaging sequences
- Post-contrast, mild enhancement of the parenchymal surface of the collection is commonly observed. This may be related to the inflammatory process itself or underlying cortical infarction. More extensive enhancement should raise the possibility of a complicating subdural empyema.

Treatment

- Antibiotics are indicated to treat the underlying meningitis

- Subdural effusions usually resolve spontaneously as meningitis resolves, but may require subdural taps. Specific therapy is not indicated in patients who are otherwise improving.

Prognosis

Neurological complications occur in ~30% of cases of *H. influenzae* meningitis, ranging from severe brain damage to milder sequelae such as sensorineural hearing loss

Suggested Readings

Castillo M. Magnetic resonance imaging of meningitis and its complications. *Topics Magn Res Imag* 6:53–58, 1994.

Friedland IR, Paris MM, Rinderknecht S, McCracken GH Jr. Cranial computed tomographic scans have little impact on management of bacterial meningitis. *Am J Dis Child* 146:1484–1487, 1992.

Zimmerman RD, Leeds N, Danziger A. Subdural empyema: CT findings. *Radiology* 150:417–422, 1984.

Case 43

Clinical Presentation

A 2-year-old girl born to an intravenous drug-abusing mother presents with developmental delay.

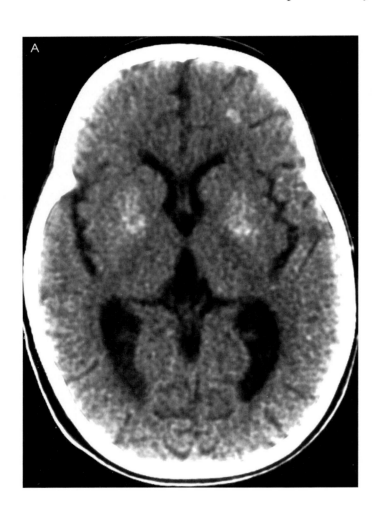 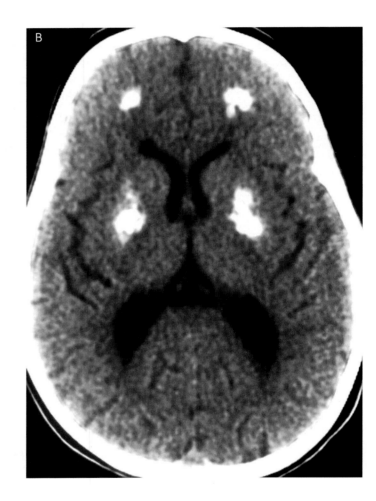

Radiologic Findings

An axial non-contrast CT scan (Fig. A) demonstrates mild global prominence of ventricles and sulci. In addition, calcification is identified within the basal ganglia and the left frontal subcortical white matter. A non-contrast CT scan obtained at a comparable level 1 year later (Fig. B) demonstrates progressive calcification in the basal ganglia and subcortical white matter.

Diagnosis

Congenital HIV infection (pediatric AIDS)

Differential Diagnosis

• Iatrogenic, i.e., radiation or intrathecal chemotherapy (clinical history)
• Disorder of calcium-phosphate metabolism (clinical history, laboratory analysis)
• Idiopathic familial basal ganglia calcification (may be identical)
• Fahr's disease (familial cerebrovascular ferrocalcinosis)
• Other congenital infection, i.e., cytomegalovirus or toxoplasmosis (different pattern of calcification, see Cases 38 and 39)

Discussion

Background

Congenital HIV infection occurs in ~30% of infants born to HIV-infected women, and the risk of infection varies with maternal plasma titers of the HIV virus. Neurologic signs rarely manifest in neonatal period. Intracranial calcification occurs in ~50% of HIV-infected children, is usually observed after 1 year of age, and characteristically affects the basal ganglia and the frontal subcortical white matter. All HIV-positive children who demonstrate intracranial calcifications are developmentally delayed. Basal ganglia calcifications in an adult are most commonly idiopathic and benign.

Etiology

The calcification is of uncertain etiology and may represent a direct effect of HIV infection or may be mediated by soluble factors.

Clinical Findings

Pediatric HIV infection is often dominated by nonspecific systemic symptoms and signs such as failure to thrive, lymphadenopathy, diarrhea, and hepatosplenomegaly. Neurologic disease is the presenting manifestation in ~18% of children and may take the form of a static (characterized by failure to develop beyond a certain point) or progressive (characterized by loss of previously achieved milestones) encephalopathy.

Complications

Neoplastic and infectious complications are rare in children with AIDS as compared with adults: lymphoma occurs in <5% of infected children, and toxoplasmosis is relatively uncommon in the pediatric population. Progressive multifocal leukoencephalopathy (PML) is the most common secondary CNS infection in pediatric AIDS. Intracranial hemorrhage and infarction may complicate pediatric AIDS probably due to an HIV-associated vasculopathy.

Pathology

Calcification may be parenchymal, may surround small- and medium-sized arteries, and/or may be present in vessel walls themselves.

Imaging Findings

Cerebral atrophy is the most common finding on both CT and MR

CT

- Calcification occurs in the basal ganglia and often the subcortical white matter of the frontal lobes as well
- Focal white matter lesions may be present as well

MR

- Calcification may be difficult to appreciate unless a gradient-echo sequence is done
- Demonstrates more extensive white matter signal abnormalities than CT

Treatment

No specific treatment is directed at the calcifications. Antiretroviral agents are typically given.

Prognosis

The calcification of the basal ganglia and subcortical white matter is seen only in patients who were infected in utero and who are already encephalopathic from the disease, so it is a relatively poor prognostic indicator. However, the development of new antiretroviral agents may alter the prognosis.

Suggested Readings

Belman AL, Lantos G, Horoupian D, et al. AIDS: calcification of the basal ganglia in infants and children. *Neurology* 36:1192–1199, 1986.

Dickson DW, Llena JF, Nelson SJ, Weidenheim KM. Central nervous system pathology in pediatric AIDS. *Ann NY Acad Sci* 693:93–106, 1993.

Kauffman WM, Sivit CJ, Fitz CR, et al. CT and MR evaluation of intracranial involvement in pediatric HIV infection: a clinical-imaging correlation. *AJNR* 13:949–957, 1992.

Case 44

Clinical Presentation

A 3-year-old boy presents with the acute onset of vomiting and ataxia.

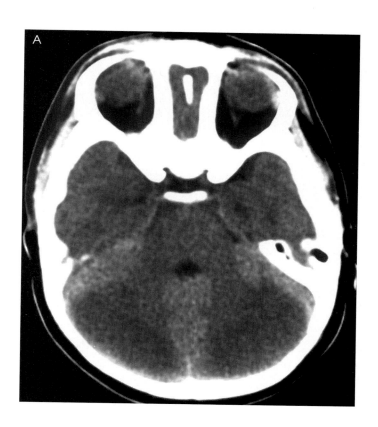 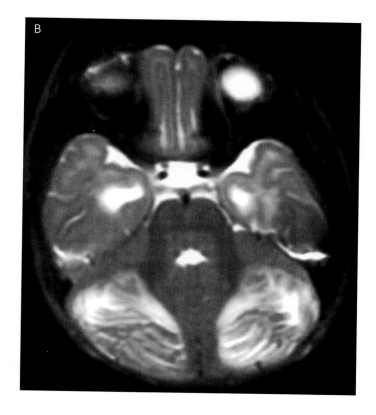

Radiologic Findings

A non-contrast CT scan (Fig. A) shows low density in the cerebellar hemispheres bilaterally. Abnormal cerebellar hyperintensity is present on a T2-WI (Fig. B).

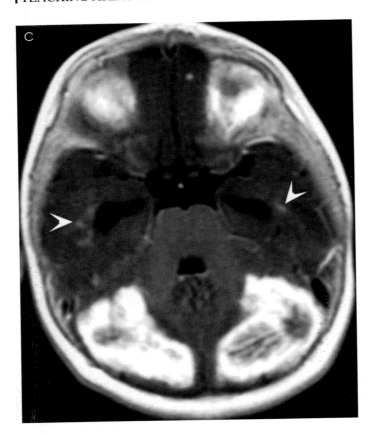

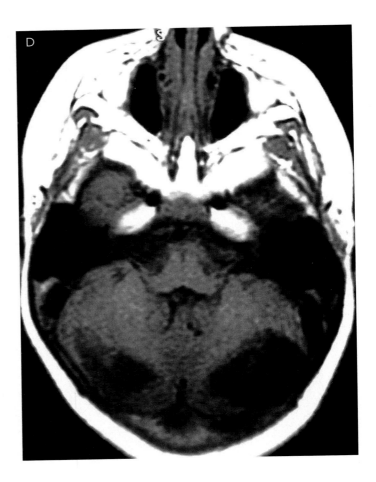

A post-gadolinium T1-WI (Fig. C) shows intense enhancement in the cerebellar hemispheres bilaterally. There is also minimal enhancement adjacent to the temporal horns bilaterally (*arrowheads*). The mild enlargement of the temporal horns is consistent with hydrocephalus. On more cephalad images (not shown), patchy T2 prolongation and enhancement were present in the hemispheric white matter. An axial T1-WI from a follow-up scan performed 1 year later (Fig. D) shows cystic encephalomalacia within the cerebellar hemispheres bilaterally. Clinically, the patient had mild residual ataxia.

Diagnosis

Acute cerebellitis

Differential Diagnosis

- Metabolic leukoencephalopathy (often recurrent episodes, may have a positive family history)
- Toxin exposure (clinical history)
- Vasculitis (usually infra- and supratentorial involvement, may be accompanied by systemic signs and symptoms, more common in adults)
- Paraneoplastic cerebellitis (more often in adults, usually occurs in the context of a known primary neoplasm, particularly lung or breast cancer)

Discussion

Background

Acute cerebellitis is characterized by the acute onset of cerebellar dysfunction and is considered by most to be of viral etiology. The process may be either infectious or more often parainfectious, occurring anywhere from hours to weeks after a viral illness. Fever and meningismus are typically absent in the parainfectious cases, and the condition usually resolves spontaneously within weeks or months. Acute cerebellitis may be a variant of acute disseminated encephalomyelitis (ADEM). Although patients with ADEM may be shown to have involvement of the cerebellum either clinically or by MR, acute parainfectious cerebellitis occurring in the absence of cerebral hemispheric involvement is extremely rare.

Clinical Findings

Patients present with headache, nausea, vomiting, and ataxia. Tremor and nystagmus are variably present. CSF often shows elevated protein and a mononuclear pleocytosis.

Complications

Complications include noncommunicating hydrocephalus due to mass effect on the fourth ventricle and tonsillar and/or upward transtentorial herniation due to cerebellar swelling.

Pathology

Material from a limited biopsy has been shown to contain lymphocytes and macrophages, as well as edema and patchy loss of Purkinje cells.

Imaging Findings

CT

• Diffuse low attenuation throughout the cerebellar hemispheres
• Effacement of the fourth ventricle and prepontine cisterns
• Hydrocephalus of a variable degree, often severe

MR

• Patchy areas of T1 and T2 prolongation in the cerebellum
• Parenchymal enhancement is variable. However, there may be prominent vascular or leptomeningeal enhancement related to contrast stasis.
• Late scans typically show cerebellar atrophy

Treatment

• Supportive care
• CSF diversion to treat hydrocephalus
• Steroids to reduce swelling

Prognosis

• This syndrome is rarely fatal, though acute hydrocephalus may lead to brain herniation and death

- Most patients recover completely or are left with mild unsteadiness or intention tremor, but some patients show permanent major neurologic deficits including severe intention tremor, hypotonia, severe gait disturbance, and dysarthria

Suggested Readings

Asenbauer B, McConachle NS, Allcutt D, et al. Acute near-fatal parainfectious cerebellar swelling with favorable outcome. *Neuropediatrics* 28:122–125, 1997.

Hayakawa H, Katoh T. Severe cerebellar atrophy following acute cerebellitis. *Pediatr Neurol* 12:159–161, 1995.

Horowitz MB, Pang D, Hirsch W. Acute cerebellitis: case report and review. *Pediatr Neurosurg* 17:142–145, 1991-92.

Case 45

Clinical Presentation

A 14-year-old girl who underwent a dental procedure 10 weeks earlier presents with headache and mild right-sided weakness.

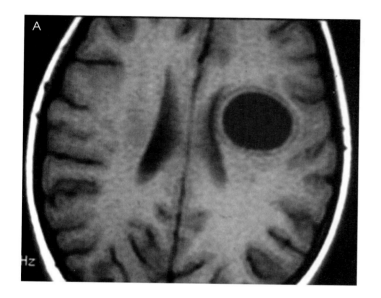

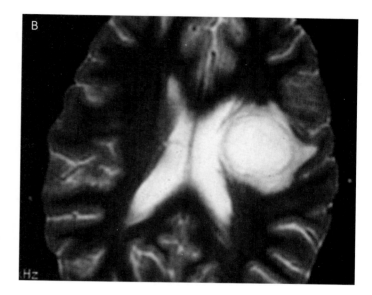

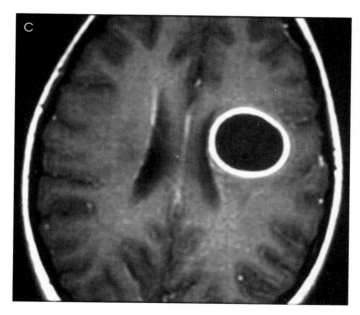

Radiologic Findings

An axial T1-WI (Fig. A) demonstrates a well-circumscribed rounded mass lesion centered in the left frontal white matter. The center of the lesion is isointense to CSF, while the periphery shows an inner rim that is slightly hyperintense to gray

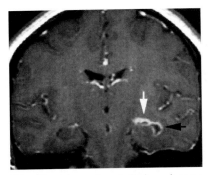

Fig. D. A post-gadolinium image demonstrates a left temporal lobe abscess (*black arrow*) which has ruptured into the temporal horn (*white arrow*). There is moderate ependymal enhancement.

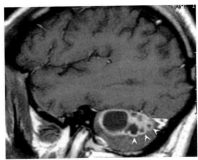

Fig. E. A parasagittal post-gadolinium T1-WI in a patient with Wegener's granulomatosis who is being treated with steroids and Cytoxan shows a large cerebellar lesion with multiple adjacent "daughter" lesions (*arrowheads*). Ten cc's of pus was aspirated at surgery.

matter and an outer rim that is hypointense. A T2-WI (Fig. B) demonstrates central hyperintensity, with a thin peripheral rim of hypointensity. Mild vasogenic edema surrounds the lesion. Following administration of gadolinium (Fig. C), there is intense smooth and linear enhancement of a peripheral rim of intermediate thickness.

Diagnosis

Brain abscess secondary to *Streptococcus pneumoniae*

Differential Diagnosis

- Brain abscess secondary to other pathogens (generally indistinguishable) (Table 1)
- Cystic primary or metastatic neoplasm (often has a thicker, more irregular wall)
- Resolving hematoma (history of trauma or stroke, blood products present)
- Tumefactive demyelination (little mass effect for the size of the lesion)
- Neuroepithelial cyst (thin rim, no edema, nonenhancing)

Discussion

Background

Brain abscesses are relatively rare in developed countries. When they do occur, they are most commonly due to pyogenic bacteria and they are more common supratentorially than infratentorially. Abscesses evolve from focal cerebritis, which may either resolve or progress to frank abscess formation. There are several major routes by which causative organisms gain access to the CNS: hematogenous spread from an extracranial site of infection, right-to-left shunts from congenital cardiac malformations or pulmonary arteriovenous fistulas, direct extension from infected paranasal sinuses or mastoid air cells (this is particularly common in children) and direct implantation of organisms into the CNS in the setting of surgery or trauma.

Etiology

Brain abscesses are most commonly caused by streptococcal and staphylococcal species, but anaerobes are also common, especially in patients with poor oral hygiene. In the immunocompromised host, think of *Pseudomonas aeruginosa* and fungi.

Clinical Findings

Headache, fever, and focal neurological signs related to edema and mass effect are the most common presenting features.

Complications

Rupture into the ventricle leads to ventriculitis, which carries a high mortality (Fig. D). Rupture into the subarachnoid space leads to acute meningitis. Choroid plexitis, formation of daughter abscesses (Fig. E) and progression of the lesion may also occur.

Pearls

Pearls

- MR is more specific for the diagnosis of abscess versus other ring-enhancing lesions (such as glioblastoma) if the characteristic appearance of the capsule is present.

- The abscess wall is usually thinner medially than laterally (the abscess "points" to the ventricle). This is attributed to the relatively poor vascular supply of white matter versus gray matter, with deficient capsule formation medially.

- There is mounting evidence that MR spectroscopy can assist in the noninvasive diagnosis of brain abscess, with pyogenic abscesses consistently demonstrating lactate and amino acids.

Pitfalls

- The imaging appearance of brain abscess may be altered in immunocompromised patients. Steroids are known to reduce edema, mass effect, and the intensity of capsular enhancement. Even in the absence of steroids, the capsule is often poorly formed in the immunocompromised patient, and enhancement may be minimal or absent.

- In neonates and young infants, abscesses tend to be large and show poor capsule formation.

Table 1. Common Causative Organisms in Brain Abscesses

Patient Population	Organisms
Neonate	*Pseudomonas*, *Serratia*, and *Proteus* species
Adult	*Staphylococcus*, and *Streptococcus* species
Posttransplant patient	Nocardia, Aspergillus, Candida species
AIDS patient	*Toxoplasmoa gondii Mycobacterium Tuberculosis*

Pathology

Brain abscesses are most commonly located at the gray-white junction in the frontal or parietal lobes and undergo an evolution from cerebritis to capsule formation:

- Cerebritis stage: initially an unencapsulated zone of congested vessels, inflammatory cells, and edema; necrotic foci gradually coalesce and the process becomes more focal. This stage evolves over ~2 weeks.
- Capsule stage: a well-defined capsule gradually develops around the necrotic core; as the capsule matures, edema and mass effect subside. Over weeks to months the abscess cavity gradually involutes as the process heals.

Imaging Findings

Vary with the stage of disease.

Cerebritis stage

- Both CT and MR show an ill-defined region of edema and mass effect
- Postcontrast, an ill-defined peripheral zone of enhancement may be seen

Capsule stage

- *CT:* thin, well-defined rim-enhancing mass with hypodense center and surrounding edema
- *MR:* the capsule is usually visible prior to contrast administration as a thin rim that is hyperintense on T1-WI and hypointense on T2-WI. Surrounding vasogenic edema is visible. Post-gadolinium studies show smooth peripheral rim enhancement.

Complications

- MR is more sensitive to complications such as ventriculitis (enhancement of the ependymal surface, often fluid-debris layer in ventricle) or choroid plexitis (enlarged, intensely enhancing plexus)

Treatment

- Antibiotics alone may be adequate for small (<2 cm) lesions
- Steroids are often given for severe brain edema
- Stereotactic aspiration is used for both diagnosis and treatment of large lesions. If an abscess enlarges on follow-up examination, repeat aspiration should be performed.

Prognosis

- Variable depending upon comorbidities and immune status

- Mortality has historically been 50 to 70%. Currently it is <5% if a patient is immunocompetent and appropriately treated, but it is as high as 80 to 90% in the posttransplant population.

Suggested Readings

Enzmann DR, Britt RH, Placone R. Staging of human brain abscess by computed tomography. *Radiology* 146:703–708, 1983.

Selby R, Ramirez CB, Singh R, et al. Brain abscess in solid organ transplant recipients receiving cyclosporine-based immunosuppression. *Arch Surg* 132:304–310, 1997.

Yang SY, Zhao CS. Review of 140 patients with brain abscess. *Surg Neurol* 39:290–296, 1993.

Case 46

Clinical Presentation

A 66-year-old woman was brought to the emergency room at an outside hospital following a motor vehicle accident. Because of persistent confusion, a CT scan of the brain was obtained.

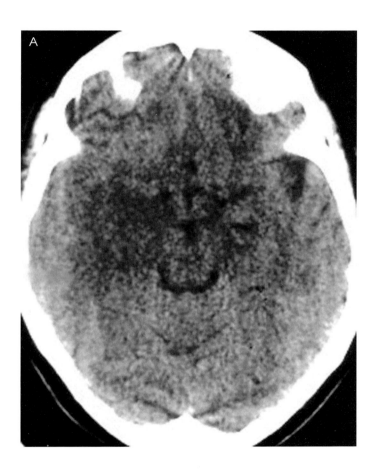

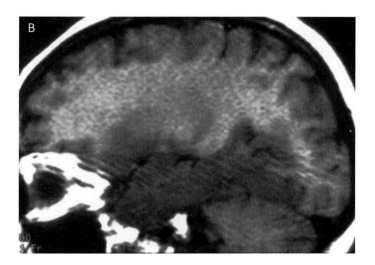

Radiologic Findings

A non-contrast CT scan of the brain (Fig. A) demonstrates an irregular zone of hypodensity involving the right medial temporal lobe. An MR scan was obtained for further evaluation. A sagittal T1-WI (Fig. B) demonstrates low-signal intensity throughout the right temporal lobe.

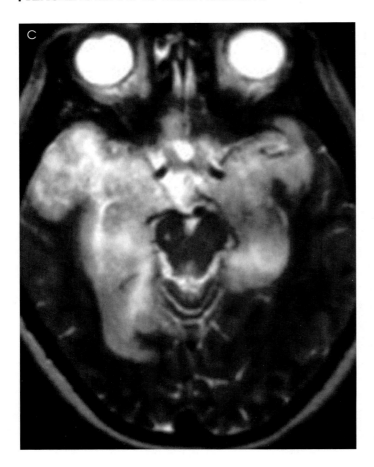

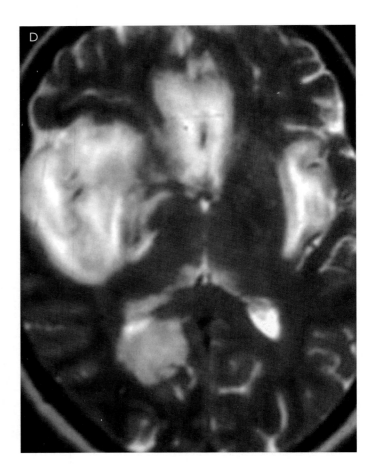

An axial T2-WI at the level of the midbrain (Fig. C) demonstrates T2 prolongation in the anterior and medial temporal lobes bilaterally, right greater than left, while a T2-WI at the level of the third ventricle (Fig. D) demonstrates asymmetric T2 prolongation involving the insular regions bilaterally, the medial frontal lobes, and the posteromedial right temporal lobe.

Diagnosis

Herpes simplex virus type 1 (HSV1) encephalitis

Differential Diagnosis

- Other viral encephalitides (generally lack temporal lobe predilection)
- Acute disseminated encephalomyelitis (usually predominant white matter involvement)
- Vasculitis (often more widespread changes, with gray and white matter infarcts)
- Infarction (should be a vascular territorial distribution)
- Gliomatosis cerebri (insidious onset of symptoms, often extensive white matter infiltration)

Pearls

- MR is significantly more sensitive than CT in the diagnosis of HSV1 encephalitis, and coronal T1- and T2-weighted images are very helpful to assess the temporal lobes (Figs. E and F)
- Suspect herpes encephalitis in the setting of a T2-prolonging lesion in the temporal lobe(s) in a patient presenting with altered mental status, seizures, and/or fever.

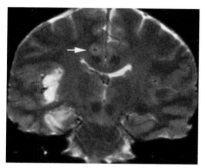

Fig. E. A coronal T2-WI demonstrates high-signal intensity involving the right insula and right medial temporal lobe, as well as subtle high signal in the right cingulum (*arrow*).

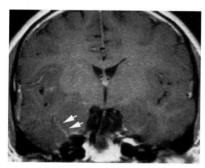

Fig. F. A post-gadolinium T1-WI (same patient as Fig. E) demonstrates edema in the right insular region and temporal lobe, as well as minimal leptomeningeal enhancement (*arrows*).

Discussion

Background

HSV1 causes a hemorrhagic necrotizing meningoencephalitis that is the most common cause of fatal sporadic encephalitis. It usually occurs in adults (~90% of cases), while infants are more commonly affected by HSV2 (see Case 40). HSV1 typically affects both temporal lobes, particularly the insular cortex, but the bilateral involvement is usually asymmetric. The inferior frontal lobes and cingulate gyri are also frequently involved.

Etiology

HSV1 is a DNA virus. HSV1 encephalitis usually occurs in the setting of reactivation of virus that lies dormant in the trigeminal ganglion. Spread from the trigeminal ganglion is thought to account for the predilection of this process for the frontal and temporal lobes.

Clinical Findings

Nonspecific findings include headache, confusion, and disorientation. Patients may be febrile and often develop seizures. Once the diagnosis is considered, therapy should be instituted promptly. The diagnosis can be effectively made using polymerase chain reaction testing of the CSF for viral DNA.

Complications

Progression to coma and death can occur even with appropriate therapy. Mesenrhombencephalitis with multiple cranial nerve palsies may develop as an isolated manifestation of HSV1 infection or in association with necrotizing meningoencephalitis.

Pathology

Hemorrhagic necrosis of both gray and white matter is observed. There is a predilection for involvement of limbic structures (cingulate gyri, temporal lobes, subfrontal areas).

Imaging Findings

CT

- Often normal early in the course of disease
- Temporal lobe edema, enhancement, and/or hemorrhage may develop after several days to a week of symptoms

MR

- Initially, subtle findings include T2 prolongation in the gray and white matter of the mesial temporal lobe(s) and mild mass effect, best seen on T1-WI
- Abnormal signal progressively involves the insula, inferior frontal lobes, and cingulate gyrus. Involvement is usually bilateral but asymmetric. The basal ganglia are typically spared. T1-WI may show cortical petechial hemorrhage and cortical laminar necrosis. Post-contrast studies show a linear cortical pattern of enhancement in affected areas.
- Late sequelae include atrophy and dystrophic calcification

Pitfalls

• This diagnosis requires a high index of suspicion as therapy is most effective when instituted promptly.

• Infiltrating glioma may mimic herpes encephalitis but usually has a more indolent presentation.

Treatment

Antiviral therapy: acyclovir

Prognosis

Early treatment significantly improves prognosis (20% vs. 70% mortality)

Suggested Readings

Demaerel P, Wilms G, Robberecht W, et al. MRI of herpes simplex encephalitis. *Neuro-radiology* 34:490–493, 1992.

Schroth G, Gawehn J, Thron A, et al. Early diagnosis of herpes simplex encephalitis by MRI. *Neurology* 37:179–183, 1987.

Tien RD, Felsberg GJ, Osumi AK. Herpesvirus infections of the CNS: MR findings. *AJR* 161:167–176, 1993.

Case 47

Clinical Presentation

A 25-year-old Mexican immigrant presents following a seizure.

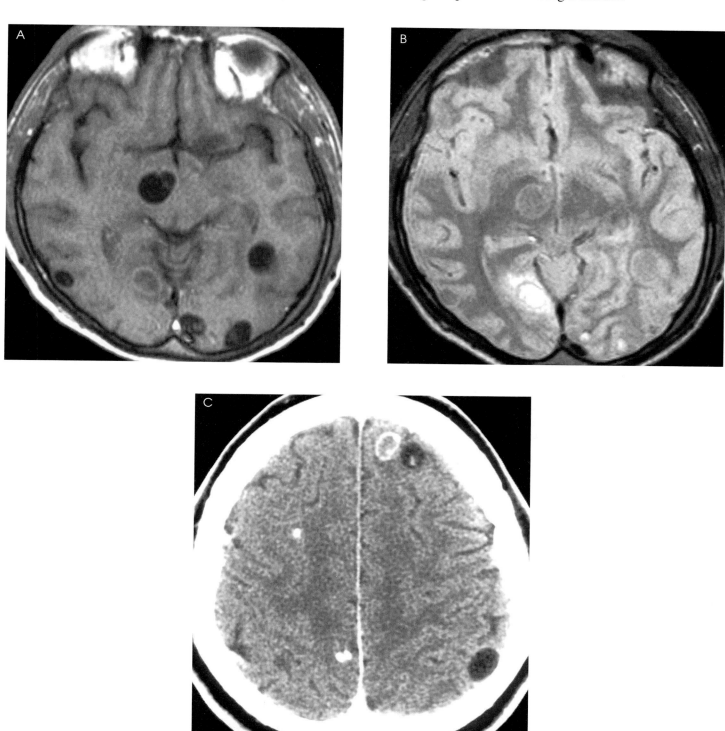

Radiologic Findings

An axial post-gadolinium T1-WI (Fig. A) demonstrates multiple well-circumscribed cystic appearing lesions in the temporal and occipital lobes, as well as in the right cerebral peduncle. A right occipital lesion shows mild peripheral enhancement. In addition, the center of the right occipital lesion is not isointense to CSF. Note that gadolinium enhancement is only very mild as this examination was performed on a low-field system. The accompanying PD-WI (Fig. B) shows that the majority of lesions contain fluid that is isointense to CSF. The right occipital lesion is hyperintense compared with CSF, and mild surrounding edema can be seen. In addition, two focal areas of T2 prolongation in the left occipital lobe are noted, likely corresponding to scolices. A CT scan in the same patient (Fig. C) shows well-circumscribed cysts as well as focal areas of calcification.

Diagnosis

Neurocysticercosis

Differential Diagnosis

- Brain abscesses (typically more surrounding edema, more symptomatic patient)
- Tuberculomas (usually not cystic)
- Metastases (more edema, can be cystic but this is relatively uncommon)

Discussion

Background

Cysticercosis is the most common parasitic infection of the CNS. It is particularly prevalent in Mexico, Central and South America, and parts of Asia and Africa, but it has become increasingly common in the United States due to immigration and foreign travel. It is the most common cause of seizures in young adults in endemic areas.

Etiology

The porcine tapeworm *Taenia solium* infects humans via two modes: the viable larval form and from viable eggs.

- Larval form (taeniasis): viable larva are ingested in undercooked pork and are released in the stomach and small bowel. The larva attach to the jejunal mucosa and cause gastrointestinal symptoms. In this case, man is the definitive host.
- Cysticercosis: viable eggs are ingested in water or food that is contaminated with human or porcine feces. In this case, humans are the intermediate hosts. As the eggs mature, some transform into oncospheres that penetrate the intestinal wall and are hematogenously disseminated to target organs such as the CNS, muscle, and eye. The oncosphere contains a larval organism that lodges in the extragastrointestinal tissue and begins to form a cyst around itself. There is minimal local reaction to a viable cyst, but when the larva dies, an intense inflammatory reaction ensues.

Clinical Findings

Symptoms vary with the stage of disease. Early infection is usually asymptomatic. Parasite death leads to symptoms due to the surrounding inflammatory host reaction. Symptoms include seizures, focal neurological deficits, and headache. Late stages present most commonly with seizures.

Complications

Hydrocephalus may occur secondary to acute meningeal exudate, chronic meningeal fibrosis, or obstructing cyst(s) in the ventricles or subarachnoid space. Rarely a massive infestation may cause severe diffuse encephalitis and death.

Pathology

Neurocysticercosis may affect the brain parenchyma, subarachnoid spaces, ventricles, and spinal cord.

Brain parenchyma

Four stages are defined which evolve over months to years

- Vesicular stage: the viable organism exists as a thin-walled vesicle ≤20 mm in size containing CSF-like fluid and a mural nodule representing the scolex. Inflammatory response is minimal or absent. This stage may last 2 to 10 years.
- Colloid stage: the viable cyst dies, the cyst fluid becomes a turbid colloid suspension, and antigenic material leaks across the cyst wall. An inflammatory reaction leads to breakdown of the blood-brain barrier.
- Nodular granular stage: the lesion undergoes involution and begins to calcify
- Calcified stage: the lesion is shrunken and completely mineralized

Subarachnoid space

Multiple vesicles which are often of large size and lack a scolex (racemose form) are present within the basal cisterns

- Progression to the colloid stage leads to exudative inflammation of the meninges and eventual fibrosis. This stage may be complicated by arteritis leading to parenchymal infarction.
- Calcification is usually not seen in this form

Intraventricular

Usually one or several thin-walled cysts

- A scolex is often visible. Obstruction usually occurs at the level of the fourth ventricle, but may occur at the foramen of Monro or the aqueduct of Sylvius. Movement of the cyst through the ventricular system may occur.

Imaging Findings

The spectrum of imaging findings depends on the number and location of parasites, the stage of evolution of a given lesion, and the host response to the infestation. Lesions in varying stages often coexist in the same patient.

Parenchymal lesions

These are typically at the gray-white junction, and are usually multiple

- *Vesicular stage*: CT and MR show thin-walled cysts without associated edema or contrast enhancement. Cyst fluid parallels the CSF. The scolex is often visible as a 2 to 4-mm nodule.

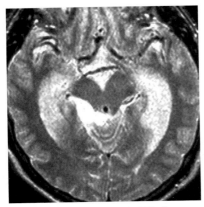

Fig. D. An axial T2-WI demonstrates asymmetric enlargement of the right ambient and quadrigeminal plate cisterns.

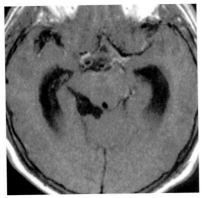

Fig. E. Cysticercal cysts within the basal cisterns are nonenhancing in the patient in Figure D, though there is some enhancement of the basal meninges in the suprasellar cistern. There is evidence of obstructive hydrocephalus, with dilatation of the temporal horns.

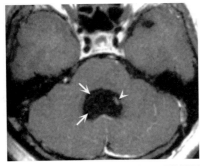

Fig. F. A post-gadolinium T1-WI shows a subtle cystic lesion expanding the fourth ventricle (*arrows*). The scolex is present on the left (*arrowhead*).

- Colloidal stage: the dying cyst incites an inflammatory response. Fluid becomes more proteinaceous, higher in density and signal. The lesion demonstrates surrounding edema and peripheral enhancement (abscesslike).
- Nodular granular stage: lesions often isodense on unenhanced CT. Postcontrast, a solid nodule or thick ring of enhancement is visible. Less edema and less mass effect occur in this stage compared with the colloidal stage.
- Calcified stage: completely mineralized lesion which may be difficult to see on MR even with gradient-echo imaging

Subarachnoid lesions

- Usually multiple cysts containing CSF-like fluid and lacking a scolex (Figs. D and E)
- May show associated meningeal inflammation and enhancement
- The cysts may form grape-like clusters ("racemose form")

Intraventricular lesions

May be subtle and difficult to identify if the cyst contents are identical to CSF (Fig. F)

Treatment

- Antihelminthic drugs such as praziquantel and albendazole
- Concomitant corticosteroids may be useful to limit acute inflammatory response
- Surgery may be required for intraventricular lesions

Prognosis

Good

Suggested Readings

Creasy JL, Alarcon JJ. Magnetic resonance imaging of neurocysticercosis. *Topics Magn Res Imag* 6:59–68, 1994.

Martinez HR, Rangel-Guerra R, Elizondo G, et al. MR imaging in neurocysticercosis: a study of 56 cases. *AJNR* 10:1011–1019, 1989.

Teitelbaum GP, Otto RJ, Lin M, et al. MR imaging of neurocysticercosis. *AJNR* 10:709–718, 1989.

Case 48

Clinical Presentation

A 5-year-old Chinese boy was brought to the emergency room following a seizure. He complained of a headache and had a low-grade fever. Meningeal signs were absent.

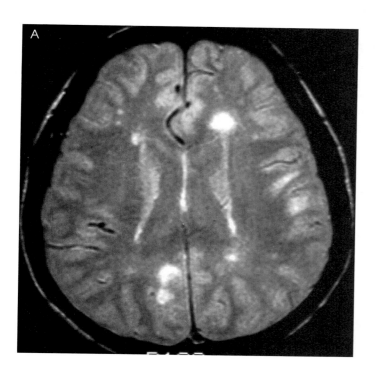

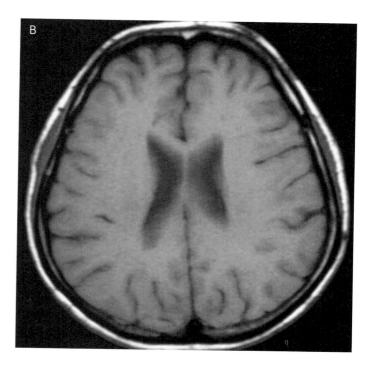

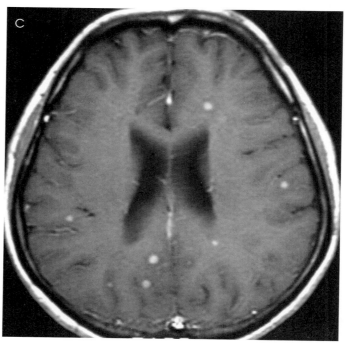

Radiologic Findings

An axial PD-WI (Fig. A) demonstrates multiple variably-sized rounded areas of parenchymal high-signal intensity, while an axial T1-WI at the same level (Fig. B) is relatively unremarkable. An axial post-gadolinium T1-WI (Fig. C) demonstrates multiple small nodular areas of enhancement that are predominantly located at the gray-white junction.

Diagnosis

Miliary tuberculosis (TB)

Differential Diagnosis

- Miliary brain metastases (may see more edema, usually an adult patient)
- Other infectious etiologies (usually more heterogeneous lesions, more edema)
- Sarcoidosis (rare cause of multiple parenchymal nodules, usually associated with dural and/or leptomeningeal disease)

Discussion

Background

TB has been on the rise since 1986, after a long period of decline. The resurgence of the disease has been due in large part to the AIDS epidemic, as ~30% of TB patients are HIV-positive. CNS involvement occurs in 2 to 5% of all patients with TB and in 10% of patients with AIDS-related TB. It may take several forms, including meningitis, tuberculous granulomas (tuberculomas, which may be intracranial and/or spinal), tuberculous abscess formation (relatively rare, more common in HIV positive patients than immunocompetent hosts), and osteomyelitis of the skull or spine, often with associated epidural abscess.

Etiology

Tuberculosis is caused by the acid-fast bacillus *Mycobacterium tuberculosis*. Other mycobacteria such as *M. avium-intracellulare* rarely affect the CNS.

Pathophysiology

From a pulmonary source, the bacilli disseminate hematogenously to the cerebrum, often lodging at the gray-white matter junction, and forming tuberculous granulomas. Tuberculous abscess formation with central liquefaction is rare, reflecting a poor host immune response: it is indistinguishable from pyogenic abscess and is more common in HIV-positive patients. If a subependymal or subpial focus ruptures into the CSF, tuberculous meningitis may result. Alternatively, direct penetration of the walls of meningeal vessels by hematogenously spread organisms may occur. Therefore parenchymal disease can occur with or without coexistent meningitis and vice-versa.

Clinical Findings

The presentation varies with the form of the disease: Meningitis leads to headache, malaise, and low-grade fever. Later complications include cranial neuropathy and hydrocephalus. Tuberculoma or tuberculous abscess formation leads to focal neurologic deficits and seizures; fever is variably present. These forms may coexist or occur independently. CSF examination often shows strikingly low glucose levels in TB meningitis, which can be a helpful diagnostic feature.

Pathology

- Tuberculoma: four stages in its evolution are recognized: (1) nonspecific focal cerebritis, (2) granulomatous, solid, noncaseating reaction with early collagenous capsule formation and variable perilesional edema, (3) central caseation, and (4) involution with coarse nodular calcification
- Tuberculous abscess: in contrast to the solid caseation seen in the granuloma, the abscess is formed by semiliquid pus containing large numbers of organisms. This makes it larger than typical tuberculoma, with a more accelerated clinical course

Complications

Hydrocephalus is common and may be communicating or noncommunicating. CNS infarction may occur due to inflammation of perforating vessels.

Imaging Findings

Tuberculoma

- Cerebritis stage: nonspecific edema, ill-defined enhancement
- Solid granulomatous stage: enhancing nodules with surrounding edema. There is usually central hyperintensity but may be peripheral hypointensity on T2-WI due to collagenous capsule formation.
- Central caseation stage: marked by central hypointensity on T2-WI. Enhancement is usually peripheral at this stage.
- Involution stage: shows multiple calcified nodules on CT scan

Tuberculous abscess

- Usually larger than a tuberculoma, may be multiloculated, and has a greater degree of surrounding edema
- May be indistinguishable from typical bacterial abscess

Tuberculous meningitis

- Typically causes a thick basilar exudate that is associated with meningeal enhancement, communicating hydrocephalus, and infarctions in the territories of perforator vessels.

Treatment

- Multidrug treatment regimen
- Serial imaging useful to assess response to therapy

Prognosis

Variable: mortality as high as 30% among HIV-negative, 79% among HIV-positive

---

Pearls

- The combination of meningeal enhancement and parenchymal nodules is highly suggestive of TB.
- Central T2 hypointensity should suggest tuberculous or fungal disease.

Pitfalls

- A dural tuberculoma may a mimic meningioma.
- More diffuse dural involvement may mimic dural metastases (Fig. D)

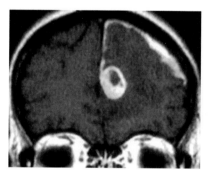

Fig. D. A coronal post-gadolinium T1-WI demonstrates dural and leptomeningeal thickening overlying the left frontal lobe. In addition, an enhancing parenchymal mass lesion is identified. An open biopsy demonstrated caseating granulomas and acid-fast bacilli.

Suggested Readings

Bargallo N, Berenguer J, Tomas X, et al. Intracranial tuberculosis: CT and MR. *Eur Radiol* 3:123–128, 1993.

Gee DT, Bazan C III, Jinkins JR. Miliary tuberculosis involving the brain: MR findings. *AJR* 159:1075–1076, 1992.

Whiteman MLH. Neuroimaging of central nervous system tuberculosis in HIV-infected patients. *Neuroimag Clin North Am* 7:199–214, 1997.

Case 49

Clinical Presentation

A 57-year-old woman developed left cranial nerve V and VII palsies. The patient is an avid hiker.

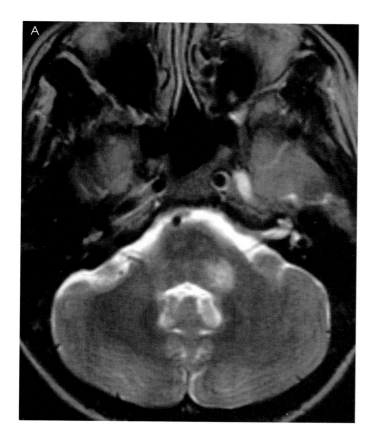

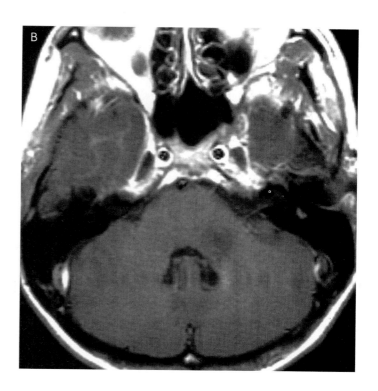

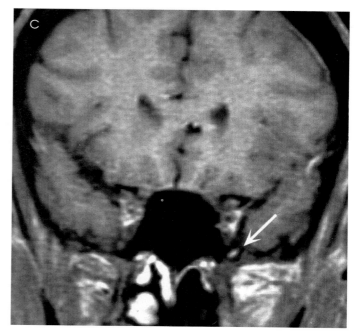

Radiologic Findings

An axial T2-WI (Fig. A) shows an area of T2 prolongation within the left middle cerebellar peduncle. On a post-gadolinium T1-WI (Fig. B), no enhancement of this lesion or mass effect is noted. On a coronal post-gadolinium image (Fig. C), asymmetric enhancement of the second division of the fifth cranial nerve is identified within foramen rotundum (*arrow*). *(Case courtesy of Erik Gaensler, M.D., San Francisco, CA.)*

Diagnosis

Lyme disease

Differential Diagnosis

- Multiple sclerosis (evidence of lesions separated in time and space, frequent involvement of the corpus callosum, enhancement of cranial nerves not expected except cranial nerve II)
- Acute disseminated encephalomyelitis (multiple asymmetric supra- and infratentorial white matter lesions)
- Vasculitis (may be indistinguishable as Lyme disease may in fact cause a vasculitis)
- Sarcoidosis (brain lesions typically enhance, as do involved cranial nerves)
- Lymphoma (brain lesions typically enhance intensely)

Discussion

Background

Lyme disease is a multisystem inflammatory disease that is caused by the spirochete *Borrelia burgdorferi*. It is a tick-borne pathogen, with the common vector being the deer tick *Ixodes dammini*. Infection is most common in children and young adults. If the disease goes undiagnosed and untreated, patients will typically progress through three clinical stages (see below). Between 10 and 15% of patients with Lyme disease develop CNS abnormalities. Diagnosis can be difficult as only 50% of patients with stage I disease (see below) have positive serologies, though the measurement of intrathecal production of specific antibodies is highly sensitive and specific.

Clinical Findings

Three stages of the disease are differentiated:

1. Stage I: 2 days to 1 month following exposure. Flulike symptoms and a characteristic expanding skin lesion (erythema chronicum migrans) are seen in 60 to 80% of patients.
2. Stage II: 1 to 4 months following infection. Cardiac and neurologic abnormalities occur.
3. Stage III: months to years following infection. Arthritis and chronic neurologic symptoms develop in ~60% of untreated patients.

Routine CSF analysis demonstrates elevated white cell count with lymphocyte predominance and elevated protein in stages II and III. In some cases the organism can be cultured from CSF or can be detected by polymerase chain reaction analysis.

Complications

Neurological symptoms may include peripheral neuropathy, radiculopathy, myelopathy, encephalitis, lymphocytic meningitis, cranial nerve palsies, pain syndromes, cerebellar signs, cognitive dysfunction, and movement disorders. Headache and blurred vision are also common.

Pathophysiology

The spirochete is transmitted through tick saliva or fecal debris. The mechanism of CNS involvement is unclear: spirochetes are often found in affected tissues, but immunologic mechanisms and vasculitis may also play a role.

Pathology

Microscopic examination of brain tissue shows perivascular or vascular lymphocytic infiltration, as well as areas of demyelination.

Imaging Findings

CT

• Often normal
• May demonstrate low-attenuation lesions in the cerebral white matter with variable enhancement

MR

• Patchy white matter lesions with variable enhancement, most commonly within the frontal and parietal subcortical white matter but also affecting the deep gray nuclei and the brain stem
• Leptomeningeal enhancement
• Cranial nerve enhancement

Treatment

• Antibiotics: choices include tetracycline, doxycycline, and ceftriaxone
• Steroids may also be given

Prognosis

Excellent with prompt diagnosis and initiation of appropriate therapy

Suggested Readings

Demaerel P, Wilms G, Van Lierde S, Delanote J, Baert AL. Lyme disease in childhood presenting as primary leptomeningeal enhancement without parenchymal findings on MR. *AJNR* 15:302–304, 1994.

Fernandez RE, Rothberg M, Ferencz G, Wujack D. Lyme disease of the CNS: MR imaging findings in 14 cases. *AJNR* 11:479–481, 1990.

Rafto SE, Milton WJ, Galetta SL, Grossman RI. Biopsy-confirmed CNS Lyme disease: MR appearance at 1.5 T. *AJNR* 11:482–484, 1990.

Case 50

Clinical Presentation

A 53-year-old man status post renal transplant complains of increasing headache and experiences a generalized seizure.

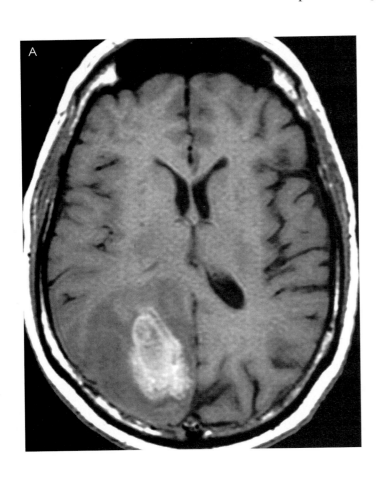
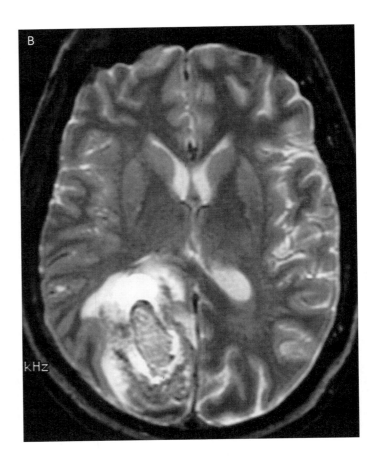

Radiologic Findings

An axial T1-WI (Fig. A) demonstrates an area of high signal consistent with hemorrhage in the right occipital lobe, with surrounding vasogenic edema. There is mass effect on adjacent sulci and the posterior right lateral ventricle. An axial T2-WI (Fig. B) demonstrates low signal within the right occipital lobe lesion consistent with acute hemorrhage.

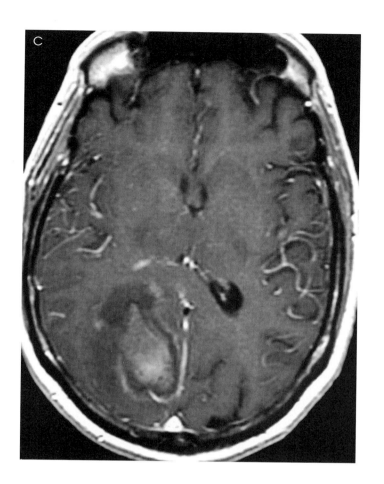

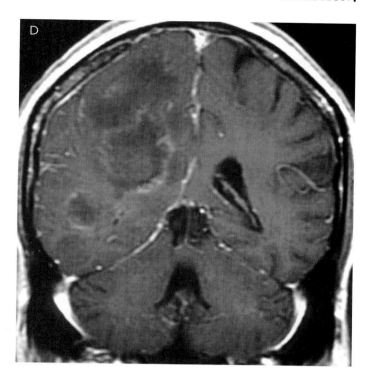

An axial post-gadolinium T1-WI (Fig. C) shows minimal enhancement around the periphery of the right occipital lobe hematoma. On the coronal post-gadolinium T1-WI image (Fig. D), a right temporal lobe lesion is also seen which demonstrates minimal enhancement and mild surrounding edema. There is mild right to left shift of the midline, as well as prominent enhancement of the tentorium and dura on the right, presumably related to local edema, inflammation, and venous stasis.

Diagnosis

CNS aspergillosis

Differential Diagnosis

- Brain abscesses due to pyogenic organisms (may be indistinguishable, but usually not hemorrhagic)
- Brain abscesses due to other opportunistic pathogens such as the *Mucoraceae* family and *Nocardia asteroides* (may be indistinguishable)
- Metastatic disease (less fulminant clinical presenation, more enhancement)
- Vasculitis (gray and white matter infarcts, ill-defined areas of enhancement)

Pearls

- Suspect aspergillosis in an immunocompromised host who develops paranasal sinusitis, proptosis, mastoiditis, unexplained infarction, and/or cerebral abscesses which fail to enhance.
- In patients with paranasal sinus Aspergillus infection, dural enhancement indicates intracranial extension and is a very poor prognostic sign.
- Patients who are immunocompromised or on steroids may manifest little or no enhancement of parenchymal fungal abscesses

Pitfall

- Aspergillus infection of the paranasal sinuses is generally very destructive in the immunocompromised host and may mimic malignant neoplasm, tuberculosis, or Wegener's granulomatosis.

Discussion

Background

The various species of Aspergillus are common contaminants of the upper respiratory tract. In immunocompromised hosts, disseminated aspergillosis and secondary cerebral aspergillosis may cause significant morbidity and mortality, with CNS infection developing in 20 to 40% of patients with disseminated disease. Patients at particular risk include organ transplant recipients, patients with hematologic malignancy, diabetics, and patients receiving corticosteroids or chemotherapy. CNS aspergillosis also occurs in the AIDS population, but it is relatively uncommon compared with infections such as toxoplasmosis or cryptococcosis. Diagnosis of CNS aspergillosis generally requires biopsy with histopathologic examination and culture.

Etiology

Infection is usually caused by *Aspergillus fumigatus*, but may also be due to other pathogenic species including *A. flavus* and *A. niger*. The organism may spread to the CNS via the bloodstream from a primary site of infection in the lungs or may infect the paranasal sinuses and then extend directly to the orbit and/or CNS.

Clinical Findings

Fever, headache, malaise, and focal neurologic signs are common.

Complications

Infarction (sterile or septic) and/or mycotic aneurysm formation are related to the organism's angioinvasive behavior. Petrous apicitis/skull base osteomyelitis may also occur.

Pathology

- *Aspergillus* species are characterized by acutely branching septate hyphae
- Aspergillosis has several patterns in the brain: (1) abscesses, with hemorrhagic necrosis surrounded by granulomatous inflammation, (2) angioinvasion, resulting in large-vessel thrombosis and/or mycotic aneurysm formation, and leading to stroke and/or subarachnoid hemorrhage, and (3) meningitis with leptomeningeal inflammation

Imaging Findings

CT and MR

- Fungal abscesses present as multiple ring-enhancing lesions. On T2-weighted MR images, the lesions are often hypointense, which is attributed to hemorrhage and/or concentration of heavy metal ions which are essential to fungal amino acid metabolism (iron, manganese, magnesium).
- Infarcts cause cortical and subcortical hypodensity on CT and T2 hyperintensity on MR and may be complicated by hemorrhage or infection (septic infarction)

Angiography

- May be useful to demonstrate mycotic aneurysms

Treatment

- Long-term therapy with intravenous or intrathecal amphotericin B
- A second agent such as oral ketoconazole may also be used in conjunction

Prognosis

Very poor – Aspergillus brain abscesses have a mortality rate of 85 to 100%

Suggested Readings

Ashdown BC, Tien RD, Felsberg GJ. Aspergillosis of the brain and paranasal sinuses in immunocompromised patients: CT and MR findings. *AJR* 162:155–159, 1994.

Cox J, Murtagh FR, Wilfong A, Brenner J. Cerebral aspergillosis: MR imaging and histopathologic correlation. *AJNR* 13:1489–1492, 1992.

Harris DE, Enterline DS. Fungal infections of the central nervous system. *Neuroimag Clin North Am* 7:187–198, 1997.

Case 51

Clinical Presentation

A 36-year-old HIV-positive female presents with progressive decline in cognitive function.

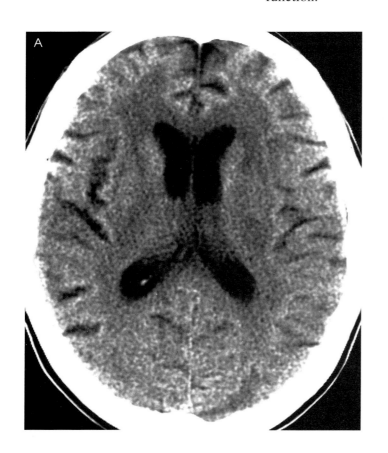

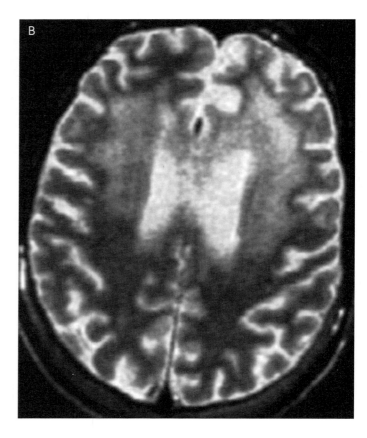

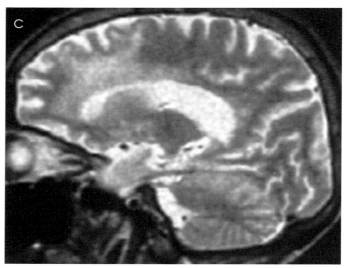

Radiologic Findings

A non-contrast CT scan (Fig. A) shows evidence of parenchymal volume loss, with prominence of the ventricles and sulci for the patient's age. In addition, mild low density is noted in the frontal white matter bilaterally, extending across the genu of the corpus callosum. There is no associated mass effect. Subcortical "U" fibers are relatively spared. An axial T2-WI (Fig. B) in the same patient demonstrates confluent, symmetric T2 prolongation in the deep frontal white matter. A sagittal T2-WI (Fig. C) also demonstrates the frontal predominance of the white matter process and the lack of mass effect. No enhancement was seen on post-gadolinium images (not shown).

Diagnosis

HIV (human immunodeficiency virus) encephalopathy

Differential Diagnosis

- Progressive multifocal leukoencephalopathy (PML) (usually more patchy and asymmetric, typically affects subcortical U fibers)
- Vasculitis (also typically more patchy and asymmetric, may show areas of enhancement and mass effect)
- Toxic, radiation, or metabolic leukoencephalopathy (clinical history essential)

Discussion

Background

HIV is the etiologic agent of AIDS. CNS symptoms are the presenting complaint in ~10% of patients with AIDS, and neurologic complications will eventually develop in ~30 to 40% of these patients. CNS involvement in patients with AIDS may be due to primary HIV infection itself or to the opportunistic infections and neoplasms that occur in the setting of severe immune dysfunction. Primary CNS involvement may lead to HIV encephalopathy, which is characterized by progressive cognitive decline and dementia. The strongest predictors of HIV encephalopathy are a CD4 count of <100 cells/µl and an AIDS-defining illness, anemia, or both. On rare occasions, seroconversion may be accompanied by a fulminant encephalopathy with changes resembling acute demyelinating perivenous encephalitis.

Etiology

HIV is a retrovirus that selectively infects human T lymphocytes of the helper/inducer subset. The only cell in the CNS that has been conclusively demonstrated to be infected by HIV is the microglia/monocyte. The mechanism by which HIV infection leads to striking neurologic changes remains unclear, as neurons do not appear to be directly infected.

Clinical Findings

Patients are often asymptomatic early in the course of the disease or have abnormalities only on formal neuropsychologic testing. Over time, cognitive deficits generally progress, and patients may develop severe disturbances of behavior and memory. Eventual loss of bladder and bowel control, disorientation, and frank dementia may occur.

Pathology

Neuropathologic abnormalities of varying severity are present in 80 to 100% of patients with AIDS. Patients with HIV encephalopathy often have:

Gross

- Global atrophy

Microscopic

- Accumulation of microglia/monocytes around blood vessels, especially in the leptomeninges, subependymal regions, and deep white matter
- Reactive astrocytosis
- White matter pallor, with a tendency to spare subcortical white matter

Imaging Findings

CT

- Cerebral atrophy of a variable degree
- Low density in periventricular and deep white matter

MR

- Symmetric patchy or confluent areas of high signal intensity on T2-WI are located in the periventricular and deep white matter regions, and in the centrum semiovale
- These areas are iso- or mildly hypointense on T1-WI and show no evidence of mass effect or enhancement
- MR spectroscopy has demonstrated a significant reduction in N-acetyl aspartate, a metabolic marker for neurons, in AIDS patients with dementia

Treatment

- Antiretroviral therapies may impede or in some cases even partially reverse the progression of neurologic changes and the white matter signal changes

Prognosis

- HIV encephalopathy is generally slowly progressive
- The median survival after onset of dementia is on the order of 6 months

Suggested Readings

Lizerbram EK, Hesselink JR. Viral infections. *Neuroimag Clin North Am* 7:261–280, 1997.

Post MJD, Berger JR, Quencer RM. Asymptomatic and neurologically symptomatic HIV-seropositive individuals: prospective evaluation with cranial MR imaging. *Radiology* 178:131–139, 1991.

Trotot PM, Gray F. Diagnostic imaging contribution in the early stages of HIV infection of the brain. *Neuroimag Clin North Am* 7:243–260, 1997.

Case 52

Clinical Presentation

A 29-year-old HIV-positive patient presents with progressive visual changes.

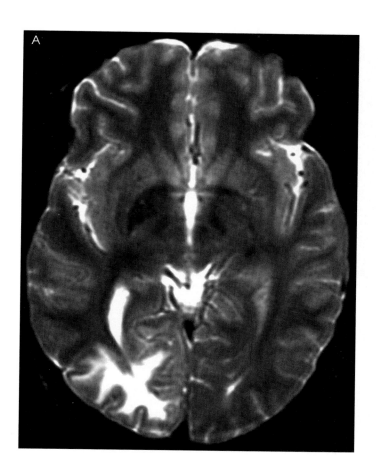

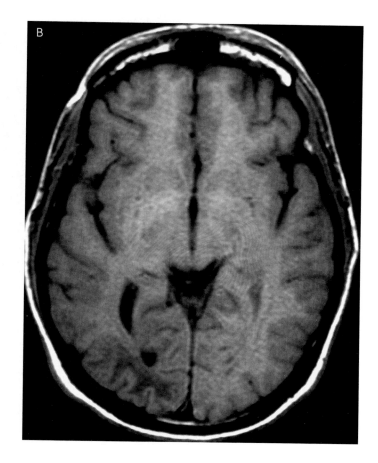

Radiologic Findings

An axial T2-WI (Fig. A) demonstrates a confluent area of T2 prolongation involving the subcortical white matter of the right occipital lobe. A T1-WI (Fig. B) demonstrates corresponding hypointensity in the right occipital lobe. Note the absence of mass effect on adjacent sulci and ventricle.

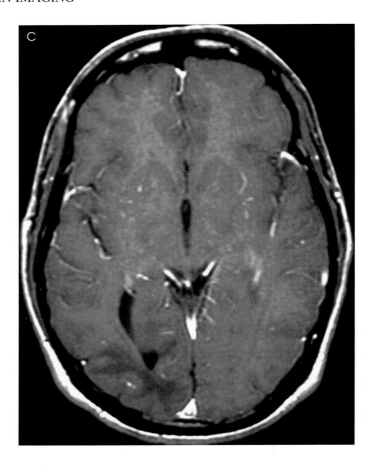

A post-gadolinium T1-WI (Fig. C) shows no associated enhancement.

Diagnosis

Progressive multifocal leukoencephalopathy (PML)

Differential Diagnosis

- HIV encephalitis (often more symmetric, spares subcortical white matter)
- Cytomegalovirus encephalitis (predilection for ependymal and periventricular regions, may cause linear periventricular enhancement)
- Toxoplasmosis (focal-enhancing mass lesion(s) with surrounding vasogenic edema)
- Lymphoma (usually enhances, usually has mass effect, is typically hypo- or isointense on T2-WI)

Discussion

Background

PML is a progressive demyelinating disorder resulting from CNS infection with the JC virus. The JC virus is believed to infect up to 80% of the human population prior to adulthood without producing obvious illness. This virus is commonly latent in the CNS, but reactivates in the setting of immune compromise

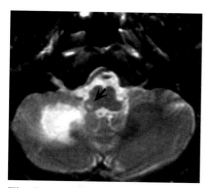

Fig. D. A T2-WI demonstrates an area of confluent T2 prolongation in the white matter of the right cerebellar hemisphere, as well as a focus of T2 prolongation in the right dorsolateral medulla (*arrow*).

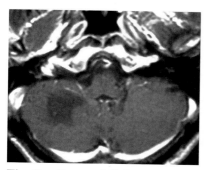

Fig. E. Post-gadolinium, a T1-WI (same patient as Fig. D) shows no evidence of associated enhancement. Note also the absence of mass effect.

Table 1. HIV encephalitis versus PML

Finding	HIV encephalitis	PML
White matter lesions	symmetric	asymmetric
Subcortical U-fibers involved	uncommon	common
Posterior fossa involvement	uncommon	common
Mass effect	never	may occur, usually mild
Enhancement	never	may occur, usually mild
Hemorrhage	never	occasional
Signal intensity on T1-WI	usually isointense	commonly hypointense

(AIDS, organ transplantation, hematologic malignancy). In the setting of AIDS, PML is found in ~5% of autopsy specimens.

Etiology

The etiologic agent of PML is a papovavirus designated "JC" after the patient from whom it was initially isolated. Oligodendrocytes infected with the virus are unable to maintain myelin, and thus focal demyelination occurs. Brain biopsy was previously required for definitive diagnosis, but viral DNA may now be detected in CSF using the polymerase chain reaction method.

Clinical Findings

PML typically results in progressive neurologic decline with altered mental status, personality change, cognitive impairment, visual changes, and motor and sensory changes. Seizures and progressive dementia may also occur.

Pathology

Gross

• Volume loss and focal myelin pallor

Microscopic

• Intranuclear inclusions within large, swollen oligodendrocytes; demyelination; astrocytosis

Imaging Findings

CT

• Asymmetric, focal, often well-demarcated zones of hypodensity are typically seen in the periventricular and/or subcortical white matter

MR

• Asymmetric, multifocal areas of T1 and T2 prolongation in the periventricular and/or peripheral white matter
• Involvement of the subcortical U-fibers (arcuate fibers) is common, giving a "scalloped" appearance to the lateral margin of the process
• Parieto-occipital involvement is classically described, but lesions may affect any lobe of the cerebrum as well as the basal ganglia, brainstem, and cerebellum (Figs. D and E)
• Mass effect, hemorrhage, and enhancement are usually absent or are mild if present
• Volume loss occurs in the chronic phase

Treatment and Prognosis

There is no specific therapy for PML, and it was previously felt that death inevitably ensued within 6 to 12 months of the onset of symptoms. New combination therapies for HIV (antiretroviral drugs, protease inhibitors, cytarabine) seem to be improving the course and prognosis of PML, with survivals of several years now reported.

Suggested Readings

Garrels K, Kucharczyk W, Wortzman G, Shandling M. Progressive multifocal leukoencephalopathy: clinical and MR response to treatment. *AJNR* 17:597–600, 1996.

Wheeler AL, Truwit CL, Kleinschmidt-DeMasters BK, et al. Progressive multifocal leukoencephalopathy: contrast enhancement on CT scans and MR images. *AJR* 161: 1049–1051, 1993.

Whiteman MLH, Post MJD, Berger JR, et al. Progressive multifocal leukoencephalopathy in 47 HIV-seropositive patients: neuroimaging with clinical and pathologic correlation. *Radiology* 187:233–240, 1993.

Case 53

Clinical Presentation

A 38-year-old HIV-positive patient presents to the emergency room following a seizure. When he has recovered, he complains of headache and visual difficulties.

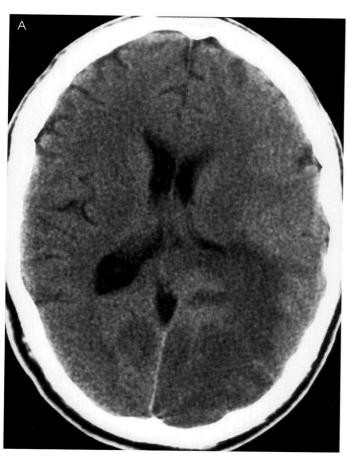 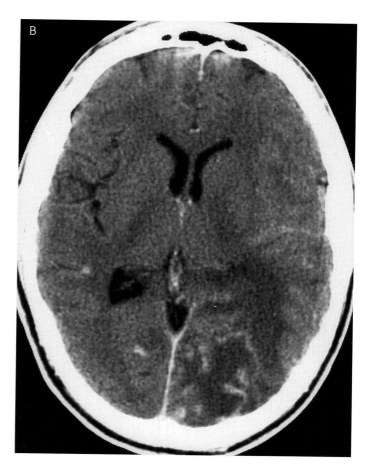

Radiologic Findings

A non-contrast head CT (Fig. A) shows edema in the left occipital and temporal lobes, extending into the splenium of the corpus callosum. A smaller area of edema is present in the right occipital lobe. Following administration of contrast (Fig. B), irregular linear enhancement is identified in the left occipital lobe. In addition, nodular foci of enhancement are identified in the right occipital and right temporal lobes.

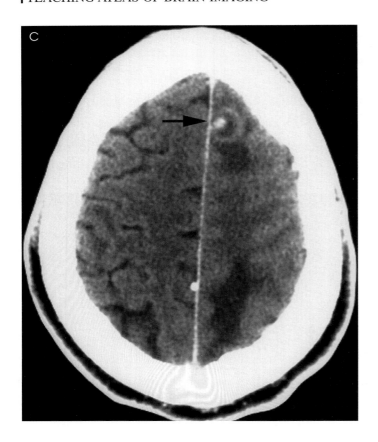

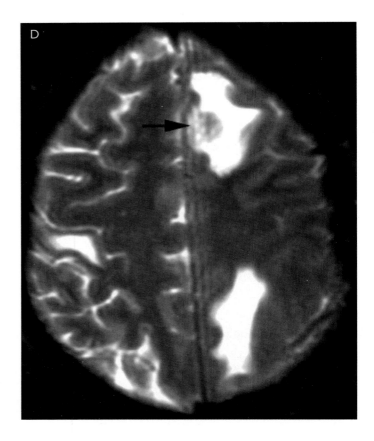

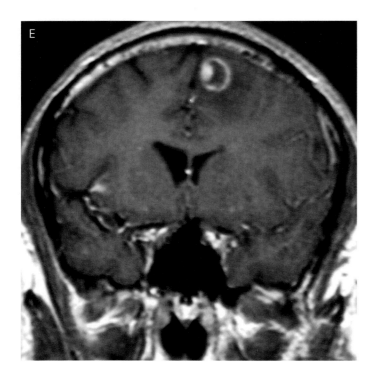

An axial post-contrast scan at a higher level (Fig. C) demonstrates a peripherally enhancing lesion in the left frontal lobe, associated with an eccentric nodular area of enhancement (*arrow*). This is consistent with the so-called "eccentric target sign." An axial T2-WI (Fig. D) from an MR in the same patient demonstrates multiple areas of vasogenic edema in the subcortical white matter bilaterally. In the left frontal lobe, a rounded area that is isointense to gray matter is identified (*arrow*). A coronal post-gadolinium T1-WI (Fig. E) demonstrates the "eccentric target sign" in the left frontal lesion.

Pearls

- CT is often used for initial diagnosis at the time of acute presentation, but MR is generally more helpful in differentiating toxoplasmosis from lymphoma. MR much better demonstrates ependymal or subarachnoid spread of disease, findings which highly favor lymphoma. If a CT scan is done, hyperattenuation on non-contrast CT favors lymphoma as well.

- The "eccentric target sign" is highly suggestive of toxoplasmosis, but it is relatively insensitive, being seen in <30% of cases. The pathologic correlate of this sign is not known but may be related to infoldings of membrane.

- Clinical and radiographic response to therapy usually occur within 7 to 10 days, and alternative diagnoses should be considered if a patient fails to respond or progresses in this time frame.

Pitfalls

- A toxoplasmosis lesion may have unusual imaging appearances: it may be hemorrhagic, it may involve the corpus callosum and mimic glioblastoma multiforme, and previously treated lesions may calcify.

- HIV-positive patients may have coexistent pathologies, (e.g., toxoplasmosis and lymphoma).

- Both toxoplasmosis and lymphoma may appear intermediate in signal intensity on T2-WI (Fig. D).

Diagnosis

CNS toxoplasmosis

Differential Diagnosis

- Primary CNS lymphoma (may be indistinguishable, but may see ependymal or subarachnoid spread of disease; lacks the eccentric target sign)
- Abscesses secondary to other organisms (fungal, pyogenic) (may be indistinguishable)
- Metastatic disease (patients often have a known primary lesion, more common in older patients)
- Primary glial neoplasm (typically causes a single lesion, but may be multifocal)

Discussion

Background

Toxoplasmosis is the most common cause of CNS mass lesion(s) in the HIV-positive patient. Positive antibody titers that reflect exposure to toxoplasmosis vary geographically. In France 75 to 90% of healthy adults are seropositive for *T. gondii*, while this drops to 20 to 35% in the United States. Up to 20% of HIV-positive patients who are seropositive for toxoplasma will develop toxoplasmic encephalitis. Congenital toxoplasmosis is a result of intrauterine infection and is discussed in Case 39.

Etiology

Toxoplasmosis is caused by the obligate intracellular protozoan parasite *Toxoplasma gondii*.

Pathophysiology

Toxoplasmosis is usually acquired from food contaminated with infectious cat feces (cats are the most important disease reservoir for this organism), but may also be acquired via direct ingestion (this usually occurs when children play in contaminated sandboxes or playgrounds). In an immune competent host, infection is usually controlled, and the organisms remain dormant for the lifetime of the host. When the immune system is compromised, as by HIV infection, the toxoplasmic infection may either progress primarily or recrudesce, leading to tissue necrosis and reactive inflammation.

Clinical Findings

CNS symptoms include fever, headache, confusion, focal neurologic signs, and seizures. Other systemic manifestations include hepatosplenomegaly, pneumonitis, rash, myositis, and myocarditis.

Complications

CNS toxoplasmosis may progress to coma and death if not appropriately treated.

Imaging Findings

CT and **MR** demonstrate similar findings.

- Typically multifocal lesions with significant surrounding edema; may affect any area, though the basal ganglia are a favored site; a lesion may be solitary in ~30% of cases
- Post-contrast: small lesions often enhance in a nodular fashion; larger lesions enhance peripherally, with a rim of variable thickness. The "eccentric target sign" may be seen–this refers to an eccentric enhancing nodule adjacent to the peripherally enhancing rim of the lesion.
- Post-therapy, lesions may completely regress or may calcify

Treatment

Generally empiric therapy with pyrimethamine and sulfadiazine. Lifelong suppressive therapy is necessary to prevent relapse.

Prognosis

Good: with appropriate therapy, clinical improvement and radiologic response should be seen within 7 to 10 days. If there is a poor response to therapy, brain biopsy may be indicated to exclude an alternative diagnosis.

Suggested Readings

Dina TS. Primary central nervous sytem lymphoma versus toxoplasmosis in AIDS. *Radiology* 179:823–828, 1991.

Ramsey RG, Gean AD. Central nervous system toxoplasmosis. *Neuroimag Clin North Am* 7:171–186, 1997.

Ramsey RG, Geremia GK. CNS complications of AIDS: CT and MR findings. *AJR* 151:449–454, 1988.

Case 54

Clinical Presentation

A 28-year-old HIV-positive patient presents with persistent headache.

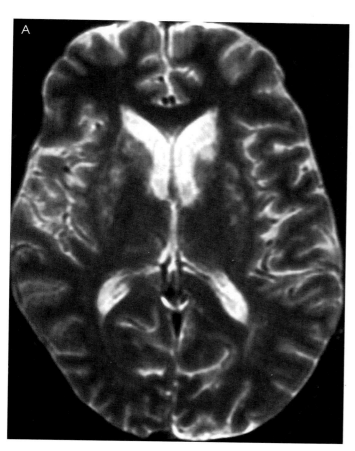 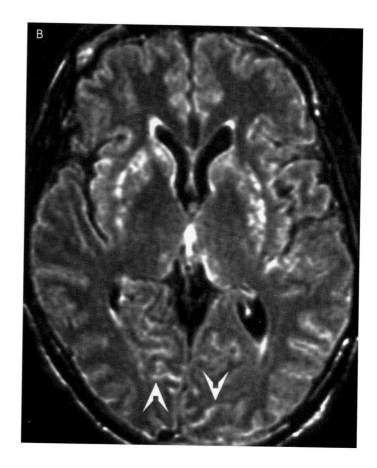

Radiologic Findings

Axial T2-weighted (Fig. A) and fluid-attenuated inversion recovery (FLAIR) (Fig. B) images demonstrates multiple punctate areas of T2 prolongation in the caudate nuclei, putamina, and thalami bilaterally. In some areas, the CSF has abnormal high signal on the FLAIR image (*arrows*), consistent with accompanying meningitis and altered protein content in the CSF.

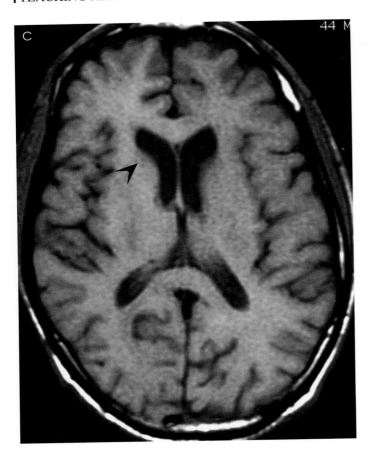

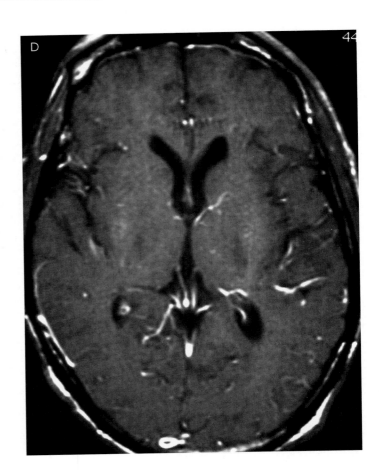

An axial T1-WI (Fig. C) shows questionable hypointensity in the right caudate nucleus (*arrowhead*) but is otherwise essentially unremarkable. No abnormal enhancement is present on a post-gadolinium T1-WI (Fig. D). A diagnosis was made based on characteristic imaging findings and CSF analysis.

Diagnosis

Cryptococcal meningitis with gelatinous pseudocysts in an HIV-positive patient

Differential Diagnosis

The differential diagnosis varies with the form of cryptococcal infection.

Gelatinous pseudocysts:

- Prominent perivascular spaces (should follow CSF on all sequences)
- Lacunar infarction (usually an older patient, often a history of hypertension)

Cryptococcal meningitis:

- Other fungal, viral or bacterial meningitides (patient often more acutely ill, usually a basilar meningitis in setting of tuberculosis)

Focal cryptococcoma:

- Tuberculoma, other fungal granuloma, lymphoma

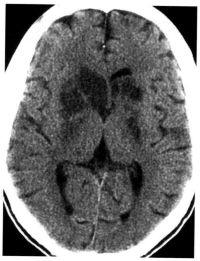

Fig. E. Non-contrast CT image of an HIV-positive patient with cryptococcus infection demonstrates extensive low attenuation in the basal ganglia consistent with gelatinous pseudocysts.

Discussion

Background

Cryptococcosis is the most common fungal infection of the CNS. HIV-positive patients are at high risk of the disease (~5% will develop CNS cryptococcosis), and they tend to present with disseminated infection. Cryptococcus ranks third after HIV itself and toxoplasmosis as causes of CNS infection in AIDS. CNS cryptococcosis primarily manifests as an acute or chronic meningitis, although mass lesions may be seen. Cryptococcal antigen ("CrAg") levels are typically increased in both serum and CSF, which is useful in confirming this diagnosis.

Etiology

Cryptococcal disease is caused by the yeastlike fungus *Cryptococcus neoformans* which is ubiquitous in the environment and produces a polysaccharide capsule that shields it from attack by the immune system. This fungus is found in soil and bird droppings.

Pathophysiology/Pathology

Inhalation of the organism is followed by hematogenous dissemination to the CNS. The organism penetrates the walls of the meningeal vessels and enters the CSF. It also colonizes the perivascular spaces. Pathologic changes include:

• Meningitis: results in leptomeningeal thickening due to inflammation
• Gelatinous pseudocysts: expansion of perivascular spaces occurs due to an accumulation of mucinous material, inflammatory cells, and organisms
• Cryptococcomas: occur when the blood-brain barrier is disrupted and the organisms extend from the perivascular space into the brain parenchyma. These irregularly marginated lesions replace brain parenchyma and contain mucinous material, inflammatory cells, and organisms.

Clinical Findings

Symptoms are usually non-specific such as headache, fever, malaise, and vomiting. Focal parenchymal lesions may cause focal neurologic signs and seizures. In 10 to 20% of cases patients with cryptococcal CNS infection have no signs or symptoms of CNS disease. CSF analysis typically shows decreased glucose, elevated protein, and lymphocytosis. India ink smear may reveal the encapsulated organism.

Complications

Complications include communicating hydrocephalus and focal cerebritis/cryptococcoma formation.

Imaging Findings

CT

• Frequently normal or shows mild communicating hydrocephalus
• May see multiple small round focal or confluent hypodensities (Fig. E), most numerous in the basal ganglia and thalami, representing gelatinous pseudocysts

Pitfalls

- Leptomeningeal enhancement due to cryptococcal infection, if present at all, may be located over the convexity surfaces and mimic the gyral enhancement of infarction.

- CNS cryptococcosis may uncommonly manifest as an intraventricular cystic lesion or as miliary nodules.

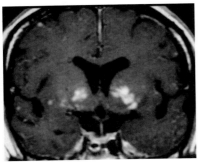

Fig. F. Post-gadolinium T1-WI obtained in an immunocompetent woman who presented with headache, fever, and stiff neck after cleaning out a trailer filled with pigeon droppings. Nodular areas of enhancement are identified in the lentiform nuclei bilaterally, consistent with cryptococcomas in this immunocompetent host.

MR

- Meningitis may lead to leptomeningeal enhancement and/or communicating hydrocephalus
- Gelatinous pseudocysts appear as punctate (<3 mm) hyperintensities on T2-WI which are usually iso- to hypointense on T1-WI. They are usually nonenhancing – but enhancement has been described – and are most commonly seen in the basal ganglia and midbrain, although they may be found throughout the brain, including the cerebellum.
- Cryptococcomas: variable appearance, but may demonstrate surrounding vasogenic edema and nodular enhancement due to compromise of the blood-brain barrier. Cryptococcomas are more likely to enhance in an immunocompetent host, since a more effective chronic granulomatous inflammatory response is mounted (Fig. F).

Treatment

Amphotericin B, with or without fluconazole or flucytosine

Prognosis

30% of patients fail to respond to therapy, and some require chronic lifelong suppression

Suggested Readings

Harris DE, Enterline DS. Fungal infections of the central nervous system. *Neuroimag Clin North Am* 7:187–198, 1997.

Mathews VP, Alo PL, Glass JD, et al. AIDS-related CNS cryptococcosis: radiologic-pathologic correlation. *AJNR* 13:1477–1486, 1992.

Tien RD, Chu PK, Hesselink JR, et al. Intracranial cryptococcosis in immunocompromised patients: CT and MR findings in 29 cases. *AJNR* 12:283–289, 1991.

Case 55

Clinical Presentation

A 35-year-old HIV-positive woman presents with headache, low-grade fever, and altered mental status.

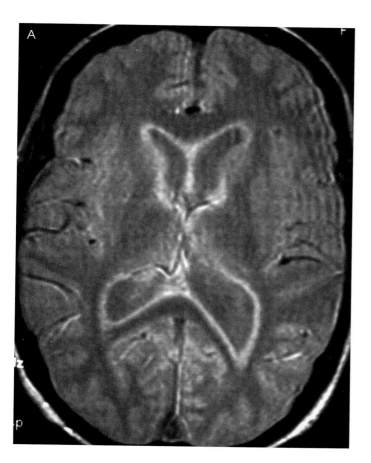

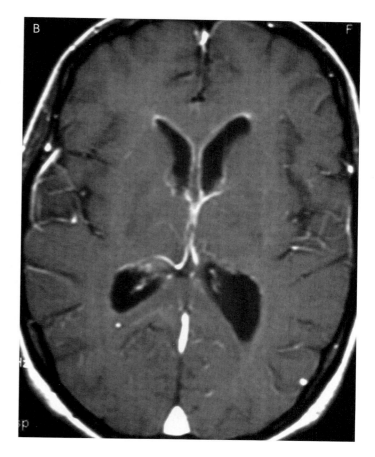

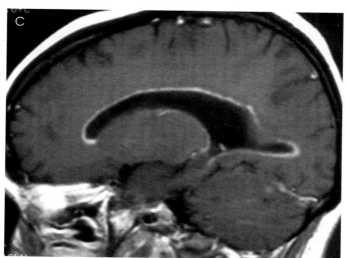

Pearls

- The characteristic rim of periventricular hyperintensity is most apparent on proton density-weighted or fluid-attenuated inversion recovery (FLAIR) (Fig. D) images.

- Ependymal/subependymal enhancement is never normal.

Pitfalls

- CNS lymphoma may occasionally demonstrate thin, regular periventricular enhancement similar to CMV.

- CMV may rarely present as a ring-enhancing space-occupying lesion that mimics a CNS tumor or abscess.

- Coexistent pathologies are common, including other viruses such as HIV itself, herpes simplex virus type 1 or 2, or varicella zoster virus.

- FLAIR images often show a thin band of periventricular high signal in normal patients (Fig. E). Thick, irregular, or asymmetric (Fig. D) high signal is abnormal.

Radiologic Findings

An axial PD-WI (Fig. A) demonstrates a thin linear rim of high signal intensity involving the ependymal/subependymal region. An axial post-gadolinium T1-WI (Fig. B) demonstrates smooth, linear enhancement around the ventricular margin. A sagittal post-gadolinium T1-WI acquired after a short time delay (Fig. C) shows more intense periventricular enhancement.

Diagnosis

Cytomegalovirus (CMV) ventriculitis

Differential Diagnosis

- Bacterial ventriculitis (patients are typically acutely ill, a fluid-debris level may be present in the ventricle)
- Lymphoma (ependymal enhancement is often more nodular and irregular)
- HIV encephalitis (nonenhancing symmetric diffuse white matter abnormality)
- Progressive multifocal leukoencephalopathy (patchy, asymmetric, often subcortical white matter hyperintensity on T2-WIs, usually nonenhancing)

Discussion

Background

CMV infection of the CNS usually affects immunosuppressed patients such as HIV-positive and organ transplant populations. The virus exists in a latent form in the general population and reactivates in the setting of immune compromise. Common sites of involvement include the CNS, respiratory system, gastrointestinal and genitourinary tracts, and hematopoietic system. CNS infection generally takes the form of meningoencephalitis and/or ventriculitis, but myelitis, polyradiculitis, and retinitis are other potential manifestations. Two cases of CMV presenting as a focal brain mass have recently been reported.

Etiology

CMV is a member of the herpesvirus family. Despite the fact that CMV infection of the CNS is diagnosed in up to 40% of autopsies of AIDS patients, the diagnosis of CMV encephalitis has been very difficult to make antemortem. Recent advances in molecular biology have facilitated the diagnosis using the polymerase chain reaction (PCR) to isolate viral DNA from CSF. The sensitivity of PCR is close to 79%, with a specificity of 95%.

Clinical Findings

CMV ventriculoencephalitis presents with nonspecific symptoms and signs such as headache, fever, altered mental status, memory impairment, seizures, and cranial nerve palsies. CSF typically shows neutrophilic pleocytosis, elevated protein, and low glucose.

Complications

Fulminant CMV ventriculoencephalitis may result in death days to weeks after the onset of clinical symptoms.

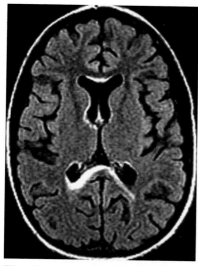

Fig. D. Axial FLAIR image in a 10-year-old AIDS patient with CSF positive for CMV demonstrates asymmetric, irregular high signal in the periventricular region.

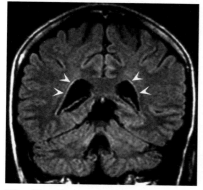

Fig. E. Coronal FLAIR image in a normal volunteer demonstrates a thin, regular rim of high signal around the margins of the ventricles (*arrowheads*).

Pathology

Gross

- Extensive destruction of both gray and white matter as well as the ventricular ependymal lining

Microscopic

- Characteristic intranuclear inclusions give an "owl's eye" appearance in ependymal cells, subependymal astrocytes, oligodendrocytes, endothelial cells and neurons

Imaging Findings

CT

- Relatively insensitive
- May demonstrate white matter hypodensity or ependymal enhancement

MR

- T2-WI: focal or diffuse hyperintensities in the white matter; ependymal/subependymal periventricular hyperintensity
- Post-gadolinium: thin, linear enhancement along the ventricular margin in ~20 to 30% of cases; rarely a focal peripherally enhancing mass lesion may be seen

Treatment

- Ganciclovir (a nucleoside analogue)
- Foscarnet sodium (a pyrophosphate analogue)

Prognosis

- Historically poor, though the prognosis is improving with the ability to make earlier diagnosis and institute therapy
- Quantitative PCR of CSF may be useful in monitoring response to therapy

Suggested Readings

Ketonen LM, Arya S, Van Epps K, et al. MR findings of autopsy-proved cytomegalovirus encephalitis in AIDS. Presented at the 35th Annual Meeting of the American Society of Neuroradiology, Toronto, Canada, 1997.

Miller RF, Lucas SB, Hall-Craggs MA, et al. Comparison of magnetic resonance imaging with neuropathological findings in the diagnosis of HIV and CMV associated CNS disease in AIDS. *J Neurol Neurosurg Psych* 62:346–351, 1997.

Post MJD, Hensley GT, Moskowitz LB, Fischl M. Cytomegalic inclusion virus encephalitis in patients with AIDS: CT, clinical and pathologic correlation. *AJNR* 7:275–280, 1986.

Case 56

Clinical Presentation

A 38-year-old HIV-positive patient presents with progressive alteration in mental status, increasing somnolence, and rigidity.

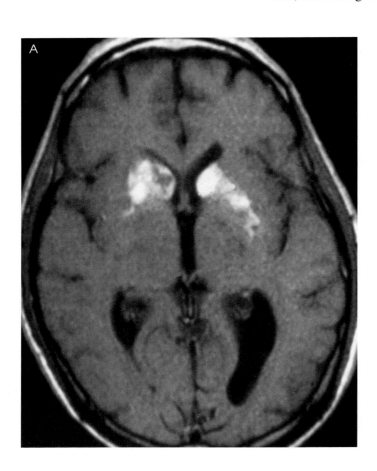
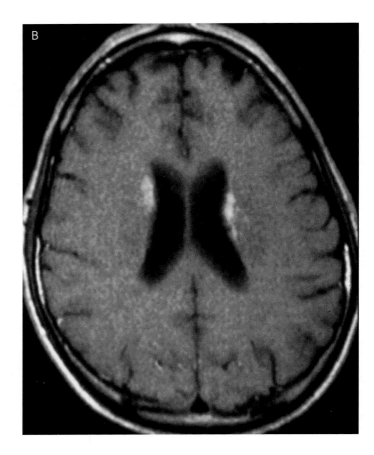

Radiologic Findings

Axial post-gadolinium T1-WIs (Figs. A and B) show patchy and confluent areas of irregular parenchymal enhancement involving the the caudate nuclei and putamina bilaterally. As these abnormalities are in the distribution of the medial and lateral lenticulostriate arteries and are concerning for infarction, an angiogram was performed for further evaluation.

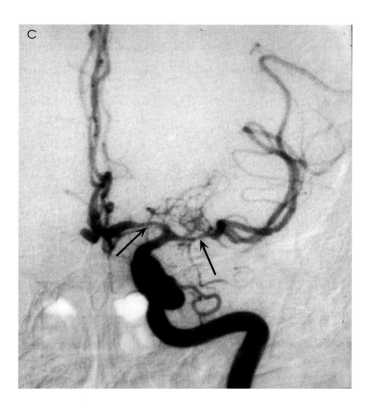
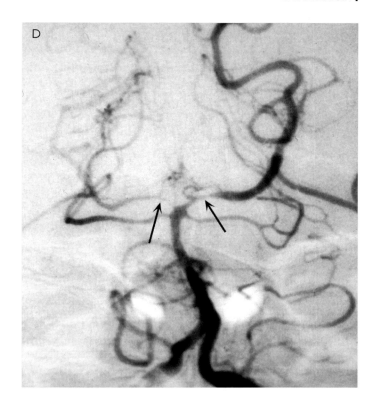

A frontal projection from a left internal carotid artery injection (Fig. C) shows irregular stenosis of the proximal left M-1 and A-1 segments (*arrows*). Examination of the posterior circulation (Fig. D) shows irregular narrowing of the proximal posterior cerebral arteries bilaterally (*arrows*). *(Figures courtesy of Alisa D. Gean, M.D., San Francisco.)*

Diagnosis

Neurosyphilis

Differential Diagnosis

Varies with the particular manifestations of disease (see below).

- Meningeal enhancement: fungal or bacterial meningitis, carcinomatus meningitis
- Gumma: focal-enhancing mass lesion(s) such as toxoplasmosis, lymphoma, and tuberculosis
- Infarction: causes of basal ganglia infarction include atherosclerosis, hypertension, vasculitis (infectious or noninfectious), vasospasm, and moya-moya

Discussion

Background

Neurosyphilis affects both the immunocompetent and the immunocompromised. The AIDS epidemic has contributed significantly to the resurgence of syphilis. It occurs in ~1.5% of the AIDS population and has a more aggressive course than in the general population. Invasion of the CNS may occur at any stage of syphilitic

Pearls

- Contrast-enhanced MR is more sensitive than CT to meningeal and perivascular inflammation. MRA may demonstrate vascular stenoses and/or occlusions.
- Gummas are typically located peripherally in the cortex of the cerebral hemispheres.
- Meningovascular syphilis should always be in the differential diagnosis when an HIV-positive patient presents with a cerebral infarction.

Pitfalls

- HIV itself may cause an arteriopathy, but syphilis should be included in the differential diagnosis and appropriate testing should be performed.

infection, but it eventually occurs in 5 to 10% of untreated patients. In the HIV-positive host, there is a shorter latent period for progression to clinically evident neurologic disease. In the CNS, syphilis may cause arteritis and cerebral infarction, nonspecific white matter lesions, focal mass lesions (cerebral gummas), and leptomeningeal inflammation.

Etiology

Syphilis is caused by the spirochete *Treponema pallidum*. Syphilis is usually acquired via sexual contact, but the fetus may be affected transplacentally (congenital syphilis). The diagnosis is established by positive CSF Venereal Disease Research Laboratories (VDRL) test, positive treponemal antibody test, or by detection of the organism itself.

Stages of Disease

- *Primary syphilis*: characterized by an ulcer or sore ("chancre") at the site of inoculation, as well as regional adenopathy
- *Secondary syphilis*: occurs 2 to 8 weeks after chancre formation if treatment is not instituted and represents hematogenous dissemination. It classically manifests as a maculopapular rash involving the palms and soles and general lymphadenopathy. CNS symptomatology may occur in the secondary stage, typically a syphilitic meningitis with headache and cranial nerve palsies
- *Tertiary syphilis*: usually seen at least 5 years after primary disease, but this progression is shortened in the AIDS population. One third of patients will develop CNS symptoms, one third develop cardiovascular symptoms, and one third have a more benign form manifested in skin, bones, joints, and mucous membranes. Later stage CNS symptoms include acute vascular events, personality change, and eventually dementia. Spinal cord symptoms (tabes dorsalis) may develop as well, with loss of pain and proprioceptive sensation.

Clinical Findings

Patients with neurosyphilis are often asymptomatic in the early stages of the disease but eventually may present with symptoms referable to meningeal inflammation, a mass lesion (gumma), or cerebral infarction. Symptoms include altered mental status, headache, fever, seizures, hemiparesis, visual changes, and gait abnormality.

Complications

Complications include acute or chronic hydrocephalus and cranial nerve palsies. Infectious vasculitis may lead to cerebral ischemia/infarction. After 10-20 years, "general paresis of the insane" may develop, with insidious impairment of attention and cognition.

Pathology

CNS involvement typically results in a meningovasculitis with meningeal thickening due to lymphocyte and plasma cell infiltration as well as perivascular inflammatory infiltration. Syphilitic gummas represent focal circumscribed masses of inflammatory tissue with granuloma formation–these arise from the dura and/or pia mater and extend into the peripheral brain parenchyma.

Imaging Findings

Imaging studies may be normal or may show only nonspecific atrophy which is more likely related to HIV-coinfection itself. Other potential findings include:

CT

- May see signs of cerebral infarction involving perforator or large vessels
- Cerebral gummas appear as mass lesions that are usually isodense on non-contrast CT and shows intense enhancement postcontrast

MR

- Nonspecific deep white matter T2 hyperintensities are frequent
- Gummas present as parenchymal masses that are hypo- or isointense on T1-WI, iso- or hyperintense on T2-WI, and enhance intensely and homogeneously post-contrast. Gummas are usually peripherally located and are associated with overlying leptomeningeal enhancement.
- Evidence of infarcts of varying age involving both perforator vessels (pontine and deep gray nuclear infarcts) or hemispheric territories. This reflects the meningovascular form of the disease and is often associated with focal leptomeningeal enhancement around arteries of the circle of Willis.

Conventional angiography or MR angiography (MRA)

Segmental arterial narrowing and irregularity favoring large and medium-sized vessels around the circle of Willis

Treatment

High-dose penicillin is the standard therapy

Prognosis

Generally good but varies with the promptness of diagnosis and the extent of infarction, if present

Suggested Readings

Brightbill TC, Ihmeidan IH, Post MJD, et al. Neurosyphilis in HIV-positive and HIV-negative patients: neuroimaging findings. *AJNR* 16:703–711, 1995.

Harris DE, Enterline DS, Tien RD. Neurosyphilis in patients with AIDS. *Neuroimag Clin North Am* 7:215–221, 1997.

Tien RD, Gean-Marton AD, Mark AS. Neurosyphilis in HIV carriers: MR findings in six patients. *AJR* 158:1325–1328, 1992.

Case 57

Clinical Presentation

A 14-year-old girl with a history of sinusitis presents with severe headache and fever.

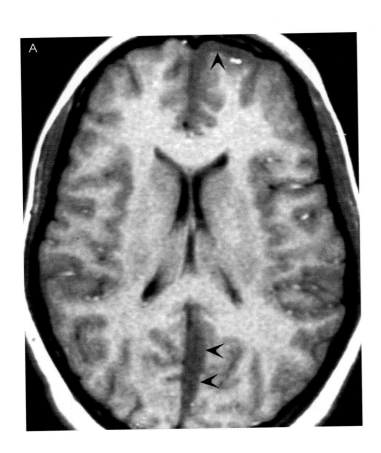 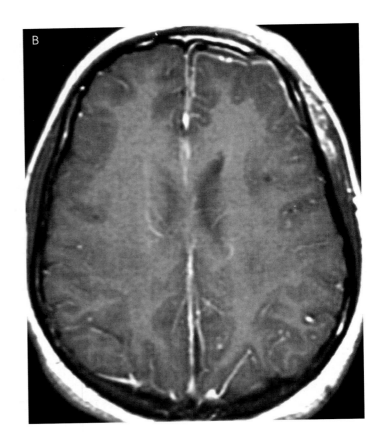

Radiologic Findings

An axial T1-WI (Fig. A) demonstrates subtle extra-axial collections along the posterior falx and over the left frontal lobe (black *arrowheads*) which are hyperintense compared to CSF. Note mild mass effect on the left frontal lobe. Postgadolinium, an axial T1-WI (Fig. B) demonstrates peripheral enhancement around the margins of these collections.

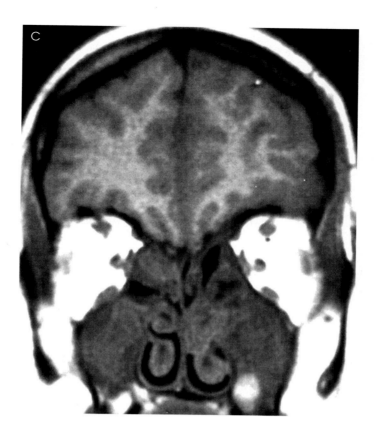

A coronal T1-WI in this patient (Fig. C) demonstrates marked mucosal thickening in the maxillary and ethmoid sinuses bilaterally.

Diagnosis

Subdural empyema secondary to paranasal sinus infection

Differential Diagnosis

• Epidural empyema (dura displaced from the inner table of the skull)
• Subdural effusion (usually bilateral, usually nonenhancing, CSF intensity)
• Subdural hematoma (imaging characteristics consistent with blood)

Discussion

Background

An empyema is a loculated collection of pus within a membrane-bound space. Intracranially, empyema can occur in the subdural or epidural space, and may involve both spaces. Subdural empyema is more common than epidural empyema, although both are uncommon infections. Both entities most commonly occur as a complication of paranasal sinus infection. Other causes include fractures involving the paranasal sinuses, mastoiditis, and intracranial surgery. Postoperative empyemas tend to be more indolent because a well-formed limiting membrane restricts the spread of the inflammatory collection. Infection may also complicate a pre-existing posttraumatic extra-axial hematoma, leading to empyema formation. In infants, secondary infection of a meningitis-related subdural

Pitfalls

- Subdural and epidural empyemas may cause significant clinical symptoms even when they appear quite small.
- Small empyemas adjacent to the calvarium are easily overlooked on CT scans.
- Empyemas along the subfrontal region of the brain may be easily missed on axial scans.
- Empyemas can rarely occur infratentorially (3 to 10% of subdural empyemas), with the usual setting being chronic otomastoiditis.

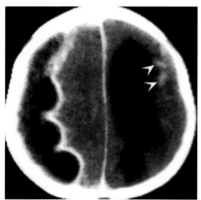

Fig D. A contrast-enhanced CT demonstrates a loculated, peripherally enhancing right holo-hemispheric extra-axial collection consistent with subdural empyema. There is severe obstructive hydrocephalus as evidenced by the markedly enlarged left lateral ventricle. In addition, focal areas of parenchymal enhancement consistent with cerebritis/early abscess formation are present (*arrowheads*).

effusion is most common cause of subdural empyema. Empyemas may be unilateral or bilateral. When bilateral, they are usually asymmetric.

Etiology

Anaerobic or microaerophilic organisms such as *Streptococcus* and *Bacteroides* species which are found in the paranasal sinuses are common pathogens.

Clinical Findings

Fever and headache are common. Sinusitis is often present. Focal neurological signs may be seen if the collection is large enough to cause mass effect. Cranial neuropathy may ensue if the paracavernous regions are affected.

Complications

Complications include thrombosis of cortical veins or dural sinuses with secondary venous infarction and parenchymal abscess formation. Seizures, hemiparesis, coma, and death may occur if treatment is delayed.

Pathophysiology

Bacterial organisms typically gain access to the subdural space from paranasal sinus and otitic infections by way of retrograde spread via bridging emissary veins.

Imaging Findings

CT

- Subdural collection that is usually isodense but may be mildly hyperdense compared with CSF
- Abnormal peripheral enhancement following contrast administration (Fig. D)

MR

- Variable-sized extra-axial fluid collection which is usually hyperintense to CSF on T1- and PD-WI, and isointense to CSF on T2-WI
- Post-contrast: abnormal enhancement of the margins of collection
- Associated cerebritis/brain abscess may occur, with parenchymal edema and focal enhancement

Treatment

- Intracranial empyema generally requires emergent drainage via burr holes or craniotomy
- Antibiotic coverage should include anaerobic organisms

Prognosis

- Good with early diagnosis and prompt therapy
- Without prompt diagnosis and treatment, morbidity ranges from 25 to 40% and mortality from 8 to 12%

Suggested Readings

Borovich B, Johnston E, Spagnuolo E. Infratentorial subdural empyema: clinical and computerized tomography findings. *J Neurosurg* 72:299–301, 1990.

Chanalet S, Gense de Beaufort D, Greselle JF, Louail C, Padovani B, Caille JM. Clinical and radiological aspects of extracerebral empyemas: 39 cases. *Neuroradiology* 33: 225–228, 1991.

Weingarten K, Zimmerman RD, Becker RD, et al. Subdural and epidural empyemas: MR imaging. *AJNR* 10:81–87, 1989.

Section III

Dural/Leptomeningeal Processes

Case 58

Clinical Presentation

A 54-year-old woman presents with progressive right-sided weakness.

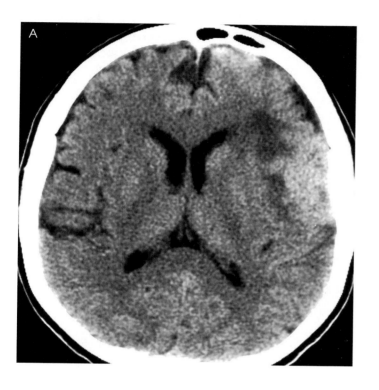

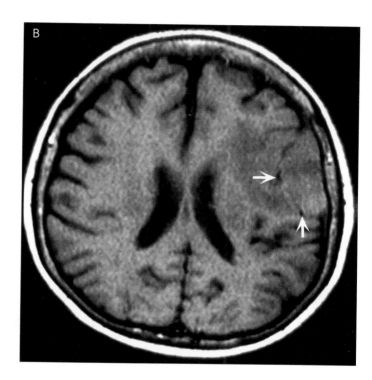

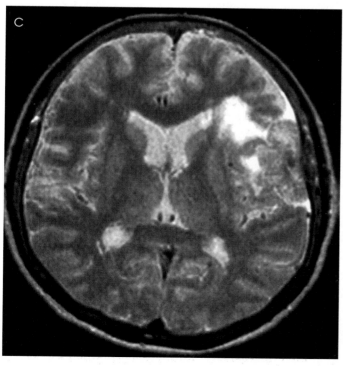

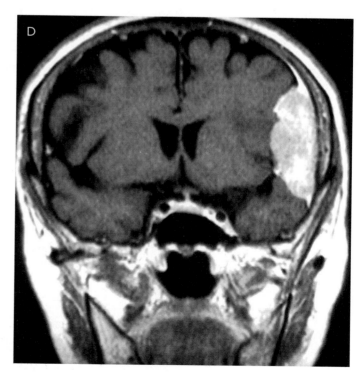

Radiologic Findings

A non-contrast CT scan (Fig. A) demonstrates a hyperdense mass in the left frontal region. Associated vasogenic edema is present. This mass appears to be displacing cortex away from it, suggesting that it is extra-axial. An MR scan was obtained to better evaluate the lesion. An axial T1-WI (Fig. B) demonstrates that the mass is isointense to gray matter. The extra-axial nature is supported by the fact that vessels (*arrows*) are identified between the brain surface and the mass. On a T2-WI (Fig. C), the mass is slightly heterogenous but mostly isointense to cortex. Vasogenic edema is noted in the subcortical white matter. Following administration of gadolinium (Fig. D), a coronal T1-WI demonstrates intense and fairly homogeneous enhancement of the mass. Enhancement extends along the adjacent dura, consistent with a "dural tail."

Diagnosis

Meningioma, benign

Differential Diagnosis

- Malignant meningioma (may be indistinguishable)
- Dural metastasis (brain invasion, brain edema, and/or calvarial erosion more likely)
- Other dural neoplasm such as hemangiopericytoma or desmoid tumor (may be indistinguishable)
- Sarcoid (often more plaquelike and infiltrative, often darker on T2-WI)

Discussion

Background

Meningiomas are extra-axial neoplasms that represent 15 to 20% of primary intracranial neoplasms. They have a peak between ages 40 to 60 years, and more commonly affect women than men. Most meningiomas arise from arachnoidal cells on the inner surface of the dura and therefore grow inward toward the brain to form bulky intradural tumor masses. Most meningiomas are benign, but ~6% of meningiomas are "atypical" or "aggressive," and 1 to 2% are frankly malignant. Common locations for meningiomas include the cerebral convexity, parasagittal region, sphenoid wing, olfactory groove, tuberculum sella, posterior fossa, and cavernous sinus. Meningiomas frequently express hormone binding sites; a statistically increased incidence of meningiomas is described in patients with breast cancer, and vice versa.

Etiology

Meningiomas arise from arachnoid "cap" cells associated with arachnoid granulations. Many meningiomas show loss of portions of tumor-suppressor genes on chromosome 22 (the same chromosome implicated in neurofibromatosis type 2).

Clinical Findings

Symptoms are related to mass effect with compression of underlying or adjacent structures and depend greatly on size and location of lesion. Patients with significant brain edema may present with headaches or seizures.

Pearls

- Meningiomas are often isointense to gray matter on all sequences and may be missed on non-contrast spin-echo imaging.
- Meningiomas may grow in an "en plaque" fashion, cloaking the inner surface of the skull and infiltrating bone and dura.
- Low signal in bone marrow is an indication of "hyperostosis".
- Calcified meningiomas are rarely malignant.

Pitfalls

- Meningiomas may be multiple in 16% of cases (even in the absence of neurofibromatosis type 2), so look carefully for additional lesions.
- Meningiomas may rarely arise extradurally (<1%). Sites of origin include the intradiploic space, outer table of skull, skin, paranasal sinuses, parotid gland, and parapharyngeal space.
- Benign, atypical, and malignant meningiomas may appear identical on imaging, although malignant tumors are more likely to demonstrate significant brain edema, brain invasion and "mushrooming" into the brain.
- Approximately 15% of meningiomas exhibit atypical imaging features including heterogeneous enhancement, cyst formation, hemorrhage, and/or fatty degeneration.

Complications

- Brain edema may be seen with benign or malignant meningiomas and is most common with convexity and sphenoid wing lesions. The mechanism is unclear but likely relates to vasoactive substances produced by the tumor, tumor parasitization of cortical vasculature, and/or impaired venous drainage.
- Encasement and narrowing of arterial structures may lead to transient ischemic attack or stroke.
- Invasion of an adjacent dural sinus may prevent complete resection.
- Acute hemorrhage is rare.
- Malignant transformation occurs in <1% of benign meningiomas.
- Blindness caused by parasellar or optic nerve/optic canal lesions can occur.

Pathology

Meningiomas typically have a lamellar internal structure with a firm central core at the dural attachment and a surrounding vascular mass at the periphery.

Gross

- Meningiomas may have a broad dural attachment ("sessile") or narrow attachment ("pedunculated")
- Usually a sharply defined brain-tumor interface
- The interface is less well-defined if the meningioma grows into the subarachnoid space or invades the brain

Microscopic

- Meningiomas have historically been divided into four subtypes: transitional, fibroblastic, angioblastic, and syncytial. These have distinctive cytoarchitecture.
- Criteria for diagnosing a malignant meningioma include hypercellularity, loss of architecture, nuclear pleomorphism, mitotic index, tumor necrosis and brain invasion

Imaging Findings

CT

- Extra-axial mass with a smooth interface with brain
- Homogeneous hyperattenuation prior to contrast
- Intense homogeneous enhancement post-contrast
- Hyperostosis
- Calcification is observed in 15 to 20% of cases
- Pneumosinus dilatans (abnormally expanded aerated sinus adjacent to a meningioma)

MR

- Well-circumscribed extra-axial mass displacing cortex inward
- Hypo- to isointense on T1-WI, iso- to hyperintense on T2-WI
- Homogeneous intense enhancement post-gadolinium
- "Dural tail" (thickening and intense enhancement of adjacent dura) is frequent but nonspecific

Treatment

- Complete surgical excision if possible

- Radiation therapy if the meningioma is malignant or if residual benign disease demonstrates progression
- Surgically inaccessible lesions may be treated with external beam radiation therapy or with gamma knife radiosurgery

Prognosis

- Excellent for benign convexity lesions. Parasagittal and skull base lesions often cannot be completely resected, so the prognosis is therefore more guarded, and radiation therapy is often required.
- Malignant lesions have high recurrence rate (~66% at 10 years)

Suggested Readings

Buetow MP, Buetow PC, Smirniotopoulos JG. Typical, atypical and misleading features in meningioma. *Radiographics* 11:1087–1106, 1991.

Elster AD, Challa VR, Gilbert TH, et al. Meningiomas: MR and histopathologic features. *Radiology* 170:857–862, 1989.

Goldsher D, Litt AW, Pinto RS, et al. Dural "tail" associated with meningiomas on Gd-DTPA-enhanced MR images: characteristics, differential diagnostic value, and possible implications for treatment. *Radiology* 176:447–450, 1990.

Case 59

Clinical Presentation

A 75-year-old woman with a history of breast cancer presents with increasing headache and confusion.

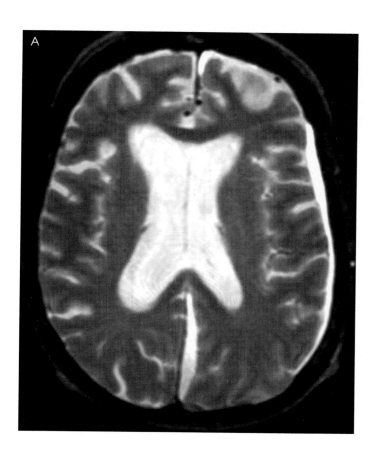

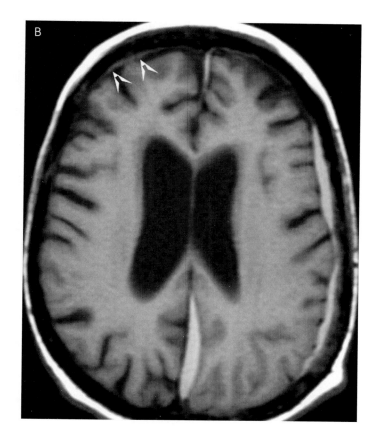

Radiologic Findings

An axial T2-WI (Fig. A) demonstrates a crescentic extra-axial fluid collection which is mildly hyperintense to CSF along the left frontoparietal convexity and the posterior falx. The extra-axial collection is hyperintense on a T1-WI (Fig. B). These findings are consistent with a subacute subdural hematoma. In addition, the dura over the right frontal lobe appears slightly thickened (*arrowheads*), and the calvarial marrow signal is somewhat heterogeneous.

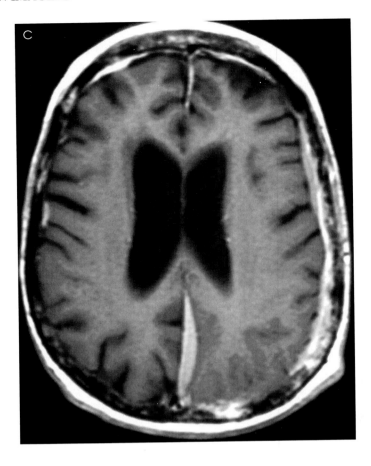

Pearls

- MR is more likely than CT to demonstrate features that suggest the diagnosis of dural metastases (nodular dural enhancement, other metastatic foci).

- Small spontaneous (nontraumatic) subdural hematomas in an older patient that fail to evolve/resolve as expected should raise possibility of hemorrhagic dural metastases and a contrast-enhanced MR should be obtained.

- Diffuse dural metastases may cause subdural effusion rather than hematoma.

Following gadolinium administration (Fig. C), a T1-WI demonstrates that the dura overlying the frontal lobes enhances intensely and is also somewhat thickened and nodular. In addition, there is heterogeneous enhancement of the calvarial marrow, most pronounced in the left parietal bone.

Diagnosis

Dural metastases complicated by subdural hematomas (pachymeningitis interna hemorrhagica)

Differential Diagnosis

- Post-traumatic subdural hematoma (post-contrast images, if done, show no nodularity)
- Spontaneous intracranial hypotension (postural headache is prominent, dural enhancement is diffuse and linear)
- Post-shunt or postoperative dural enhancement (evidence of prior procedure, dural enhancement is diffuse and linear)

Discussion

Background

Metastatic infiltration of the dura is unusual, representing ~5 to 10% of all intracranial metastases. Dural metastases most commonly appear as enhancing dural-

Pitfall

• An isolated dural metastasis may mimic a meningioma (Figs. D and E). However, dural metastases do not typically demonstrate hyperostosis, more often invade brain parenchyma and incite brain edema, and often show concurrent calvarial or brain parenchymal metastases.

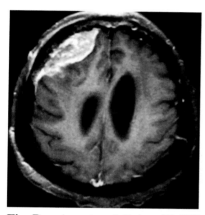

Fig. D. A post-gadolinium T1-WI demonstrates an enhancing extraaxial dural-based mass adjacent to the right frontal bone.

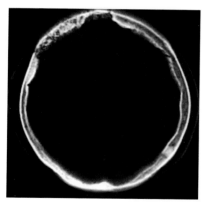

Fig. E. A CT scan in the patient in Fig. D shows a mixed lytic-sclerotic pattern in the right frontal bone. This is uncommon with meningioma but common with dural and calvarial metastatic disease. Metastatic carcinoma was confirmed surgically.

based mass(es) that may mimic meningioma. However, dural metastases are more commonly multiple than are meningiomas, and they more frequently invade the underlying brain parenchyma. They also tend to involve the overlying calvarium. Subdural hematoma formation is an uncommon complication of diffuse dural metastases and is usually seen secondary to adenocarcinomas of the breast or prostate.

Clinical Findings

Headache, seizure, and/or focal neurologic deficits secondary to mass effect are the typical presenting features.

Complications

A subdural hematoma may expand and cause brain herniation.

Pathophysiology

Mechanisms of dural metastases include direct infiltration of the dura by calvarial metastases and hematogenous dissemination. There are several theories of the origin of subdural hematoma associated with dural metastases:

• Obstruction of veins and capillaries in the outer dura with dilatation and rupture of capillaries in the inner dural layer
• Bleeding or hemorrhagic effusion from the tumor itself
• Angiogenetic response of the inner layer of the dura secondary to tumor invasion

Pathology

Gross

• Diffuse thickening of dura which appears hemorrhagic on inner surface

Microscopic

• Tumor deposits in dura
• Vascular granulation tissue enclosing organizing clot in the subdural space

Imaging Findings

CT

• Enhancing dural-based mass(es)
• Spontaneous subdural hematoma(s), which are often bilateral and heterogeneous
• Calvarial metastases may be present

MR

• Heterogeneous subdural collections with signal characteristics that vary with the age of hemorrhage
• Irregular and nodular dural enhancement
• Other metastatic foci (calvarium, brain parenchyma)

Treatment

• Radiation therapy is most commonly used
• The need for surgery is determined by the size of the subdural collections

Prognosis

Poor

Suggested Readings

Ambiavager PC, Sher J. Subdural hematoma secondary to metastatic neoplasm. Report of two cases and review of the literature. *Cancer* 42:2015–2018, 1978.

McKenzie CR, Rengachary SS, McGregor DH, et al. Subdural hematoma associated with metastatic neoplasms. *Neurosurgery* 27:619–625, 1990.

Turner DM, Graf CJ. Nontraumatic subdural hematoma secondary to dural metastasis: case report and review of the literature. *Neurosurgery* 11:678–680, 1982.

Case 60

Clinical Presentation

A 40-year-old African-American female with progressive headaches presents for evaluation.

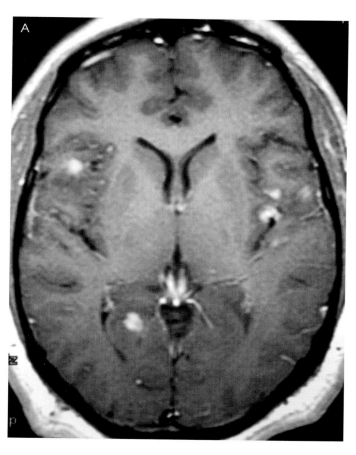

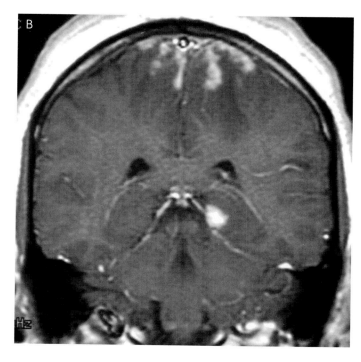

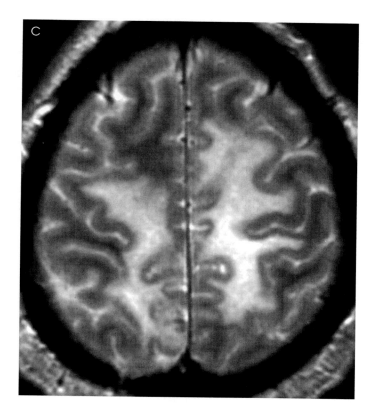

Radiologic Findings

A post-gadolinium axial T1-WI (Fig. A) demonstrates multiple enhancing nodules located peripherally within the cortex or arising from the leptomeninges. A post-gadolinium coronal T1-WI (Fig. B) demonstrates irregular, nodular dural and leptomeningeal enhancement overlying the superomedial aspect of the hemispheres bilaterally. Another focus of nodular enhancement is identified along the posteromedial temporal lobe. An axial T2-WI at the vertex (Fig. C) demonstrates striking T2 prolongation within the subcortical white matter, but a relative lack of mass effect.

Diagnosis

Neuro-sarcoidosis

Differential Diagnosis

- Dural or leptomeningeal metastases (may be indistinguishable)
- En plaque meningioma (older patient, hyperostosis, dural-based)
- Langerhans cell histiocytosis (usually in younger patients)
- Other granulomatous processes such as Wegener's granulomatosis or tuberculosis (patients often much more ill, but may be indistinguishable on imaging)

Discussion

Background

Sarcoidosis is a noninfectious multisystem granulomatous disease that is worldwide in distribution and has a prevalence of ~10 to 40 cases per 100,000 persons in the United States. It occurs more commonly in females than in males and is significantly more common in blacks than in whites. The disease is also more frequently acute and more severe in blacks. Symptomatic CNS involvement occurs in ~5% of cases, but pathologic CNS involvement is found in 10 to 15% of patients at autopsy.

Etiology

The etiology is unknown, although it seems that genetically predisposed hosts have an exaggerated cellular immune response to as yet undefined antigens, which leads to granuloma formation.

Clinical Findings

Patients can present with chronic headache (dural involvement), cranial neuropathy (leptomeningeal involvement), seizures or focal neurological findings (parenchymal involvement), or diabetes insipidus (involvement of infundibulum). The diagnosis of sarcoidosis is usually confirmed by tissue sampling, though measurement of serum or CSF angiotensin-converting enzyme (ACE) levels may be useful. ACE is elevated in 70 to 80% of patients with pulmonary sarcoidosis.

Pathology

Microscopic examination shows noncaseating granulomata that contain macrophages, epithelioid cells, and multinucleated giant cells.

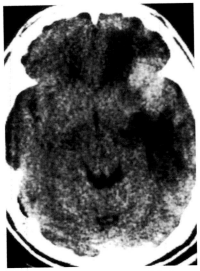

Fig D. A non-contrast CT shows an intrinsically dense mass involving the left sylvian region. Edema is noted in the adjacent brain parenchyma. Sarcoidosis.

Pearls

- Sarcoid masses are often hypointense on T2-WIs.

- Enhancement may course along the perivascular (Virchow-Robin) spaces (Figs. E and F).
(continued)

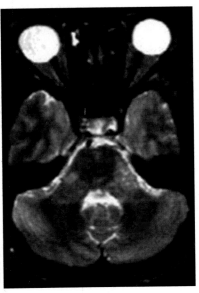

Fig. E. An axial T2-WI in a patient with known sarcoidosis shows high signal in the middle cerebellar peduncles bilaterally.

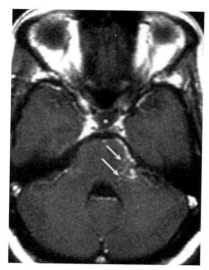

Fig. F. Postcontrast, an axial T1-WI (same patient as Fig. E) shows enhancement over the surface of the pons and the cerebellar peduncles. Enhancement appears to extend into the parenchyma (*arrows*), along perivascular spaces.

- MR is significantly more sensitive than CT in the detection of dural and leptomeningeal pathology.

Pitfalls

- Sarcoid is a great mimic: enhancing lesions may involve dura, leptomeninges, brain parenchyma, hypothalamic-pituitary axis, and cranial nerves (Fig. G).

- Rarely, patients with neurosarcoidosis will have no evidence of systemic disease.

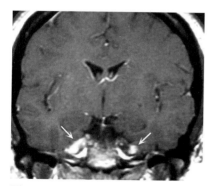

Fig. G. A coronal post-gadolinium T1-WI in a different patient with sarcoidosis shows intense enhancement in the region of the fifth nerve ganglia bilaterally (*arrows*), right greater than left.

Imaging Findings

CT

- Plaquelike or masslike dural thicking
- Often intrinsically dense (Fig. D), with homogeneous enhancement
- Generally no calcification or hemorrhage

MR

- Dural plaques are usually isointense on T1-WI and are frequently hypointense on T2-WI
- Homogeneous enhancement of involved dura and leptomeninges follows gadolinium administration
- Underlying brain parenchyma may be edematous
- Parenchymal lesions generally show nodular enhancement

Treatment

- Steroids
- Cytotoxic agents, radiation therapy, and/or surgical debulking may be required if there is a poor response to steroids alone

Prognosis

- Variable response
- Patients are at risk of complications of steroid and cytotoxic therapy

Suggested Readings

Seltzer S, Mark AS, Atlas SW. CNS sarcoidosis: evaluation with contrast-enhanced MR imaging. *AJNR* 12:1227–1233, 1991.

Stern BJ, Krumholz A, Johns C, et al. Sarcoidosis and its neurological manifestations. *Arch Neurol* 42:909–917, 1985.

Zouaoui A, Maillard JC, Dormont D, et al. MRI in neurosarcoidosis. *J Neuroradiol* 19:271–284, 1992.

Case 61

Clinical Presentation

A 44-year-old otherwise healthy female presents with severe postural headaches.

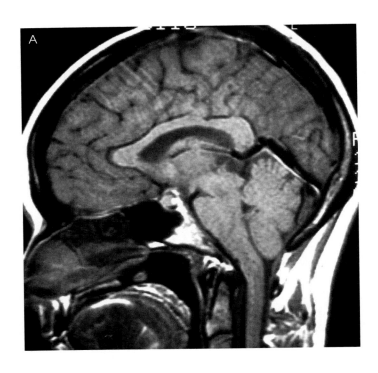

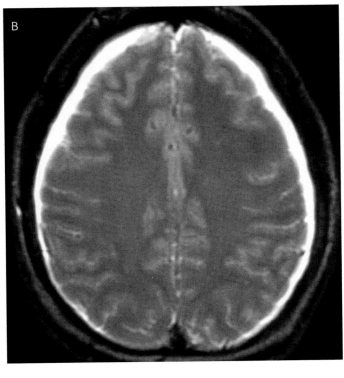

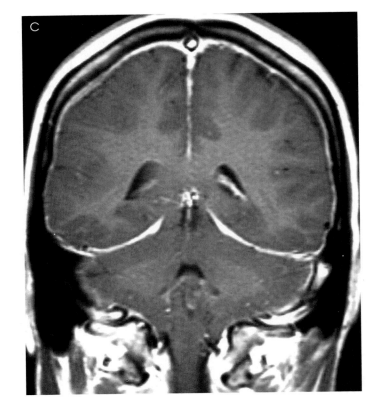

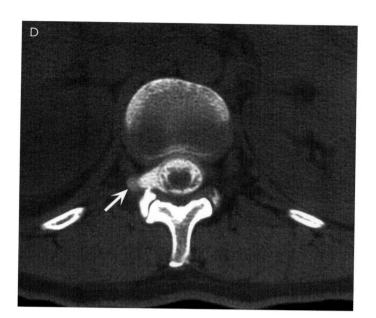

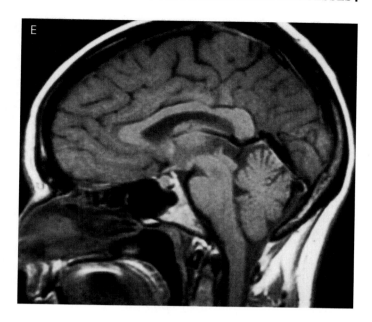

Radiologic Findings

A sagittal T1-WI (Fig. A) demonstrates mild downward displacement of the cerebellar tonsils, flattening of the pons against the dorsal clivus, draping of the optic chiasm over the sella, and prominence of the superior sagittal and straight sinuses. An axial T2-WI (Fig. B) shows small bilateral convexity subdural hematomas. Following gadolinium administration, a coronal T1-WI (Fig. C) shows diffuse, intense, smooth enhancement of the dura. A CT myelogram (Fig. D) performed for further evaluation of the patient's condition demonstrates a lower thoracic perineural cyst that is leaking into adjacent tissues (*arrow*). A follow-up scan after surgical ligation of the cyst (Fig. E) shows that the cerebellar tonsils have resumed a more normal position, and the pons is no longer flattened against the clivus.

Diagnosis

Spontaneous intracranial hypotension (SIH) due to rupture of a spinal perineural cyst

Differential Diagnosis

Of diffuse dural enhancement:

- Post-operative/post-shunt dural enhancement (clinical history essential)
- Dural metastases (less linear, more irregular and asymmetric)
- Sarcoid (more nodular dural enhancement; systemic features of disease)
- Wegener's granulomatosis (uncommonly involves the dura; associated sinopulmonary and/or renal symptoms)

Of low-lying cerebellar tonsils:

- Chiari I malformation (history of exertional or cough headache, lacks dural enhancement)
- Intracranial hypertension (often small ventricles, papilledema, effacement of dural venous sinuses)
- Tonsillar herniation (usually occurs in the setting of a posterior fossa mass)

Discussion

Background

The syndrome of intracranial hypotension results when CSF volume is lowered by leakage or by withdrawal of CSF in greater amounts than can be replenished by normal production. The syndrome is designated "spontaneous" in the absence of prior violation of the dura.

Etiology

Intracranial hypotension may be primary or secondary. Primary hypotension results from occult leakage of CSF, mainly from spinal sources in areas of intrinsic dural deficiency (e.g., perineural cyst). Secondary hypotension is associated with overt trauma which is often iatrogenic (arachnoid penetration during surgery, spinal anesthesia, or lumbar puncture). Severe dehydration (inadequate CSF production) has also been implicated in some cases.

Clinical Findings

Postural headache is elicited or exacerbated by upright positioning. Patients may also experience various cranial nerve deficits including diplopia, vertigo, and hearing loss. Severe cases may lead to altered mental status and even coma. CSF opening pressure is usually ≤ 40 mm H_2O in patients with the full-blown syndrome but may be normal. CSF analysis often shows mildly elevated protein and mild pleocytosis.

Pathology

Very few cases have correlative pathology, but dural thickening and fibrosis have been described.

Imaging Findings

CT

- Often normal
- Downward coning of midbrain and tonsillar herniation may be appreciated in severe cases
- Thickened enhancing dura post-contrast

MR

- Downward displacement of cerebellar tonsils (70%) and midbrain (70 to 80%) with elongation in the anteroposterior dimension
- Flattening of the pons against the dorsal clivus
- Draping of the optic chiasm over the sella
- Prominent upward convexity of the pituitary gland
- Distension of major dural venous sinuses
- Uniform, diffuse enhancement of the dura
- Subdural hematomas due to downward tension on the dura and rupture of bridging veins

Treatment

- May resolve spontaneously

- An epidural blood patch is frequently useful. Several attempts with large-volume ($\geq$20 cc) patches may be required. Performing the epidural blood patch under fluoroscopic guidance may be helpful if one or two attempts at empiric treatment have failed. This procedure involves mixing a few ccs of contrast with blood (1 cc contrast per 10 cc blood) and using real-time fluoroscopy to insure instillation into the epidural space near the suspected site of the leak.
- Cases of SIH that do not respond to empiric treatment with epidural blood patch require intensive radiologic evaluation to localize source of leak. Helpful studies include total spine imaging in multiple planes with T2-weighted fast spin-echo images with fat saturation, conventional myelography with bilateral decubitus views, total spine CT myelography, and nuclear cisternography.
- Cases refractory to epidural patch are often due to perineural cysts which leak into an epidural cystlike collection. These may require surgical repair if they can be located.

Prognosis

Excellent with careful attention to localizing the source of refractory leaks

Suggested Readings

Fishman RA, Dillon WP. Dural enhancement and cerebral displacement secondary to intracranial hypotension. *Neurology* 43:609–611, 1993.

Mokri B, Piepgras DG, Miller GM. Syndrome of orthostatic headache and diffuse pachymeningeal gadolinium enhancement. *Mayo Clin Proc* 72:400–413, 1997.

Rando TA, Fishman RA. Spontaneous intracranial hypotension: report of two cases and review of the literature. *Neurology* 42:481–487, 1992.

Case 62

Clinical Presentation

A 45-year-old woman with known breast cancer presents with worsening headache.

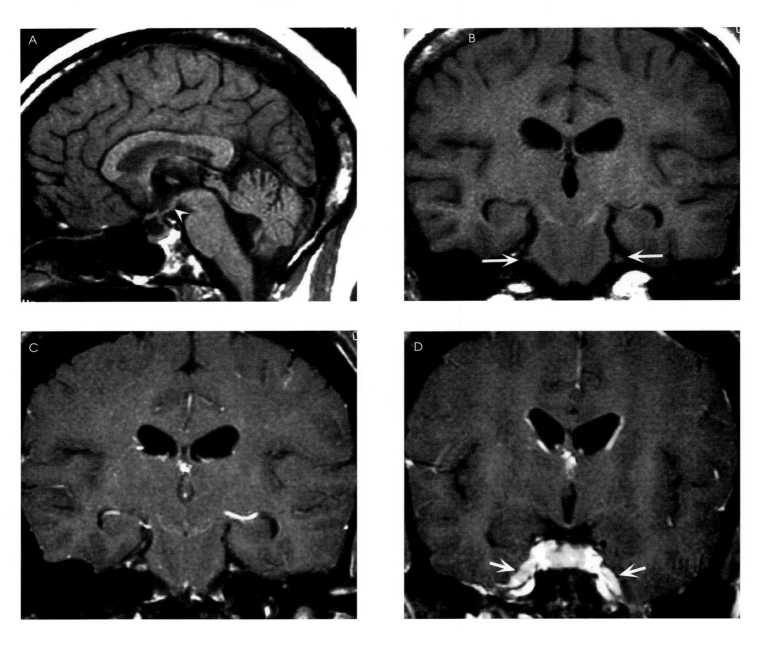

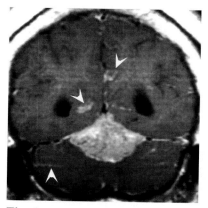

Fig. E. A post-gadolinium T1-WI in a patient with a history of breast cancer demonstrates a large dural-based mass, as well as extensive leptomeningeal enhancement (*arrowheads*). Dural and leptomeningeal metastases.

Pearls

- Contrast-enhanced MR is much more sensitive than CT to leptomeningeal pathology.

- The leptomeninges insinuate into the cerebral sulci, a feature which helps distinguish a leptomeningeal process from a dural process.

- Subarachnoid tumor may be detected early by careful examination of the cisternal segment of cranial nerve V and the intracanalicular portion of cranial nerves VII and VIII.

Radiologic Findings

A sagittal T1-WI (Fig. A) demonstrates heterogeneous signal within the clivus, consistent with bony metastatic disease. In addition, the third ventricle is dilated as evidenced by its floor of the third ventricle being convex downward (*arrowhead*). The aqueduct of Sylvius is also prominent, as is the fourth ventricle, and these findings suggest a degree of communicating hydrocephalus. A coronal T1-WI (Fig. B) shows slight prominence of the third ventricle and temporal horns, also consistent with communicating hydrocephalus. The cisternal segments of the fifth cranial nerves bilaterally (*arrows*) are unremarkable. Post-gadolinium coronal T1-WIs demonstrate abnormal enhancement along the cisternal segments of the fifth cranial nerves bilaterally (Fig. C) and also within Meckel's cave bilaterally (Fig. D, *arrows*). A lumbar puncture performed following the MR scan demonstrated an opening pressure of 200 mm of water, as well as markedly elevated protein. CSF cytology showed malignant cells.

Diagnosis

Carcinomatous meningitis secondary to breast cancer

Differential Diagnosis

- Lymphomatous meningitis (may be identical)
- Sarcoidosis (may be identical, need to correlate with CSF cytology and other studies such as chest x-ray)
- Fungal or tuberculous meningitis (often a dense basilar exudate)
- Severe leptomeningeal irritation secondary to subarachnoid hemorrhage or intrathecal chemotherapy (clinical history and cytologic examination helpful)
- Dural metastases (enhancement does not follow sulci or perivascular spaces)

Discussion

Background

Historically, meningeal carcinomatosis has been considered rare. It is now identified with increasing frequency because patients with systemic tumor are living longer due to advances in cancer treatment, and diagnostic methods have advanced (improved CSF cytology, gadolinium-enhanced MRI). At the present time, leptomeningeal metastases are thought to occur in ~8% of patients with CNS metastases. Leptomeningeal metastases are more common than dural metastases, though the two may coexist (Fig. E).

Etiology

Common primary neoplasms that cause carcinomatous meningitis include those of the breast, lung, and skin (melanoma). Tumor cells may reach the leptomeninges by several routes: hematogenous spread to small meningeal vessels or to the choroid plexus with subsequent shedding of tumor cells into the CSF, or direct extension of peripheral parenchymal metastases into the CSF space.

Clinical Findings

Carcinomatous meningitis presents as a low-grade meningitis syndrome with headache, nuchal rigidity, papilledema, and/or cranial nerve dysfunction.

Pitfalls

- MR findings suggestive of carcinomatous meningitis should be correlated with lumbar puncture and CSF cytology, as MR is abnormal in only 33 to 66% of cases of carcinomatous meningitis.

- The yield of cytology in the setting of carcinomatous meningitis is only 45% for the first tap but as high as 95% after six taps.

- *Dural* enhancement should not be confused with *leptomeningeal* enhancement, as the clinical implications are quite different.

- Contrast administration is essential to detect leptomeningeal carcinomatosis.

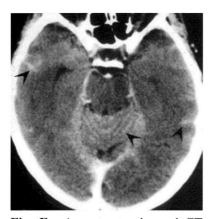

Fig. F. A contrast-enhanced CT scan in another patient with a history of breast cancer demonstrates abnormal leptomeningeal thickening and enhancement (*arrowheads*).

Complications

Communicating hydrocephalus secondary to blockage of CSF resorptive pathways is common.

Pathology

Gross

- Diffuse opaque thicking of leptomeninges

Microscopic

- Cellular infiltration of pia-arachnoid with reactive inflammatory changes in leptomeninges and often extension along perivascular spaces into brain parenchyma

Imaging Findings

CT

- Insensitive, may see leptomeningeal thickening and enhancement in severe cases (Fig. F)

MR

- T1- and T2-WIs often appear normal, but there may be loss of normal low-signal CSF in the subarachnoid space on T1-WI, and the subarachnoid space may appear abnormally bright on PD-WI or on the fluid-attenuated inversion recovery sequence (FLAIR)
- Post-gadolinium T1-WIs often show linear or nodular enhancement of the leptomeninges

Treatment

Systemic and intrathecal chemotherapy

Prognosis

Very poor

Suggested Readings

Sze G. Diseases of the intracranial meninges: MR imaging features. *AJR* 160:727–733, 1993.

Sze G, Soletsky S, Bronen R, Krol G. MR imaging of the cranial meninges with emphasis on contrast enhancement and meningeal carcinomatosis. *AJNR* 10:965–975, 1989.

Yousem DM, Patrone PM, Grossman RI. Leptomeningeal metastases: MR evaluation. *J Comput Assist Tomogr* 14:255–261, 1990.

Case 63

Clinical Presentation

A 45-year-old intravenous drug abuser presents with fever and altered mental status.

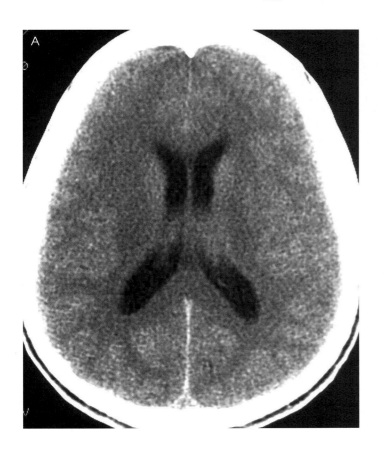 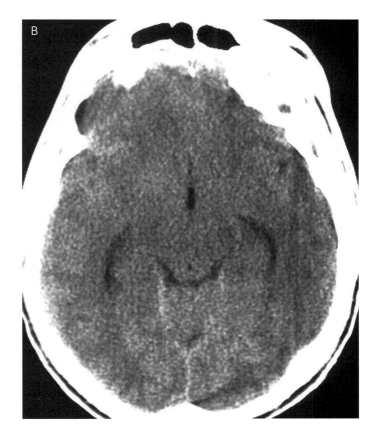

Radiologic Findings

A non-contrast CT scan (Fig. A) shows prominence of the lateral ventricles and poor visualization of cortical sulci. A more inferior image (Fig. B) shows slight prominence of the anterior recess of the third ventricle and the temporal horns. Visualization of sulci remains poor. The fourth ventricle is unremarkable (not shown), and these findings are consistent with communicating hydrocephalus.

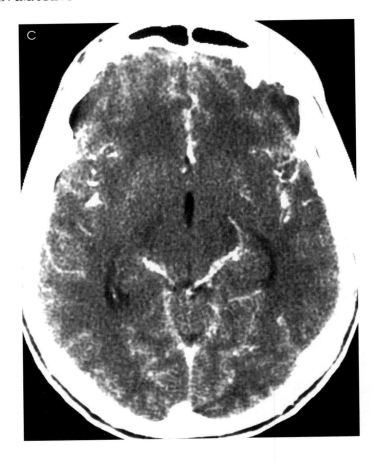

Following administration of contrast (Fig. C), there is intense linear enhancement over the brain surface, consistent with leptomeningeal enhancement.

Diagnosis

Pneumococcal meningitis

Differential Diagnosis

- Carcinomatous or lymphomatous meningitis (less acute clinical presentation, often a known underlying malignancy)
- Aseptic meningitis (need CSF to differentiate from bacterial meningitis)
- Tuberculous or fungal meningitis (usually more intense basal meningeal enhancement)
- Meningeal sarcoidosis (less fulminant clinical presentation, often known systemic sarcoidosis)

Discussion

Background

Bacterial meningitis is a purulent infection of the leptomeninges that generally presents acutely and may be fatal if not rapidly diagnosed and treated. Infectious organisms reach the meninges by a number of different routes: hematogenous spread, including spread to the choroid plexus; rupture of a cortical abscess into

Pearls

- The diagnosis of meningitis is made by lumbar puncture, with imaging indicated to assess for the compications of meningitis.
- Contrast-enhanced MR is much more sensitive than CT to certain complications such as ventriculitis (look for ependymal enhancement), venous thrombosis (may be cortical venous or dural venous sinus), and subdural or epidural empyema (especially if at the base of the skull).

Pitfalls

- A normal enhanced scan in no way excludes the diagnosis of meningitis.
- CT scans are often ordered to "see if patient can be tapped," but unfortunately, no CT findings definitively answer this question.
- Though there are some reports that lumbar puncture may cause brain herniation, the diagnosis of bacterial meningitis must be established. In some settings (such as a trapped fourth ventricle), a ventricular tap rather than a lumbar puncture may be indicated. If a patient has a mass lesion at initial presentation (abscess, empyema) then the diagnosis should be established with surgical intervention.
- Prominent vascular enhancement may be confused with leptomeningeal enhancement.

the subarachnoid space; penetrating trauma (which may be iatrogenic); and contiguous extension (sinusitis; otitis media).

Etiology

Common causative organisms vary with the age of the patient and include:

- Neonate: Group B streptococci, *Escherichia coli*, *Listeria monocytogenes*
- Child: *Hemophilus influenzae*, *Neisseria meningitidis*, *Streptococcus pneumoniae*
- Adult: *Streptococcus pneumoniae*, *Neisseria meningitidis*
- Elderly: *Listeria monocytogenes*, gram negative rods

Clinical Findings

Headache, fever, nuchal rigidity, papilledema, and nausea/vomiting are often present. Patients may progress rapidly to seizure, coma, and death. Neutrophilic pleocytosis, elevated protein, and decreased glucose are commonly seen on CSF analysis.

Complications

Complications include communicating or noncommunicating hydrocephalus, ventriculitis, brain abscess, subdural or epidural empyema, ischemia/infarction secondary to infectious vasculitis, and venous thrombosis.

Pathology

The meninges are lined by a purulent exudate that involves the base of the brain and may extend over the cerebral convexities. Perivascular inflammation is often prominent.

Imaging Findings

The findings vary with whether meningitis is uncomplicated or complicated

CT

- Frequently normal in the acute phase
- If abnormal, the most common finding is communicating hydrocephalus
- Complications of meningitis as outlined above may be seen

MR

- Frequently normal in the acute phase
- Leptomeningeal enhancement and communicating hydrocephalus are the most common findings

Treatment

- Antibiotics with high CSF penetration
- Surgery may be indicated to treat complications (abscess, empyema, hydrocephalus)

Prognosis

Variable: depends on underlying condition of patient and rapidity with which therapy is instituted

Suggested Readings

Castillo M. Magnetic resonance imaging of meningitis and its complications. *Topics Magn Res Imag* 6:53–58, 1994.

Harris TM, Edwards MK. Meningitis. *Neuroimag Clin North Am* 1:39–56, 1991.

Mellor DH. The place of computed tomography and lumbar puncture in suspected bacterial meningitis. *Arch Dis Child* 67:1417–1419, 1992.

Case 64

Clinical Presentation

A 20-year-old male is evaluated for headache and progressive obtundation.

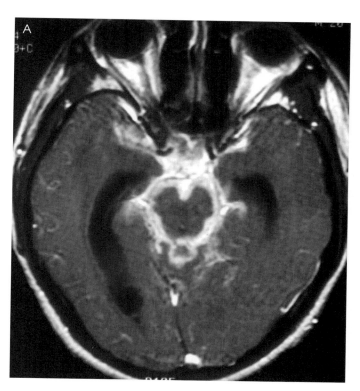

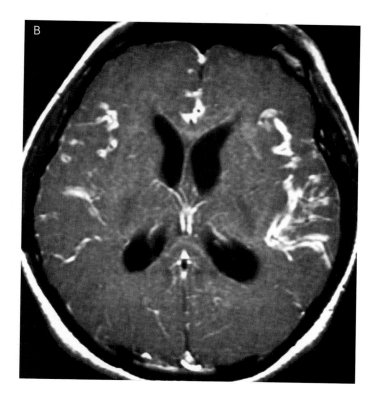

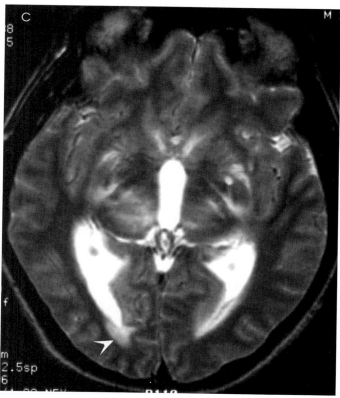

Radiologic Findings

An axial post-gadolinium T1-WI (Fig. A) demonstrates intense enhancement of the basal cisterns, as well as evidence of hydrocephalus. A more superior gadolinium-enhanced T1-WI (Fig. B) shows intense leptomeningeal enhancement involving the sylvian and interhemispheric cisterns. A T2-WI (Fig. C) demonstrates high signal likely related to ischemic change in the thalami and putamina bilaterally. There is also periventricular high signal (*arrowhead*), presumably due to transependymal flow of CSF.

Diagnosis

Meningitis secondary to *Coccidioides immitis* ("cocci" meningitis)

Differential Diagnosis

- Tuberculous meningitis (indistinguishable)
- Carcinomatous meningitis (often a less striking basal predominance)
- Bacterial meningitis (does not favor basal meninges, leptomeningeal enhancement is typically far more mild)
- Sarcoidosis (usually not such a thick, confluent basal meningitis)

Discussion

Background

Coccidioidomycosis is due to infection with the soil fungus *Coccidioides immitis*, which is endemic in parts of California and Arizona. Infection usually begins in the lungs and causes a mild self-limited respiratory infection. In ~0.5% of affected patients, the fungus may disseminate hematogenously to the CNS. Extrapulmonary dissemination is uncommon in whites (≤1% of cases) and is more common in blacks, Filipinos, and the immunosuppressed. Typically, the CNS involvement manifests as a basilar meningitis, but encephalitis and parenchymal granulomas and abscesses may be seen.

Etiology

C. immitis is a dimorphic fungus. In its mycelial phase, it grows in dry, dusty soil as branched septate hyphae. When mechanically disrupted, a portion of the hypha breaks off and becomes airborne. Once it enters host lung, it shifts into its parasitic phase and forms spherules filled with endospores. Rupture of spherules and release of endospores propagate the infection.

Clinical Findings

Chronic headache and symptoms of elevated intracranial pressure are the common presenting symptoms. The process may progress to seizures, focal neurological findings, coma, and death.

Complications

Complications include cranial neuropathy, vascular occlusions (less common than with TB), meningoencephalitis, meningomyelitis, and focal brain abscess (rare).

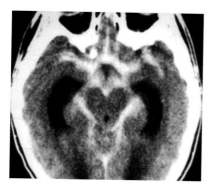

Fig. D. Post-contrast CT scan in a patient with coccidioidal meningitis demonstrates intense leptomeningeal enhancement in the basal cisterns, as well as severe hydrocephalus.

Pathology

Host response may be granulomatous, suppurative, or a combination of the two.

Imaging Findings

CT

- Communicating hydrocephalus
- Post-contrast scans show intense enhancement of the basal meninges (Fig. D)

MR

- Communicating hydrocephalus
- Thickening of the leptomeninges and obliteration of the cisternal spaces, which appear isointense on T1-WI and hyperintense on PD-WI and fluid-attenuated inversion recovery images
- Post-contrast scans show intense enhancement of basal meninges

Treatment

- Intrathecal amphotericin B
- Oral azoles such as fluconazole are given adjunctively and for chronic suppression

Prognosis

- With no therapy, 10% survival at 1 year; survival is >60% with amphotericin B
- Patients with cocci meningitis require chronic lifelong suppression with oral azoles: discontinuation of antifungal therapy may result in relapse and death

Suggested Readings

Dewsnup DH, Galgiani JN, Graybill JR, et al. Is it ever safe to stop azole therapy for Coccidioides immitis meningitis? *Ann Int Med* 124:305–310, 1996.

Mischel PS, Vinters HV. Coccidioidomycosis of the central nervous system: neuropathological and vasculopathic manifestations and clinical correlates. *Clin Infec Dis* 20:400–405, 1995.

Wrobel CJ, Meyer S, Johnson RH, Hesselink JR. MR findings in acute and chronic coccidioidomycosis meningitis. *AJNR* 13:1241–1245, 1992.

Case 65

Clinical Presentation

A 35-year-old man with a history of surgery for a "posterior fossa cyst" in childhood presents with ataxia and hearing loss.

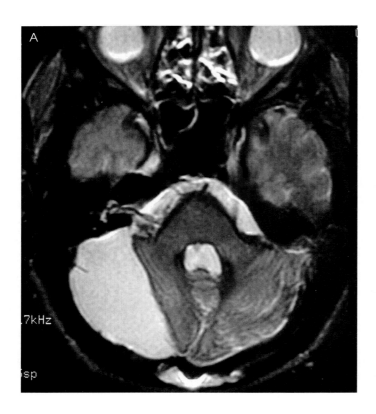

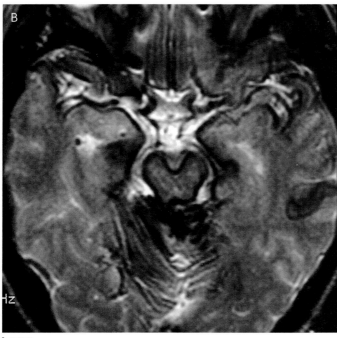

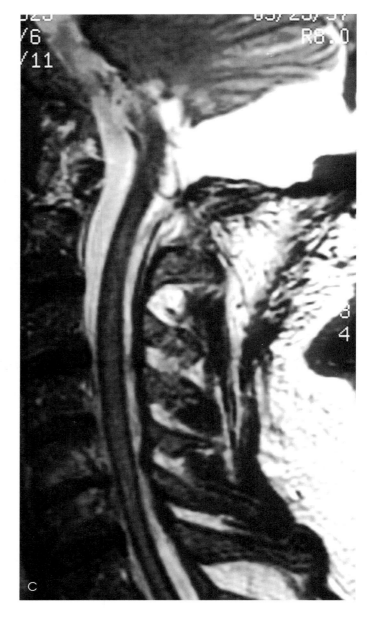

Pearls

- MR is much more sensitive than CT to the diagnosis, and the findings are more apparent with increasing field strength or with gradient echo-based sequences which enhance magnetic susceptibility effects.

- The location of siderosis corresponds to the extent of central myelin. Therefore, cranial nerves (CN) I, II, and VIII are preferentially affected because CN I and II are enveloped by central myelin over their entire cisternal course and CN VIII presents its transition point from central to peripheral myelin quite peripherally near the internal acoustic meatus, while other CNs have their transition points closer to the brain stem.

- CSF usually shows xanthochromia and elevated protein.

Pitfall

- If no etiology of chronic bleeding is identified intracranially by MR or cerebral angiography, MR of the spine should be performed to exclude a chronically bleeding spinal neoplasm such as an ependymoma or a paraganglioma.

Radiologic Findings

An axial T2-WI (Fig. A) shows a right posterior fossa cyst. In addition, there is striking hypointensity over the surface of the pons and cerebellar peduncles, and also along the right eighth nerve. A more superior T2-WI (Fig. B) demonstrates striking linear hypointensity around the midbrain, the vermian folia, and the medial temporal lobes. Similar hypointensity extends along the surface of the cervical spinal cord on a sagittal T2-WI (Fig. C). In addition, there is mild hyperintensity in the cord parenchyma.

Diagnosis

Superficial siderosis

Differential Diagnosis

None: this is a pathognomonic appearance. The only differential issue is the etiology of the siderosis.

Discussion

Background

Superficial siderosis is a rare condition characterized by deposition of hemosiderin in the leptomeninges and on the surface of the inferior cerebral hemispheres, cerebellum, brain stem, cranial nerves, and spinal cord. This entity was first described in 1940. Prior to the availability of MR imaging, this diagnosis could only be made at autopsy.

Etiology

The deposition of hemosiderin in the leptomeninges is secondary to massive or repetitive subarachnoid or intraventricular hemorrhage. Important causes include tumor-related hemorrhages (notably spinal ependymomas), vascular malformations, chronic subdural hematomas, spinal pseudomeningoceles, and friable posthemispherectomy membranes. In 25% of cases, no cause of bleeding is found, even at autopsy.

Clinical Findings

Symptoms include progressive bilateral hearing loss, ataxia, anosmia, long tract signs, and dementia. Over time, brain atrophy will ensue in severe cases.

Pathology

Gross

- Diffuse yellow-brown or orange discoloration of the leptomeninges and subpial surface of affected areas

Microscopic

- Leptomeningeal fibrosis and accumulation of hemosiderin-laden macrophages and fibroblasts

Imaging Findings

CT

- Usually normal but may rarely see mild hyperdensity around the brainstem
- Vermian atrophy may be apparent

MR

- A rim of hypointensity on T2-WI is present on the surface of the brainstem, cerebellum, inferior cerebral hemispheres, and upper cervical cord. This hypointensity may extend along cranial nerves, especially cranial nerves I, II, and VIII.
- Atrophy of the vermis and cerebellar hemispheres is common
- Enhancement of the thickened meninges may be seen

Treatment

- Removal of bleeding source if possible
- Iron-chelating agents may be useful

Prognosis

Usually slow progression of sensorineural hearing loss and ataxia if the source of the bleeding not removed

Suggested Readings

Bourgouin PM, Tampieri D, Melancon D, et al. Superficial siderosis of the brain following unexplained subarachnoid hemorrhage: MRI diagnosis and clinical significance. *Neuroradiology* 34:407–410, 1992.

Pyhtinen J, Paakko E, Ilkko E. Superficial siderosis in the central nervous system. *Neuroradiology* 37:127–128, 1995.

Section IV

Vascular/Ischemic

Case 66

Clinical Presentation

An 81-year-old woman presents with sudden onset of the worst headache of her life.

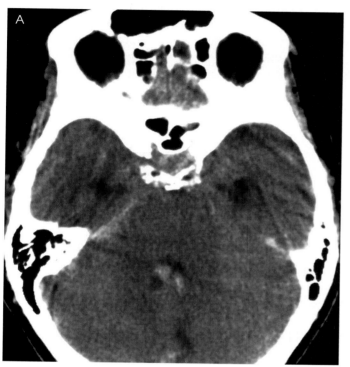

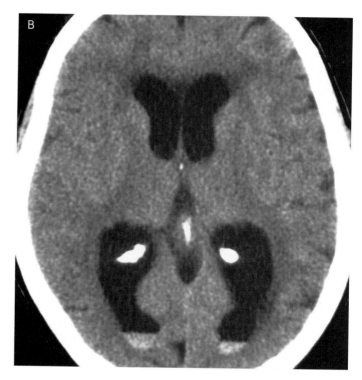

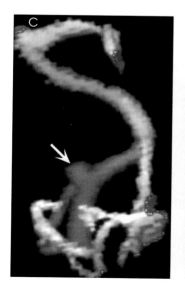

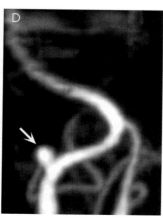

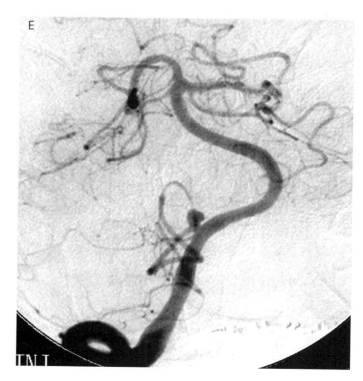

Radiologic Findings

A non-contrast CT scan (Fig. A) demonstrates blood within the fourth ventricle. In addition, the peripontine cisterns are poorly visualized due to subarachnoid blood. A more cephalad image (Fig. B) demonstrates blood within dilated third and lateral ventricles. The ventricles are enlarged out of proportion to the sulci, consistent with obstructive hydrocephalus. A CT angiogram was performed for further evaluation. Figures C and D represent postprocessed projection images, with Figure C representing a shaded surface display and Figure D representing a maximum intensity projection image. Both demonstrate a saccular aneurysm at the origin of the right posterior inferior cerebellar artery (PICA) (*arrows*). This finding was confirmed with conventional catheter angiography. An anteposterior (AP) projection from a right vertebral artery injection (Fig. E) demonstrates a slightly irregular saccular aneurysm at the origin of the right PICA.

Diagnosis

Subarachnoid hemorrhage (SAH) and intraventricular hemorrhage (IVH) due to ruptured saccular aneurysm arising at PICA origin

Differential Diagnosis

- Post-traumatic SAH/IVH (no history of trauma; not classic location for post-traumatic SAH, which is typically seen in the quadrigeminal plate cistern and the posterior sylvian cistern or over the cerebral convexity)
- SAH/IVH due to extension of parenchymal hematoma into CSF spaces (expect a parenchymal hemorrhage)
- Vascular malformation with bleeding exclusively into CSF spaces (could lead to these findings on non-contrast CT; an arteriovenous malformation would be appropriately assessed with CT angiography and/or conventional angiography, but a cryptic malformation would be missed and would be best assessed with MR)

Discussion

Background

Each year in the United States, there are 25,000 new cases of subarachnoid hemorrhage due to rupture of an intracranial aneurysm. Autopsy studies suggest that there is a 2 to 5% prevalence of intracranial aneurysms in the general population. This figure is increased in patients with conditions that predispose to intracranial aneurysm formation such as adult polycystic kidney disease, Marfan syndrome, Ehlers-Danlos syndrome, and fibromuscular dysplasia. There is also an increased risk of intracranial aneurysm in people who have first-degree relatives who have suffered aneurysmal rupture, and intracranial aneurysms will be multiple in 20 to 30% of cases. Additionally, aneurysm formation has been described as a complication associated with carotid ligation or carotid balloon occlusion, presumably on the basis of altered hemodynamic stresses in the remaining cerebral vasculature. Aneurysmal SAH is uncommon in children and is more frequently associated with trauma or infection than in adults.

• An initial angiogram may be negative in cases of SAH that later turn out to be aneurysmal in origin. This may be related to temporary thrombosis, compression by hematoma, or technical factors.

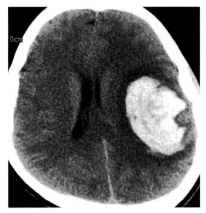

Fig. F. A non-contrast CT scan in a 23-year-old woman with bacterial endocarditis shows a large left frontoparietal parenchymal hematoma with surrounding edema and mass effect.

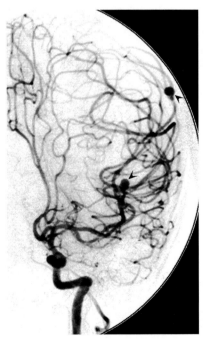

Fig. G. AP projection of a left internal carotid artery injection (same patient as Fig. F) demonstrates two saccular aneurysms arising from middle cerebral artery (MCA) branches (*arrowheads*). The more inferior aneurysm is quite irregular and was considered to be the cause of the hemorrhage. Mycotic aneurysms.

Etiology

Both congenital and acquired factors are implicated in the development of saccular or "berry" aneurysms. Defects in the media of the arterial wall as well as defects in the internal elastic lamina are found in certain locations such as arterial bifurcations and sites of involution of embryonic vessels. Trauma and infection (Figs. F and G) may predispose to aneurysm formation by damaging and weakening vessel walls.

Clinical Findings

Headache (often severe and of precipitous onset), nuchal rigidity, drowsiness, and nausea and vomiting are associated with SAH. Patients are typically graded using the system of Hunt and Hess (Table 1). A not-yet-ruptured but enlarging aneurysm may cause symptoms by compressing adjacent structures (i.e., a posterior communicating artery aneurysm may present with a cranial nerve III palsy).

Table 1. Hunt and Hess Assessment of Patients with SAH

Grade 1	Asymptomatic, or minimal headache and slight nuchal ridigity
Grade 2	Moderate to severe headache, nuchal rigidity, no neurologic deficit other than cranial nerve palsy
Grade 3	Drowsiness, confusion, or mild focal deficit
Grade 4	Stupor, moderate to severe hemiparesis, possibly early decerebrate rigidity and vegetative disturbances
Grade 5	Deep coma, decerebrate rigidity, moribund appearance

Complications

Complications include hydrocephalus, which may be communicating or noncommunicating, and coma. Vasospasm typically occurs 4 to 12 days after SAH and may lead to cerebral infarction.

Pathology

Gross

• Saccular aneurysms are typically located in the circle of Willis, especially the anterior communicating artery (30 to 35%), posterior communicating artery (30 to 35%), and middle cerebral artery trifurcation (20%)
• The posterior circulation is affected in 10 to 15% of cases, typically the top of the basilar artery (10%) or less commonly the posterior inferior cerebellar artery origin (<3%)
• More distally located aneurysms are associated with trauma and infection

Microscopic

• Defect in muscularis media or absence of internal elastic lamina
• Thinning of arterial wall

Imaging Findings

CT

• High-density blood within subarachnoid space
• May be associated with IVH or parenchymal hematoma

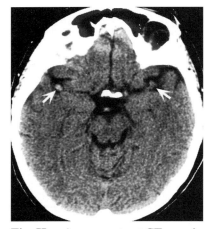

Fig. H. A non-contrast CT scan in a 54-year-old woman with headaches was suggestive, but not diagnostic, of bilateral MCA trifurcation aneurysms (*arrows*).

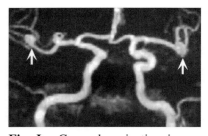

Fig. I. Coronal projection image from an MR angiogram (same patient as Fig. H) confirms the presence of the bilateral MCA trifurcation aneurysms (*arrows*) that were suggested on the CT scan.

- The pattern of hemorrhage may give a clue to the location of the ruptured aneurysm, with typical patterns being:
    1. Anterior communicating artery: interhemispheric fissure
    2. Posterior communicating artery: ipsilateral basal cisterns
    3. MCA trifurcation: sylvian fissure
    4. Basilar tip: interpeduncular fossa, intraventricular
    5. PICA: posterior fossa cisterns, intraventricular
- Routine CT may rarely demonstrate an unruptured saccular aneurysm (Figs. H and I)
- CT angiography may directly demonstrate an aneurysm

MR

- Not usually indicated in the evaluation of acute, typical SAH
- If performed, may detect subarachnoid blood as showing increased signal compared with CSF on proton-density and fluid-attenuated inversion recovery (FLAIR) sequences
- MR angiography may demonstrate the offending aneurysm

Conventional arteriography

Demonstrates a saccular outpouching, typically at an arterial bifurcation

Treatment

- Supportive care, with managment of complications such as hydrocephalus and vasospasm
- Surgical clipping for definitive therapy
- Endovascular coiling in patients who are poor surgical candidates because of the location of the aneurysm or medical factors. However, in many institutions, this technique is becoming a mainstay of acute treatment.
- Wide-necked aneurysms may need to be treated by excluding them from the circulation surgically or by endovascular methods

Prognosis

- Sixty to 75% of patients with aneurysmal SAH will die or have severe disability as a result of their initial hemorrhage. Twenty-five to 35% of patients will die of rehemorrhage if they go untreated.
- Unruptured aneurysms are thought to have a risk of rupture of approximately 2.3% per year. The cumulative rate of bleeding for unruptured aneurysms is estimated to be approximately 20% at 10 years and 35% at 15 years.

Suggested Readings

Camarata PJ, Latchaw RE, Rufenacht DA, Heros RC. Intracranial aneurysms. *Investig Radiol* 28:373–382, 1993.

Hunt WE, Hess RM. Surgical risk as related to time of intervention in the repair of intracranial aneurysms. *J Neurosurg* 28:14–20, 1968.

Yasui N, Suzuki A, Nishimura H, Suzuki K, Abe T. Long-term follow-up study of unruptured intracranial aneurysms. *Neurosurgery* 40:1155–1160, 1997.

Case 67

Clinical Presentation

A 63-year-old woman with recent onset of a left third nerve palsy presents for evaluation.

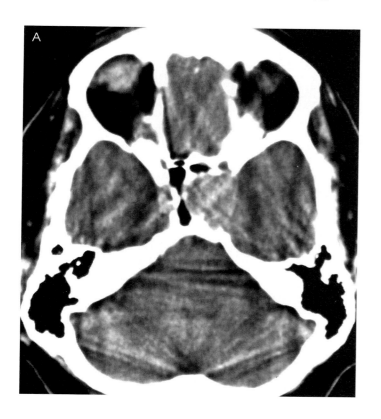

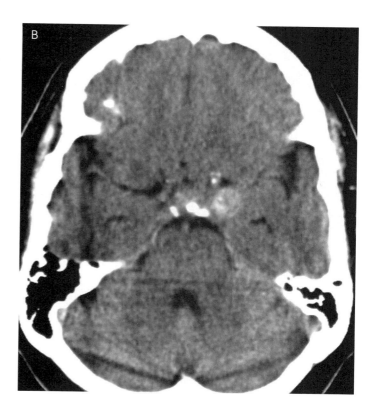

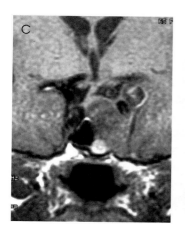

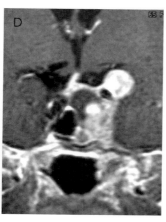

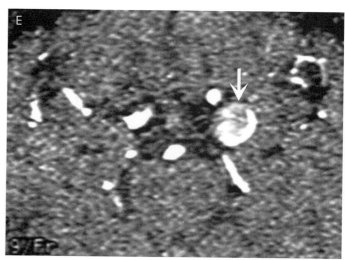

Pearl

- The identification of phase artifact on MR images is very helpful in suggesting the diagnosis of aneurysm (Fig. G). Visualization of phase artifact can be facilitated by viewing a sequence with wide windows.

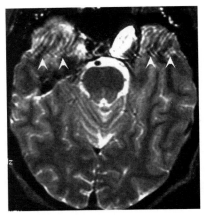

Fig. G. An axial T2-WI in a 45-year-old man demonstrates a mass lesion centered in the left cavernous sinus, with areas of mixed high and low intensity. Note the prominent phase artifact extending across the image (*arrowheads*) from this large aneurysm.

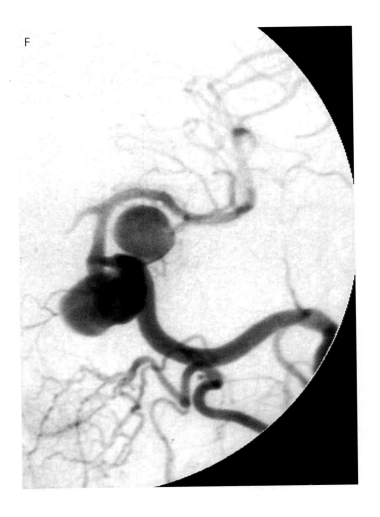

F

Radiologic Findings

A non-contrast CT scan at the level of the cavernous sinus (Fig. A) demonstrates a rounded mass which remodels the left sphenoid bone and appears slightly hyperdense compared with adjacent brain parenchyma. Slightly superior, a rounded hyperdense mass is identified to the left of the dorsum sella (Fig. B). A coronal T1-WI from an MR scan (Fig. C) demonstrates a heterogeneous ovoid soft tissue mass remodeling the left sphenoid sinus and deviating the pituitary stalk to the right. A second somewhat heterogeneous mass lesion is identified superolateral to the left cavernous carotid artery. Following administration of gadolinium (Fig. D), a T1-WI demonstrates partial, heterogeneous enhancement of the more inferomedial mass. The superolateral lesion enhances intensely and more homogeneously. An axial partition image from an MR angiogram obtained prior to administration of gadolinium (Fig. E) shows flow-related enhancement within one of the two mass lesions (*arrow*). A catheter angiogram was performed. An anteroposterior projection from a left common carotid artery injection (Fig. F) demonstrates filling of a bilobed lesion projecting inferiorly and medially from the cavernous carotid artery. A second rounded, contrast-filled structure projects superiorly from the posterior aspect of the left cavernous segment.

Diagnosis

Large and giant aneurysms of the internal carotid artery

Pitfalls

- Methemoglobin within a thrombosed aneurysm may mimic flow on time-of-flight MR angiography because of "shine-through" due to the clot's intrinsic high-signal intensity. However, phase-contrast MR angiography techniques will resolve this problem.

- Giant serpentine aneurysm is a subgroup of giant aneurysm that is often associated with progressive neurologic deficits, edema, and mass effect, and can be mistaken for a neoplasm on routine imaging studies.

- Giant cavernous aneurysms can erode through the skull base and mimic a skull base or infratemporal fossa neoplasm. Biopsy can have disastrous consequences in these cases.

- Angiography may underestimate the size of a giant aneurysm because it only demonstrates the patent lumen. Therefore, CT and/or MR are complementary to angiography.

Differential Diagnosis

- Schwannoma of cavernous sinus (no phase artifact, no flow on MRA)
- Meningioma of cavernous sinus (no phase artifact, often extends back along the tentorium)
- Cavernous hemangioma of cavernous sinus (intensely enhancing, bright on T2-WI, no phase artifact)

Discussion

Background

Aneurysms are classified according to size as small (<15 mm in diameter), large (15 to 25 mm), and giant (>25 mm). Giant aneurysms represent 5 to 7% of aneurysms in most series. Giant aneurysms present with subarachnoid hemorrhage as frequently as smaller aneurysms, but they may also present with symptoms and signs of an expanding mass lesion. Giant aneurysms most frequently occur in the cavernous and supraclinoid carotid segments, and less commonly arise from the vertebral artery (approximately 5% of intracranial giant aneurysms) or intracranial carotid segments.

Clinical Findings

There are two main presentations of giant aneurysms. Subarachnoid hemorrhage presents with sudden headache, nuchal rigidity, focal neurologic deficit, and/or coma. Mass effect presents with headache, cranial neuropathy, and symptoms of brainstem compression.

Complications

A giant aneurysm may rupture into the subdural space. Embolic events may be related to thrombus formation within the lumen of giant aneurysms.

Pathology

Gross

- Rounded mass often with peripheral calcification
- Layers of thrombus of varying ages

Microscopic

- Wall consists primarily of adventitia, thinned or defective media, and thickened intima with fibrocollagenous tissue and areas of calcification
- The internal elastic lamina is deficient or absent

Imaging Findings

CT

- Mass lesion that is typically intrinsically dense prior to contrast and has peripheral calcification
- Post-contrast, there may be enhancement of a patent lumen

MR

- Mass lesion that usually contains lamellated thrombus and is visualized as alternating layers of bright, intermediate, and dark material on all sequences. If there is no thrombus, the lesion will appear as a homogeneous flow void on all sequences.

- Phase artifact is usually visible if there is flow within a residual lumen
- MR angiography may directly demonstrate flow within a residual lumen

Angiography

- May not demonstrate the lesion if the aneurysm is completely thrombosed
- These lesions are often wide necked and incorporate branch vessels into the mouth of the aneurysm

Treatment

- Surgical clipping
  1. Multiple clips may be required to adequately exclude the aneurysm from the circulation. In addition, the parent artery must often be reconstructed with part of the aneurysmal wall itself.
  2. Giant aneurysms are often debulked after they have been completely eliminated from the circulation in order to decrease mass effect
- Endovascular management
  1. Coil embolization: small-necked aneurysms are best suited to this method
  2. Parent artery occlusion: a balloon test occlusion with hypotensive challenge is generally performed preoperatively in order to minimize the risk of post-occlusion hemispheric infarction
  3. A combination of endovascular and surgical techniques may be useful in some cases

Prognosis

The prognosis of untreated giant intracranial aneurysm is dismal as a result of hemorrhage, thromboembolism, and compression of vital structures

Suggested Readings

Camarata PJ, Latchaw RE, Rufenacht DA, Heros RC. Intracranial aneurysms. *Investig Radiol* 28:373–382, 1993.

Lawton MT, Spetzler RF. Surgical management of giant intracranial aneurysms: experience with 171 patients. *Clin Neurosurg* 42:245–266, 1995.

Standard SC, Guterman LR, Chavis TD, Fronckowiak MD, Gibbons KJ, Hopkins LN. Endovascular management of giant intracranial aneurysms. *Clin Neurosurg* 42:267–293, 1995.

Case 68

Clinical Presentation

A 43-year-old male presents with sudden onset of the worst headache of his life.

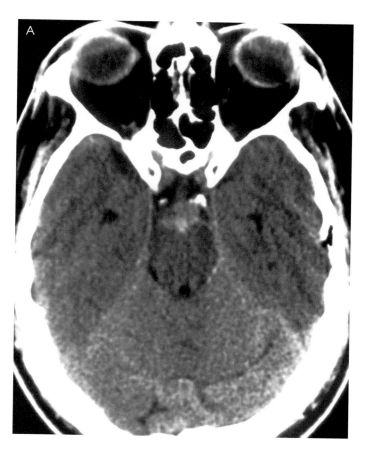

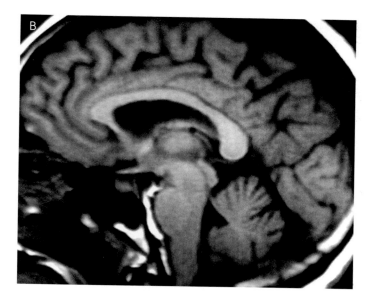

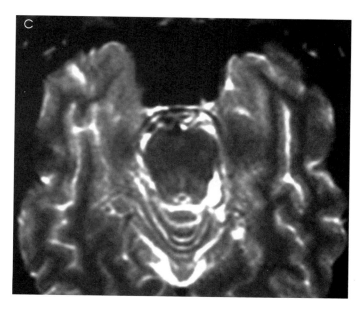

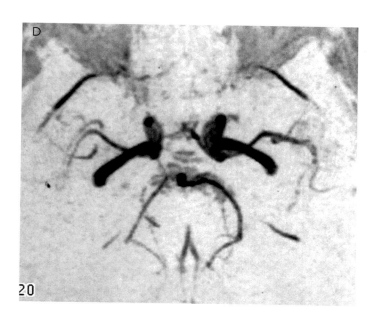

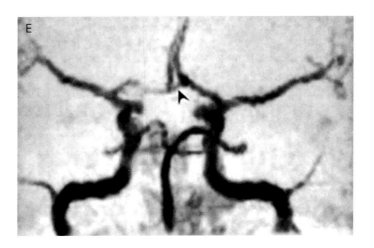

Radiologic Findings

A non-contrast CT scan (Fig. A) demonstrates high-density material within the interpeduncular cistern. MR imaging/angiography was performed to rule out aneurysm. A sagittal T1-WI (Fig. B) demonstrates high-signal intensity material in the prepontine and premedullary cisterns. On a T2-WI (Fig. C), this material is hypointense. A collapsed view from intracranial MR angiography (Fig. D) and a coronal maximum intensity projection from the MR angiogram (Fig. E) show no evidence of aneurysm. Note the excellent visualization of the anterior communicating artery (*arrowhead*). The individual partition images were also unremarkable. A conventional four-vessel catheter angiogram (not shown) was negative as well.

Diagnosis

Perimesencephalic nonaneurysmal subarachnoid hemorrhage (PNSH, also known as benign perimesencephalic hemorrhage)

Differential Diagnosis

- Aneurysmal subarachnoid hemorrhage (often more blood in basal cisterns, usually a positive angiogram)
- Post-traumatic SAH (history of trauma; typically seen in sylvian fissures and ambient cisterns, as well as over the cerebral convexities)
- Intracranial arterial dissection with rupture of a dissecting aneurysm (evident angiographically)
- Pituitary apoplexy with SAH (sellar/suprasellar mass with evidence of hemorrhage)

Discussion

Background

Approximately 15% of patients presenting with SAH will have no lesion revealed by an initial four-vessel cerebral angiogram. Some of these cases are due to occult aneurysms or arteriovenous malformations that are concealed by vasospasm, adjacent hematoma with mass effect, thrombosis (partial or complete), small size, or a technically inadequate study. These occurrences have led to the common practice of repetition of cerebral angiography, which yields pathologic findings in 2 to 24% of cases. However, a substantial number of cases will remain idiopathic. It is estimated that as many as 60 to 70% of cases of angiogram-negative SAH are accounted for by PNSH.

Etiology

PNSH is, by definition, nonaneurysmal and has the center of the hemorrhage located immediately anterior to the midbrain or within the prepontine cistern (which in some cases may be the only site of hemorrhage). Extension of blood to the anterior part of the ambient cistern or to the basal part of the sylvian fissure may occur. Frank intraventricular hemorrhage is absent. The hemorrhage is located posterior to the membrane of Liliequist. Blood that has transgressed the membrane of Liliequist and passed into the chiasmatic or interhemispheric cisterns is more likely to be aneurysmal in origin The source of the bleeding in PNSH is considered to be venous, although there is no direct evidence to support this. A recent case report shows PNSH associated with a capillary telangiectasia.

Clinical Findings

Patients with PNSH tend to be younger, less hypertensive, and predominantly male as compared with patients with aneurysmal SAH. Symptoms are similar to those of aneurysmal SAH: sudden onset of headache, meningismus, photophobia, and nausea. Most patients are Hunt and Hess Grade 1 or 2 at presentation (see Case 66 for a discussion of grading).

Complications

Angiogram-negative SAH is associated with a subsequent bleeding rate of 2 to 5%, while rebleeding complicates less than 1% of cases of PNSH. Minor transient ventricular enlargement is common, but shunts are rarely required. The frequency of clinical vasospasm is low in PNSH, but follow-up angiography will show angiographic spasm in as many as 42% of patients.

Imaging Findings

CT

- Typically shows blood in perimesencephalic cisterns
- Communicating hydrocephalus, usually mild, may be present

MR

- May also demonstrate subarachnoid blood, particularly on proton density-weighted and fluid-attenuated inversion recovery (FLAIR) sequences
- May be more sensitive than CT to subacute (>3 days old) blood

Angiography

- No aneurysm is demonstrated
- Mild vasospasm may be detected, usually on follow-up studies at 10 to 24 days posthemorrhage

Treatment

- Supportive care

- Management of complications such as hydrocephalus or vasospasm (uncommon)

Prognosis

PNSH has a good outcome in close to 100% of cases, without delayed cerebral ischemia or rehemorrhage. This is in contrast to good outcomes of 88% in other patients with negative angiographic findings and 64% for those with aneurysms.

Suggested Readings

Kallmes DF, Clark HP, Dix JE, et al. Ruptured vertebrobasilar aneurysms: frequency of the nonaneurysmal perimesencephalic pattern of hemorrhage on CT scans. *Radiology* 201:657–660, 1996.

Rinkel GJE, Wijdicks EFM, Vermeulen M, et al. Nonaneurysmal perimesencephalic subarachnoid hemorrhage: CT and MR patterns that differ from aneurysmal rupture. *AJNR* 12:829–834, 1991.

Schwartz TH, Solomon RA. Perimesencephalic nonaneurysmal subarachnoid hemorrhage: review of the literature. *Neurosurgery* 39:433–440, 1996.

Case 69

Clinical Presentation

A 46-year-old man presents with acute onset of left hemiparesis.

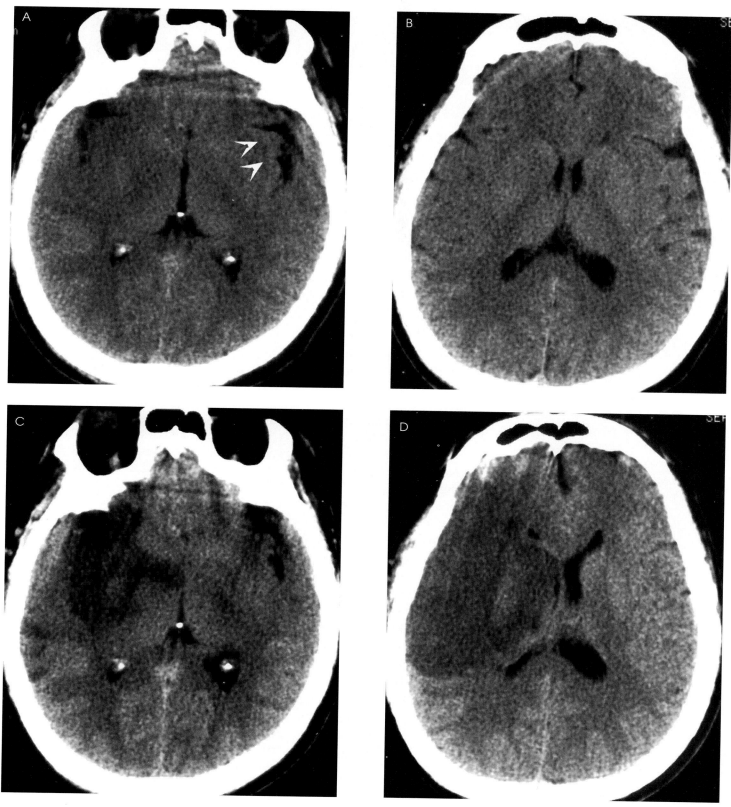

Radiologic Findings

A non-contrast CT scan obtained 3 hours after the onset of symptoms (Fig. A) demonstrates loss of the normal cortical insular ribbon on the right. Compare with the normal-appearing insular ribbon on the left (*arrowheads*). At a slightly more superior level (Fig. B), sulci are mildly effaced in the right sylvian region as compared with the left. In addition, the right putamen appears mildly hypodense as compared with the left. Follow-up images obtained 24 hours after the onset of symptoms (Figs. C and D) demonstrate clear-cut low density involving the right insular region, right frontal lobe, right putamen, and portions of the right caudate nucleus. There is accompanying sulcal effacement and mass effect on the right lateral ventricle. A medical evaluation in this patient was remarkable for a patent foramen ovale demonstrated by echocardiography.

Diagnosis

Acute infarction in the territory of the right middle cerebral artery (MCA)

Differential Diagnosis

- Herpes simplex virus type I encephalitis (typically involves the insula, but clinical presentation is quite different)
- Infiltrative glioma (subacute rather than abrupt onset, stable on short interval follow-up scans)

Discussion

Background

The term "stroke" refers to the acute onset of an irreversible focal neurologic deficit. Stroke is the third leading cause of death in the United States and is the major cause of serious long-term disability among adults. CT is generally the study of choice in the acute setting in order to exclude nonstroke etiologies (such as a subdural hematoma or neoplasm) as the cause of the patient's deficit, to define the type of stroke (ischemic or hemorrhagic), and to define the extent of the infarction. Large vessel occlusions account for most cases of cerebral infarction, and the territory of the MCA is most commonly involved. In patients with acute ischemic infarction, CT scans may be normal early on, unless a hyperdense MCA is present. After several hours, clear signs of an ischemic infarct may become evident: loss of the insular ribbon, obscuration of the lentiform nucleus, mild mass effect manifested as sulcal asymmetry, and loss of gray matter-white matter differentiation. MR is more sensitive to hyperacute infarction than CT, as it allows direct visualization of an absent flow void and arterial enhancement. CT and MR are both sensitive to subacute and chronic infarctions, but MR is the study of choice to assess brainstem and cerebellar infarctions. New MR techniques such as diffusion and perfusion imaging will offer further insight into the early diagnosis of ischemic stroke and pathophysiological mechanisms.

Etiology

Strokes are broadly divided into those that are ischemic (80%) and those that are due to primary intracerebral hemorrhage (15%). Ischemic stroke is further subdivided into thrombotic or embolic events. Large vessel thromboembolic events oc-

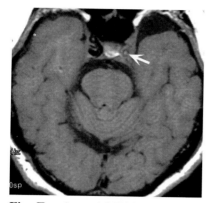

Fig. E. An axial T1-WI in a 78-year-old man with acute onset of aphasia demonstrates slow flow or occlusion of the left cavernous carotid artery (*arrow*).

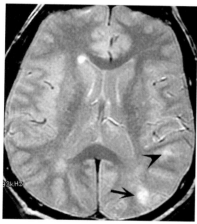

Fig. F. An axial proton density-weighted image (same patient as Fig. E) shows a focus of T2 prolongation in the left posterior parieto-occipital region that did not explain the patient's symptoms (*arrow*). A questionable focus was identified slightly more anteriorly (*arrowhead*).

cur in 50% of cases, perforator vessel (lacunar) infarcts in 25%, cardiogenic emboli in 15 to 20%, and vasculitis/vasculopathy in 5%. Intracranial hemorrhage may be caused by hypertension, amyloid angiopathy, tumors, and vascular malformations. Non-traumatic subarachnoid hemorrhage accounts for approximately 5% of "strokes." Venous infarction accounts for a small percentage of strokes as well.

Pathophysiology

Ischemic infarction results when cerebral blood flow falls below 10 ml/100 g brain tissue/min, at which point cells lose their ability to maintain intracellular ion concentrations (energy failure). Normal gray matter requires 60 to 80 ml/100 g/min, and normal white matter requires 20 to 25 ml/100 g/min. At 15 to 18 ml/100 g/min, electrical failure ensues (reversible if blood flow is restored). At levels below 10 ml/100 g/min for several minutes, cells will die even if blood flow is restored. Between "electrical failure" and "energy failure" the cells may survive for several hours and function will normalize if blood flow is restored–this state defines the so-called ischemic penumbra.

Clinical Findings

The presentation varies with the territory involved. Patients present with contralateral hemiparesis and sensory loss, and possibly homonymous hemianopia, if the MCA is involved. Aphasia occurs if the infarction is in the dominant hemisphere, while confusion or neglect occurs if the infarction is in the nondominant hemisphere.

Anterior cerebral artery infarction presents with contralateral leg weakness and hemisensory loss. Bilateral infarctions present with akinetic mutism and incontinence.

Unilateral involvement of the posterior cerebral artery presents with hemianopia, while bilateral involvement presents with cortical blindness and memory loss. If the involvement is at the "top of the basilar," the presentation is thalamic sensory deficits, impaired arousal, and cranial nerve deficits.

Cerebellar involvement presents with ataxia and dysmetria. Crossed motor and sensory deficits, cranial nerve dysfunction, ataxia, and somnolence are seen with brain stem involvement.

Complications

Complications include hemorrhagic transformation and brain herniation with secondary infarction and/or hydrocephalus (Figs. I and J). Petechial hemorrhage is usually confined to gray matter and is not necessarily accompanied by clinical deterioration. Parenchymal hematoma is a confluent collection of blood which may dissect tissue planes widely and exert mass effect, and is often accompanied by clinical deterioration.

Pathology

Gross

- Edema and blurring of the gray-white junction occur acutely and subacutely
- Volume loss and gliosis are seen in the chronic stage
- Calcification and hemosiderin staining may be visible

Microscopic

- Neuronal loss and astroglial reaction
- Neuronal eosinophilia with pylenosis occurs

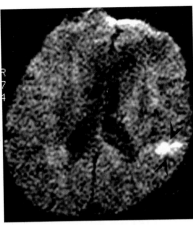

Fig. G. An axial DWI (same patient as Figs. E and F) shows focal hyperintensity on the left (*arrowheads*), consistent with the reduced diffusion characteristic of acute infarction.

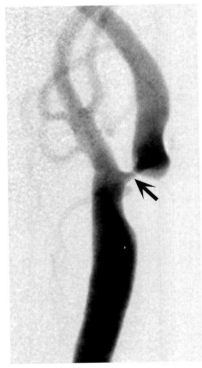

Fig. H. A left common carotid artery angiogram (same patient as Figs. E, F, and G) demonstrates a focal high-grade stenosis at the origin of the left internal carotid artery (*arrow*). Subsequent carotid endarterectomy was performed.

Imaging Findings

Imaging of MCA stroke:

HYPERACUTE (<6 hours)

CT   • Often normal except for hyperdense MCA sign or subtle obscuration of the insular ribbon

MR   • Absent flow void
- Vascular enhancement
- Abnormalities of diffusion (Figs. K and L) and perfusion

ACUTE (6 to 24 hours)

CT   • Loss of the insular ribbon
- Obscuration of the lentiform nucleus
- Sulcal asymmetry
- Loss of gray-white matter differentiation

MR   • Sulcal effacement
- Progressive T1 and T2 prolongation in gray matter > white matter

EARLY SUBACUTE (1 to 7 days)

Hemorrhagic transformation and secondary infarction may occur, maximum mass effect at 3 to 7 days

CT   • Progressive swelling
- Onset of parenchymal enhancement

MR   • Progressive swelling
- Onset of parenchymal +/– meningeal enhancement
- Resolution of vascular enhancement

LATE SUBACUTE (1 to 6 weeks)

CT and MR   • Swelling gradually resolves
- "Fogging" effect may occur
- Contrast enhancement peaks

CHRONIC (> 6 weeks)

CT and MR   • Resolution of mass effect
- Resolution of parenchymal enhancement
- Presence of volume loss
- Evidence of Wallerian degeneration

Treatment

In evolution:

- In the absence of hemorrhage or other contraindications, ischemic infarcts less than 3 hours old may be treated with intravenous tissue plasminogen activator. Intra-arterial thrombolysis using pro-urokinase delivered via a microcatheter in the MCA is still under investigation
- Neuroprotective agents
- Supportive care for completed infarcts

Prognosis

- Varies significantly with patient's underlying condition, extent of infarction, and presence or absence of complicating hemorrhage

Pitfalls

• The hyperdense MCA sign is seen in only 15 to 20% of patients and is not useful in patients with heavily calcified arteries.

• The "fogging effect" refers to an increase in the density of infarcted tissue toward isodensity as a consequence of capillary ingrowth, macrophage invasion, and/or small petechial hemorrhages. A subacute infarct may therefore be invisible on a non-contrast CT scan, although the administration of contrast facilitates detection of a subacute infarct in this setting.

• Patients who survive a large MCA stroke are severely disabled in approximately 50% of cases

• In general, there is an 8 to 20% chance of death within the first 30 days following ischemic stroke. For hemorrhagic stroke, the case fatality rate is in the 30 to 80% range

Suggested Readings

Lutsep HL, Albers GW, DeCrespigny A, Kamat GN, Marks MP, Moseley ME. Clinical utility of diffusion-weighted magnetic resonance imaging in the assessment of stroke. *Ann Neurol* 41:574–580, 1997.

Moulin T, Cattin F, Crepin-Leblond T, et al. Early CT signs in acute middle cerebral artery infarction: predictive value for subsequent infarct locations and outcome. *Neurology* 47:366–375, 1996.

Truwit CL, Barkovich AJ, Gean-Marton AD, Hibri N, Norman D. Loss of the insular ribbon: another early CT sign of acute middle cerebral artery infarction. *Radiology* 176:801–806, 1990.

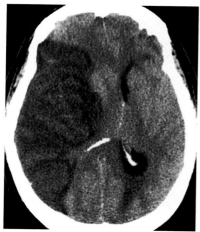

Fig. I. A 63-year-old woman 3 days status post-MCA infarction "blows her pupil" and becomes progressively obtunded. Geographic hypodensity in the right MCA territory is consistent with a large infarction. There is significant midline shift, as well as trapping of the left lateral ventricle and transependymal flow of CSF.

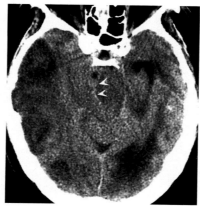

Fig. J. A more inferior image (same patient as Fig. I) demonstrates striking uncal herniation (*arrowheads*) and brainstem compression. The left temporal horn is enlarged, and transependymal flow of CSF is again identified on the left.

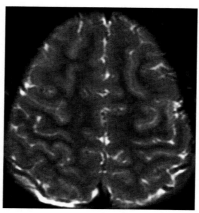

Fig. K. An axial T2-WI in a child with sudden onset of right hand weakness is normal 1 hour following symptom onset.

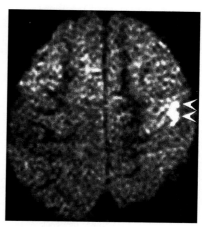

Fig. L. An axial diffusion-weighted image (same patient as Fig. K) shows a focal area of high signal (*arrowheads*) consistent with reduced diffusion and acute cortical infarction.

Case 70

Clinical Presentation

A 43-year-old man who suffered a gastrointestinal bleed complicated by severe hypotension 2 weeks earlier is noted to have confusion and bilateral upper extremity weakness, right greater than the left, as well as bilateral upgoing toes and lower extremity hyperreflexia.

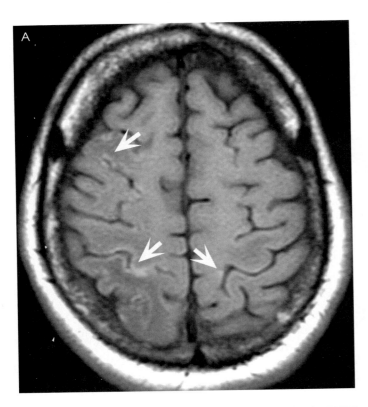

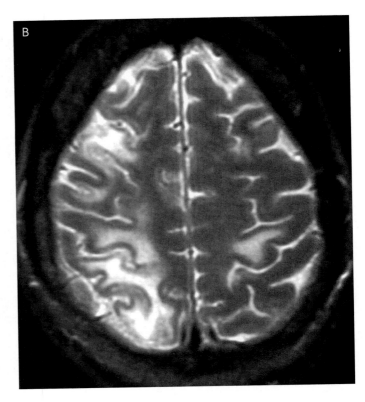

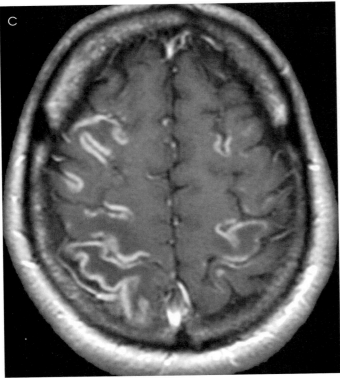

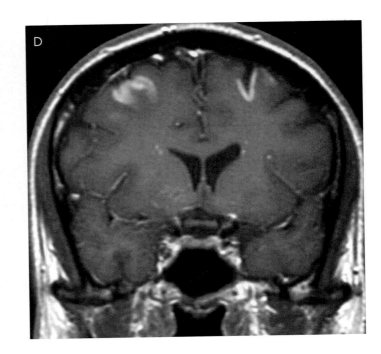

Pearl

- Observing an apparently narrow lumen or slow flow in the intracranial carotid artery supports a proximal cause of unilateral watershed infarction (Figs. E through G).

Pitfalls

- Watershed infarcts are more likely to be clinically silent than nonborderzone infarcts and may first be identified on imaging studies.

- Watershed infarction may mimic tumor (Figs. H and I). Follow-up studies are very helpful in making this distinction, and diffusion-weighted sequences (if obtained less than approximately 10 days following symptom onset) are also very helpful as neoplasm does not demonstrate the pattern of severely decreased diffusion that is seen with acute stroke.

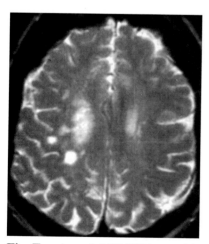

Fig. E. An axial T2-WI in an elderly woman with episodic left-sided weakness demonstrates asymmetric T2 prolongation in the right frontal white matter.

Radiologic Findings

An axial T1-WI (Fig. A) demonstrates abnormal hypointensity and mild gyral swelling in the right frontal and parietal and left frontal regions. Linear T1 shortening is observed in multiple areas of cortex (*arrows*). A corresponding T2-WI (Fig. B) shows abnormal T2 prolongation in the subcortical white matter. Post-gadolinium, an axial T1-WI (Fig. C) shows striking linear enhancement of multiple regions of cortex, the right greater than the left. A coronal post-gadolinium T1-WI (Fig. D) shows similar findings and emphasizes the parasagittal distribution of the abnormality.

Diagnosis

Bilateral watershed infarctions due to global hypoperfusion

Differential Diagnosis

- Multiple embolic infarctions (would not affect only borderzone territories)
- Anoxic injury (frequently affects deep gray nuclei, affects cortex diffusely)
- Venous infarction (often hemorrhagic, typically located in temporal lobe or parasagittal region, cortex often relatively spared)

Discussion

Background

Cerebral watershed or borderzone infarction affects the boundary zones between major cerebral arterial territories. Watershed infarcts are typically divided into several subtypes: anterior watershed infarcts, located between the territories of the anterior and middle cerebral arteries; posterior watershed infarcts, located between the territories of the middle and posterior cerebral arteries; and internal junctional infarcts, located between the deep and superficial territories of the middle cerebral artery. Overall, watershed infarction accounts for approximately 10% of cases of ischemic stroke. In affected patients, vascular risk factors such as hypertension, diabetes mellitus, and hypercholesterolemia are common.

Etiology

The majority of bilateral watershed infarcts are caused by decreased perfusion of distal arteries. This occurs in the setting of systemic hypotension due to orthostasis, perioperative complications, myocardial ischemia/infarction, or cardiac arrhythmia. Watershed infarcts may be unilateral in the setting of preexisting ipsilateral vascular disease and only mild or moderate hypotension. The extent of infarction is determined by the severity and duration of hypoperfusion, the location and severity of occlusive vascular disease, and the adequacy of collateral blood supply.

Some cases of watershed infarction appear to be caused by small cerebral emboli (~200 μm) that are selectively propagated to the distal branches of arteries located in the watershed zone rather than diverging into small caliber branches which arise along the way.

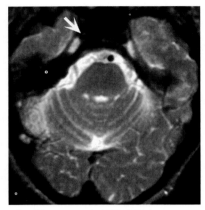

Fig. F. An axial T2-WI (same patient as Fig. E) at the level of the cavernous carotid arteries demonstrates marked asymmetry of the arterial flow voids, with the right being significantly smaller than the left (*arrow*). This finding and the asymmetric T2 abnormality suggest a proximal flow-limiting carotid lesion.

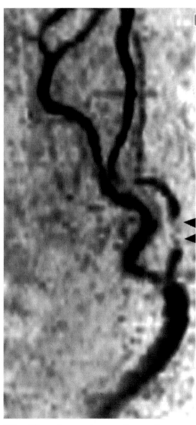

Fig. G. A maximum intensity projection image from a carotid MR angiogram (same patient as Figs. E and F) demonstrates a high-grade proximal stenosis (*arrowheads*) in the right internal carotid artery.

Clinical Findings

Watershed infarction is frequently associated with syncope, focal convulsions, and headache. Symptoms are related to the site of infarction.

- Anterior infarction causes mainly crural hemiparesis, often associated with transcortical motor aphasia (dominant hemisphere) or mood disturbances (nondominant hemisphere).
- Posterior infarction commonly causes hemianopia, often in association with transcortical sensory aphasia (dominant hemisphere) or neglect (nondominant hemisphere).
- Subcortical infarction is associated with hemiparesis and noncortical hemisensory deficits.

Complications

Hemorrhagic transformation may occur but is generally asymptomatic. Parenchymal hematoma formation is unusual in the setting of watershed infarction.

Pathology

Gross

- Edematous, congested brain in watershed territories

Microscopic

- Coagulative necrosis

Imaging Findings

CT

- May be normal acutely
- Focal triangular regions of hypodensity are observed in the frontoparietal (ACA-MCA) and/or temporo-occipital (MCA-PCA) territories
- Linear or rounded areas of hypodensity may be seen in the corona radiata and centrum semiovale (internal junctional infarcts), often with a chainlike pattern

MR

- Areas of T1 and T2 prolongation may be identified in regions as described above
- Areas of cortical T1 shortening may be seen, representing petechial hemorrhage or laminar necrosis
- May see narrowed lumen or evidence of slow flow or occlusion in the intracranial segment of internal carotid artery
- Diffusion-weighted imaging may demonstrate zones of restricted diffusion before CT or conventional MR sequences show any abnormality
- Perfusion imaging may demonstrate decreased hemispheric perfusion or delay in peak arrival time of contrast in the setting of a flow-limiting carotid artery lesion

Note: The evolution of cerebral infarction on CT and MR is reviewed in detail in Case 69.

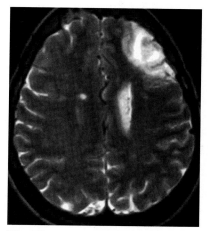

Fig. H. An axial T2-WI in a patient with altered mental status demonstrates abnormal T2 prolongation involving a wedge-shaped region of the left frontal cortex and subcortical white matter.

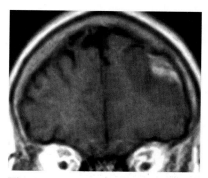

Fig. I. A coronal post-gadolinium T1-WI (same patient as Fig. H) demonstrates predominantly peripheral enhancement of this process. The patient was taken to surgery for a suspected diagnosis of brain tumor. Brain biopsy was consistent with subacute infarction, and the lesion gradually regressed over time (not shown).

Treatment

- Supportive care
- Management of cardiovascular risk factors
- Unilateral watershed infarction may indicate the need for carotid endarterectomy

Prognosis

- Relatively poor overall due to frequent cardiovascular comorbidities, with a death rate as high as 9.9% per year
- In the setting of watershed infarction due to intraoperative hypotension, prognosis is generally much better

Suggested Readings

Bogousslavsky J, Regli F. Unilateral watershed cerebral infarcts. *Neurology* 36:373–377, 1986.

Mounier-Vehier F, Leys D, Godefroy O, Rondepierre P, Marchau M, Pruvo JP. Borderzone infarct subtypes: preliminary study of the presumed mechanism. *Eur Neurol* 34:11–15, 1994.

Mull M, Schwarz M, Thron A. Cerebral hemisphere low-flow infarcts in arterial occlusive disease: lesion patterns and angiomorphological conditions. *Stroke* 28:118–123, 1997.

Case 71

Clinical Presentation

A 65-year-old woman began to vomit and then passed out during her morning yoga class. She was brought to the emergency room where she was intubated and sent for CT scan.

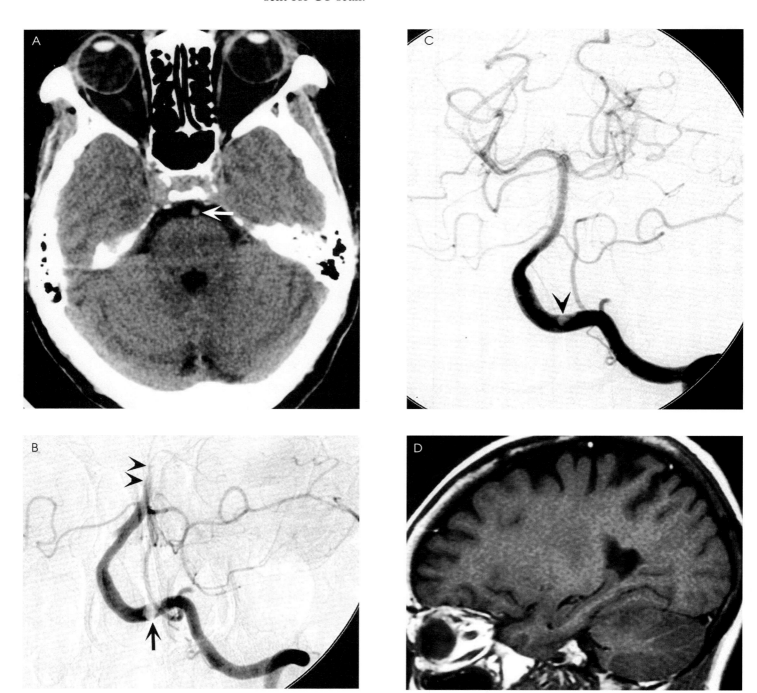

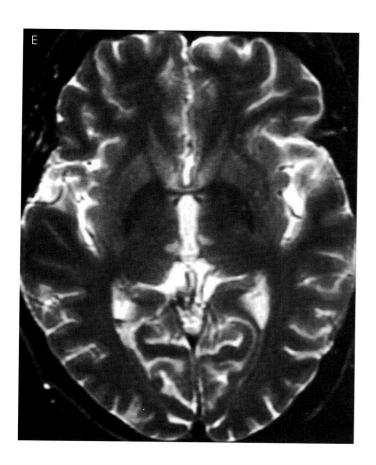

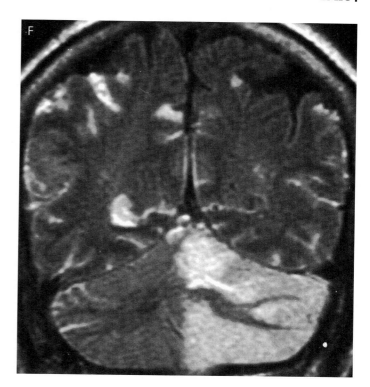

Radiologic Findings

A non-contrast CT scan through the posterior fossa (Fig. A) is essentially unremarkable, although the basilar artery may be slightly dense (*arrow*). Because of a clinical concern for basilar artery thrombosis, the patient was brought immediately for angiography. A frontal projection from a left vetebral artery injection (Fig. B) demonstrates a rounded filling defect in the distal vertebral artery (*arrow*). In addition, only minimal filling of the basilar artery beyond the level of the anterior inferior cerebellar arteries is seen (*arrowheads*). There is also poor visualization of the proximal left posterior inferior cerebellar artery. Emergent thrombolysis was performed. At the conclusion of the procedure, injection of the vertebral artery (Fig. C) shows that good flow has been restored in the basilar artery. A small filling defect is still present in the distal left vertebral artery (*arrowhead*). A sagittal T1-WI from an MR scan performed 1 day later (Fig. D) demonstrates edema in the cerebellum, involving the territories of the posterior inferior cerebellar artery and superior cerebellar artery. An axial T2-WI (Fig. E) demonstrates focal areas of hyperintensity in the medial thalami bilaterally. A coronal fluid-attenuated inversion recovery image (Fig. F) nicely demonstrates the infarction of the left cerebellum, which respects the midline. Note also multiple areas of high-signal intensity within cortical sulci, representing subarachnoid hemorrhage that complicated the thrombolysis procedure.

Diagnosis

Basilar artery thromboembolic occlusion with cerebellar and bithalamic infarction

Differential Diagnosis

Of bithalamic hyperintensities:

- Deep venous thrombosis (evidence of occlusion of straight sinus/vein of Galen)
- Wernicke's encephalopathy (clinical setting, does not involve cerebellum)
- Extrapontine myelinolysis (clinical setting, often accompanied by central pontine myelinolysis)
- Bithalamic tumors (mass effect, more infiltrative, less symmetric)

Of the constellation of findings:

- None

Discussion

Background

The basilar artery is formed by the junction of the right and left vertebral arteries. Major branches of the basilar artery include the paired anterior inferior cerebellar arteries and superior cerebellar arteries. Terminally, the basilar artery divides into the posterior cerebral arteries. Small penetrating branches of the basilar artery supply the pons, portions of the midbrain, and the posteroinferior thalami. Patients with basilar artery occlusion typically have a sudden, dramatic clinical presentation due to infarction in any or all of the above distribution. In some cases, only bithalamic infarction will be present. This may be due to occlusion (typically embolic) of the small perforating arteries that supply the paramedian thalami bilaterally, the so-called arteries of Percheron.

Etiology

Risk factors for basilar artery occlusion include atherosclerosis, cardiac arrhythmia with emboli, vertebral artery dissection, cocaine use, and oral contraceptive use.

Clinical Findings

The so-called "top of the basilar syndrome" includes oculomotor dysfunction, with third nerve and vertical gaze palsies; hemiataxia and mild weakness; and altered level of consciousness, including hypersomnia, akinetic mutism, amnestic state, obtundation, and/or deep coma. If cerebellar infarction is present, patients may present acutely with nausea, vomiting, and vertigo; seizures may be present as well.

Complications

A "locked in" state (in which the patient is alert but is incapable of voluntary movement except for vertical eye movements) may ensue from large ventral pontine infarcts. Hemorrhagic transformation of infarctions may occur, usually postthrombolysis.

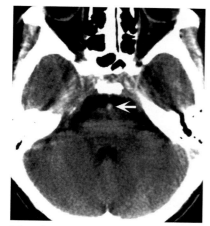

Fig. G. A non-enhanced CT in a young woman with a known hypercoagulable condition who presented with progressive obtundation shows a strikingly dense basilar artery (*arrow*). Basilar artery thrombosis was confirmed angiographically.

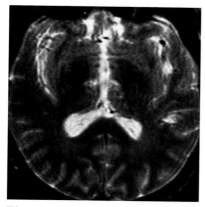

Fig. H. An axial T2-WI in a young man 4 days status post-thrombolysis for basilar artery thrombosis demonstrates bithalamic T2 hyperintensity.

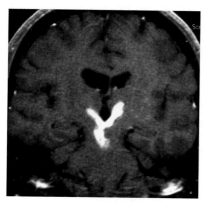

Fig. I. A coronal post-gadolinium T1-WI (same patient as Fig. G) demonstrates striking enhancement in the thalami bilaterally, extending down into the midbrain, consistent with a several day-old infarct.

Imaging Findings

CT

- The basilar artery may appear abnormally dense (Fig. G)
- In the acute phase, subtle hypodensity may be seen in the thalami, brainstem and cerebellum, and/or occipital lobes

MR

- T2 hyperintensity is variably present in the thalami, midbrain, pons, cerebellum, and/or occipital lobes
- Often mild corresponding T1 hypointensity in these areas in the acute/subacute phase
- Post-gadolinium enhancement may be present after several days (Figs. H and I)
- Absence of a normal flow void in the basilar artery and/or vertebral arteries is typically seen

Treatment

- Anticoagulation
- Emergent thrombolysis in appropriate candidates. This has an immediate recanalization rate of 44 to 75%

Prognosis

- Mortality without thrombolysis is as high as 80 to 100%
- With thrombolysis, 3-month survival in patients with distal basilar clot is approximately 70%, while in patients with proximal or midbasilar clot, it is approximately 15%. Survivors may be left with severe residual neurologic deficits.

Suggested Readings

Bell DA, Davis WL, Osborn AG, Harnsberger HR. Bithalamic hyperintensity on T2-weighted MR: vascular causes and evaluation with MR angiography. *AJNR* 15:893–899, 1994.

Cross DT III, Moran CJ, Akins PT, Angtuaco EE, Diringer MN. Relationship between clot location and outcome after basilar artery thrombolysis. *AJNR* 18:1221–1228, 1997.

Tatemichi TK, Steinke W, Duncan C, et al. Paramedian thalamopeduncular infarction: clinical syndromes and magnetic resonance imaging. *Ann Neurol* 32:162–171, 1992.

Case 72

Clinical Presentation

A 43-year-old man presents with neck pain and transient left-sided weakness following a motor vehicle accident.

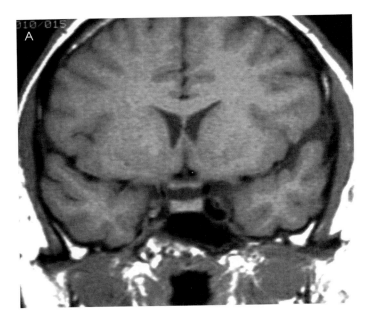

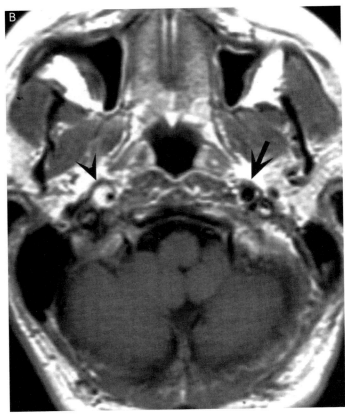

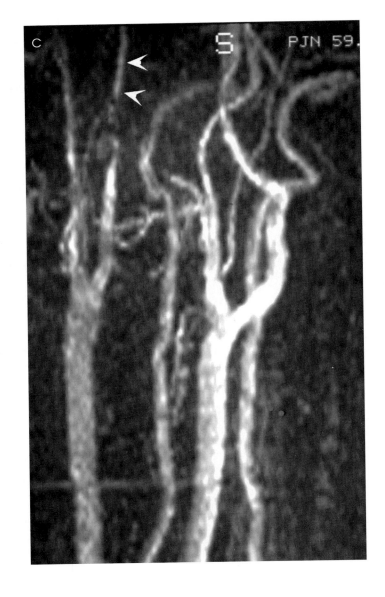

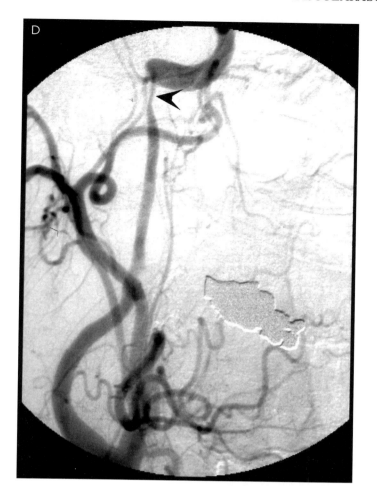

Radiologic Findings

A coronal T1-WI (Fig. A) demonstrates asymmetry in caliber of the cavernous carotid arteries, with the right being significantly reduced compared with the left. An axial T1-WI (Fig. B) shows that the lumen of the right internal carotid artery (ICA) is reduced in size, and a crescent of high-signal intensity material is noted around the eccentrically located lumen (*arrowhead*). Compare the normal contralateral distal cervical ICA (*arrow*). A maximum intensity projection image from a two-dimensional time-of-flight MR angiogram through the cervical vessels (Fig. C) demonstrates segmental narrowing of the right ICA (*arrowheads*). A conventional angiogram was performed and an anteroposterior projection from a right common carotid artery injection (Fig. D) demonstrates segmental narrowing of the distal cervical ICA (*arrowhead*), which returns to a more normal caliber above the level of the skull base.

Diagnosis

Dissection of the internal carotid artery

Differential Diagnosis

None

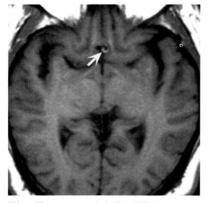

Fig. E. An axial T1-WI in a patient with acute onset of right leg weakness demonstrates a narrow and eccentric lumen of the left anterior cerebral artery with a surrounding crescent of hyperintensity (*arrow*).

Discussion

Background

ICA dissection has been increasingly recognized as an important cause of ischemic stroke in young patients. The term "dissection" refers to the extrusion of blood into the vessel wall in the setting of an intimal tear, with blood dissecting along the vessel wall in the subintimal, medial, and/or subadventitial layers. Pseudoaneurysm formation may accompany dissection. Associated infarction may occur secondary to a low-flow state induced by luminal compromise or to vascular thrombotic and/or embolic events. The typical extracranial ICA dissection extends from just beyond the carotid bulb to the level of the carotid canal, but ICA dissection may involve the cranial base and intracranial segments of the vessel as well (Fig. E). Vertebral artery dissections typically involve the distal segment, extending from C2 to the skull base.

Etiology

Many cases are apparently "spontaneous." Trauma is an important cause of arterial dissection. Other predisposing factors include underlying vessel diseases such as Marfan syndrome, fibromuscular dysplasia, or Ehlers-Danlos syndrome, hypertension, kinking or coiling of the ICA, family history of dissection and intracranial aneurysms, and upper respiratory tract infection.

Clinical Findings

Symptoms include ipsilateral neck pain and/or headache, oculosympathetic paresis (Horner's syndrome), lower cranial nerve symptoms, and transient ischemic attacks.

Complications

If infarction accompanies dissection, focal neurologic findings may be observed.

Imaging Findings

CT

- Often normal, although a lack of vascular enhancement may be observed post-contrast
- Low-density acute hemorrhage may surround the patent lumen of the carotid
- Signs of complicating cerebral infarction may be identified

MR

- Classically, there is a narrowed eccentric flow void surrounded by semilunar hyperintense signal that represents the intramural hematoma. The signal characteristics of the hematoma vary with its age, but it is typically hyperintense on both T1- and T2-WIs (extracellular methemoglobin).
- In some cases, the vessel may be occluded rather than simply narrowed, and the normal flow void is absent
- The hematoma may "spiral" around the vascular lumen on serial slices
- MR angiography shows luminal narrowing or possibly occlusion

Conventional Angiography

- Flame-shaped tapering of distal carotid bulb at proximal aspect of dissection
- Long-segment high-grade stenosis of the vascular lumen

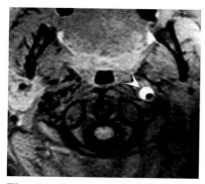

Fig. F. An axial T1-WI with fat saturation at the C1-2 level clearly demonstrates the intramural hematoma (*arrowhead*) in this left internal carotid artery dissection.

Treatment

- Heparin to decrease the risk of thromboembolic complications. This may be contraindicated with intracranial dissection.
- Possibly long-term anticoagulation with Coumadin

Prognosis

Generally good if anticoagulation therapy is instituted promptly and cerebral infarction has not occurred

Suggested Readings

Goldberg HI, Grossman RI, Gomori JM, Asbury AK, Bilaniuk LT, Zimmerman RA. Cervical internal carotid artery dissecting hemorrhage: diagnosis using MR. *Radiology* 158:157–161, 1986.

Ozdoba C, Sturzenegger M, Schroth G. Internal carotid artery dissection: MR imaging features and clinical-radiologic correlation. *Radiology* 199:191–198, 1996.

Pacini R, Simon J, Ketonen L, Kido D, Kieburtz K. Chemical-shift imaging of a spontaneous internal carotid artery dissection: case report. *AJNR* 12:360–362, 1991.

Case 73

Clinical Presentation

A 49-year-old woman with a history of hypertension presents with the acute onset of left hemiparesis.

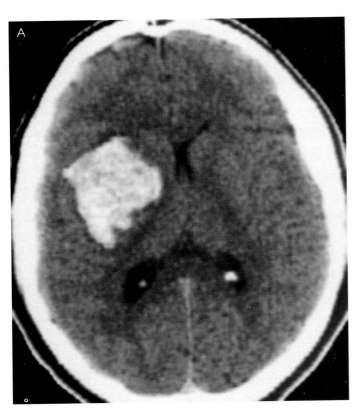

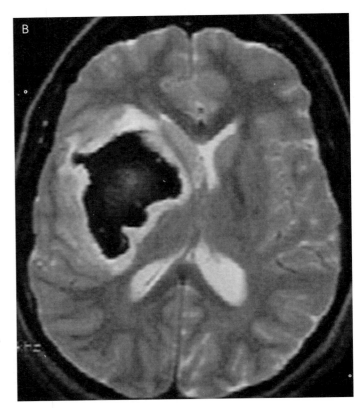

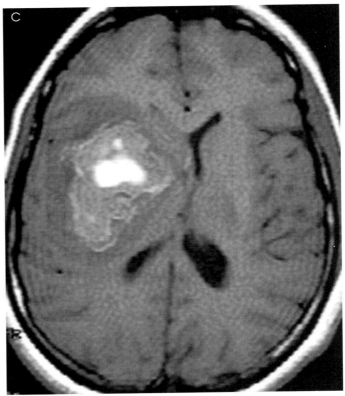

Radiologic Findings

A non-contrast CT scan (Fig. A) shows a large, somewhat irregular hematoma centered in the right putamen. On this scan obtained 1 hour after the onset of symptoms, there is minimal if any surrounding edema and very mild mass effect on the right lateral ventricle. An MR scan was performed 24 hours later. An axial T2-WI (Fig. B) shows that the hematoma is largely hypointense, with mild central hyperintensity. Surrounding vasogenic edema is noted, with increased mass effect on the right lateral ventricle as compared with the CT scan. An axial T1-WI (Fig. C) shows that the hematoma is centrally very hyperintense and peripherally relatively isointense. These characteristics are most consistent with a mix of deoxyhemoglobin and intracellular methemoglobin. Note that the T1-WI is mildly motion degraded.

Diagnosis

Putaminal hemorrhage secondary to hypertension

Differential Diagnosis

Parenchymal hematoma due to:

• Underlying vascular malformation (may see enlarged feeding or draining vessels, parenchymal calcification)
• Metastatic lesion (history of a primary lesion, often multiple lesions)
• Primary tumor (evidence for an associated mass)
• Amyloid angiopathy (typically lobar hemorrhages, evidence for amyloid on MR, usually over age 65)
• Trauma (clinical history, evidence of scalp injury, deep gray nuclei are uncommonly affected except with extensive severe injuries)
• Bleeding diathesis (clinical history, often multiple hemorrhages)

Discussion

Background

Intracerebral hemorrhage accounts for 10 to 15% of all strokes, and 50% of primary parenchymal hemorrhages are secondary to hypertension. Hypertensive hemorrhages typically occur in areas supplied by penetrating branches of the middle cerebral artery, posterior cerebral artery, and basilar artery. Therefore, common sites include the putamen (65%), thalamus (20%), pons (10%), cerebellum (5%), and subcortical white matter (~1%).

Etiology

Systemic hypertension damages and weakens vessel walls, which then may rupture in the setting of an acute elevation of blood pressure. Some implicate Charcot-Bouchard aneurysms (microaneurysms of deep perforating vessels) in the genesis of hypertensive hemorrhages, but this is controversial.

Pathophysiology

Active bleeding is typically acute and lasts less than an hour. Cerebral edema then ensues and progresses over 1 to 3 days. Because hematomas dissect brain

Table 1. MR Appearance of Evolving Parenchymal Hemorrhage

Stage	Time posthemorrhage	Physical state of blood	T1-WI*	T2-WI*
Hyperacute	<24 hours	Oxyhemoglobin	Iso	Hyper
Acute	1-3 days	Deoxyhemoglobin	Iso to hypo	Very hypo
Early subacute	4-7 days	Intracellular methemoglobin	Hyper	Very hypo
Late subacute	7-14 days	Extracellular methemoglobin	Hyper	Hyper
Chronic	>2 weeks	Hemosiderin/ferritin	Mildly hypo	Very hypo

*MR signal characteristics are compared with brain parenchyma; Iso, isointense; Hyper, hyperintense; Hypo, hypointense

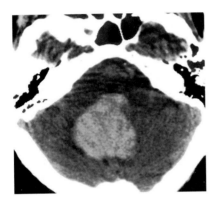

Fig. D. A 67-year-old male with a history of hypertension presents with acute ataxia. A non-contrast CT scan shows a large cerebellar hematoma extending anteriorly into the fourth ventricle.

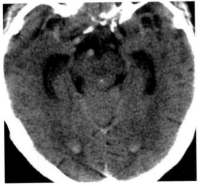

Fig. E. A more cephalad image (same patient as Fig. D) demonstrates mild upward transtentorial herniation of the cerebellar vermis, blood within the occipital horns bilaterally, and evidence for obstructive hydrocephalus with enlargement of the temporal horns.

rather than causing infarction and tissue necrosis, remote hypertensive bleeds typically appear as slitlike cavities with hemosiderin staining.

Clinical Findings

The presentation varies with location. If the hemorrhage is in the cerebellum, the findings are ataxia, nausea/vomiting, and dysequilibrium. If it is in the putamen or thalamus, the presentation is hemiparesis and confusion. Cranial nerve symptoms and coma are the presentation when the hemorrhage is in the pons.

Complications

Brain herniation may lead to secondary infarction, coma or death. Large hematomas may rupture into the ventricular system and cause communicating or noncommunicating hydrocephalus. Cerebellar hematomas may cause noncommunicating hydrocephalus by compressing the fourth ventricle or the aqueduct of Sylvius (Figs. D and E). Rehemorrhage or rapid expansion of the hematoma may occur with persistent hypertension.

Imaging Findings

CT

- Focal high-density lesion located in deep gray nuclei (especially the putamen and thalamus), pons, or cerebellum
- Surrounding edema

MR

- Focal hematoma in a typical location as above; the appearance varies with the stage of the hemorrhage (see Table 1)
- Variable degree of surrounding edema and associated mass effect

Treatment

- Supportive care in most cases, with medical management of hypertension
- Surgical evacuation of hematoma if there is severe mass effect/herniation. This is particularly relevant in the posterior fossa.
- Management of hydrocephalus

Prognosis

- Highly variable depending on size and location of the bleed

- Overall approximately 25% of patients will die within the first 48 hours of bleeding
- Thirty percent of survivors are functionally incapacitated

Suggested Readings

Bradley WG Jr. MR appearance of hemorrhage in the brain. *Radiology* 189:15–26, 1993.

Challa VR, Moody DM, Bell MA. The Charcot-Bouchard aneurysm controversy: impact of a new histologic technique. *J Neuropath Exp Neurol* 51:264–271, 1992.

Wityk RJ, Caplan LR. Hypertensive intracerebral hemorrhage. Epidemiology and clinical pathology. *Neurosurg Clin North Am* 3:521–532, 1992.

Case 74

Clinical Presentation

A 3-year-old previously abused child was under the care of foster parents when she went into status epilepticus. She had been seizing for at least 20 minutes when the paramedics arrived and transported her to the hospital.

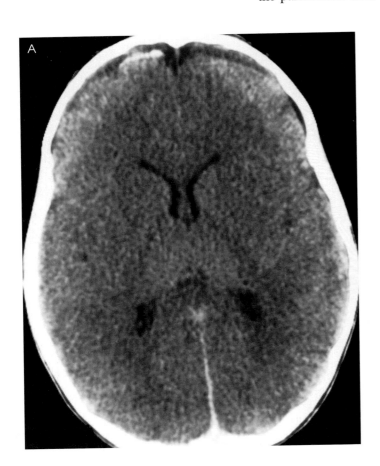
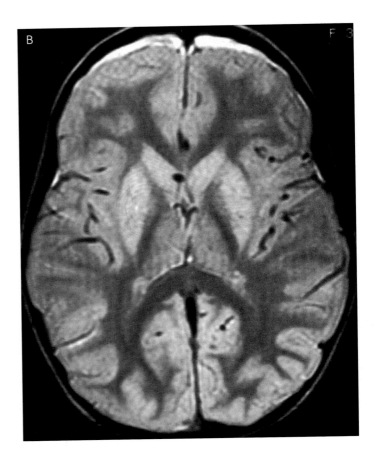

Radiologic Findings

A non-contrast CT scan obtained at the time of admission (Fig. A) demonstrates bifrontal extra-axial collections, with a small amount of hyperdense material identified within the right frontal collection. In addition, there is thickening and increased density along the posterior falx. These findings are consistent with subdural hematomas of varying ages. There is also abnormal hypodensity in the basal ganglia, as well as subtle loss of the normal sharp distinction between cortical gray matter and underlying white matter. An MR scan was obtained 2 days later. An axial proton density-weighted image (Fig. B) demonstrates abnormal high signal in the caudate nuclei and putamina bilaterally. The bifrontal subdural collections are again identified. The cortex appears slightly hyperintense in the posterior temporal and occipital regions.

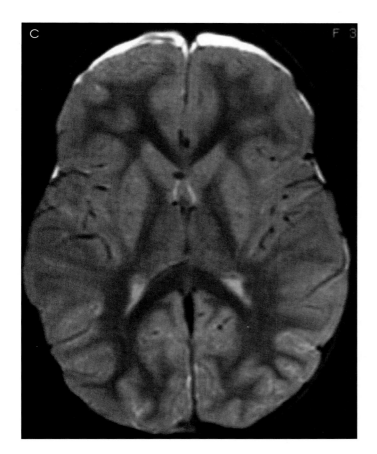
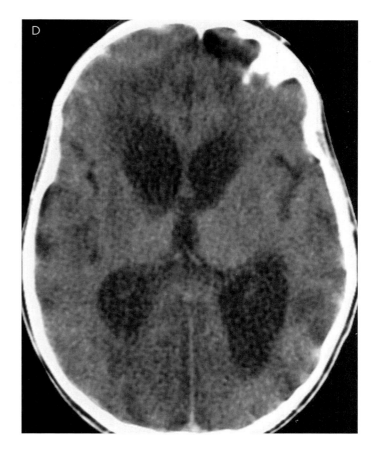

The corresponding T2-WI (Fig. C) demonstrates similar findings. A follow-up CT scan was obtained 2 months later (Fig. D). In this interval, the ventricles have markedly enlarged, and the basal ganglia have atrophied. In addition, extensive areas of abnormal cortical low attenuation are identified, most prominent in the occipital lobes bilaterally.

Diagnosis

Diffuse anoxic brain injury

Differential Diagnosis

- Arterial infarction (should correspond to a vascular distribution)
- Venous infarction (often extensive subcortical edema, often hemorrhagic)
- Toxic/metabolic process (often affects white matter more than cortex, appropriate clinical history)
- Severe trauma (appropriate history, external evidence of trauma)

Discussion

Background

The manifestations of anoxia or a severe hypoxic/ischemic insult are different in older children and adults than in neonates and young children. These insults often occur in the setting of cardiorespiratory arrest, near drowning, drug overdose, status epilepticus, or trauma. If an insult results predominantly in hypotension, changes related to borderzone ischemia and watershed infarction are seen. With a

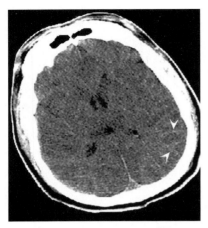

Fig. E. A non-contrast CT scan in a patient who suffered severe trauma and respiratory arrest demonstrates diffuse hypodensity of the cortex and basal ganglia. White matter appears more dense than adjacent cortex (*arrowheads*).

Pearls

• A curvilinear stripe of T2 prolongation at the gray matter-white matter interface may be seen, likely representing cortical laminar necrosis (Fig. F).

• The "reversal sign," an indicator of severe brain injury, is seen as dense white matter compared to gray matter on CT. The thalami, brainstem, and cerebellum ("white cerebellum sign," Fig. G) often appear abnormally dense as well. While the cause is uncertain, considerations include relative preservation of brain tissue in certain locations, petechial hemorrhage, and mineralization of neurons.

• The "reversal sign" is far more common in children than in adults.

• In cases of profound asphyxia, the caudate nuclei and putamina are affected more significantly than the thalami (the reverse is true in neonates).

more profound anoxic insult, generalized gray matter injury results. However, findings are quite variable in individual cases.

Clinical Findings

Patients typically present after resuscitation from cardiorespiratory arrest, near drowning, or drug overdose. Most do not regain consciousness after the insult.

Complications

Cerebral swelling, brain herniation, and death.

Pathophysiology

Gray matter is more profoundly affected than white matter by anoxic insults as it has higher blood flow and a higher metabolic rate than white matter. In cases of anoxia or profound hypoxic/ischemic insults, the third, fifth, and sixth layers of the cortex are predominantly affected and show laminar necrosis pathologically. The caudate nuclei and putamina are also profoundly affected. Intracellular cytotoxic edema occurs initially, followed by superimposed vasogenic edema.

Imaging Findings

CT is generally the initial study of choice in a patient who has suffered an anoxic or hypoxic-ischemic insult.

CT

- Early (<24 hours)
  1. Mild hypoattenuation of basal ganglia and cortex
  2. Effacement of perimesencephalic cisterns due to brain swelling
- Later (>24 hours)
  1. Loss of gray matter-white matter differentiation
  2. Complete effacement of cortical sulci and basal cisterns
  3. Petechial hemorrhage may be seen in cortex and basal ganglia
  4. "Reversal sign": hemispheric white matter is more dense than cortex (Fig. E)
- Late (weeks to months)
  1. Global parenchymal volume loss
  2. Shrunken basal ganglia

MR

- T1-WI: hypointensity of cortex and basal ganglia
- T2-WI: hyperintensity of cortex and basal ganglia
- Petechial hemorrhage may be present
- Effacement of sulci and basal cisterns as edema evolves

Treatment

- Supportive care
- Correction of inciting factors and metabolic abnormalities
- In the future, there may be a role for neuroprotective agents

Prognosis

- Poor, with most patients dying of cerebral swelling and brain herniation
- Survivors have profound neurologic deficits

Pitfalls

- Early MR findings of anoxic injury are very subtle in the first 24 to 48 hours.

- The reversal sign may not be evident on the initial scan, but appears 2 days to several weeks later, and may become chronic.

- Hyperdensity of vascular structures and dural reflections in patients with global anoxic injury may mimic subarachnoid or subdural hemorrhage (Figs. H and I). This hyperdensity is presumably due to venous stasis; the high density of blood-filled structures contrasts sharply with the hypodense parenchyma.

Suggested Readings

Barkovich AJ. Ischemic injury in older children. In: Barkovich AJ. *Pediatric Neuroimaging*, 2nd ed. New York, Raven Press, pp. 138–140, 1995.

Bird CR, Drayer BP, Gilles FH. Pathophysiology of "reverse" edema in global cerebral ischemia. *AJNR* 10:95–98, 1989.

Han BK, Towbin RB, De Courten-Myers G, McLaurin RL, Ball WS Jr. Reversal sign on CT: effect of anoxic/ischemic cerebral injury in children. *AJNR* 10:1191–1198, 1989.

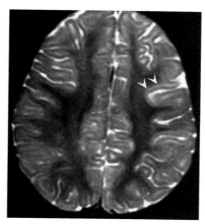

Fig. F. An axial T2-WI in a child who was strangled demonstrates a stripe of increased signal intensity at the gray matter/white matter junction (*arrowheads*).

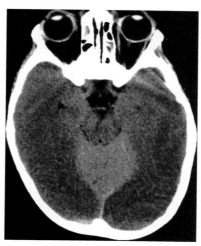

Fig. G. A non-contrast CT scan in a 5-year-old male status post-complicated cardiac surgery demonstrates a dense-appearing cerebellum, in contrast to diffuse hypodensity in the temporal and occipital lobes.

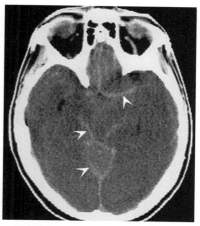

Fig. H. A non-contrast CT scan in a patient who became profoundly hypoxic in the setting of cardiac arrest demonstrates diffuse loss of gray-white differentiation, as well as effacement of sulci and basal cisterns due to cerebral edema. Vascular structures and dural reflections appear abnormally dense (*arrowheads*), which may mimic subarachnoid or subdural hemorrhage to the unwary observer.

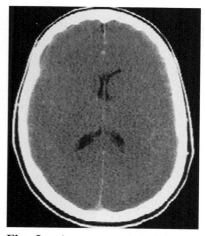

Fig. I. A more cephalad image from the patient in Figure G also demonstrates complete loss of distinction among deep gray nuclei, white matter, and cortex. Sulci are globally effaced.

Case 75

Clinical Presentation

A 45-year-old woman presents with the acute onset of ataxia.

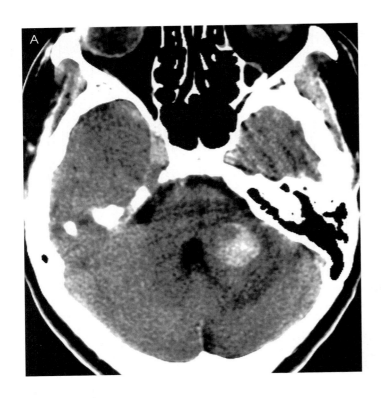

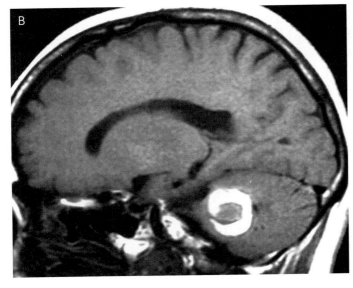

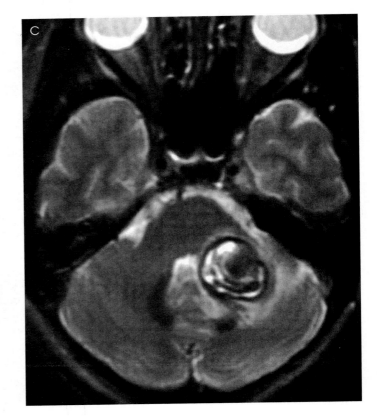

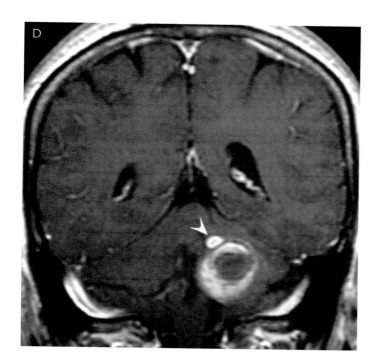

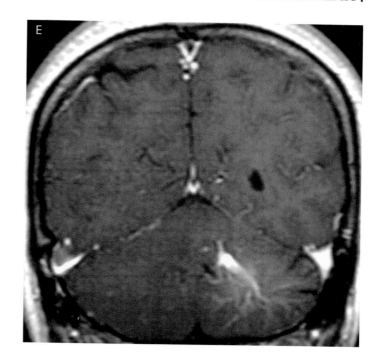

- When a presumed cavernous malformation is identified, it is important to administer gadolinium to look for an associated venous malformation. The presence and location of anomalous veins may affect the surgical approach, as venous malformations drain normal brain parenchyma and their ligation may lead to venous infarction.

- Venous malformations also occur in association with cavernous malformations of the spinal cord.

- A gradient-echo sequence should be performed to look for subtle areas of hemorrhage and additional lesions.

- Cavernous malformations may appear to "grow" over time because of reendothelialization of hemorrhagic cavities and the proliferation of granulation tissue.

Radiologic Findings

A non-contrast CT scan (Fig. A) demonstrates a round, intrinsically dense lesion centered in the left middle cerebellar peduncle. Mild surrounding edema is present. A sagittal T1-WI (Fig. B) demonstrates that the mass lesion is peripherally hyperintense and centrally isointense to brain parenchyma. A T2-WI (Fig. C) shows that the lesion is centrally more hypointense and peripherally relatively hyperintense, with a surrounding complete hemosiderin ring. Vasogenic edema is noted in the adjacent brain parenchyma. A post-gadolinium coronal T1-WI (Fig. D) demonstrates an enhancing structure adjacent to the mass lesion (*arrowhead*). A slightly more posterior post-gadolinium coronal T1-WI (Fig. E) demonstrates the classic "Medusa head" appearance of a large venous malformation that is draining the left cerebellar hemisphere. The patient was taken to surgery, where a hematoma was encountered and evacuated. Underlying the hematoma, a cavernous malformation was identified and removed, leaving the venous malformation intact.

Diagnosis

Cavernous malformation of the left middle cerebellar peduncle associated with a venous malformation and parenchymal hematoma

Differential Diagnosis

- Arteriovenous malformation (dilated arteries and veins, arteriovenous shunting)
- Thrombosed arteriovenous malformation (may be impossible to differentiate from a cavernous malformation, but the distinction may not be clinically significant and these are rare)
- Capillary telangiectasia (typically pontine, often only visible on post-contrast or gradient-echo images not usually associated with hematoma)

Pitfalls

- Hemorrhagic neoplasms may mimic cavernous malformations, so a follow-up examination may be useful if any imaging features are atypical for cavernous malformation and in patients at risk for metastatic disease.

- Overlap or transitional forms of vascular malformations may occur that give rise to intermediate or atypical imaging patterns.

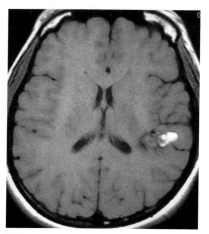

Fig F. An axial T1-WI in a young woman with medically refractory epilepsy demonstrates a multilobulated lesion with intrinsic high-signal intensity. Medial to the lesion is an area of irregular low-signal intensity consistent with hemosiderin or calcification.

- Hemorrhagic neoplasm (may occasionally appear identical to cavernous angioma, but lesions are often multiple and associated with edema; hemorrhagic neoplasms are not usually associated with venous malformations)
- Traumatic hematoma (very unusual location, no history of trauma)

Discussion

Background

A cavernous malformation (also commonly referred to as a cavernous angioma or cavernoma) is an angiographically occult vascular malformation that consists of a collection of vascular spaces lined by thin walls devoid of smooth muscle. The incidence of this lesion in an unselected autopsy population is approximately 0.5%. Cavernous malformations are typically isolated vascular malformations, but they may be multiple and familial. Multiple lesions are more common in patients of Hispanic extraction and have been linked to a mutation in a gene on 7q in some cases. Isolated cavernous malformations are associated with a visible venous malformation in approximately 30 to 50% of cases.

Etiology

The etiology/pathogenesis of these lesions is uncertain. In some cases, cavernous malformations have been shown to arise *de novo* in the vicinity of a venous malformation. It is theorized that in these cases regional venous hypertension may facilitate formation of cavernous malformations via red blood cell diapedesis and angiogenic growth factor release. In familial cases, the actual gene and gene product involved with the development of multiple cavernous malformations have not yet been identified.

Clinical Findings

Patients usually present between the ages of 30 and 60 years, most frequently with seizures, focal neurologic deficits, or headache. These lesions may also be detected incidentally on routine imaging studies.

Complications

Hemorrhage may be catastrophic, particularly if the lesion is located in the brainstem or other eloquent areas. Overt hemorrhage seems to be more common in females than in males and is prone to occur during pregnancy.

Pathology

Gross

- Lesions are most commonly located in the frontal and temporal lobes
- Mulberry-like multilobulated appearance, typically blue-black in color

Microscopic

- Cavernous spaces are lined by thin walls consisting of endothelium and collagen and devoid of smooth muscle
- Typically no brain tissue intervenes between the vascular channels, except toward the periphery of the lesion
- Surrounding brain parenchyma is often hemosiderin-stained and gliotic

Table 1. Features of Intracranial Vascular Malformations

Malformation	Pathology	CT Appearance	MR Appearance
Arteriovenous malformation	Cluster of hypertrophied arteries and arterialized veins lacking an intervening capillary bed. Minimal intervening gliotic brain tissue.	Intrinsically dense serpiginous structures that enhance intensely post-contrast. Calcification of adjacent parenchyma is frequent.	Cluster of flow-voids represents the nidus. Adjacent areas of gliosis and hemosiderin-staining are frequently identified.
Cavernous malformation	Clusters of sinusoidal channels with thin walls devoid of elastin and smooth muscle. Caverns filled with blood and/or thrombus at varying stages of organization, no intervening brain tissue except at the periphery of the lesion.	Often hyperdense due to calcification and/or hemorrhage. May show enhancement post-contrast. Typically no mass effect or edema unless there has been recent hemorrhage.	Round or multilobulated lesion that often shows "popcornlike" pattern of central high signal on T1- and T2-WIs. Surrounding hemosiderin rim. "Blooming" on gradient-echo sequences.
Venous malformation	Collections of histologically normal small veins clustering around one or more larger veins. Normal brain tissue intervenes between vessels.	Usually occult on non-contrast scan. Post-contrast, may see a tuft of small vessels draining into a dilated vein, often a subependymal or subpial vein.	"Medusa head" appearance of small radicles draining into a larger vein, best seen on post-gadolinium images. Adjacent brain may be normal or show gliotic changes.
Capillary telangiectasia	Cluster of dilated capillaries intermixed with normal brain tissue. Typically located in the pons.	Non-contrast study may be normal or show subtle calcification. A faint blush may be seen post-contrast.	Routine T1- and T2-WIs are often normal. Post-gadolinium, a faint blush of contrast is seen. Gradient-echo sequence often shows mild hypointensity.

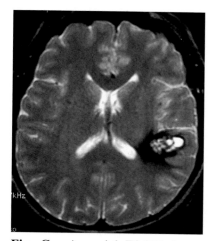

Fig. G. An axial T2-WI (same patient as Fig. F) demonstrates a "mulberry" or "popcornlike" bright lesion surrounded by a low-signal intensity hemosiderin rim of variable thickness. A cavernous malformation was removed at surgery.

Imaging Findings (Table 1)

CT

- Lesions are frequently calcified
- Mass effect is minimal or absent in the absence of recent hemorrhage
- Only a hematoma may be appreciated if the lesion has recently bled

MR

- Round or lobulated lesion with a mixed-signal intensity core that typically includes multiple round areas that are bright on both T1- and T2-WIs. These rounded deposits give rise to the so-called "popcorn" appearance of many of these lesions (Figs. F and G)
- Low-signal intensity rim of hemosiderin which may be smooth and thin or slightly thicker and more diffuse
- Post-contrast images may show partial enhancement of the lesion as well as an associated venous malformation

Angiography

- Typically negative, although a subtle vascular blush may occur
- An associated venous malformation may be visible

Treatment

- Surgical removal in symptomatic patients is recommended if clinically feasible
- Radiosurgery is being applied to some of these lesions, but its role is not yet established

Prognosis

While most lesions exhibit evidence of occult bleeding by MR imaging, overt hemorrhage occurs at a rate of only 0.7 to 2% per year

Suggested Readings

Rigamonti D, Drayer BP, Johnson PC, et al. The MRI appearance of cavernous malformations (angiomas). *J Neurosurg* 67: 518–524, 1987.

Robinson JR, Awad IA, Little JR. Natural history of the cavernous angioma. *J Neurosurg* 75:709–714, 1991.

Wilson CB. Cryptic vascular malformations. *Clin Neurosurg* 38:49–84, 1992.

Case 76

Clinical Presentation

A 25-year-old pregnant female presents with acute onset of severe headache and right hemiparesis.

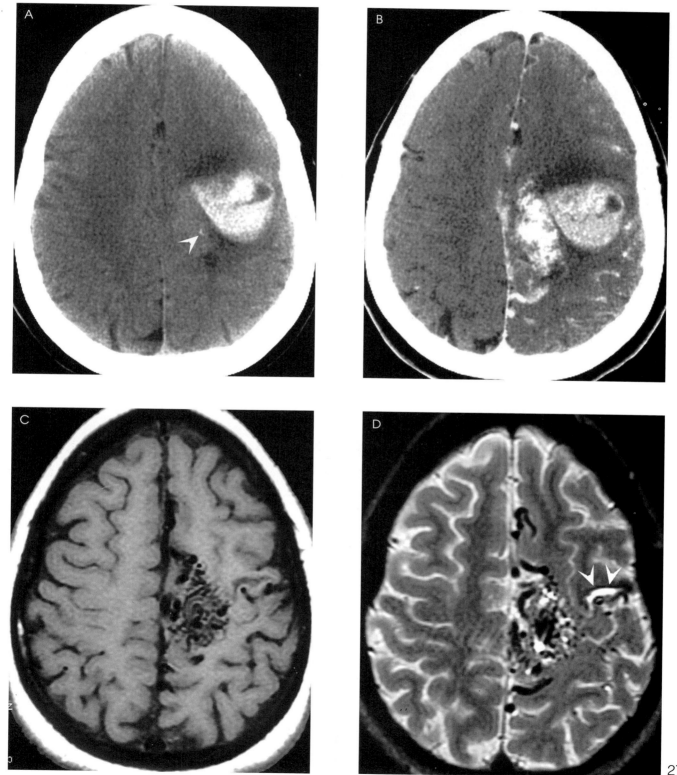

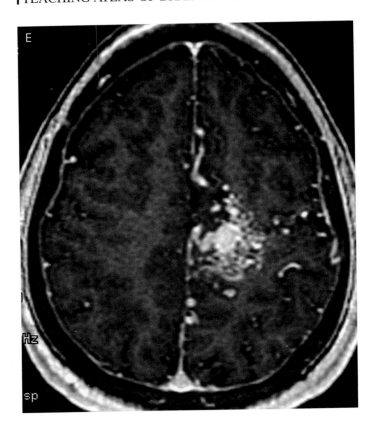

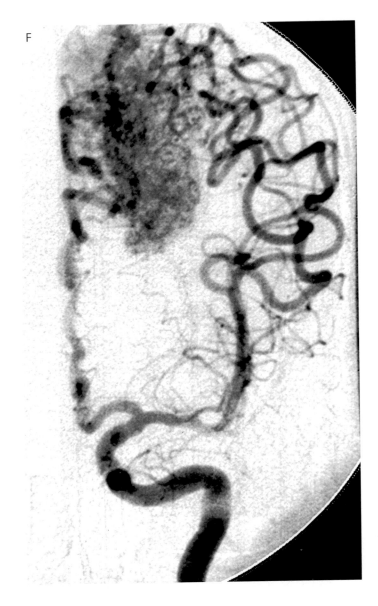

Radiologic Findings

A non-contrast CT scan (Fig. A) shows a left posterior frontal parenchymal hematoma with surrounding edema. Subtle lobulated increased density is noted medial to the hematoma, as well as a questionable focus of calcification (*arrowhead*). Following contrast administration (Fig. B), multiple linear and rounded serpiginous areas of enhancement are identified deep to the hematoma, as well as over the cerebral convexity. Several months later, following delivery of her child, the patient returned for preoperative evaluation. An axial T1-WI from an MR scan (Fig. C) shows a tangle of linear hypointensities consistent with flow voids in the left posterior frontal paramedian region. These vessels are seen to good advantage on an axial T2-WI (Fig. D). Note also the hemosiderin-stained cleft (*arrowheads*) representing the residuum of the prior hematoma. An axial partition image from a three-dimensional time-of-flight MR angiogram (Fig. E) shows flow-related enhancement within these vascular structures. A conventional angiogram was performed. A frontal view from a conventional angiogram during left internal carotid injection (Fig. F) shows a vascular nidus supplied by enlarged branches of the left anterior and middle cerebral arteries.

Diagnosis

Arteriovenous malformation (AVM)

Differential Diagnosis

Of a focus of abnormal vessels with arteriovenous shunting:

- None

Of a parenchymal hematoma:

- Hypertensive hemorrhage (history of hypertension typical location)
- Cavernous malformation (typical MR appearance, angiographically occult)
- Underlying neoplasm (may see other brain lesions or suspicious enhancement)
- Amyloid angiopathy (elderly patient, foci of hemosiderin on T2-WI or gradient-echo sequence)
- Trauma (history, evidence of scalp injury)
- Dural sinus thrombosis (evidence of occluded venous sinus)
- Mycotic aneurysm with rupture (often associated with subarachnoid hemorrhage, often a history of endocarditis)

Discussion

Background

Intracranial vascular malformations are typically divided into four major categories: AVMs, cavernous malformations, venous malformations, and capillary telangiectasias. AVMs are located within brain parenchyma and are congenital lesions consisting of abnormal networks of arterial supply and venous drainage that bypass the normal capillary bed of the brain. AVMs are located supratentorially in approximately 85% of cases. Hemorrhage occurs at a rate of approximately 2 to 3% per year and is the most devastating complication of AVM. Hemorrhages are more common with increasing age and in women in their fertile years. Anatomic risk factors that increase the rate of cerebral hemorrhage include central venous drainage, periventricular or intraventricular location of the AVM, and intranidal aneurysm. Hypertension is also a risk factor for hemorrhage from an AVM. AVMs are typically graded according to the Spetzler-Martin classification system (see Table 1).

Clinical Findings

AVMs typically present in adult life, generally between the ages of 20 and 40. Approximately 50% of patients present with symptoms of hemorrhage. Other common presenting symptoms include seizures, headache, and progressive neurologic deficit.

Complications

The hemorrhage rate increases to 6 to 18% in the year following a first hemorrhage, with the rate gradually returning to 2 to 3% per year over time. The mortality rate of a first hemorrhage is approximately 10%.

Table 1. Grading System for AVMs (Spetzler and Martin, 1986)

Feature	Score
Size of nidus	
Small (<3 cm)	1
Moderate (3-6 cm)	2
Large (>6 cm)	3
Located in eloquent region	
No	0
Yes	1
Venous drainage	
Superficial	0
Deep	1

- Grade = sum of points for size, eloquence, and venous drainage
  - A Grade I lesion is small (1 point), located in a non-eloquent region (0 points), and has only superficial drainage (0 points)
  - A Grade V lesion is larger than 6 cm (3 points), located within or immediately adjacent to eloquent brain (1 point), and has at least partial drainage into the deep venous system (1 point)
  - Various combinations of lesion size, location, and venous drainage result in the intermediate grades of AVM
  - There is also a "Grade VI" category that includes inoperable lesions, i.e., lesions whose resection would be associated with a totally disabling deficit or death. This includes extremely large diffuse AVMs that are dispersed through eloquent areas, or malformations with a diffuse nidus that encompasses critical structures such as the hypothalamus or brainstem.
- Eloquent areas may be superficial (primary motor and sensory cortex, speech and auditory areas, visual cortex) or deep (thalamus, internal capsule, brainstem)

Pathology

Gross

- Complex tightly packed nidus of abnormal vascular channels
- A large direct arteriovenous fistula may rarely occur
- Normal brain parenchyma does not intervene between the abnormal vessels within the vascular nidus

Microscopic

- No capillary bed is interposed between arteries and veins
- Adjacent brain may demonstrate calcification, hemosiderin staining, and encephalomalacia

Imaging Findings

CT

- Dense serpiginous structures consistent with dilated veins may be seen
- Post-contrast, an abnormal tangle of vessels may be identified
- Areas of parenchymal calcification are common
- Hematoma is seen in the setting of acute hemorrhage

MR

- Abnormal tightly packed parenchymal nidus with low-signal intensity flow voids
- Areas of encephalomalacia and hemosiderin deposition are common in the adjacent brain parenchyma
- MR angiography (particularly the thin partition images) will generally show the abnormal vessels and is useful for radiosurgical planning

Angiography

- Tightly packed mass of enlarged feeding arteries and tortuous, dilated draining veins
- Arteriovenous shunting, with visualization of "early" draining veins
- Feeding arteries and draining veins may show thrombosis and/or stenosis
- Intranidal or feeding arterial aneurysms may be identified

Treatment

- Complete obliteration of the AVM nidus is the goal of treatment
- Several options are available which may be used independently or in combination: surgical excision, radiosurgery, and intravascular embolization
  1. Surgical excision is limited by the location of the AVM
  2. Radiosurgery carries inherent risks of radionecrosis and bleeding during the latency period between the time of treatment and the time of obliteration of the AVM
  3. Embolization is rarely curative as it is limited by increasing angioarchitectural complexity, but may be useful as an adjunct to surgery or radiosurgery

Prognosis

- Treatment-associated morbidity and mortality generally increase with the Spetzler-Martin grade of the lesion
- Treatment of a Grade I or II lesion generally carries a mortality rate of 0 to 1% and a morbidity rate of 5 to 10%

Suggested Readings

Marks MP, Lane B, Steinberg GK, Chang PJ. Hemorrhage into intracerebral arteriovenous malformations: angiographic determinants. *Radiology* 176:807–813, 1990.

Schaller C, Schramm J. Microsurgical results for small arteriovenous malformations accessible for radiosurgical or embolization treatment. *Neurosurgery* 40:664–674, 1997.

Spetzler RF, Martin NA. A proposed grading system for arteriovenous malformations. *J Neurosurg* 65:476–483, 1986.

Case 77

Clinical Presentation

A 23-year-old man presents for evaluation of chronic headache.

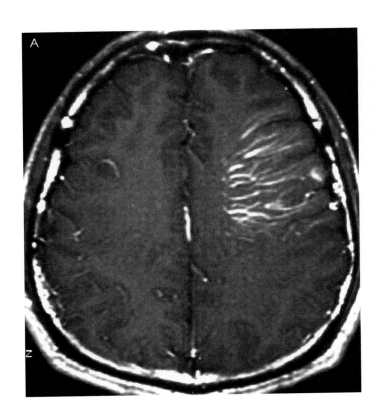

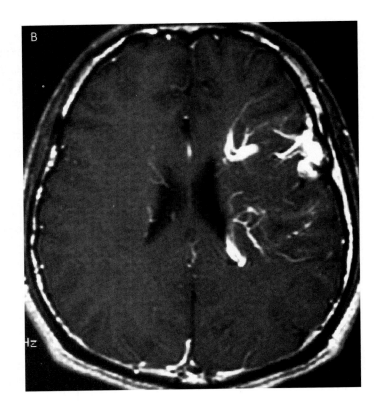

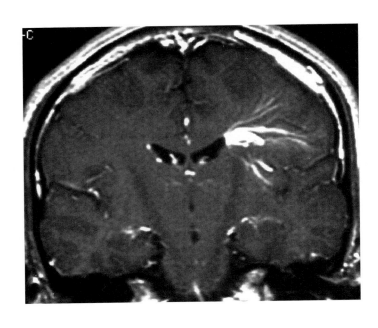

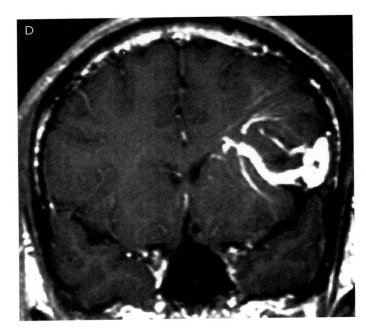

Pearls

- VMs occur in all parts of the brain but are most common in the frontal lobes and the posterior fossa.

- It is important to identify any VM occurring in association with a cavernous malformation so that the neurosurgeon can avoid injuring the VM (which drains normal brain parenchyma) during any surgery on the cavernous malformation.

- Focal anomalies of neuronal migration may uncommonly be associated with VMs.

Pitfalls

- Many VMs may only be detected if contrast material is administered.

- Some lesions may have a transitional morphology, with features of both VM and arteriovenous shunting suggestive of arteriovenous malformation. This is likely a consequence of chronically elevated pressures in the VM with eventual development of arteriovenous shunting at the precapillary level.

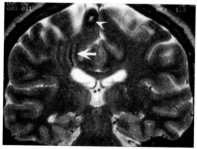

Fig. E. A coronal fast spin-echo T2-WI demonstrates spatial misregistration artifact due to a venous malformation (*arrow*), as well as an associated cavernous malformation (*arrowhead*).

Radiologic Findings

An axial post-gadolinium T1-WI (Fig. A) demonstrates multiple linear enhancing structures in the left frontal lobe. There is no associated mass effect. A more inferior post-gadolinium T1-WI (Fig. B) demonstrates two large serpiginous enhancing structures in the subependymal region on the left, as well as a serpigious enhancing structure at the superior aspect of the left sylvian fissure. In the coronal plane, post-gadolinium T1-WIs (Figs. C and D) demonstrate multiple linear enhancing structures converging on larger central draining structures that then join with a torturous serpiginous enhancing structure in the left sylvian fissure.

Diagnosis

Venous malformation (VM), a.k.a. developmental venous anomaly

Differential Diagnosis

- Arteriovenous malformation (arteriovenous shunting, central "nidus" of vessels, arterial phase as well as venous phase abnormalities on angiography)
- Capillary telangiectasia (lacks characteristic "Medusa head" pattern, typically found in pons although it may occur in cerebral hemispheres)

Discussion

Background

VMs (also referred to as venous angiomas or developmental venous anomalies) are quite common, being found in up to 3% of autopsies. VMs provide anomalous venous drainage of normal brain parenchyma. They are most commonly small, but range in size from holohemispheric to microscopic. These lesions are often quite subtle angiographically unless large and are far more easily recognized on contrast-enhanced CT or MR scans. In approximately 7% of cases, a cavernous malformation is identified in association with the distal radicles of a VM (Figs. E and F), likely arising in the setting of elevated venous pressures due to venous stenosis. Conversely, as many as 30% of solitary cavernous malformations are intimately associated with an MR-visible VM.

Etiology

VMs are thought to arise from an arrest of venous development after arterial development is complete. This arrest could then result in the retention of primitive medullary veins that drain in a single large anomalous draining vein.

Clinical Findings

VMs are most commonly identified incidentally on contrast-enhanced imaging studies of the brain. Headache is common, although the causal relationship with the VM is unclear. Some patients may experience focal neurological deficits related to stenosis of the VM, with resultant venous hypertension and chronic parenchymal ischemia. Seizures may occur, also likely related to chronic ischemia with resultant parenchymal encephalomalacia and/or calcification. Cerebellar VMs have been associated with ataxia, diplopia, and dizziness, even in the absence of hemorrhage.

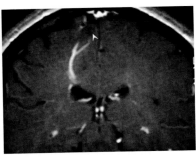

Fig. F. A coronal post-gadolinium T1-WI (same patient as Fig. E) better demonstrates a venous malformation draining toward subependymal veins. The associated cavernous malformation (*arrowhead*) is less well seen on this sequence.

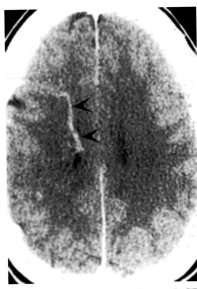

Fig. G. A contrast-enhanced CT scan demonstrates an anomalous enhancing vein coursing toward the ventricular surface (*arrowheads*).

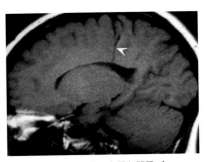

Fig. H. A sagittal T1-WI demonstrates a flow void due to an anomalous vein coursing toward the ventricular surface (*arrowhead*).

Complications

Hemorrhage may occur from either an associated cavernous malformation or rarely from the VM itself.

Pathology

Gross
- Radially arranged anomalous medullary veins converge on a larger central draining vein, which in turn empties into a subependymal vein, cortical vein, or dural sinus

Microscopic
- The walls of the veins are typically slightly thickened and hyalinized
- The venous radicles are separated by normal intervening brain parenchyma

Imaging Findings

CT
- Non-contrast CT is typically normal unless there is calcification or hemorrhage related to an associated cavernous malformation or calcification related to chronic ischemia
- Contrast-enhanced CT scan shows small anomalous enhancing veins coursing toward a larger draining vein (Fig. G)

MR
- Flow voids (Fig. H) and spatial misregistration artifact (Fig. E) may be appreciated on pre-contrast studies
- Post-contrast, the characteristic "Medusa head" appearance of venous radicles converging on a larger central draining vein is seen
- T2 prolongation may be present in adjacent tissues if there is venous hypertension and venous ischemia

Angiography
- Anomalous venous structures converge on a larger central draining vein (Fig. I)

Treatment

None

Prognosis

- Generally excellent, unless there is venous stenosis or an associated cavernous malformation, in which case there is an increased rate of hemorrhage
- If venous stenosis complicated by chronic ischemia develops, there are unfortunately few options as the VM cannot be resected and the venous radicles are generally inaccessible to any endovascular approach

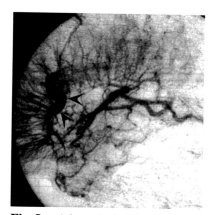

Fig. I. A lateral view from the late phase of a carotid angiogram demonstrates a frontal venous malformation with multiple radicles converging on an anomalous dilated central vein (*arrowheads*).

Suggested Readings

Dillon WP. Cryptic vascular malformations: controversies in terminology, diagnosis, pathophysiology, and treatment. *AJNR* 18:1839–1846, 1997.

Rigamonti D, Spetzler RF, Medina M, et al. Cerebral venous malformations. *J Neurosurg* 73:560–564, 1998.

Truwit CL. Venous angioma of the brain: history, significance, and imaging findings. *AJR* 159:1299–1307, 1992.

Case 78

Clinical Presentation

A 45-year-old woman who had been involved in a motor vehicle accident several weeks earlier presents with right-sided proptosis and diplopia.

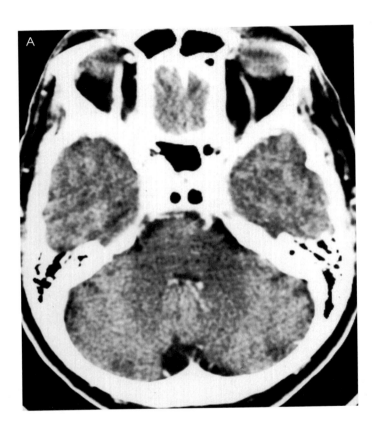

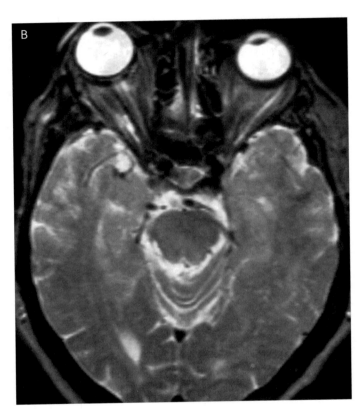

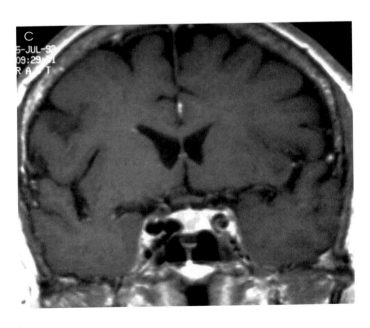

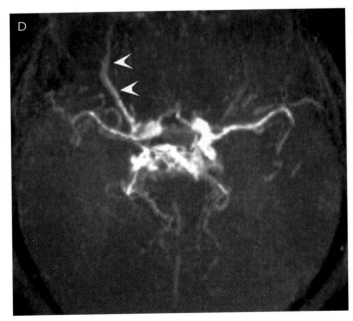

Pearls

- Direct visualization of the intercavernous sinuses (which connect the two cavernous sinuses along the back of the clivus) on contrast-enhanced MR images may be an ancillary sign of CCF.

- During angiography, compression of the ipsilateral carotid artery below the catheter injection site may slow arterial flow and help to better localize the fistula site. Rapid filming is also essential.

- If the SOV is patent and dilated, this represents a possible therapeutic access route to the cavernous sinus if the inferior petrosal sinus is occluded. However, surgical exposure of the vessel is usually required.

Pitfalls

- Cortical venous drainage may be present even if the normal drainage routes (SOV, IPS) are patent.

- The actual CCF may be contralateral to the dilated SOV.

- Anomalous intracranial venous drainage may mimic a CCF; bilateral sigmoid sinus aplasia/hypoplasia may result in the majority of cerebral venous drainage occurring through the cavernous sinus and SOV.

- Abrupt closure of a large fistula may result in massive cerebral edema, since the cerebral vasculature may be unable to tolerate the reestablishment of normal cerebral perfusion ("normal perfusion pressure breakthrough"). This complication can be avoided with staged or slow occlusion.

E

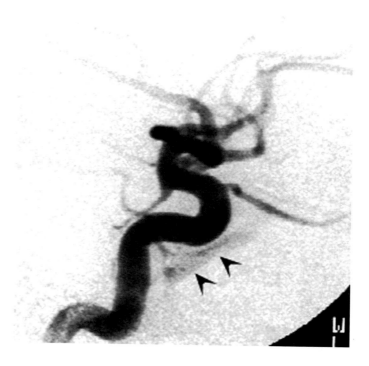

Radiologic Findings

A contrast-enhanced CT scan (Fig. A) demonstrates asymmetry of the superior ophthalmic veins, with the right larger than the left. An axial T2-WI from an MR scan (Fig. B) shows significant right-sided proptosis. A coronal T1-WI (Fig. C) demonstrates asymmetric enlargement of the right cavernous carotid artery, as well as prominent flow voids in the right cavernous sinus. A collapsed image from an intracranial three-dimensional time-of-flight MR angiogram (Fig. D) demonstrates abnormal vascular structures in the region of the cavernous sinuses bilaterally, as well as striking prominence of the right superior ophthalmic vein (*arrowheads*). A lateral view of a right internal carotid angiogram (Fig. E) obtained during the early arterial phase shows abnormal filling of the right cavernous sinus (*arrowheads*) via a direct communication.

Diagnosis

Carotid cavernous fistula (CCF)

Differential Diagnosis

- Anomalous intracranial venous drainage (may mimic CCF, diagnosis established by angiography)
- Cavernous sinus thrombosis (may clinically mimic CCF, but can be differentiated with MR or angiography)

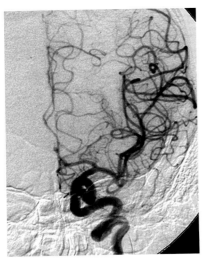

Fig. F. A frontal projection from a left internal carotid angiogram in a 52-year-old man with proptosis and chemosis of the left eye is unremarkable.

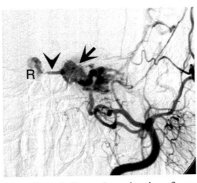

Fig. G. A frontal projection from a left external carotid angiogram (same patient as Fig. F) demonstrates hypertrophy of the accessory meningeal artery and filling of the left cavernous sinus (*arrow*) via fistulous communications. The right cavernous sinus (R) is filling via the intercavernous sinus (*arrowhead*).

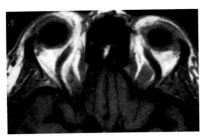

Fig. H. An axial T1-WI in a 79-year-old woman with bilateral pulsatile exophthalmos demonstrates marked enlargement of the superior ophthalmic veins bilaterally.

Discussion

Background

CCF refers to an abnormal communication between the carotid artery or its branches and the cavernous sinus. A CCF may be direct, when the internal carotid artery (ICA) itself communicates with the cavernous sinus, or indirect, when meningeal branches of the ICA and/or external carotid artery (ECA) communicate with the cavernous sinus. Direct CCFs are usually due to trauma or to intracavernous rupture of an ICA aneurysm and are high-flow lesions. Indirect or dural CCFs usually occur spontaneously as a result of multiple small dural arterial connections between meningeal branches of the ICA siphon, the ECA (Figs. F and G), or both with the cavernous sinus(es) and are usually relatively low-flow lesions.

Clinical Findings

Classic symptoms of a CCF are pulsatile exophthalmos, bruit, and conjunctival chemosis. However, symptoms may also be nonspecific, with blurred vision, headache, and proptosis. Cranial nerve palsies may also be present (usually III, IV, and VI).

Complications

Visual loss due to elevated intraocular pressure and elevated intracranial pressure are complications of CCFs. Intracranial hemorrhage (parenchymal or subarachnoid) may occur when cortical venous drainage is present. Cerebral ischemia is related to elevated venous pressures or steal of blood by the fistula.

Pathophysiology

The cavernous sinus usually receives venous blood from the superior and inferior ophthalmic veins and the sphenoparietal sinus. Blood then flows from the cavernous sinus into the jugular vein via the inferior petrosal sinus (IPS). The cavernous sinuses may communicate with each other via the intercavernous sinus, and the cavernous sinuses may also communicate with cortical veins. Classically, a CCF results in reversal of flow through an enlarged superior ophthalmic vein (SOV). Some cases may additionally demonstrate abnormal retrograde flow in dilated cortical veins.

Imaging Findings

CT

- Prominent SOV(s) may be seen
- Contrast-enhanced CT may show marked dilatation and enhancement of the cavernous sinus

MR

- Enlargement of the cavernous sinus is usually seen
- Abnormal flow voids in the cavernous sinus are typically present
- Prominent SOV is commonly seen either unilaterally or bilaterally. The reversal of flow away from the cavernous sinus may be demonstrable with phase-contrast MR angiography (Figs. H and I).

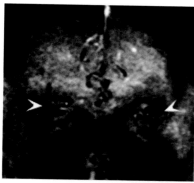

Fig. I. A coronal view from a phase-contrast MR angiogram sensitized to flow in the anterior-posterior direction (same patient as Fig. F) shows reversal of flow (i.e., posterior to anterior) in the superior ophthalmic veins bilaterally (*arrowheads*), manifest as low-signal intensity instead of the expected high-signal intensity in the vessels.

Angiography

- Direct fistula: single-hole communication between the ICA and the cavernous sinus, with rapid opacification of the cavernous sinus during the arterial phase
- Indirect fistula: multiple small meningeal branches from internal and/or external carotid arteries which supply the dura of the cavernous sinus empty through abnormal communications into the cavernous sinus

Treatment

- Indirect (dural) CCFs have a high rate of spontaneous cures or disappearance of symptoms. They may also respond to carotid compression therapy. When the clinical course is progressive, transarterial (rare) or transvenous (common) therapy may be indicated. Transvenous occlusive methods include detachable balloons, coil embolization, fibrin glue, and other materials.
- Direct CCFs are typically high-flow lesions that require acute treatment through transarterial and/or transvenous routes. Transarterial balloon embolization is the treatment of choice. Transarterial coil embolization may also play a role, particularly in difficult cases where a balloon cannot be manipulated into the necessary position. When transarterial routes are unsuccessful, transvenous embolization may be indicated.

Prognosis

Successful treatment is accomplished in more than 90% of cases

Suggested Readings

Elster AD, Chen MYM, Richardson DM, Yeatts PR. Dilated intercavernous sinuses: an MR sign of carotid-cavernous and carotid-dural fistulas. *AJNR* 12:641–645, 1991.

Halbach VV, Higashida RT, Barnwell SL, Dowd CF, Hieshima GB. Transarterial platinum coil embolization of carotid-cavernous fistulas. *AJNR* 12:429–433, 1991.

Halbach VV, Higashida RT, Hieshima GB, Norman D. Normal perfusion pressure breakthrough occurring during treatment of carotid and vertebral fistulas. *AJNR* 8:8751–756, 1987.

Case 79

Clinical Presentation

An 85-year-old woman complains of right-sided pulsatile tinnitus and vague left hemisensory changes.

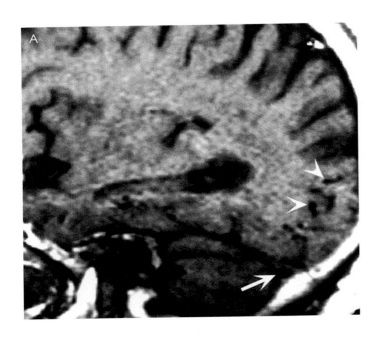

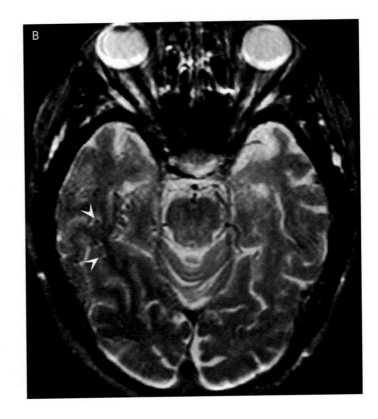

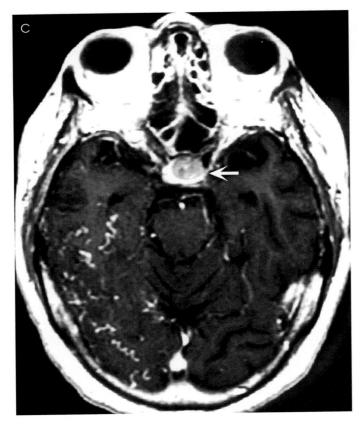

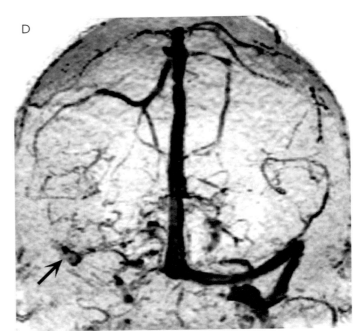

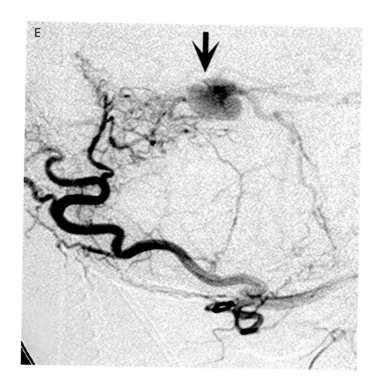

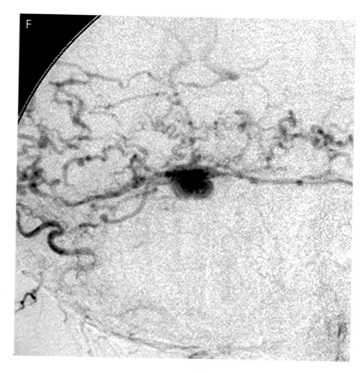

Radiologic Findings

A sagittal T1-WI (Fig. A) demonstrates prominent flow voids in the left occipital lobe (*arrowheads*). In addition, abnormal signal intensity is present in the right transverse sinus (*arrow*), consistent with slow flow or occlusion. An axial T2-WI (Fig. B) demonstrates prominent flow voids in the right temporal lobe (*arrowheads*). Parenchymal signal intensity is normal. An axial post-gadolinium T1-WI (Fig. C) demonstrates serpiginous enhancing structures in the right occipital and temporal lobes, most consistent with abnormal vascular structures. Incidental note is made of an enhancing sellar mass (*arrow*) consistent with a pituitary macroadenoma. A coronal maximum intensity projection from an MR venogram (Fig. D) demonstrates absence of flow in the right transverse and sigmoid sinuses, except for a focal area of flow-related enhancement at the transverse-sigmoid junction (*arrow*). Note also the prominence of small vascular structures projecting superior to the expected position of the right transverse sinus. A lateral view from a right occipital artery angiogram (Fig. E) demonstrates supply to multiple small irregular arterial channels, consistent with a dural arteriovenous fistula. A focal area of contrast accumulation (*arrow*) corresponds to focal filling at the right transverse-sigmoid junction, but the transverse and sigmoid sinuses are otherwise occluded. A later image from the same angiographic injection (Fig. F) demonstrates extensive filling of dilated cortical veins, corresponding to the finding on contrast-enhanced MRI.

Diagnosis

Dural arteriovenous fistula (DAVF)

Differential Diagnosis

- Arteriovenous malformation (a nidus is present, supply is from pial vessels)
- Venous malformation (generally asymptomatic, normal arterial phase at angiography, characteristic "Medusa head" appearance)

- Venous sinus thrombosis (this alone would not account for the pattern of multiple vessels in the right temporal and occipital regions)

Discussion

Background

DAVFs account for 10 to 15% of all intracranial arteriovenous lesions. These are thought to be acquired lesions, related in many cases to previous thrombosis of a dural sinus. DAVFs consist of abnormal arteriovenous connections that are located within the dura mater, usually within the wall of a dural sinus or involving an adjacent draining vein. Approximately 95% of DAVFs are fed by meningeal arteries and only 5% by both meningeal arteries and cortical branches. As DAVFs are most common in the posterior fossa, the occipital artery commonly supplies these lesions. DAVFs are classified by their pattern of venous drainage (Table 1). The most common locations include the transverse sinus at the transverse-sigmoid junction, the cavernous sinus, the tentorium cerebelli, and the superior sagittal sinus.

Etiology

Etiology is unknown, although they seem to be acquired lesions in most cases. Predisposing factors for the development of DAVF include cranial trauma, neurologic surgery, and clinical states associated with hypercoagulability (infection, pregnancy, oral contraceptives).

Clinical Findings

Patients most commonly present in the fourth to seventh decade. Symptoms are highly variable and depend to some extent on the location of the fistula. Posterior fossa lesions may present with pulsatile tinnitus. Cavernous carotid fistulas (see Case 78) may present with proptosis, chemosis, and retro-orbital pain. A lesion in any location may present with headache or papilledema due to elevated intracranial pressure, cranial bruit, and fixed or reversible focal neurologic deficits due to venous hypertension or venous infarction. Symptoms may also be due to parenchymal, subarachnoid, or subdural hemorrhage.

Complications

Hemorrhage is the major complication.

Table 1. Classification of Dural Arteriovenous Fistulas*

Type	Description
I	Drains into a sinus with normal antegrade flow.
II	Drains into a sinus with insufficient antegrade venous drainage. The insufficiency may be due to stenosis or occlusion of the sinus into which a DAVF with moderate flow rate drains or to a DAVF with very high flow rate that cannot drain into a normal or even an enlarged sinus. Retrograde drainage may be into sinus(es) only and/or into cortical vein(s).
III	Drains directly into cortical vein(s), without venous ectasia.
IV	Drains into a cortical vein with venous ectasia larger than 5 mm in diameter and 3x larger than the diameter of the draining vein.
V	Drains into spinal perimedullary veins despite its intracranial location.

*As described by Cognard et al. (1995)

Pathology

Gross

- Thickening of walls of involved arteries and veins
- The presence of sinus thrombosis is variable
- A discrete nidus is generally not present

Microscopic

- Direct communications between dural arteries and dilated venules without intervening capillaries are present in the walls of the involved venous sinuses

Imaging Findings

CT

- Frequently normal unless a complicating hemorrhage has occurred

MR

- May be normal
- May show white matter signal abnormalities with T2 hyperintensity
- Multiple enlarged vascular channels may be present
- Dural sinuses may show slow flow or occlusion

Angiography

- Abnormal communication between external carotid artery branches or between dural branches of the internal carotid or vertebral arteries and the dural sinuses are present

Treatment

Obliteration of the fistulous communication via endovascular and/or surgical methods. Type I fistulas are often simply followed and in some cases may spontaneously close. Symptomatic lesions may respond to compression of the ipsilateral carotid or occipital artery.

Prognosis

Varies tremendously with the type of fistula:

- Type I fistulas generally have a benign course
- Types II-IV have a progressively increasing incidence of intracranial hypertension and intracranial hemorrhage
- Type V fistulas frequently results in progressive myelopathy

Suggested Readings

Cognard C, Gobin YP, Pierot L, et al. Cerebral dural arteriovenous fistulas: clinical and angiographic correlation with a revised classification of venous drainage. *Radiology* 194:671–680, 1995.

Hamada Y, Goto K, Inoue T, et al. Histopathological aspects of dural arteriovenous fistulas in the transverse-sigmoid sinus region in nine patients. *Neurosurgery* 40:452–458, 1997.

Zeidman SM, Monsein LH, Arosarena O, et al. Reversibility of white matter changes and dementia after treatment of dural fistulas. *AJNR* 16:1080–1083, 1995.

Case 80

Clinical Presentation

A 40-year-old woman became increasingly confused over the course of several days. Soon after being admitted to the hospital, she progressed to coma.

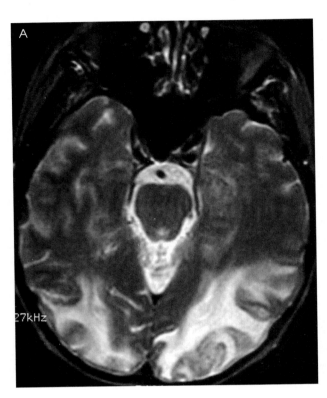

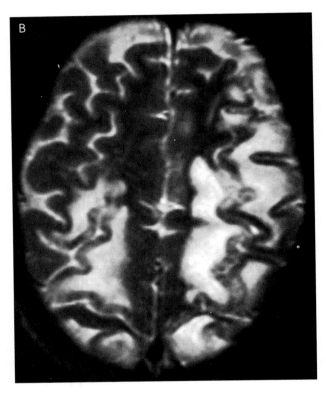

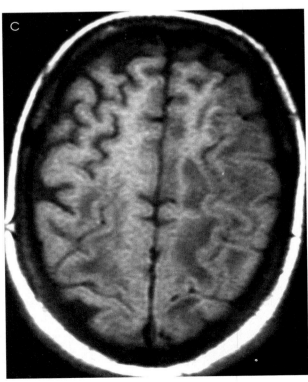

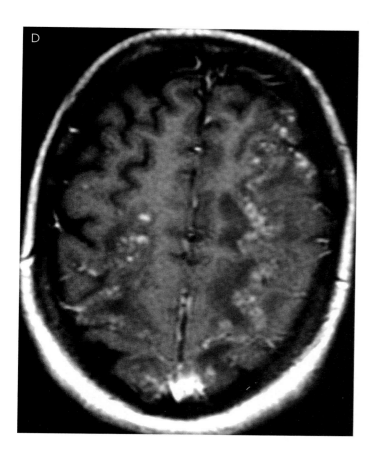
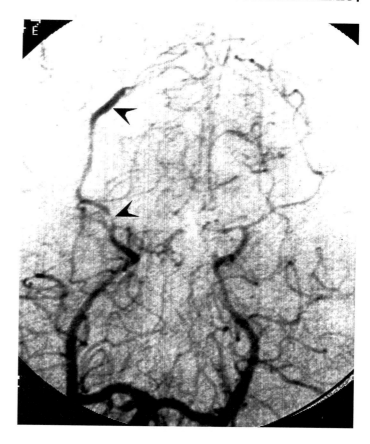

Radiologic Findings

An axial T2-WI (Fig. A) demonstrates high-signal intensity involving the occipital cortex and subcortical white matter. A more cephalad image (Fig. B) demonstrates abnormal high signal intensity in the cortex and subcortical white matter of the frontal and parietal lobes, left greater than right. A corresponding axial T1-WI (Fig. C) shows mild parenchymal swelling, with associated sulcal effacement. The subcortical white matter is hypointense. An axial T1-WI following administration of gadolinium (Fig. D) demonstrates nodular enhancement predominantly involving the cortex and immediate subcortical white matter. A diagnostic angiogram was performed. A Towne's projection from a left vetebral artery injection (Fig. E) demonstrates areas of irregular narrowing and dilatation involving the right posterior cerebral artery (*arrowheads*).

Diagnosis

Primary angiitis of the CNS (PACNS)

Differential Diagnosis

- Other causes of CNS vasculitis (clinical and laboratory features)
- Encephalitis (fever, acute onset)
- Postictal changes or hypertensive encephalopathy (appropriate clinical history)
- Gliomatosis or lymphomatosis cerebri (more mass effect, insidious onset)
- Intravascular lymphoma ("malignant angioendotheliomatosis," indistinguishable from CNS vasculitis but very rare)

• Acute disseminated encephalomyelitis (typically younger patient, often history of antecedent vaccination or upper respiratory illness, normal angiogram)
• Toxic leukoencephalopathy (clinical history essential, often very symmetric)
• Metabolic disease (unusual to present in an adult patient, usually symmetric)

Discussion

Background

CNS vasculitis occurs in three settings: as an isolated entity (PACNS), as a complication of rheumatic or vasculitic disorders such as systemic lupus erythematosus or Wegener's granulomatosis, or as a consequence of diverse insults such as infection and toxin exposure. PACNS is a rare disease of unknown cause. The disease most commonly affects small leptomeningeal and cortical arteries, arterioles, and veins. Because involvement may be segmental, this diagnosis may be missed antemortem on biopsy. The principal clinical manifestation is progressive cerebral dysfunction, with development of focal or multifocal areas of cerebral infarction. The disease has a slight male predominance, and the mean age of onset is 45 years. A variant designated "benign angiopathy of the CNS" describes a subset of young women who present with acute symptoms, a bland CSF, and positive angiography who often have a self-limiting course and may not require treatment with cytotoxic agents or even steroids.

Etiology

The etiology is unknown but may result from a viral-induced immune reaction. Histologically similar changes in vessel walls have been described with Hodgkin's disease and varicella zoster infection.

Clinical Findings

PACNS is not associated with systemic illness. Early symptoms include headache, confusion, intellectual deterioration, memory loss, and malaise. This may progress to seizures, focal neurologic deficits, and coma. Lumbar puncture may demonstrate elevated protein and a mononuclear cell predominance, but CSF analysis is insensitive and nonspecific.

Complications

Subarachnoid hemorrhage and multiple parenchymal hematomas have been described with PACNS. Survivors frequently have residual neurologic deficits. Patients are at risk of infectious complications due to treatment with steroids and cytotoxic agents.

Pathology

Gross

• Multifocal cerebral infarcts
• Intraparenchymal or subarachnoid hemorrhage due to focal necrosis of vessel walls may be present

Microscopic

- Granuloma formation in the walls of leptomeningeal and parenchymal arteries and veins with focal fibrinoid necrosis. Infiltration by polymorphonuclear leukocytes, lymphocytes, epithelioid cells, and multinucleated giant cells.

Imaging Findings

CT

- May be normal
- Areas of decreased attenuation with a white matter predominance
- Rarely subarachnoid or intraparenchymal hemorrhage

MR

- Examination may be normal
- Usually multifocal areas of T2 prolongation in the deep white matter and often the cortex as well. These lesions may exert mass effect, presumably due to vasogenic edema caused by increased vascular permeability.
- Some parenchymal lesions demonstrate gadolinium enhancement
- Diffuse leptomeningeal enhancement has been reported

Angiography

- Segmental narrowing or beading of vessels with multiple areas of involvement
- Typically affects more than one vascular territory

Treatment

Prednisone, often in combination with cyclophosphamide

Prognosis

- PACNS has a broad clinical spectrum that ranges from death in days to weeks to spontaneous remission. Treatment with steroids and cytotoxic agents improves outcome.
- Overall mortality is 10 to 20%, with 25 to 35% of patients making an incomplete recovery and 50 to 60% of patients making a complete recovery

Suggested Readings

Ozawa T, Sasaki O, Sorimachi T, Tanaka R. Primary angiitis of the central nervous system: report of two cases and review of the literature. *Neurosurgery* 36:173–179, 1995.

Shoemaker EI, Lin ZS, Rae-Grant AD, Little B. Primary angiitis of the central nervous system: unusual MR appearance. *AJNR* 15:331–334, 1994.

Stone JH, Pomper MG, Roubenoff R, Miller TJ, Hellman DB. Sensitivities of noninvasive tests for central nervous system vasculitis: a comparison of lumbar puncture, computed tomography, and magnetic resonance imaging. *J Rheumatol* 21:1277–1282, 1994.

Case 81

Clinical Presentation

A 47-year-old woman presents with left-sided weakness.

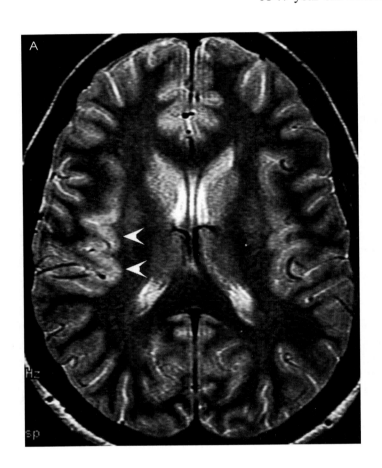 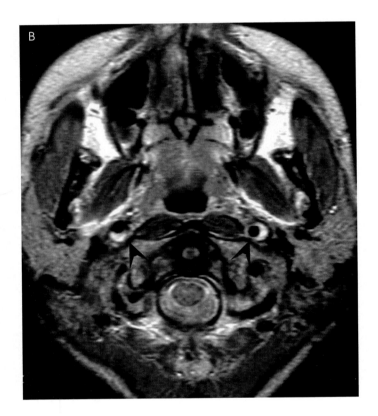

Radiologic Findings

An axial T2-WI (Fig. A) demonstrates subtle abnormal T2 prolongation in the right insular cortex (*arrowheads*). An axial PD-WI (Fig. B) at the level of C1 demonstrates crescentic high signal eccentric to the lumina of the distal cervical internal carotid arteries bilaterally (*arrowheads*), consistent with subintimal hematoma and bilateral dissection.

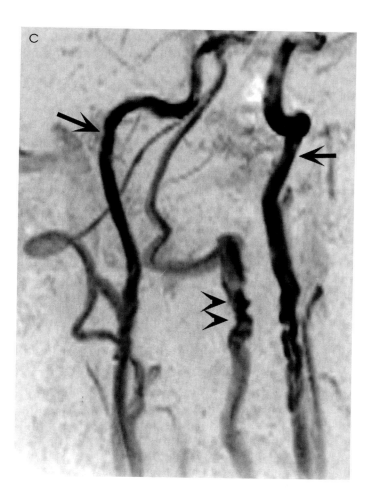

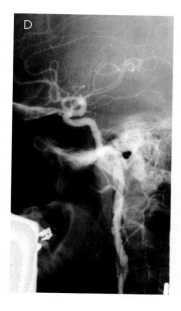

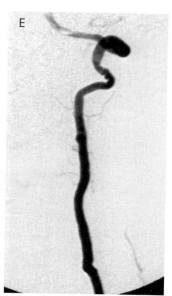

An oblique coronal maximum intensity projection image from a cervical MR angiogram (Fig. C) demonstrates irregularity of the proximal cervical internal carotid arteries bilaterally, as well as irregularity of the distal cervical left vertebral artery (*arrowheads*). Note also the mild irregularity and narrowing of the distal cervical internal carotid arteries (*arrows*), with extension into the petrous segment on the right. A lateral view from a conventional catheter angiogram (Fig. D) confirms the "string of beads" appearance of the cervical internal carotid artery. A digital subtraction image from a left vertebral angiogram (Fig. E) similarly shows a "string of beads" appearance of the distal cervical vertebral artery, corresponding to the appearance on MR angiography.

Diagnosis

Fibromuscular dysplasia (FMD)

Differential Diagnosis

- Takayasu arteritis (typically involves the common carotid artery, long-segment stenosis, systemic symptoms, decreased or absent peripheral pulses)
- Atherosclerosis (eccentric irregular stenosis, predilection for carotid bulb)
- Dissection (may coexist with FMD, or be spontaneous or secondary to trauma; isolated dissection usually causes a smooth narrowing)
- Catheter-induced spasm (reversible)

- FMD usually spares vascular origins, which is helpful in differentiating these lesions from atherosclerosis.
- Severe stenoses are uncommon in FMD, and complete occlusions are rare.
- Complete cerebral angiography is necessary in FMD to exclude an associated intracranial aneurysm.
- The angiographic appearance of FMD may evolve over time, with transition from a string-of-beads pattern to an elongated tubulostenotic pattern.

Pitfalls

- The atypical or aneurysmal form of FMD may be difficult to distinguish from atherosclerotic aneurysm or traumatic pseudoaneurysm.
- A motion-degraded MR angiogram of the cervical carotid arteries may mimic the "string of beads" appearance of FMD.

- Stationary wave artifact (regular, evenly spaced appearance; vessel caliber normal between areas of constriction rather than dilated; appearance varies between angiographic runs)

Discussion

Background

FMD is an uncommon arteriopathy of unknown etiology that affects small- and medium-sized arteries, most commonly the renal arteries. The cervical internal carotid arteries are the second most common site of involvement, and the vertebral arteries are also frequently affected (25%). Intracranial involvement is rare. Nearly 90% of patients with cervical FMD are women, usually in their fourth or fifth decade. FMD is very uncommon in children. In the typical medial type of FMD (see below), the midcervical portion of the internal carotid artery tends to be involved, especially opposite the C2 vertebral body; the proximal 2 to 3 cm of the vessel are characteristically spared. Involvement is bilateral in 60 to 85% of cases.

Etiology

The cause is unknown, but familial occurrence and association with intracranial aneurysmal disease suggest a congenital mesenchymal disorder.

Clinical Findings

FMD is often discovered incidentally during cerebral arteriography. Focal neurologic deficits related to vascular stenosis and/or thromboembolic events may be observed. Renovascular hypertension is common.

Complications

Intracranial aneurysms are described in 20 to 50% of cases. Spontaneous carotid artery dissection, carotid aneurysm formation, and spontaneous arteriovenous fistula are described. As many as 20% of carotid dissections occur in patients with FMD.

Pathology

FMD is characterized by disorganization of the arterial wall with elastic fiber destruction, fibrous tissue proliferation, and fibroblast-like metaplasia of smooth muscle cells. Three histologic subtypes of FMD are described: medial (90% of cases), intimal, and periarterial or subadventitial.

- Medial: concentric rings of fibrous proliferation or smooth muscle hypertrophy with associated destruction of the internal and external elastic membranes. These rings may alternate with areas of arterial dilatation.
- Intimal: accumulation of irregularly arranged subendothelial mesenchymal cells within a loose matrix of fibrous connective tissue
- Subadventitial: fibrosis of adventitia and periarterial tissues, abnormal accumulation of elastic tissue between the media and adventitia

Imaging Findings

CT

- May show evidence for cerebral infarction

MR

- Imaging may be normal or show evidence of ischemia/infarction
- MRA may demonstrate areas of apparent dilatation alternating with areas of narrowing or signal loss, or areas of smooth stenosis

Angiography

- Most common pattern is segments of constriction alternating with normal-appearing or dilated segments ("string of beads" appearance). This is usually associated with the medial histologic subtype.
- A smooth concentric tubular lesion is seen in less than 10% of cases
- An "atypical" pattern consists of eccentric outpouchings that may progress to frank aneurysm formation

Treatment

- Medical: antiplatelet therapy, anticoagulation
- Surgical: angioplasty, endarterectomy, resection-anastomosis

Prognosis

- The natural history is uncertain, as lesions may be static or progressive
- Regression has not been reported

Suggested Readings

Furie DM, Tien RD. Fibromuscular dysplasia of arteries of the head and neck: imaging findings. *AJR* 162:1205–1209, 1994.

Heiserman JE, Drayer BP, Fram EK, Keller PJ. MR angiography of cervical fibromuscular dysplasia. *AJNR* 13:1454–1457, 1992.

Russo CP, Smoker WRK. Nonatheromatous carotid artery disease. *Neuroimag Clin North Am* 6:811–830, 1996.

Case 82

Clinical Presentation

A 28-year-old woman has been noting low-grade fever, malaise, and arthralgias for several months. She presents for evaluation after developing acute onset of right-sided weakness.

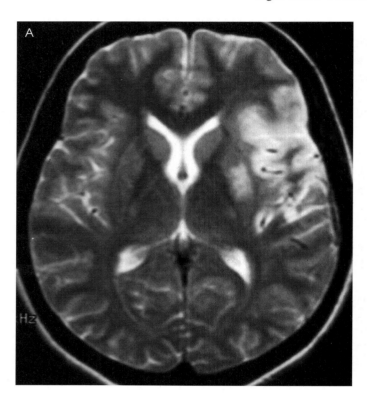

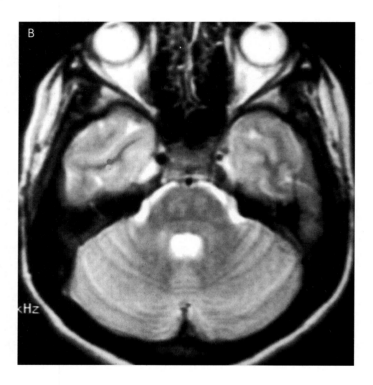

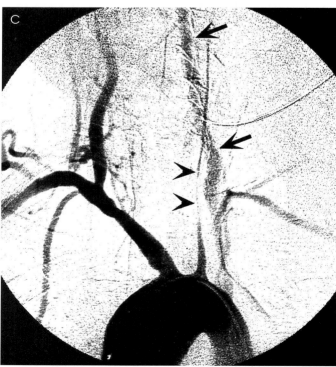

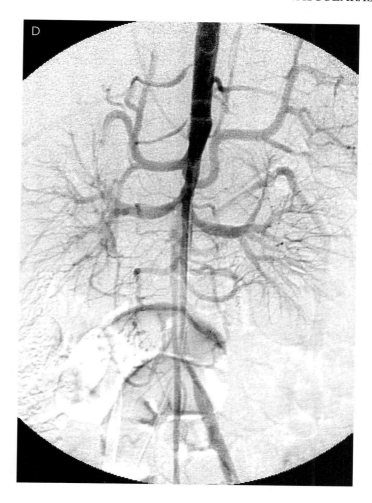

Radiologic Findings

An axial T2-WI (Fig. A) demonstrates edema in the left frontal cortex and left putamen, consistent with acute left middle cerebral artery infarction. A more inferior T2-WI (Fig. B) demonstrates marked asymmetry of the cavernous carotid arteries, with the left being significantly smaller than the right. An angiogram was performed. A right posterior oblique projection from an arch aortogram (Fig. C) demonstrates striking long-segment tubular narrowing of the left common carotid artery (*arrowheads*). The left subclavian artery is also somewhat narrow and irregular. The brachiocephalic artery is focally narrow and irregular. The right common carotid artery is patent. The left vertebral artery (*arrows*) is significantly enlarged, presumably due to increased flow in compensation for the severe left common carotid artery narrowing. A frontal projection from an abdominal aortogram (Fig. D) demonstrates marked smooth, tapered narrowing of the mid and distal abdominal aorta.

Diagnosis

Takayasu arteritis (TA)

Differential Diagnosis

• Fibromuscular dysplasia ("string of beads," irregular dilatations of vessel)

- Carotid dissection (smoothly tapering narrowing or occlusion, often a history of trauma)
- Carotid infection (uncommon, usually leads to pseudoaneurysm formation)

Discussion

Background

TA, also known as aortitis syndrome, is a chronic inflammatory arteriopathy that usually affects women in the second to fourth decade of life. The disease was initially reported in the Japanese literature, but it has a worldwide occurrence and may affect males as well. TA affects large- and medium-sized arteries such as the aortic arch and its branches. The aorta is affected in essentially all cases, while carotid involvement is seen in 60 to 70% of cases. The common carotid artery is usually the affected segment, with the internal and external carotid arteries being relatively spared. The subclavian and renal arteries are commonly involved, as are the pulmonary arteries.

Etiology

The cause is unknown but is presumed to be autoimmune. High levels of gamma globulins, immune complexes, and rheumatoid factor are observed.

Clinical Findings

Two phases of the disease are classically described. The early or systemic phase is characterized by fever, weakness, arthralgia, arthritis, myalgia, and chest and abdominal pain. The late, pulseless, or occlusive phase presents with symptoms related most often to cerebrovascular insufficiency. Asymmetrical blood pressure and absent radial pulses are common.

Complications

Complications include cerebral ischemia/infarction, renovascular hypertension, arm claudication, and aneurysm formation. Cerebral ischemia/infarction is related to progressive vascular stenosis/occlusion. Stroke is the initial presentation in 15% of cases. Aneurysm formation can lead to embolic complications, or rupture and subarachnoid hemorrhage.

Pathology

Gross

- Vessel walls are typically markedly thickened
- In some cases, when supporting tissues are severely damaged and deficient, vessels may show dilatation and focal aneurysm formation

Microscopic

- Destruction of elastic fibers in the media, cellular infiltration of the adventitia and media, and fibrosis and hyperplasia of the intima without cellular infiltration have been described

Imaging Findings

CT

- A non-contrast scan may demonstrate thickening and increased density of vessel walls
- Contrast-enhanced CT may show only irregularity of vessel walls

MR

- MR imaging demonstrates circumferential vascular wall thickening and reduction in caliber of flow voids
- Both CT and MR may demonstrate evidence of cerebral infarction or hypoperfusion
- MR angiography may demonstrate vascular stenosis, occlusion, and aneurysm formation

Ultrasound

- Homogeneous circumferential thickening of the intima-media complex
- There is often a clear-cut boundary between involved and uninvolved segments

Angiography

- Typically shows long-segment areas of arterial stenosis as well as branch vessel occlusions

Treatment

- Medical: aspirin, steroids, cytotoxic agents
- Surgical: angioplasty, vascular stenting, vascular reconstruction, bypass

Prognosis

- Response to therapy is variable and unpredictable
- Vasculopathy may progress even if systemic symptoms respond to steroids and/or cytotoxic agents
- Overall, 20% of patients never achieve remission, and 45% relapse after remission. However, premature death is uncommon unless poor outcome predictors (aneurysm, severe hypertension, cardiac involvement) are present.

Suggested Readings

Murakami R, Korogi Y, Matsuno Y, Matsukawa T, Hirai T, Takahashi M. Percutaneous transluminal angioplasty for carotid artery stenosis in Takayasu arteritis: persistent benefit over 10 years. *Cardiovasc Intervent Radiol* 20:219–221, 1997.

Yamada I, Numano F, Suzuki S. Takayasu arteritis: evaluation with MR imaging. *Radiology* 188:89–94, 1993.

Yamato M, Lecky JW, Hiramatsu K, Kohda E. Takayasu arteritis: radiographic and angiographic findings in 59 patients. *Radiology* 161:329–334, 1986.

Case 83

Clinical Presentation

A 10-month-old ex-26-week-premature infant whose course was complicated by significant cardiac arrhythmia presents for evaluation of spasticity.

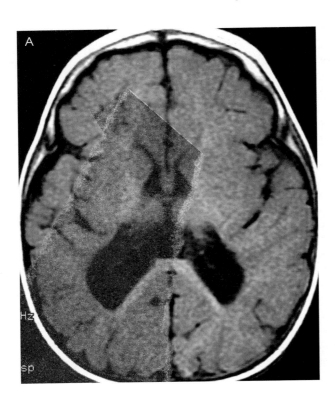

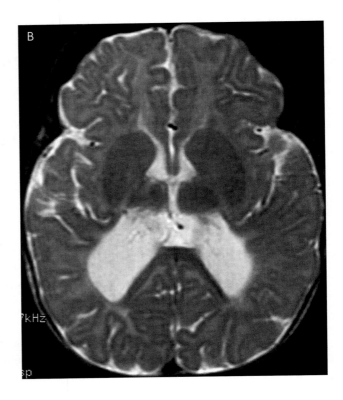

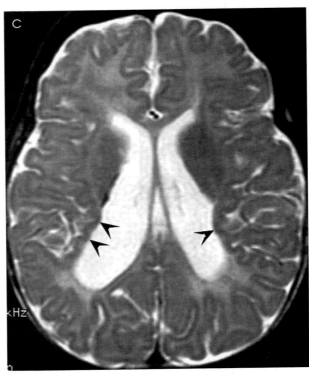

Radiologic Findings

An axial T1-WI (Fig. A) demonstrates enlargement of the trigones of the lateral ventricles. The splenium of the corpus callosum is thinned. A corresponding axial T2-WI (Fig. B) shows abnormally high signal in the posterior limbs of the internal capsules. The pattern of myelination is delayed even when the patient's age is corrected for prematurity. A T2-WI at a slightly higher level (Fig. C) demonstrates a striking paucity of parieto-occipital periventricular white matter. The cortex appears to abut the ventricular surface in multiple locations (*arrowheads*). In addition, a linear area of hypointensity along the lateral aspect of the right lateral ventricle is related to a remote subependymal hemorrhage.

Diagnosis

Periventricular leukomalacia

Differential Diagnosis

• Ventriculitis (clinical history of meningitis, often a fluid-debris level in the ventricle)
• Prenatal infectious or ischemic insult (may be indistinguishable on imaging)
• Congenital hypoplasia of the white matter (lacks history of prematurity)

Discussion

Background

Cerebral injury in the premature infant manifests primarily in two forms: germinal matrix hemorrhage and parenchymal injury. Germinal matrix hemorrhage affects 30 to 50% of premature infants and is unusual after 34 weeks of age; it is most easily diagnosed by head ultrasound. Manifestations of parenchymal injury vary depending on the nature of the insult. Ischemia, if profound, primarily affects the deep gray nuclei, brain stem nuclei, and cerebellar vermis. When the ischemia is milder, damage occurs in the periventricular "watershed" regions. The term "periventricular leukomalacia" refers to necrosis of white matter in a characteristic distribution (i.e., dorsal and lateral to the external angles of the lateral ventricles). The incidence is variably reported as affecting from 7 to 22% of infants with a gestational age of less than 35 weeks or a birth weight of less than 1500 g. A less common type of parenchymal injury seen in premature infants is venous infarction, also called periventricular hemorrhagic infarction or grade IV hemorrhage. These infarctions result in large periventricular hemorrhages that ultimately cavitate to form cystic "porencephalies" in the periventricular white matter.

Clinical Findings

The patient with PVL often has had a stormy perinatal course, although sometimes the clinical course is surprisingly benign; however, there are no specific findings in the acute phase. The chronic presentation depends on the location and severity of injury. Patients may appear completely normal if involvement is mild. Spastic diplegia or quadriplegia are common. Poor school performance and cognitive dysfunction may reflect diffuse insult. Cortical blindness and deafness may be observed.

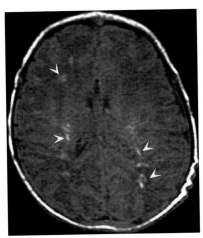

Fig. D. An axial T1-WI in a 7-day-old male born via a difficult delivery at 33 weeks demonstrates multiple foci of T1 shortening (*arrowheads*) with a periventricular distribution.

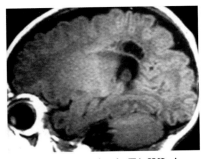

Fig E. A sagittal T1-WI in a 3-month-old male born at 27 weeks demonstrates low-signal intensity cystic areas in the periventricular white matter.

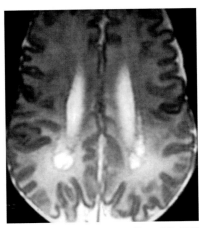

Fig. F. A corresponding T2-WI (same patient as Fig. E) demonstrates cavitation of the periventricular white matter bilaterally.

Complications

Hemorrhage, usually petechial, may complicate the acute phase of periventricular leukomalacia.

Pathophysiology

It is generally accepted that the "watershed" regions of the change evolve as the brain matures. In premature infants, the periventricular regions are perfused by penetrating arteries that extend inward from the surface of the brain. When auto-regulation is compromised (i.e., by hypoxia, ischemia, sepsis, or stress), flow through these long penetrating vessels is compromised. The periventricular regions are therefore at highest risk for damage. In older infants, the watershed regions are similar to those in adults. Another important factor may be the intrinsic vulnerability of the cerebral white matter of the premature newborn because of the sensitivity of rapidly differentiating oligodendroglial cells to glucose deprivation and the presence of lactate.

Pathology

Gross

- Acute: white spots and/or focal cavitations distributed particularly around the anterior horns and trigones of the lateral ventricles
- Chronic: myelin loss and focal ventricular dilatation, particularly the ventricular trigones

Microscopic

- Acute: foci of coagulative necrosis in the periventricular white matter, often with sparing of a thin layer of white matter just adjacent to the ventricular wall; round neuroaxonal swellings are prominent
- Chronic: oligodendroglial deficiency, myelin loss, astrocytic gliosis, involution of cystic lesions

Imaging Findings

CT

- Symmetric periventricular white matter lucency
- Cysts of varying sizes in the acute/subacute phase
- Bilateral atrial enlargement in the chronic phase

MR

- Acute/subacute
  1. Peritrigonal T2 prolongation
  2. Focal T1 (Fig. D) and T2 shortening, which may represent hemorrhage or myelin and cellular breakdown products
  3. Variable cyst formation (Figs. E and F)
- Chronic
  1. Ventricular enlargement (particularly the atria)
  2. T2 prolongation in the periventricular white matter
  3. Decreased thickness of the white matter and corpus callosum
  4. Cortical sulci appear to abut the ventricular wall, giving it a "scalloped" appearance

Ultrasound

- Periventricular increased echogenicity
- Cystic lesions that typically persist for 2 to 60 days

Treatment

None except prevention: improved prenatal care to limit premature births, improved neonatal ICU management to minimize hemodynamic shifts and stresses

Prognosis

Varies with severity of involvement

Suggested Readings

Baker LL, Stevenson DK, Enzmann DR. End-stage periventricular leukomalacia: MR evaluation. *Radiology* 168:809–815, 1988.

Flodmark O, Lupton B, Li D, Stimac GK, Roland EH, Hill A, Whitfield MF, Norman MG. MR imaging of periventricular leukomalacia in childhood. *AJR* 152:583–590, 1989.

Volpe JJ. Hypoxic-ischemic encephalopathy: neuropathology and pathogenesis. In Volpe JJ, ed. *Neurology of the Newborn*, 3rd ed. Philadelphia; W.B. Saunders Co., 1995, pp 291–299.

Case 84

Clinical Presentation

A term infant suffered birth asphyxia due to prolapse of the umbilical cord. An MR examination was obtained on day 4 of life to assess the extent of parenchymal injury.

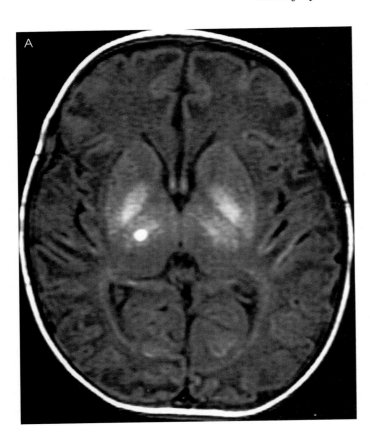
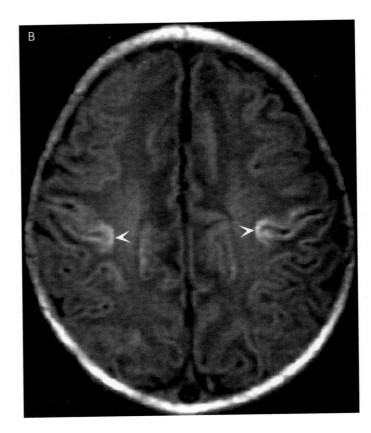

Radiologic Findings

An axial T1-WI (Fig. A) demonstrates abnormal hyperintensity in the globi pallidi as well as in the ventrolateral thalami. A more focal, rounded area of T1 shortening is present in the right ventrolateral thalamus. In addition, the posterior limb of the internal capsule is abnormally hypointense in this term infant. A more cephalad axial T1-WI (Fig. B) demonstrates abnormal hyperintensity involving the perirolandic cortex bilaterally, particularly at the depths of the sulci (*arrowheads*).

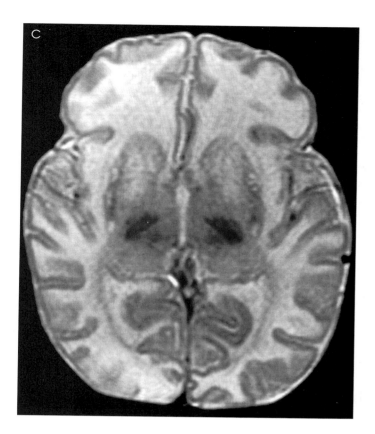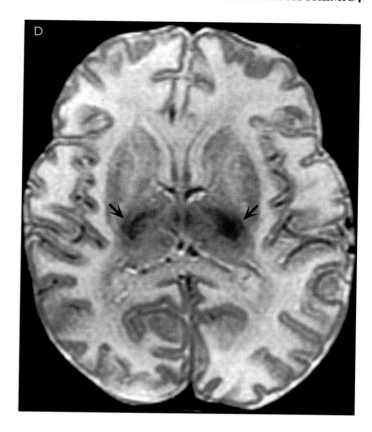

Axial T2-WIs (Figs. C and D) at the level of the deep gray nuclei demonstrate abnormal hyperintensity in the putamina and globi pallidi bilaterally. The expected focal hypointensity in the posterior limbs of the internal capsules is seen on the T2-WIs (*arrows*).

Diagnosis

Profound hypoxic-ischemic injury in a term neonate

Differential Diagnosis

- Watershed ischemia (affects watershed territories)
- Metabolic encephalopathy (typically affects lentiform nuclei more than thalami)

Discussion

Background

Hypoxic-ischemic encephalopathy results from a deficit in the supply of energy substrates and leads to neuronal injury. Severe asphyxia affects 1 in 100 to 1 in 500 term neonates. Brain injury almost always results from reduced delivery of blood to the brain parenchyma (ischemia), although hypoxemia (a diminished amount of oxygen in the blood) may be present as well. Of note, certain groups of neurons are more vulnerable to injury in the perinatal period than similar neurons in the adult. This selective vulnerability appears to be related to regional metabolic activity and to the activation of excitatory amino acid receptors in these neuronal groups; it appears to correlate with early myelination of these areas.

Pearls

- The pattern of injury in hypoxic-ischemic encephalopathy correlates with the degree of maturation of the brain (timing of the insult) and the nature of the insult (partial versus profound) (Table 1).

- The presence of moderate to high levels of lactate in the brain of asphyxiated neonates is indicative of poor outcome. This can be assessed using single-voxel proton MR spectroscopy.

- Proton density-weighted images may be more sensitive than heavily T2-WIs in the first 3 to 4 days after injury.

Pitfalls

- Hippocampal injury is difficult to identify on routine axial sequences and is best evaluated in the coronal plane.

- Cerebellar injury, even when present pathologically, is difficult to identify with imaging.

Table 1. Generalized Patterns of Hypoxic-Ischemic Injury

	Premature	Term
Partial Profound	Periventricular leukomalacia Brainstem and thalamic injury Lentiform nuclear injury by middle of third trimester	Watershed ischemia Injury to the lateral thalami, lentiform nuclei, hippocampi, and corticospinal tracts

Some differences in regional vulnerability have been identified in premature versus term newborns, although the basal ganglia/thalami and cranial nerve nuclei may be profoundly affected by hypoxic-ischemic insults in both. In term infants, areas at particular risk include Sommer's sector of the hippocampus, neurons of the calcarine cortex and the pre- and postcentral cortices (particularly in the depths of sulci), and the Purkinje cells of the cerebellum. In premature infants, areas at particular risk include the subiculum of the hippocampus, the ventral pons and the inferior olivary nuclei, and the internal granule cells of the cerebellum. When an infant suffers a reduction rather than a near-complete cessation of cerebral perfusion, the resultant pattern is that of periventricular leukomalacia in the premature infant and watershed or borderzone infarction in the term infant.

Etiology

The causes of perinatal asphyxia are many and include severe respiratory distress syndrome, congenital heart disease, cord prolapse, uterine rupture, and meconium aspiration. Hypoxic-ischemic insults may also occur in utero secondary to acute or chronic disturbances of gas exchange across the placenta (as with placental abruption or insufficiency). The assessment of fetal well-being in utero relies on the biophysical profile (fetal movement, heart rate, motor response, tone, and breathing). In term infants, insults leading to hypoxic-ischemic encephalopathy are thought to occur antepartum in 20% of cases, intrapartum in 35% of cases, intra- and antepartum in 35% of cases, and postnatally in 10% of cases.

Clinical Findings

Neonates with profound hypoxic-ischemic injury present with low Apgar scores, depressed level of consciousness, "periodic" breathing or respiratory failure, hypotonia, and seizures. Profound acidemia (arterial pH <7.0) is the hallmark of a hypoxic-ischemic insult.

Complications

Complications include coma, multiorgan system dysfunction (particularly renal), respiratory arrest, and death.

Pathology

Gross

- Early: cerebral swelling and congestion
- Late: cavitation may occur

Microscopic

- Early: cytoplasmic vacuolization, marked eosinophilia of neuronal cytoplasm, loss of Nissl substance, and nuclear condensation or fragmentation

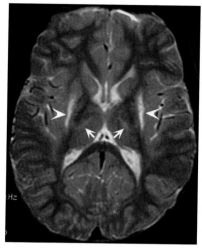

Fig. E. An axial T2-WI in a 5-year-old boy who was born at term and suffered severe asphyxia demonstrates shrunken and hyperintense putamina bilaterally (*arrows*) as well as mild hyperintensity in the ventrolateral thalami (*arrowheads*).

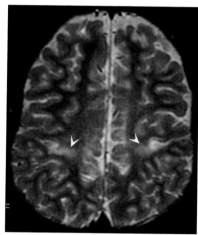

Fig. F. A more cephalad axial T2-WI (same patient as Fig. E) demonstrates abnormal hyperintensity in the perirolandic cortex and subcortical white matter (*arrowheads*). This patient suffers from spastic quadriplegia, dystonia, and seizures. He is also mentally retarded.

- Late: overt signs of cell necrosis, appearance of microglia and hypertrophic astrocytes

Note: The distribution of the neuropathological features of neonatal hypoxic-ischemic encephalopathy varies considerably with the gestational age of the infant and the nature and degree of the insult.

Imaging Findings

Acute phase (<10 days):

CT

- Low attenuation in the deep gray nuclei due to edema
- High attenuation if petechial hemorrhage is present

MR

- Imaging findings are quite consistent on T1-WI:
    1. Diffuse and homogeneous high signal in the lateral thalami, globi pallidi, and posterior putamina
    2. Variable high signal in the caudate nuclei
    3. Hypointensity of the posterior limb of the internal capsule
    4. High signal in at the depths of sulci, particularly the perirolandic region
- Imaging findings are highly variable on T2-WI:
    1. May be normal
    2. May demonstrate diffuse high-signal intensity in the lateral thalami, globi pallidi, and posterior putamina
    3. Globular hypointensity may be seen in the lateral thalami and posterior putamina
- Post-gadolinium, there is a variable degree of enhancement

Chronic phase (weeks to years):

CT

- Atrophy of thalami and putamina
- High attenuation in basal ganglia if hemorrhage or calcification is present

MR

- Abnormal T2 prolongation and atrophy in the lateral thalami and posterior putamina (Fig. E)
- Abnormal T2 prolongation in the perirolandic regions (Fig. F)
- Delayed myelination
- The globi pallidi and caudate nuclei may assume a normal appearance, perhaps due to remyelination or less severe injury

Treatment

- Prevention is the only effective method
- Supportive care includes management of seizures, control of brain swelling, and maintenance of adequate ventilation and perfusion
- Experimental evidence from a variety of perinatal hypoxic-ischemic injury models suggest that neurons may be protected from death by treatment with glutamate receptor blockers, calcium channel blockers, and/or free radical inhibitors

Prognosis

- Long-term sequelae are common in infants with moderate or severe insults and include mental retardation, spastic quadriparesis, seizure disorder, ataxia, bulbar and pseudobulbar palsies, and hyperactivity and impaired attention.
- Overall, 25% of term infants with hypoxic-ischemic injury will have significant long-term neurologic deficits and 10% will die. Of premature infants with hypoxic-ischemic injury, approximately 13% survive with significant neurologic sequelae and 60% die.

Suggested Readings

Barkovich AJ. MR and CT evaluation of profound neonatal and infantile asphyxia. *AJNR* 13:959–972, 1992.

Barkovich AJ, Westmark K, Partridge C, Sola A, Ferriero DM. Perinatal asphyxia: MR findings in the first 10 days. *AJNR* 16:427–438, 1995.

Rademakers RP, van der Knaap M, Verbeeten B Jr, Barth PG, Valk J. Central cortico-subcortical involvement: a distinct pattern of brain damage caused by perinatal and postnatal asphyxia in term infants. *J Comput Assist Tomog* 19:256–263, 1995.

Case 85

Clinical Presentation

A 14-year-old girl who has undergone a prior surgical procedure presents with episodic left-sided weakness.

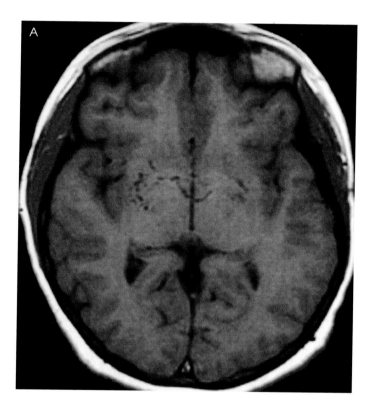

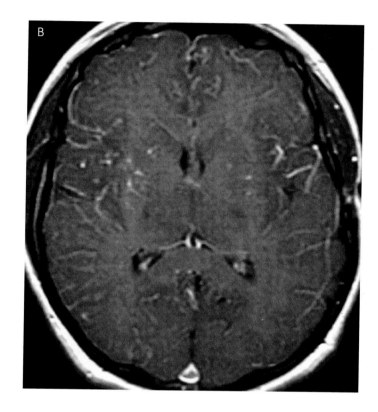

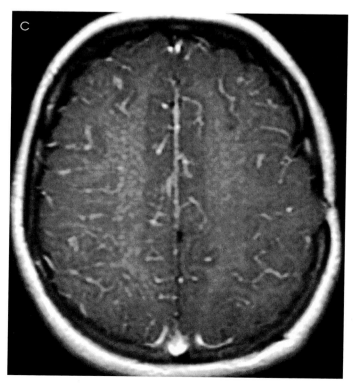

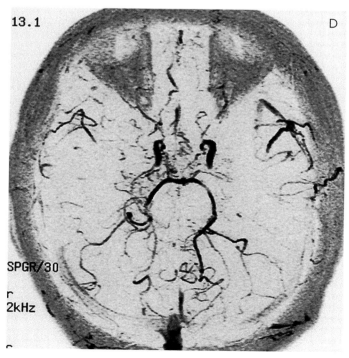

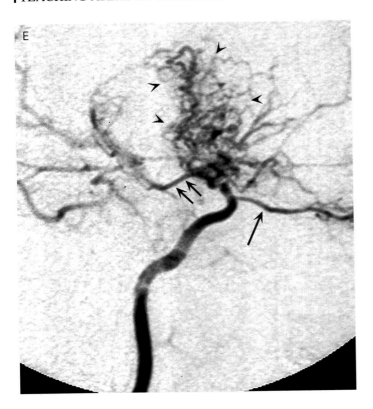

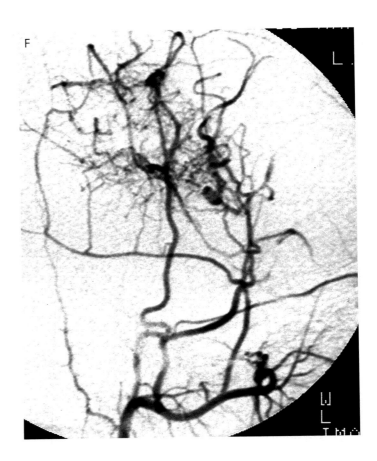

Radiologic Findings

An axial T1-WI (Fig. A) demonstrates multiple flow voids in the right lentiform nucleus, consistent with enlarged lenticulostriate vessels. Axial post-gadolinium T1-WIs (Figs. B and C) show no evidence of abnormal parenchymal enhancement. However, there is asymmetric enhancement within cortical sulci, suggesting slower arterial flow on the right as compared with the left. A collapsed maximum intensity projection image from an MR angiogram (Fig. D) demonstrates narrowing of the supraclinoid carotid arteries bilaterally, poor visualization of the M-1 and A-1 segments bilaterally, and prominent collateral vessels in the region of the posterior communicating artery and right lenticulostriate territory. A lateral projection from a right internal carotid artery angiogram (Fig. E) demonstrates a prominent ophthalmic artery (*arrow*), a prominent posterior communicating artery (*double arrow*), and a prominent lenticulostriate vascular blush (*arrowheads*). The normal middle cerebral artery and anterior cerebral artery branches are not identified. A lateral view from a left external carotid artery injection (Fig. F) shows branches of the superficial temporal artery supplying a fine network of cortical vessels. This patient has undergone a prior encephaloduralarteriosynangiosis (EDAS) revascularization procedure.

Diagnosis

Moyamoya (progressive occlusive cerebrovascular) disease

Differential Diagnosis

Other causes of moyamoya (determined by clinical history)

- Radiation vasculopathy, neurofibromatosis Type I, sickle cell anemia

Other causes of ischemia or infarction in childhood

- Hypercoagulable state
- Congenital cardiac lesions
- Carotid or vertebral arterial dissection
- Vasculitis
- Mitochondrial encephalopathy with lactic acidosis and stroke (MELAs)

Discussion

Background

Moyamoya disease is a chronic occlusive cerebrovascular disorder that is characterized by progressive stenosis of the arteries of the circle of Willis. This process initially involves the supraclinoid internal carotid arteries but progressively involves the middle, anterior, and posterior cerebral arteries. Parenchymal collateral vessels, most importantly the lenticulostriate arteries, markedly enlarge distal to the stenotic or occluded carotid arteries. Leptomeningeal and transdural collaterals may develop as well. Both primary and secondary forms of moyamoya exist. Primary moyamoya or moyamoya disease is defined as idiopathic bilateral stenosis of the arteries of the circle of Willis with collateral vascular networks demonstrated by angiography. Secondary moyamoya or moyamoya syndrome is associated with a number of underlying conditions (see below). Whether "unilateral" moyamoya disease is an early underlying form of the typical bilateral moyamoya disease remains controversial.

Etiology

Primary moyamoya is idiopathic, with a relatively high prevalence in Japan. Secondary moyamoya is associated with neurofibromatosis Type I, sickle cell anemia, prior radiation therapy with radiation vasculopathy, Down syndrome, and Williams syndrome. Atherosclerotic stenoses in adults may on occasion mimic moyamoya. A familial occurrence has been reported in up to 10% of cases.

Clinical Findings

Moyamoya has a bimodal peak but most commonly presents in children. The average age at onset of symptoms is 7 years. Children typically present with ischemic symptoms such as hemiplegia or transient and often recurrent weakness, although seizures and headache may also be presenting complaints. Adults more typically present with intracranial hemorrhage.

Complications

Left untreated, the disease typically shows a progressive course over 2 to 3 years with repeated cerebrovascular episodes that may result in permanent motor, speech, visual, and cognitive deficits. Therapy is directed at minimizing the deficits due to the progressive ischemic phase by improving cerebrovascular perfusion.

Pathology

Gross

- Thickening of the wall and narrowing of the lumen of the large intracranial arteries
- Dilatation, tortuosity, and occasionally focal aneurysm formation of the lenticulostriate vessels

Microscopic

- Marked thickening of the vascular intima with smooth muscle cells admixed with macrophages and T cells
- Increased elastin accumulation within smooth muscle cells

Imaging Findings

CT

- Multiple bilateral infarcts of varying ages
- Parenchymal hemorrhage may occur in adults

MR

- Multiple infarcts of varying ages, often in a watershed distribution
- Narrowing and reduced flow velocity of the intracranial carotid circulation and often the posterior circulation as well
- Hypertrophy of small collateral vessels with multiple flow voids present in the deep gray nuclei
- Postcontrast, there may be asymmetry of vascular enhancement depending on the severity of the underlying stenoses

Angiography (Table 1)

- Stenosis of the supraclinoid internal carotid arteries (ICAs), usually bilateral but often asymmetric
- The posterior cerebral arteries (PCA) also show steno-occlusive changes, with the frequency of PCA involvement increasing as steno-occlusive lesions of the ICAs advance
- Marked hypertrophy of the lenticulostriate and thalamoperforating vessels, resulting in a "puff of smoke" or "moyamoya" appearance

Table 1. Angiographic Classification of Moyamoya Disease (modified from Yamada et al., 1995)

Stage	Angiographic Appearance
1	Mild-moderate stenosis in the region of the distal ICA bifurcation(s) only
2	Severe stenosis of ICA bifurcation(s), appearance of moyamoya collateral vessels
3	Progression of moyamoya collaterals, occlusion of anterior and middle cerebral arteries
4	Decrease in moyamoya collaterals, occlusion of posterior cerebral arteries
5	Further decrease in moyamoya collaterals and occlusion of all major cerebral arteries
6	Disappearance of moyamoya collaterals, with blood supply only from the external carotid arteries

Treatment

- EDAS: a scalp artery along with a strip of galea is transplanted to the dura, and spontaneous anastomoses form between the scalp artery in the dural strip and the cortical arteries. A modification of this technique, the so-called pial synangiosis, involves suturing the adventitia of the donor superficial temporal artery directly to the pia. EDAS or pial synangiosis are currently the treatments of choice in moyamoya.
- Superficial temporal artery to middle cerebral artery anastomosis (difficult in children younger than age 5)
- Encephalomyosynangiosis: in this procedure, used in pediatric patients prior to the development of EDAS, temporalis muscle was placed on the surface of the brain in the hope of achieving revascularization
- Sometimes combinations of these procedures are used to revascularize multiple territories
- Medical management: calcium channel blockers have been shown to provide symptomatic relief but do not interrupt the inexorable progression of the arteriopathic process

Prognosis

- With surgical treatment, approximately 70 to 85% of patients will develop good or excellent collateralization to the middle cerebral artery circulation via the external carotid system and the progression of symptoms will be halted
- Age of onset is also important for prognosis, as irreversible neurologic deficits and intellectual deterioration are more likely to develop when the onset of disease occurs earlier than 4 years of age

Suggested Readings

Robertson RL, Burrows PE, Barnes PD, et al. Angiographic changes after pial synangiosis in childhood moyamoya disease. *AJNR* 18:837–845, 1997.

Suzuki J, Takaku A. Cerebrovascular "moyamoya" disease: disease showing abnormal net-like vessels in base of brain. *Arch Neurol* 20:288–299, 1969.

Yamada I, Himeno Y, Suzuki S, Matsushima Y. Posterior circulation in moyamoya disease: angiographic study. *Radiology* 197:239–246, 1995.

Case 86

Clinical Presentation

A 6-month-old girl is evaluated for enlarging head circumference.

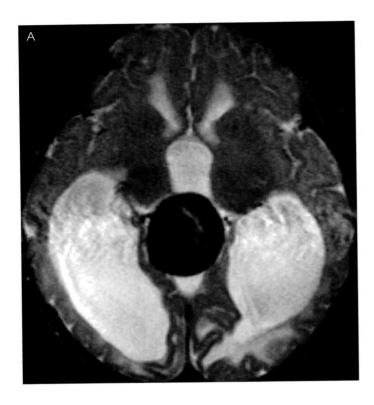

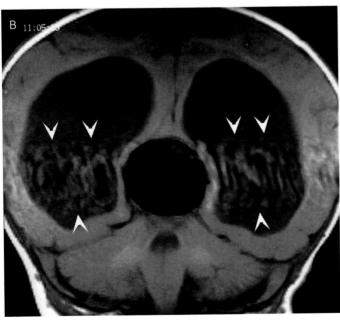

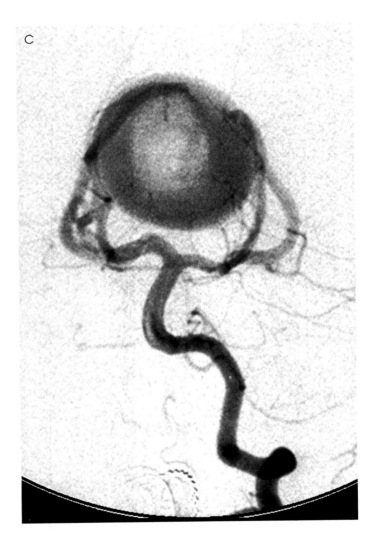

D

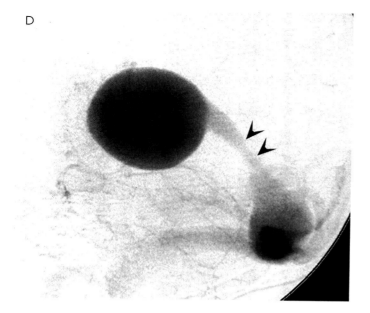

E

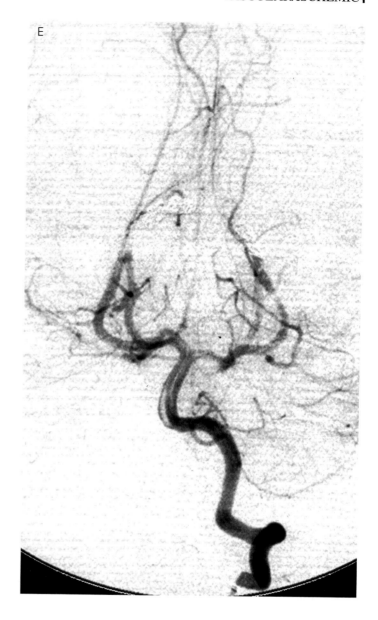

Radiologic Findings

An axial T2-WI (Fig. A) demonstrates a rounded, strikingly hypointense mass in the region of the vein of Galen. There is accompanying dilatation of the third ventricle and lateral ventricles, consistent with hydrocephalus. High signal in the periatrial white matter may be related to transependymal flow of CSF secondary to the hydrocephalus. A coronal T1-WI (Fig. B) also demonstrates aneurysmal dilatation of the vein of Galen. Note the prominent pulsation artifact arising from the mass (*arrowheads*). A frontal projection from a left vertebral artery angiogram (Fig. C) demonstrates multiple enlarged branches of the posterior cerebral arteries supplying the aneurysmally dilated vein of Galen, consistent with a mural-type vein of Galen malformation. A lateral image obtained later in the angiographic run (Fig. D) demonstrates drainage via the straight sinus. A region of stenosis is present in the midportion of the straight sinus (*arrowheads*), presumably restricting venous outflow to some extent and likely accounting for the lack of congestive heart failure in this patient. A frontal projection from a left vertebral artery angiogram obtained following coil embolization (Fig. E) demonstrates absence of shunting into the vein of Galen. Note that the coils are difficult to see on this subtracted image.

Diagnosis

Vein of Galen aneurysmal malformation (VGAM)

Differential Diagnosis

None

Discussion

Background

The VGAM is caused by an arteriovenous fistula in the wall of an embryologic precursor of the vein of Galen, the median vein of the prosencephalon. A normal vein of Galen does not exist, but is rather replaced by this persistent midline venous structure that drains only the arteriovenous fistula and does not drain normal brain. The fistula may be subclassified as choroidal or mural. A choroidal fistula usually receives bilateral arterial supply from multiple arterial feeders which normally supply choroidal structures such as the posterolateral, posteromedial, and anterior choroidal arteries; the subforniceal branch of the pericallosal artery; and subependymal branches of the thalamoperforators. A mural shunt is typically supplied by a single collicular or posterior choroidal artery. The VGAM should be distinguished from vein of Galen aneurysmal dilatation (VGAD). VGAD typically results from a parenchymal arteriovenous malformation that then drains into a normally formed but dilated vein of Galen; in the setting of venous stenosis, aneurysmal dilatation of the vein of Galen occurs.

Embryology

Normal development

By approximately 6 weeks of gestation, the development of the circle of Willis is complete. Also at this time, the median prosencephalic vein develops as the main drainage for the telencephalic choroid plexus. By week 10, the median prosencephalic vein is largely replaced by the paired internal cerebral veins. The most caudal portion of the median prosencephalic vein joins the internal cerebral veins to form the vein of Galen. Under normal circumstances, the vein of Galen serves as a bridge between the deep parenchymal venous system and the venous sinuses.

Vein of Galen aneurysmal malformation

Raybaud has proposed that the "vein of Galen aneurysm" represents dilatation of persistent median prosencephalic veins. Evidence for this includes the following:

- The true vein of Galen develops late and lacks connection to the choroidal branch of the anterior cerebral artery, an important feeder in most vein of Galen malformations
- The typical vein of Galen aneurysm drains in a pattern typical of the median prosencephalic vein, with "anomalous" veinous drainage probably representing persistent fetal drainage

Clinical Findings

Infants typically present with high-output congestive heart failure and an audible cranial bruit. This is the usual presentation of the choroidal-type fistula. Older infants and children are more likely to present with symptoms and signs of hydrocephalus, possibly with a cranial bruit, and typically have mural-type fistulae. The hydrocephalus is usually due to obstruction of the aqueduct of Sylvius by the mass effect of the aneurysm. Rarely, vein of Galen malformations may present for the first time in adulthood. These patients typically manifest headaches, exercise syncope, or subarachnoid hemorrhage.

Complications

Myocardial ischemia and death are related to right heart failure. Developmental delay is related to arterial steal, ischemia caused by compression by enlarged veins, and/or increased venous pressures after aneurysm thrombosis. Acute aneurysm thrombosis, which may be spontaneous, can result in sudden hydrocephalus or intraventricular hemorrhage. Shunting for hydrocephalus is often complicated by hemorrhage from massively dilated ependymal veins.

Imaging Findings

CT

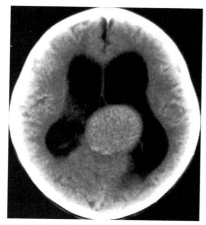

Fig. F. A non-contrast CT scan in a 3-month-old male with congestive heart failure demonstrates a rounded hyperdense mass representing an aneurysmally dilated vein of Galen.

- A round mass in the quadrigeminal cistern is typically seen (Fig. F)
- This mass is mildly dense pre-contrast and shows intense, homogeneous enhancement after contrast
- Calcification of the aneurysm wall occurs in approximately 15% of older patients but is rare in infants and young children
- Evidence of ischemic parenchymal damage (calcification, encephalomalacia) may be present

MR

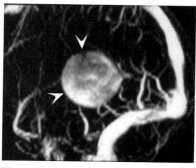

Fig. G. A sagittal maximum intensity projection from an MR venogram demonstrates flow-related enhancement within a large vein of Galen aneurysm (*arrowheads*).

- If thrombosis has not occurred, MR demonstrates a large flow void at the level of the vein of Galen, as well as pulsation artifact in the phase direction
- A thrombosed malformation will demonstrate intermediate signal and often enhances post-contrast
- Hemosiderin staining may be seen if there has been prior hemorrhage
- Parenchymal T2 prolongation may reflect ischemic damage
- An atretic or absent straight sinus (Fig. G) and anomalous falcine sinus are frequently demonstrated

Treatment

- Ideally, intensive medical management is used so that surgical or endovascular treatment can be postponed until a child is old enough to make intervention relatively safe. Endovascular approaches include transarterial, transvenous, and transtorcular embolization, often in combination.
- A neonate with congestive heart failure refractory to medical treatment may require emergent intervention. Staged treatment is often done in order to avoid the risk of normal perfusion pressure breakthrough, a situation where previously hypoperfused brain suddenly receives increased blood flow that leads to brain swelling, hemorrhage, and/or seizures. Imaging evidence of ischemic brain damage is a relative contraindication to treatment.

Prognosis

- With modern endovascular approaches, mortality ranges from 0 to 20%
- Neurologically, outcome following endovascular therapy is good in 45% of patients under 1 year of age, 65% of those ages 1 to 2 years, and 100% of those older than 2 years

Suggested Readings

Berenstein A, Lasjaunias P. Arteriovenous fistulas of the brain. In: *Surgical Neuroangiography, 4: Endovascular Treatment of Cerebral Lesions*. New York; Springer-Verlag, 1991, pp. 268–319.

Horowitz MB, Jungreis CA, Quisling RG, Pollack I. Vein of Galen aneurysms: a review and current perspective. *AJNR* 15:1486–1496, 1994.

Raybaud CA, Strother CM, Hald JK. Aneurysms of the vein of Galen: embryonic considerations and anatomical features relating to the pathogenesis of the malformation. *Neuroradiology* 31:109–128, 1989.

Case 87

Clinical Presentation

A 15-year-old male with a history of cerebral infarction presents for follow-up examination.

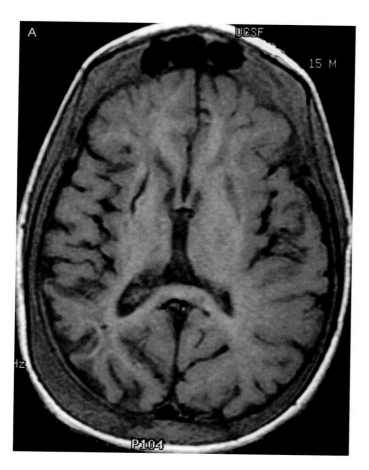

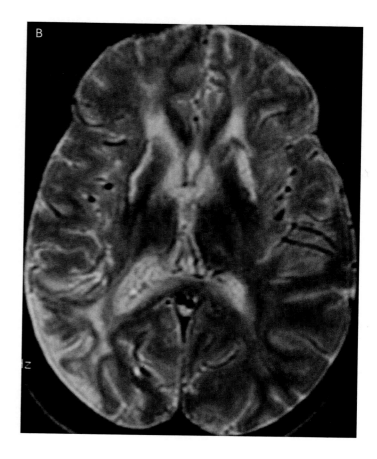

Radiologic Findings

An axial T1-WI (Fig. A) demonstrates striking expansion of the diploic space as well as hypointensity of the calvarial marrow. Parenchymal volume loss is present in the right occipital and posterior temporal regions. In addition, abnormal hypointensity is present in the putamina bilaterally, right greater than left. A corresponding axial T2-WI (Fig. B) demonstrates abnormal hyperintensity in the putamina, as well as in the deep white matter adjacent to the right ventricular atrium and adjacent to the frontal horns.

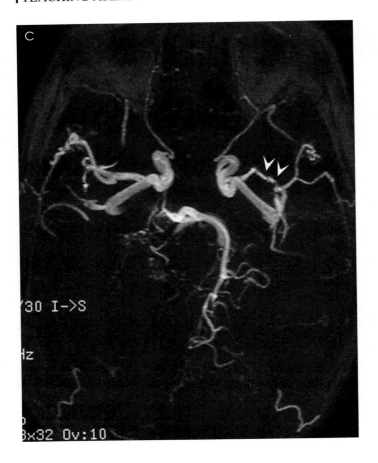

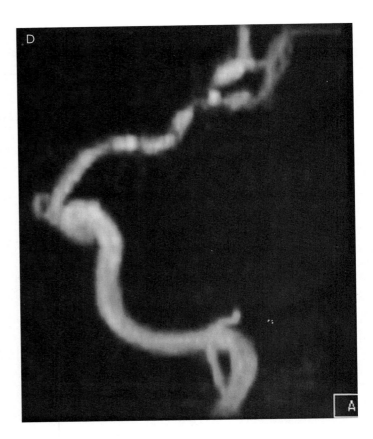

An axial collapsed image from an intracranial MR angiogram (Fig. C) demonstrates absence of the anterior cerebral arteries bilaterally, a small and irregular left middle cerebral artery (MCA) (*arrowheads*), a prominent right posterior communicating artery, and small tortuous collateral vessels in the expected region of the (occluded) right posterior cerebral artery. A frontal projection of a volume of interest around the left internal carotid artery and left middle cerebral artery (Fig. D) demonstrates marked irregularity and multifocal stenosis of the M1 and M2 segments of the left MCA, as well as absence of the anterior cerebral artery.

Diagnosis

Sickle cell disease (SCD) with associated vasculopathy

Differential Diagnosis

- Thalassemia (also causes marrow expansion and hypointensity, does not lead to vasculopathic changes and infarction)
- Fibrous dysplasia (causes marked calvarial thickening, but often more focal and more heterogeneous; underlying brain should be normal)
- Other causes of a moyamoya pattern: idiopathic, radiation therapy, neurofibromatosis Type I (these would not lead to striking marrow expansion)

Discussion

Background

SCD refers to a group of heritable disorders characterized by production of abnormal hemoglobin (Hb) and is most commonly seen in blacks of African descent. The most common types include Hb SS (homozygous) disease, sickle cell-hemoglobin C disease (Hb SC), and the sickle-beta thalassemia syndromes. The presence of the abnormal Hb in red blood cells causes them to assume an abnormal "sickle" shape, which leads to chronic hemolytic anemia as well as ischemic tissue injury due to altered blood flow. Neurologic morbidity and mortality is high in SCD, with as many as 12% of patients experiencing a stroke by age 21. Ischemic injuries may also be present in patients who do not have a clinical history of stroke, and clinically silent cerebral infarctions are commonly seen when the brains of patients with SCD are screened with MRI.

Etiology

The defect in classic sickle-cell anemia (SS disease) is inherited in an autosomal recessive fashion and is due to substitution of valine by glutamic acid in the Hb-beta chain. Another common form of SCD that is slightly less severe than SS disease is so-called SC disease, whereby the Hb molecule includes one S chain and one C chain.

Clinical Findings

SCD is characterized by anemia, susceptibility to pneumococcal and other infections, pain, multiple organ dysfunction (notably splenic and renal), and retinopathy. Neurologic presentations include focal neurologic deficits related to infarction or hemorrhage, seizures, altered levels of consciousness, and intellectual impairment. Pneumococcal meningitis may complicate pneumonia. Currently, many cases are detected by state-run newborn screening programs.

Complications

Development of a moyamoya pattern may lead to further ischemic or hemorrhagic episodes. Ischemic strokes typically occur in childhood, whereas adolescents and adults are prone to intracranial hemorrhage. Patients may experience subarachnoid hemorrhage due to the presence of microaneurysms or visible aneurysms. Venous infarction due to occlusion of dural venous sinuses has also been reported in SCD.

Pathophysiology

Neurologic morbidity is related to the fact that the sickled cells produce endothelial cell injury and luminal blockages of both large and small vessels. This leads to alterations of blood flow, chronic ischemia, and superimposed thromboembolic episodes. Pathologically, blood vessels demonstrate endothelial hyperplasia with stenosis and/or occlusion.

Imaging Findings

CT

- Calvarial thickening
- Parenchymal volume loss

- Variable presence of focal areas of infarction

MR

- Global parenchymal volume loss
- Marrow expansion and hypointensity on T1-WIs
- Localized deep white matter T2-prolonging lesions due to small vessel occlusion or borderzone ischemia/infarction
- More extensive areas of cortical and deep white matter ischemia or infarction in the distribution of a major artery
- Narrowing or occlusion of vessels of the circle of Willis, possibly associated with a "moyamoya" pattern of collateral flow
- Occasional decrease in signal intensity of basal ganglia on T2-WIs due to accelerated iron deposition

Treatment

- Management of clinically silent CNS lesions is controversial
- Neurologically symptomatic lesions are generally managed with long-term transfusion therapy
- Other interventions under investigation for SCD include bone marrow transplantation and hydroxyurea therapy

Prognosis

- Morbidity is high, but advances in transfusion therapy and antibiotic prophylaxis have considerably reduced the mortality of this condition
- 50% of patients with SCD survive beyond the fifth decade. Risk factors for early death include renal failure, acute chest syndrome, seizures, baseline white blood cell count > 15,000, and a low level of fetal Hb.

Suggested Readings

Armstrong FD, Thompson RJ Jr, Wang W, et al. Cognitive functioning and brain magnetic resonance imaging in children with sickle cell disease. *Pediatrics* 97:864–870, 1996.

Moser FG, Miller ST, Bello JA, et al. The spectrum of brain MR abnormalities in sickle-cell disease: a report from the cooperative study of sickle cell disease. *AJNR* 17:965–972, 1996.

Platt OS, Brambilla DJ, Rosse WF, et al. Mortality in sickle cell disease. *N Engl J Med* 330:1639–1644, 1994.

Case 88

Clinical Presentation

A 34-year-old woman presents complaining of 4 days of persistent right occipital headache. She is in excellent health and takes no medications except oral contraceptive pills.

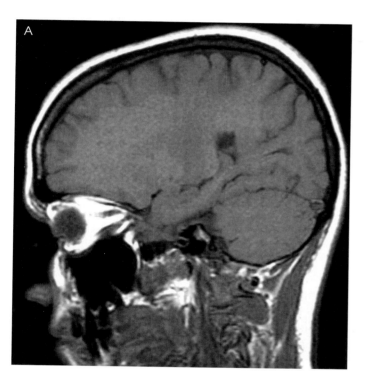

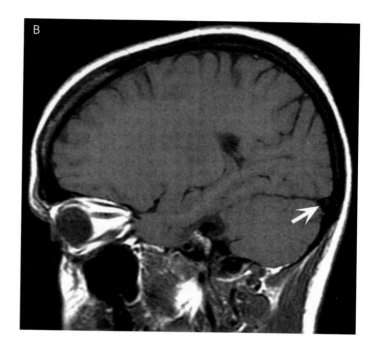

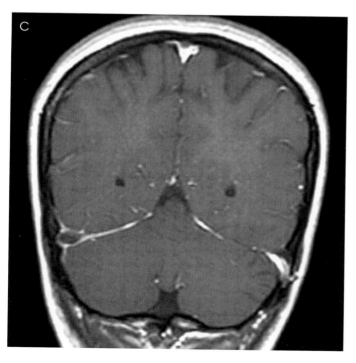

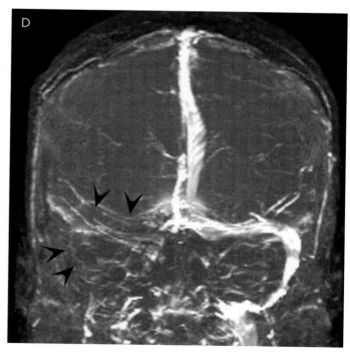

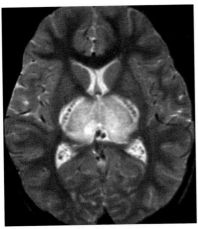

Fig. E. An axial T2-WI in a child who was severely dehydrated from viral gastroenteritis and then developed seizures and coma demonstrates abnormal T2 prolongation in the thalami and posterior limbs of the internal capsules bilaterally.

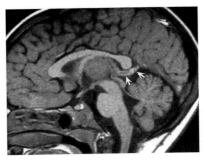

Fig. F. A sagittal T1-WI (same patient as Fig. E) demonstrates abnormal hypointensity in the thalamus. Note abnormal increased signal intensity in the vein of Galen (*arrows*), consistent with deep venous thrombosis.

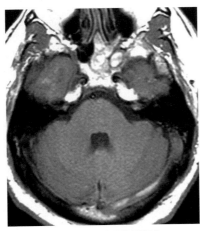

Fig. G. An axial T1-WI in a patient with protein C deficiency who presented with a seizure demonstrates abnormal increased signal intensity in the left transverse sinus consistent with venous sinus thrombosis.

Radiologic Findings

A right parasagittal T1-WI (Fig. A) demonstrates abnormal intermediate signal intensity within the right transverse sinus. The brain is unremarkable on this image. A left parasagittal T1-WI in the same patient (Fig. B) demonstrates a normal flow void in the left transverse sinus (*arrow*). A coronal post-gadolinium T1-WI (Fig. C) demonstrates a filling defect within the right transverse sinus, as well as slightly asymmetric enhancement of the tentorium and nearby vessels. A frontal projection from a two-dimensional (2-D) time-of-flight MR venogram (Fig. D) demonstrates absence of flow-related enhancement in the expected position of the right transverse sinus, right sigmoid sinus, and right jugular vein (*arrowheads*). Normal flow-related enhancement is present in the sagittal sinus, left transverse sinus, left sigmoid sinus, and left jugular vein.

Diagnosis

Transverse sinus thrombosis

Differential Diagnosis

- Slow flow in dural sinus (evidence of flow on MR venography)
- Subdural hematoma (adjacent to dural sinus rather than within it)

Discussion

Background

Dural sinus thrombosis is being detected with increasing frequency due to the widespread availability of MR imaging. Venous occlusive disease is different from arterial occlusion in that the blood-brain barrier often remains intact, signal abnormalities that are detected on neuroimaging studies are often reversible, and hemorrhage is far more common than with arterial ischemia/infarction. Unlike arterial infarction, which tends to affect discrete, well-defined territories, venous infarction does not consistently affect a given region of the brain. However, superior sagittal sinus thrombosis tends to affect the parasagittal frontal lobes, transverse sinus thrombosis tends to affect the temporal lobes, and vein of Galen/straight sinus thrombosis tends to affect the thalami (Figs. E and F). Venous infarcts are typically subcortical and hemorrhagic. Retrograde extension of thrombus into cortical or deep medullary veins occurs in approximately 40% of cases of dural sinus thrombosis (Figs. G, H and I) and can lead to stroke, coma, and/or death.

Etiology

There are many potential causes of dural sinus thrombosis, but no definite etiology is found in up to 25% of cases. Predisposing factors include hematologic disorders such as protein S or protein C deficiency, antithrombin III deficiency, diffuse intravascular coagulation, and anticardiolipin syndrome; neoplasm via paraneoplastic hypercoagulability or by direct compression or invasion of a dural sinus; dehydration, especially in infants; pregnancy/puerperium; infection such as generalized sepsis, otomastoiditis, and sinusitis; trauma; use of drugs such as oral contraceptives or L-asparaginase; dural arteriovenous fistula; and underlying inflammatory conditions such as ulcerative colitis or Behçet's disease.

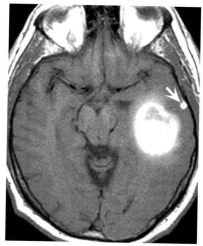

Fig. H. A T1-WI through the temporal lobe in the same patient as Figure G demonstrates a subcortical hyperintense mass with surrounding edema and mass effect on the midbrain, consistent with a hematoma. Note the rounded, peripherally located structure (*arrow*) consistent with a thrombosed cortical vein, likely the vein of Labbé.

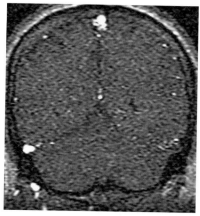

Fig. I. A coronal partition image from a 2-D time of flight MR venogram (same patient as Figs. G and H) demonstrates lack of flow-related enhancement in the left transverse sinus.

Clinical Findings

Patients may present with rapid onset of focal neurological deficits and depressed consciousness or with the more insidious development of signs of elevated intracranial pressure (headache, papilledema, cranial nerve palsies, confusion). CSF opening pressure and protein are elevated in the majority of patients. CSF pleocytosis is common.

Complications

Major complications include cerebral edema, hydrocephalus, infarction, hemorrhage, and death.

Imaging Findings

CT

- Non-contrast: the thrombosed sinus may appear as a linear density ("cord sign," Fig. J) and its walls may bulge outward
- Post-contrast: enhancement of dural collaterals in the walls of the thrombosed sinus may occur, resulting in the "empty delta" sign in 25 to 75% of cases
- Brain edema, hydrocephalus (in children), and bland or hemorrhagic venous infarcts may occur

MR

- Both the intravascular thrombus and associated parenchymal complications may be identified
- *MR imaging*: the expected signal void in the dural sinus or cortical vein is replaced by abnormal signal, the specific appearance of which varies with the age of the thrombus and the sequence parameters selected. Depending on the stage of the process, the brain may appear normal, may show swelling without T2 abnormalities, may show swelling and T2 abnormalities (usually subcortical hyperintensity representing interstitial edema), or may show the above changes plus hematoma.
- *MR venography*: may be performed with time-of-flight or phase contrast techniques. The absence of flow-related enhancement or motion-related phase shift supports the diagnosis of sinus thrombosis.

Treatment

Varies with the clinical stage of the process:

- *Stage 1* (headache, papilledema, weakness; venous pressure <20 mm Hg): anticoagulation with heparin alone
- *Stages 2–4* (focal neurologic signs, seizure, change in consciousness and progression to coma; venous pressures range from 20 to 50 mmHg): thrombolytic therapy as well as systemic heparinization
- *Stage 5* (coma, response to deep pain only; venous pressures presumed >50 mmHg): these patients have a very high mortality and the utility of treatment is controversial

Prognosis

- Patients with isolated dural sinus thrombosis have a better prognosis than patients with extension of thrombosis to the cerebral cortical veins

Pearls

- On time-of-flight MR venography, the T1-shortening effect of methemoglobin can "shine-through" and mimic a patent sinus. In this situation, phase-contrast MR venography (venc 30 to 50 cm/sec) is helpful since this is a background-subtraction technique that eliminates signal from stationary objects such as thrombus and hematomas.

- In cases of bithalamic edema, inspect the vein of Galen and straight sinus carefully for evidence of thrombosis.

- In cases of temporal lobe hematoma, carefully examine the transverse sinuses for evidence of thrombosis.

Pitfalls

- CT is relatively insensitive to cortical venous thrombosis because of beam-hardening artifact.

- On CT, a false-positive cord sign may occur in patients with elevated hematocrit (due to polycythemia, dehydration, etc.).

- On both CT and MR, enhancement of organized thrombus may result in a false-negative empty delta sign.

- A false-positive empty delta sign may result from a small subdural hematoma adjacent to a dural sinus or from a high bifurcation of the superior sagittal sinus.

- Early diagnosis and prompt institution of therapy also improve prognosis, unless the patient has already developed massive edema and/or hemorrhage
- Overall mortality figures range from 20 to 75% in the literature, with the lower numbers in more recent series

Suggested Readings

Cure JK, Van Tassel P. Congenital and acquired abnormalities of the dural venous sinuses. *Semin US, CT, MRI* 15:520–539, 1994.

Tsai FY, Wang A, Matovich VB, et al. MR staging of acute dural sinus thrombosis: correlation with venous pressure measurements and implications for treatment and prognosis. *AJNR* 16:1021–1029, 1995.

Yuh WTC, Simonson TM, Wang A, et al. Venous sinus occlusive disease: MR findings. *AJNR* 15:309–316, 1994.

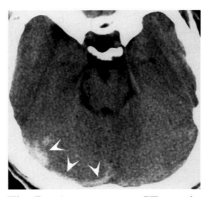

Fig. J.   A non-contrast CT scan in a patient with persistent right occipital headache demonstrates a linear "cord" of increased density (*arrowheads*) at the expected location of the right transverse sinus. Thrombosis of the sinus was confirmed with MR (not shown).

Section V

White Matter Disease/Metabolic

Case 89

Clinical Presentation

A 54-year-old woman presents with recent onset of numbness and weakness in her right leg.

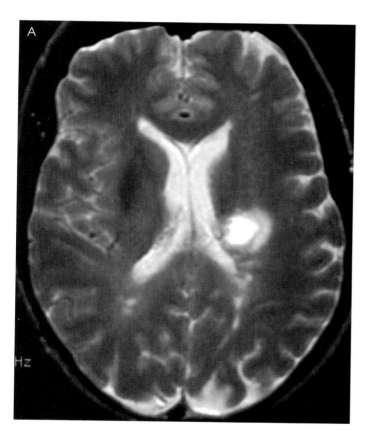

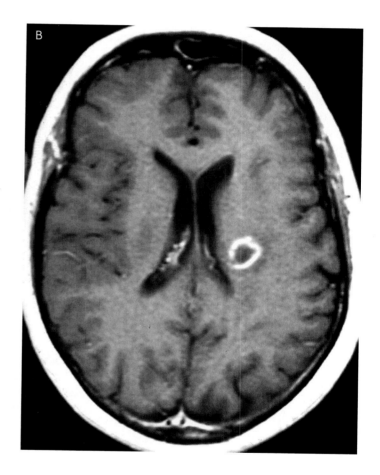

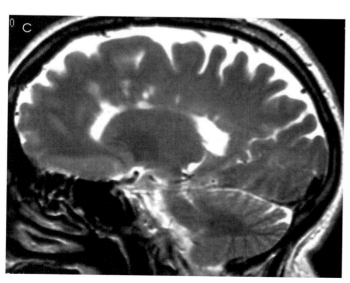

Radiologic Findings

An axial T2-WI (Fig. A) demonstrates a rounded hyperintense lesion in the left corona radiata. Note the presence of marked hyperintensity centrally, surrounded by a slightly lower signal intensity rim, and then a second zone of somewhat less intense T2 prolongation. Note also the presence of punctate foci of T2 prolongation in the periatrial white matter. An axial post-gadolinium T1-WI (Fig. B) demonstrates a fairly regular rim of contrast enhancement around the periphery of the left-sided lesion. A parasagittal fast spin-echo T2-WI (Fig. C) demonstrates multiple ovoid areas of T2 prolongation involving the corpus callosum and pericallosal white matter which have a perpendicular orientation toward the ventricular surface.

Diagnosis

Multiple sclerosis (MS)

Differential Diagnosis

- Acute disseminated encephalomyelitis (more common in children, deep gray nuclear involvement common and colossal involvement uncommon, but may be indistinguishable from the first episode of MS)
- White matter lesions of aging (older patient, typically sparing of corpus callosum and subcortical U fibers, lack of enhancement)
- Vasculitis (areas of infarction and leptomeningeal enhancement are common)
- Encephalitis (patients are typically acutely ill with fever and alteration in consciousness)
- Neurosarcoidosis (may see leptomeningeal enhancement, and the corpus callosum is not typically involved)

Discussion

Background

MS is the most common neurologic disorder in young adults, generally having its onset between 20 and 45 years of age, although 13% of cases present before age 20 and 15% after age 50. MS is more common in women than men with a ratio of 3:2. The clinical definition of MS requires that the patient demonstrate evidence of lesions separated in time and place. Separation in time requires two attacks each lasting at least 24 hours involving different parts of the CNS and separated by at least 1 month. Separation in place requires clinical evidence of distinct neurologic deficits and/or MR imaging evidence of separate CNS lesions. Pathologically, MS is a disease of oligodendroglia and results in multifocal areas of well-demarcated demyelination with little or no axonal degeneration.

Etiology

The cause is unknown, but it is likely a postinfectious autoimmune reaction in genetically susceptible individuals.

Clinical Findings

The presentation varies with the location of lesions. Focal motor or sensory deficits are typical, with headache or seizures being less common presenting symp-

• Optic neuritis may mimic an optic nerve glioma. Again, follow-up imaging may be very useful.

• MR is highly sensitive for the detection of MS lesions, but it is nonspecific. Therefore, findings must be correlated with other clinical parameters.

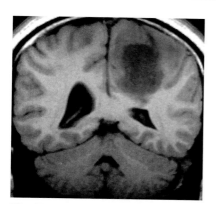

Fig. D. A coronal T1-WI in a 28-year-old man with right-sided numbness and weakness demonstrates a hypointense lesion centered in the left frontoparietal white matter. Note the mass effect on the left lateral ventricle.

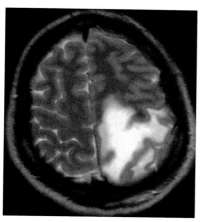

Fig. E. A corresponding T2-WI (same patient as Fig. D) demonstrates striking T2 prolongation in the subcortical white matter. Again note mass effect with sulcal effacement.

toms. Optic nerve involvement is common, and patients may present with acute visual changes due to optic neuritis. Spinal cord involvement may cause myelopathic symptoms. Most patients have a chronic relapsing and remitting course, though some patients may demonstrate steady progression of deficits.

Complications

Blindness, paralysis, dementia, and loss of sphincter control may develop as the disease progresses.

Pathology

Gross

• Acute plaques are edematous and have a pink-gray color
• Chronic plaques show atrophy and cystic change

Microscopic

• There is a variable degree of perivenular inflammation, macrophage infiltration, myelin loss, edema, and gliosis, with relative sparing of axons
• Necrosis, hemorrhage, and calcification are rare
• Cystic change may occur in large lesions

Imaging Findings

CT

• Lesions are typically isodense or hypodense on non-contrast scan
• Lesions may show enhancement post-contrast

MR

• Lesions are typically homogeneously hyperintense on T2-WI. Large acute lesions may have a "target" appearance: a hyperintense center representing demyelination with a slightly less hyperintense periphery representing vasogenic edema. A rim of hypointensity separates these two regions.
• Lesions may be iso- or hypointense on T1-WI, and may demonstrate a rim of T1 shortening attributed to free radicals in infiltrating macrophages
• Acute lesions often enhance following gadolinium administration, and the pattern may be nodular, arclike, or ringlike
• Enhancement generally lasts 1 to 2 months and then resolves
• Lesions typically affect the corpus callosum, periventricular white matter, and arcuate fibers; they may also occur in the posterior fossa and in gray matter structures such as the basal ganglia and thalami

Treatment

• Corticosteroids are a mainstay of therapy
• New therapies such as beta-interferon are under investigation

Prognosis

Highly variable depending on the form of the disease and its responsiveness to therapy

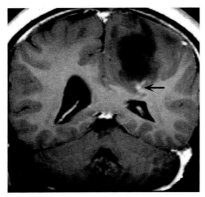

Fig. F. Post-gadolinium, a T1-WI (same patient as Figs. D and E) demonstrates minimal peripheral enhancement at the inferior aspect of the lesion (*arrow*) in this patient with tumefactive MS.

Suggested Readings

Gean-Marton AD, Vezina LG, Marton KI, et al. Abnormal corpus callosum: a sensitive and specific indicator of multiple sclerosis. *Radiology* 180:215–221, 1991.

Horowitz AL, Kaplan RD, Grewe G, et al. The ovoid lesion: a new MR observation in patients with multiple sclerosis. *AJNR* 10:303–305, 1989.

Nesbit GM, Forbes GS, Scheithauer BW, et al. Multiple sclerosis: histopathologic and MR and/or CT correlation in 37 cases at biopsy and three cases at autopsy. *Radiology* 180:467–474, 1991.

Case 90

Clinical Presentation

A 5-year-old child became increasingly irritable and then somnolent over the course of a day. He is brought to the emergency room following a generalized seizure. History is remarkable only for a viral upper respiratory infection several weeks earlier.

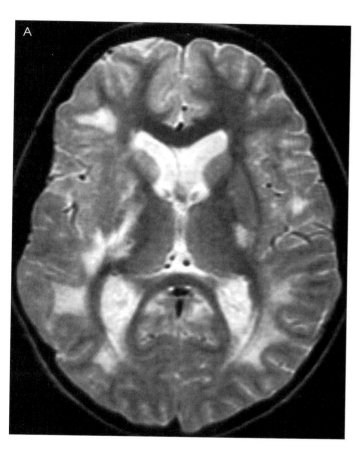

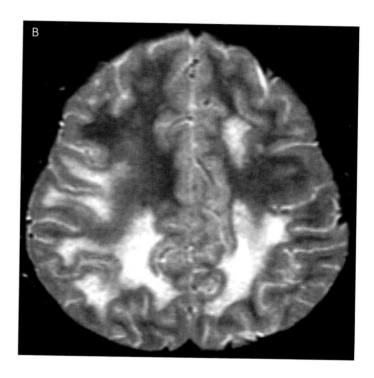

Radiologic Findings

Axial T2-WIs (Figs. A and B) demonstrate patchy and asymmetric T2 prolongation in the subcortical and periventricular white matter, as well as along the internal capsules. These areas demonstrate no significant mass effect.

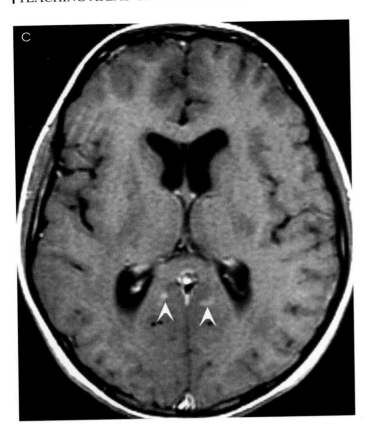

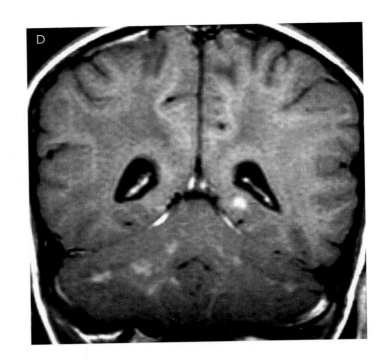

An axial post-gadolinium T1-WI (Fig. C) shows minimal enhancement in the occipital regions bilaterally (*arrowheads*). A coronal post-gadolinium T1-WI (Fig. D) demonstrates that the supratentorial white matter is abnormally hypointense. Note a focus of enhancement in the left occipital lobe, as well as irregular patchy enhancement throughout the cerebellar white matter.

Diagnosis

Acute disseminated encephalomyelitis (ADEM)

Differential Diagnosis

- Multiple sclerosis (generally a less acute presentation, not monophasic)
- Vasculitis (both gray and white matter infarctions)
- Toxic/metabolic demyelination (typically symmetric white matter lesions)
- Viral encephalitis (may be indistinguishable, but often more gray matter involvement)
- Lyme disease (may have history of tick exposure or characteristic rash, may have associated cranial nerve enhancement)

Discussion

Background

ADEM is a demyelinating disease of probable autoimmune etiology. It generally has an abrupt clinical onset 1 to 3 weeks following a viral illness or vaccination

Pearls

- Although ADEM is a monophasic illness, not all lesions will enhance at the same time because some lesions may be developing while others are resolving.
- As with other demyelinating conditions, the lesions of ADEM may exert relatively little mass effect for their size.

Pitfalls

- Vasculitis may mimic ADEM, so consider cerebral angiography because the treatment of vasculitis generally requires the addition of a cytotoxic agent.
- In some cases, definitive diagnosis may require brain biopsy.
- The initial presentation of multiple sclerosis may be fulminant and may be indistinguishable from ADEM. However, thalamic involvement is rare in multiple sclerosis but not uncommon in ADEM, which may be a helpful distinguishing feature.

and runs a monophasic course. ADEM is more common in children than adults. In some cases, it may occur in the absence of an identifiable antecedent event. Because of its sensitivity to white matter pathology, MR has significantly facilitated the diagnosis of this condition.

Etiology

The presumed pathogenetic mechanism is an immune-mediated reaction against CNS myelin triggered by viral infection or vaccination. Viral particles are not usually isolated from the nervous system of ADEM patients, ruling out a direct pathogenic role. Many viruses have been implicated, including measles, rubella, varicella zoster, mumps, influenza, parainfluenza, and Epstein-Barr.

Clinical Findings

Clinical presentation and laboratory evaluation are variable and nonspecific. Headache, meningismus, fever, irritability, and drowsiness are common. Seizures and focal neurologic deficits may occur. Cranial nerve deficits and spinal cord symptoms may also occur. CSF examination often shows a nonspecific lymphocytic pleocytosis and elevated protein.

Complications

Severe cases may progress to stupor, coma, and death. A hemorrhagic form exists that may be complicated by parenchymal hematoma.

Pathology

Gross

- Multifocal lesions of the white matter of the cerebrum, cerebellum, brainstem, and spinal cord
- Lesions may be found in gray matter as well, but are less extensive
- Petechial hemorrhages may be present

Microscopic

- Perivenular lymphocytic and monocytic infiltration and demyelination
- Loss of myelin with relative sparing of axon cylinders

Imaging Findings

CT

- Asymmetric areas of low density in the white matter may be seen

MR

- Patchy bilateral asymmetric areas of T2 prolongation in the subcortical and deep white matter of the cerebral hemispheres. Lesions are common in the cerebellum and brainstem, and deep gray matter involvement is also common, especially in children.
- May see hemorrhage superimposed on areas of demyelination
- Lesions may occasionally show central cavitation
- Post-gadolinium, there is variable enhancement of the lesions with a pattern that may be nodular, peripheral, or diffuse

Treatment

Corticosteroids and supportive care

Prognosis

- Mortality rates are as high as 10 to 30% in patients with severe disease (i.e., hemorrhagic ADEM)
- Of patients who survive, approximately 90% will recover completely, while 10% will be left with variable residual neurologic deficits

Suggested Readings

Atlas SW, Grossman RI, Goldberg HI, et al. MR diagnosis of acute disseminated encephalomyelitis. *J Comput Assist Tomogr* 10:798–801, 1986.

Baum PA, Barkovich AJ, Koch TK, Berg BO. Deep gray matter involvement in children with acute disseminated encephalomyelitis. *AJNR* 15:1275–1283, 1994.

Mader I, Stock KW, Ettlin T, Probst A. Acute disseminated encephalomyelitis: MR and CT features. *AJNR* 17:104–109, 1996.

Case 91

Clinical Presentation

A 45-year-old patient with a history of alcoholism is admitted to the hospital with progressive confusion and dysarthria.

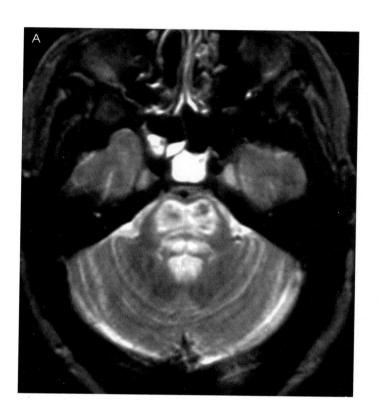 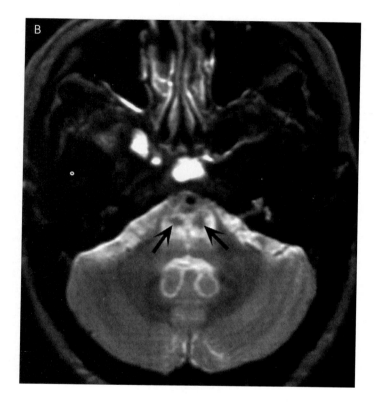

Radiologic Findings

An axial T2-WI (Fig. A) demonstrates abnormal T2 prolongation within the central pons. Note the sparing of a peripheral rim of tissue, best appreciated anteriorly and laterally. On a T2-WI at a slightly more inferior level (Fig. B), the corticospinal tracts are well seen (*arrows*) surrounded by abnormal T2 prolongation.

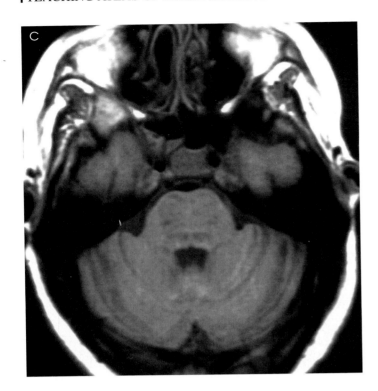

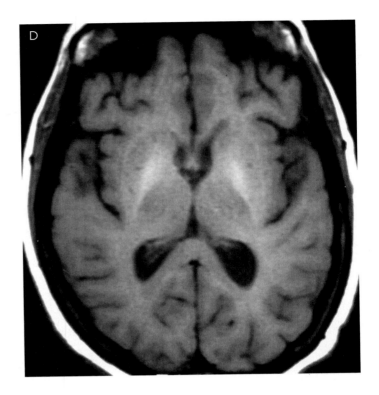

An axial T1-WI (Fig. C) shows mild hypointensity within the central pons. Note also the prominence of the cerebellar folia, presumably related to cerebellar atrophy in this chronically alcoholic patient. A more cephalad T1-WI (Fig. D) demonstrates intrinsic T1 shortening in the globi pallidi bilaterally, which is presumed related to the patients history of alcoholism and accompanying liver disease.

Diagnosis

Central pontine myelinolysis (CPM)

Differential Diagnosis

- Multiple sclerosis (callosal and periventricular lesions are common)
- Acute disseminated encephalomyelitis (lesions typically involve subcortical and deep white matter)
- Ischemia/infarction (should follow a vascular distribution)
- Infiltrating neoplasm (insidious presentation, mass effect, may enhance)

Discussion

Background

CPM is characterized by symmetric, noninflammatory demyelination of the basis pontis. There has been increasing recognition of the occurrence of extrapontine myelinolysis (EPM), which may occur with or without accompanying CPM. Extrapontine sites of involvement include the cerebellum, cerebral cortex/subcortex, putamen, caudate nucleus, and thalamus (Figs. E and F).

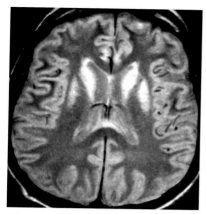

Fig. E. An axial proton density-weighted image in a patient whose hyponatremia had been rapidly corrected demonstrates abnormal high-signal intensity in the caudate nuclei and putamina bilaterally.

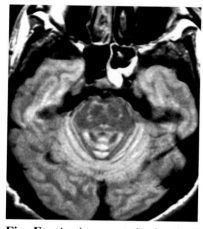

Fig. F. An image at the level of the pons in the same patient as Figure E demonstrates mild hyperintensity within the central pons, with sparing of the corticospinal tracts. Findings are consistent with CPM/EPM.

Etiology

The exact mechanism is unknown, but osmotic shifts are implicated because patients with hyponatremia which is rapidly corrected or overcorrected are at greatest risk of CPM/EPM. CPM/EPM has also been observed in chronic alcoholic and malnourished patients, and in patients undergoing orthotopic liver transplantation.

Clinical Findings

Severe cases are characterized by spastic quadriparesis, pseudobulbar palsies, and acute changes in mental status. Milder cases are characterized by weakness, confusion, and dysarthria.

Complications

CPM may progress to a "locked-in" syndrome, coma, and even death in severe cases.

Pathology

Gross

- Brain softening and loss of myelin in affected regions

Microscopic

- Characterized by regions of demyelination that are usually most prominent in the central portion of the basis pontis
- Destruction of myelin with relative sparing of neurons, axon cylinders, and blood vessels, and an absence of inflammation

Imaging Findings

CT

- Often negative as the posterior fossa is obscured by artifact

MR

- Characteristic triangular or trident-shaped area of T2 prolongation in the central pons, with sparing of a peripheral rim of tissue. The corticospinal tracts are generally spared as well.
- Extrapontine lesions are commonly observed in the putamina and thalami, but may be seen in the periventricular white matter and at the corticomedullary junction
- Lesions may be iso- or hypointense on T1-WI
- Lesions typically lack mass effect or enhancement
- Follow-up scans typically demonstrate atrophy and persistent T2 prolongation in the involved areas

Treatment

No specific therapy—supportive care

Prognosis

- Previously thought to be uniformly fatal as only severe cases were diagnosed
- In the MR era, there is increasing recognition of the variability of the condition

• Most patients survive but have varying degrees of residual neurological deficit

Suggested Readings

Koci TM, Chiang F, Chow P, et al. Thalamic extrapontine lesions in central pontine myelinolysis. *AJNR* 11:1229–1233, 1990.

Miller GM, Baker HL, Okazaki H, Whisnant JP. Central pontine myelinolysis and its imitators: MR findings. *Radiology* 168:795–802, 1988.

Yuh WTC, Simonson TM, D'Alessandro MP, et al. Temporal changes of MR findings in central pontine myelinolysis. *AJNR* 16:975–977, 1995.

Case 92

Clinical Presentation

An 18-year-old woman with liver disease and metabolic derangements suffers a series of grand mal seizures. When she is able to communicate, she complains of blindness.

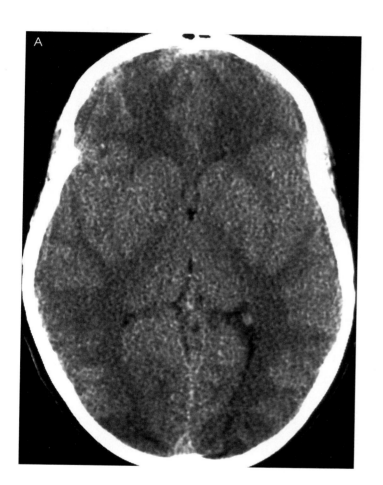

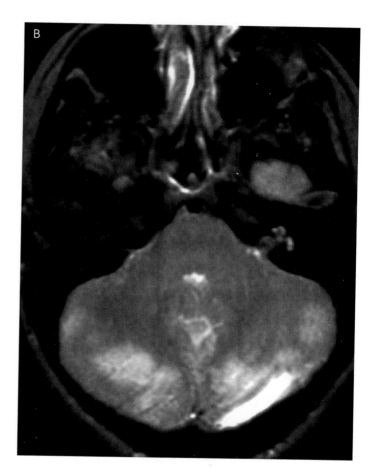

Radiologic Findings

A non-contrast CT scan (Fig. A) shows subtle hypodensity in the occipital cortex and subcortical white matter bilaterally. The patient was transferred to MR for further evaluation. An axial T2-WI through the cerebellum (Fig. B) demonstrates patchy T2 prolongation involving gray and white matter.

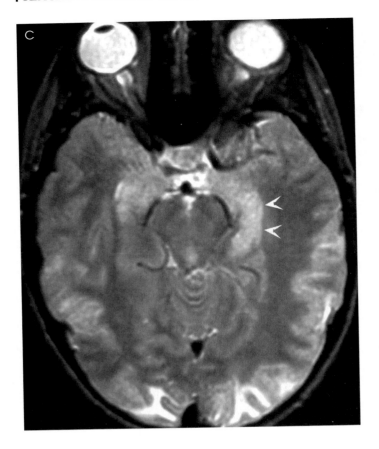

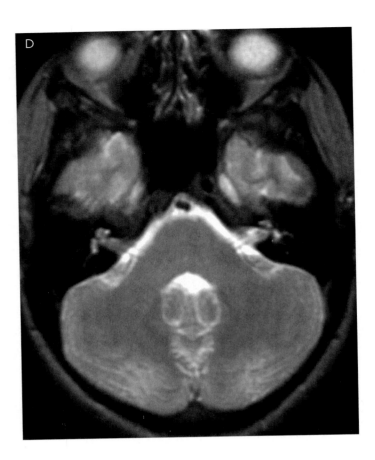

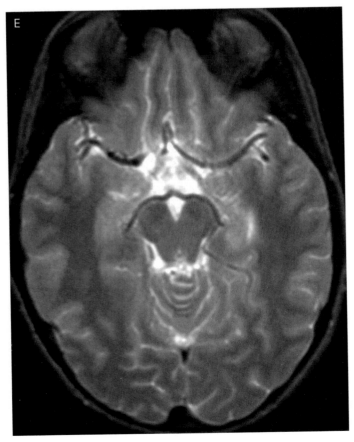

A more cephalad T2-WI (Fig. C) demonstrates hyperintensity of the occipital and posterior temporal cortex as well as intense high signal in the occipital subcortical white matter. Note also mild hyperintensity in the left hippocampus (*arrowheads*). A follow-up MRI was obtained approximately 2 weeks later, by which time the patient's blindness had completely resolved. Axial T2-WIs (Figs. D and E) show essentially complete resolution of the previously noted abnormalities.

Diagnosis

Reversible post-ictal cerebral edema

Differential Diagnosis

Predominantly parieto-occipital white matter hyperintensity

- These entities are distinguished by the clinical setting: hypertensive encephalopathy, eclampsia/preeclampsia, cyclosporine-induced neurotoxicity, watershed ischemia

More widespread signal changes

- Vasculitis (multifocal areas of infarction), acute disseminated encephalomyelitis (ADEM) (more common in children, typically multifocal lesions of white matter both supra- and infratentorially, as well as deep gray matter)

Temporal lobe hyperintensity

- Encephalitis (acute onset, often fever and personality change, often involvement of cingulum and insula), neoplasm (insidious onset, mass effect, variable enhancement)

Discussion

Background

Reversible changes on CT and MR are known to occur following status epilepticus. However, acute brain edema may also occur following a single or several seizures. In these cases, the seizures are usually generalized or focal with secondary generalization, and the imaging abnormalities have a parieto-occipital predominance. The etiology of the observed parenchymal changes is uncertain, but vasogenic edema due to focal blood-brain barrier disruption best explains the phenomenon. This is supported by the reversibility, relative lack of mass effect, absence of reduced diffusion, and white matter predominance of the transient radiologic abnormalities. The posterior predominance of the lesions may be explained by the regional variability of sympathetic vascular innervation; because less innervation exists in the vertebrobasilar circulation, it is more prone to loss of autoregulation and disruption of the blood-brain barrier. Cytotoxic edema and frank infarction due to acidosis and hypoxemia may, in some cases, complicate the picture and limit the reversibility of the changes. Associated hippocampal swelling and/or T2 prolongation may be observed.

Clinical Findings

The presentation varies with the location of the signal abnormality, but parieto-occipital abnormalities typically result in visual deficits. Postictal lethargy and confusion are common.

Pathology

- It is rare for these cases to come to pathologic analysis
- Occasionally brain biopsies are done because of clinical concern for tumor, and in these cases, normal brain tissue or mild gliosis have been found

Imaging Findings

CT

- Hypodensity of parieto-occipital white matter may be seen
- Loss of gray-white distinction if the cortex is also edematous

MR

- T2 prolongation involving gray and white matter of parieto-occipital and posterior temporal regions, but with a white matter predominance
- Usually iso- or hypointense on T1-WI
- Lacks mass effect or has only mild mass effect
- Patchy parenchymal enhancement may be seen, consistent with disruption of the blood-brain barrier

Treatment

Management of the underlying seizure disorder and control of associated hypertension, if present

Prognosis

Usually complete resolution of MR abnormalities and clinical symptoms. Rarely cortical blindness may be permanent.

Suggested Readings

Cox JE, Mathews VP, Santos CC, Elster AD. Seizure-induced transient hippocampal abnormalities on MR: correlation with positron emission tomography and electroencephalography. *AJNR* 16:1736–1738, 1995.

Dillon W, Brant-Zawadzki M, Sherry RG. Transient computed tomographic abnormalities after focal seizures. *AJNR* 5:107–109, 1984.

Yaffe K, Ferriero D, Barkovich AJ, Rowley H. Reversible MRI abnormalities following seizures. *Neurology* 45:104–108, 1995.

Case 93

Clinical Presentation

A 53-year-old man is evaluated for short-term memory loss, rigidity, and hyper-reflexia. He has a history of a suicide attempt 6 months earlier.

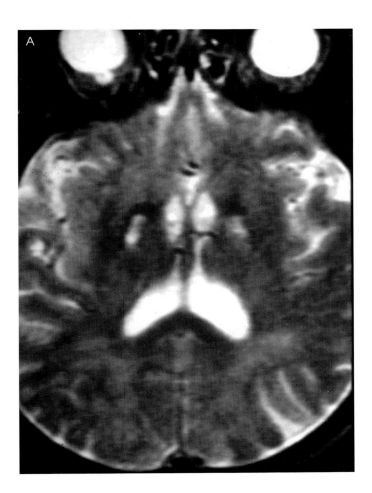

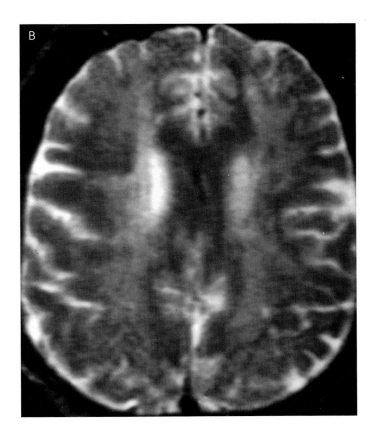

Radiologic Findings

An axial T2-WI (Fig. A) shows focal sharply circumscribed areas of T2 prolongation within the globi pallidi bilaterally. More cephalad T2-WIs through the hemispheric white matter (Figs. B and C) show diffuse and symmetric T2 prolongation within the white matter without mass effect. A coronal T1-WI (Fig. D) demonstrates focal T1 shortening in the globi pallidi bilaterally.

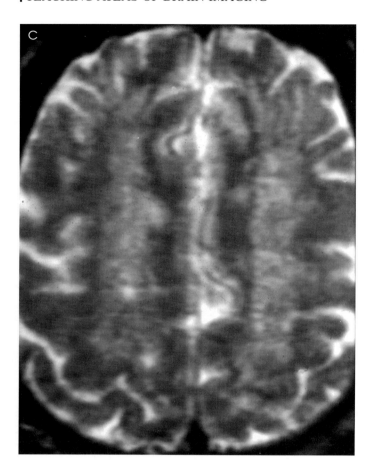

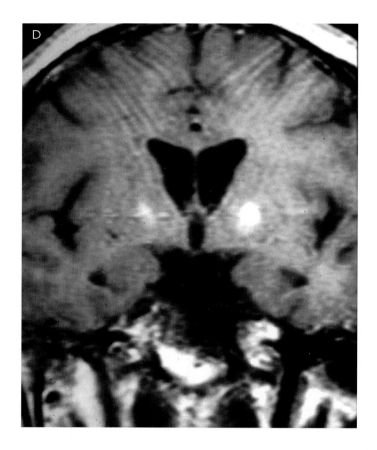

Diagnosis

Carbon monoxide (CO) poisoning

Differential Diagnosis

- Other white matter toxins such as toluene or methanol (clinical history essential)
- Other toxins that affect the globi pallidi (i.e., cyanide poisoning, which is distinguished by clinical history, cerebellar involvement, and lack of white matter changes)
- Inborn errors of metabolism such as methylmalonic acidemia or L-2-hydroxy-glutaric acidemia (typically present in childhood, need appropriate clinical history, and laboratory analysis)
- Vasculitis, acute disseminated encephalomyelitis (more patchy and asymmetric, pallidal necrosis not a feature)

Discussion

Background

CO poisoning most commonly occurs in the setting of attempted suicide or with the use of coal heaters in poorly ventilated homes. There are thought to be three mechanisms of cellular toxicity in CO poisoning: (1) the formation of carboxyhemoglobin (which cannot bind oxygen) causes hypoxia; (2) the oxyhemoglobin dissociation curve is shifted to the left, which decreases oxygen release to body tissues; and (3) a direct toxic effect on mitochondria via CO binding to cytochrome a_3 interferes with oxidative phosphorylation.

Clinical Findings

Patients are often unconscious at presentation and may remain in prolonged coma. Survivors may manifest movement disorders, hypertonia, short-term memory loss, and mental deterioration.

Complications

Cardiac arrhythmia is a frequent cause of death.

Pathology

- Bilateral necrosis of the globus pallidus is the most common lesion
- Demyelination and areas of focal necrosis may occur in the white matter

Imaging Findings

CT

- Bilateral and symmetrical low-attenuation lesions in the globus pallidus and white matter

MR

- Focal T2 prolongation in the globus pallidus
- Diffuse symmetric T2 prolongation in hemispheric white matter. Mild mass effect, if any. Nonenhancing.
- Focal T1 shortening in the globus pallidus may be seen, representing either petechial hemorrhage, dystrophic calcification, or tissue breakdown products
- Cerebellum may be involved as well as cerebrum

Treatment

Usually 100% or hyperbaric oxygen

Prognosis

- Varies with severity and duration of exposure
- Long-term neurologic sequelae often occur in survivors

Suggested Readings

Silver DA, Cross M, Fox B, Paxton RM. Computed tomography of the brain in acute carbon monoxide poisoning. *Clin Radiol* 51:480–483, 1996.

Silverman CS, Brenner J, Murtagh FR. Hemorrhagic necrosis and vascular injury in carbon monoxide poisoning: MR demonstration. *AJNR* 14:168–170, 1993.

Uchino A, Hasuo K, Shida K, et al. MRI of the brain in chronic carbon monoxide poisoning. *Neuroradiology* 36:399–401, 1994.

Case 94

Clinical Presentation

A 7-year-old boy presents with progressive difficulty walking and decline in intellectual function.

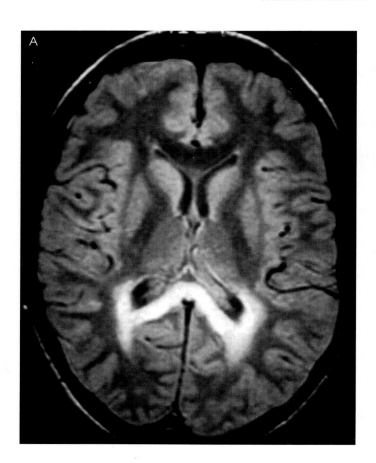

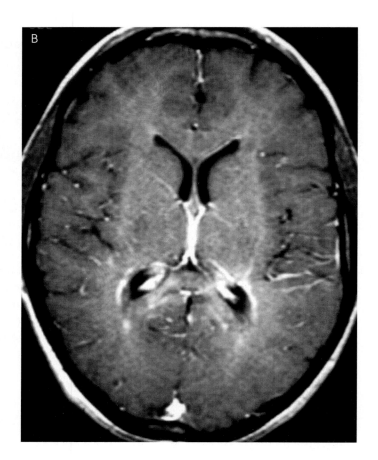

Radiologic Findings

An axial proton density-weighted image (Fig. A) demonstrates symmetric high-signal intensity involving the splenium of the corpus callosum and the periatrial white matter. There is no associated mass effect. An axial post-gadolinium T1-WI (Fig. B) demonstrates mild enhancement in the splenium of the corpus callosum, as well as at the periphery of the periatrial abnormalities.

Pearls

- Pontomedullary corticospinal tract involvement is a common finding in ALD and is unusual in other leukodystrophies. This finding is particularly useful if atypical cerebral findings are present.

- New MR techniques such as magnetization transfer imaging may be useful in tissue characterization and monitoring of response to specific therapies.

- Ten to 15% of heterozygote carriers of X-linked ALD develop overt neurologic disturbances.

Pitfall

- Atypical imaging patterns include predominantly frontal white matter changes, predominantly unilateral white matter changes, and parieto-occipital calcification.

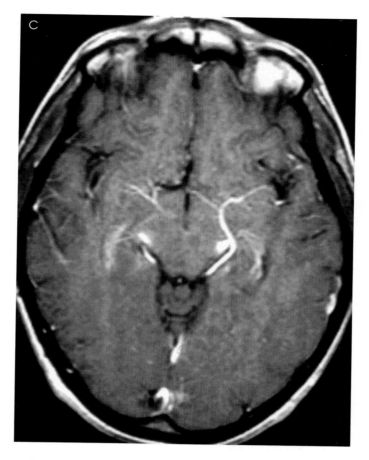

A post-gadolinium T1-WI at a more inferior level (Fig. C) demonstrates focal enhancement along the corticospinal pathways bilaterally.

Diagnosis

X-linked adrenoleukodystrophy (ALD)

Differential Diagnosis

None: this is a pathognomonic appearance

Discussion

Background

ALD encompasses two genetic disorders that cause varying degrees of malfunction of the adrenal cortex and CNS myelin, and both of which are characterized by elevated levels of very long-chain fatty acids (VLCFAs). X-linked ALD is an uncommon disorder seen exclusively in males and characterized by demyelination in the central nervous system. The hallmark of the disease is impaired peroxisomal β-oxidation of VLCFAs, and the diagnosis is established by the combination of a typical clinical presentation and the presence of elevated blood levels of very long-chain fatty acids. In X-linked ALD, peroxisomes are structurally normal. Neonatal ALD is autosomal recessive and resembles the Zellweger cerebrohepatorenal syndrome in that the number and size of peroxisomes are reduced and the function of at least five peroxisomal enzymes is impaired.

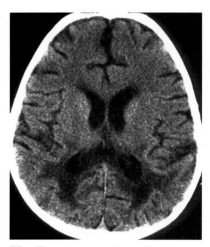

Fig. D. A non-enhanced CT scan demonstrates low attenuation in the periatrial white matter, with involvement of the splenium of the corpus callosum. Note also the generalized prominence of ventricles and sulci in this 8-year-old male with ALD.

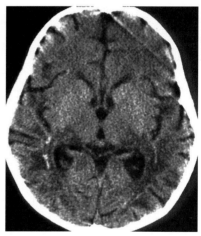

Fig. E. A non-enhanced CT scan at a more inferior level (same patient as Fig. D) demonstrates linear, irregular dystrophic calcification at the periphery of this process.

Etiology

An underlying defect exists in lignoceryl-coenzyme A ligase, a peroxisomal enzyme involved in the breakdown of VLCFAs in the CNS, adrenal cortex, and testes. The gene for this disorder has been mapped to Xq28. The mechanism of CNS damage remains unresolved. Factors include a direct toxic effect of VLCFAs, recruitment of inflammatory cells, and stimulation of inflammatory cells to initiate a cytokine cascade that leads to demyelination

Clinical Findings

X-linked ALD typically presents between ages 5 and 10 years with gait disturbance and intellectual impairment. Spinal cord and peripheral nerve involvement may occur. Adrenal insufficiency is present in greater than 90%. There may be delayed presentation with onset of symptoms in adolescence or adulthood. The disorder is then referred to as adrenomyeloneuropathy. These patients experience progressive paraparesis and sphincter disturbance over a period of decades, and 66% have adrenal insufficiency.

Complications

Progression of disease leads to hypotonia, seizures, visual changes, dysphagia, and deafness. Progressive dementia occurs. Death usually ensues 1 to 10 years from onset of symptoms.

Pathology

Gross

- Atrophy and myelin pallor, most apparent in the parieto-occipital regions

Microscopic

- Extensive diffuse demyelination, with relative sparing of U fibers
- Affected areas are divided into three distinct zones:
    1. *Central zone* of scarring and gliosis with an absence of oligodendroglia, axons, myelin, and inflammatory cells
    2. *Peripheral zone* with perivascular inflammatory cells, demyelination, and axonal preservation
    3. *Outermost zone* characterized by active destruction of the myelin sheath and lack of perivascular inflammatory cells

Imaging Findings

CT

- Classic finding is low attenuation in the occipital white matter with involvement of the splenium of the corpus callosum (Fig. D)
- Dystrophic calcification may occasionally be seen (Fig. E)

MR

- Marked symmetric T1 and T2 prolongation in the occipital white matter and splenium of the corpus callosum. Involvement of the retrolenticular portion of the posterior limb of the internal capsule is often contiguous. As the disease progresses, there is extension anteriorly to involve the frontal white matter.

- T2 prolongation involving the corticospinal tracts in the pons and medulla. The auditory pathways (lateral lemniscus, medial geniculate bodies, acoustic radiations) are involved as well.
- Post-gadolinium: enhancement of the leading edge of active demyelination is frequently observed

Treatment

- Immunosuppression has been tried to modify the inflammatory response
- Dietary therapy with specific fatty acids may have a role but is controversial
- Bone marrow transplantation may have a role in arresting progression of the disease
- Adrenal hormone replacement therapy is usually required

Prognosis

- Classic X-linked ALD has a poor prognosis with relentless progression to death
- Adrenomyeloneuropathy has a much more favorable prognosis

Suggested Readings

Barkovich AJ, Ferriero DM, Bass N, Boyer R. Involvement of the pontomedullary corticospinal tracts: a useful finding in the diagnosis of X- linked adrenoleukodystrophy. *AJNR* 18:95–100, 1997.

Korenke GC, Hunneman DH, Kohler J, et al. Glyceroltrioleate/glyceroltrierucate therapy in 16 patients with X-chromosomal adrenoleukodystrophy-adrenomyeloneuropathy: effect on clinical, biochemical and neurophysiological parameters. *Eur J Pediatr* 154:64–70, 1995.

Melhem ER, Breiter SN, Ulug AM, et al. Improved tissue characterization in adrenoleukodystrophy using magnetization transfer imaging. *AJR* 166:689–695, 1996.

Case 95

Clinical Presentation

A 10-month-old girl presents with failure to thrive, hypotonia, and infantile spasms.

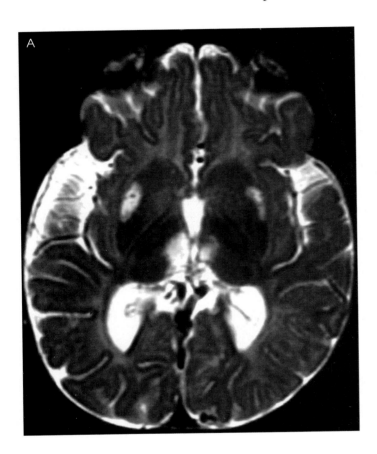

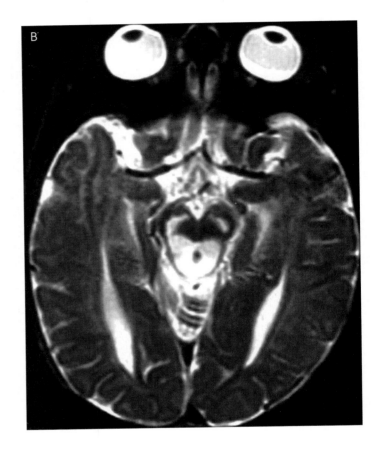

Radiologic Findings

An axial T2-WI (Fig. A) demonstrates abnormal T2 prolongation in the putamina and medial thalami bilaterally, right more extensive than left. A more inferior T2-WI (Fig. B) demonstrates extensive T2 prolongation within the midbrain.

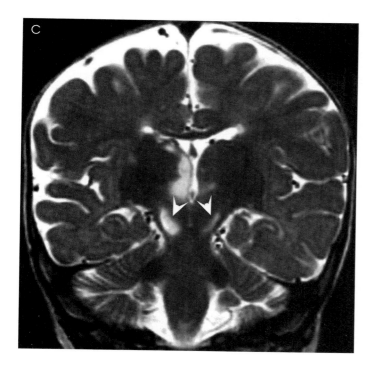

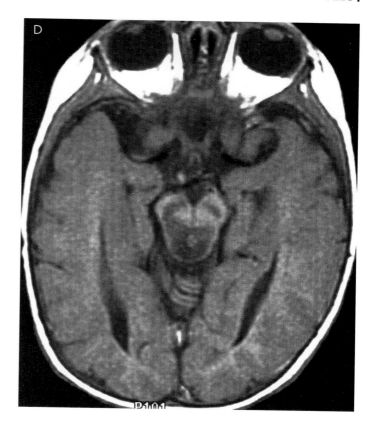

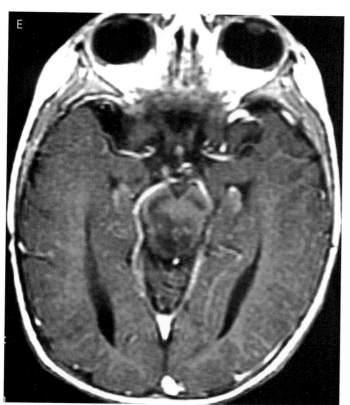

A coronal T2-WI (Fig. C) again demonstrates the medial thalamic abnormality, as well as T2 prolongation in the region of the subthalamic nuclei bilaterally (*arrowheads*). An axial T1-WI (Fig. D) through the midbrain shows that the areas of abnormal T2 prolongation are hypointense. Following administration of gadolinium (Fig. E), a T1-WI shows no evidence of abnormal enhancement.

Table 1.   Mitochondrial Disorders that Predominantly Affect the CNS

Disorder	Cardinal Clinical Manifestations
Leigh disease (subacute necrotizing encephalomyelopathy)	Present in first 2 years of life with hypotonia, ataxia, ophthalmoplegia, and brainstem dysfunction
MERRF syndrome (Myoclonus, Epilepsy, Ragged Red Fibers)	Myoclonus, seizures, ataxia, optic atrophy, hearing loss, proximal limb weakness
MELAS syndrome (Mitochondrial myopathy, Encephalopathy, Lactic Acidosis, Strokelike episodes)	Hemiparesis, hemianopsia, and other focal neurologic findings varying with the location of strokes; seizures
Kearns-Sayre syndrome	Chronic external ophthalmoplegia, retinal pigmentary abnormalities, cardiac arrhythmias, ataxia
Leber's hereditary optic neuropathy	Predominantly affects males, vision is lost between ages 18 and 40
Alpers' disease (progressive infantile poliodystrophy)	Seizures, blindness, hypotonia, liver dysfunction
Menkes' syndrome (trichopoliodystrophy) (Note that mitochondria are affected secondarily due to low copper levels which impair cytochrome c function)	Hypotonia, seizures, hypothermia, coarse and sparse hair

Diagnosis

Leigh disease

Differential Diagnosis

• Organic acidopathies (usually more white matter involvement)
• Other mitochondrial disorders (differentiated clinically, see Table 1)
• Toxic ingesion (more acute history)
• Thiamine deficiency (less lentiform nuclear involvement)

Discussion

Background

Leigh disease, also known as subacute necrotizing encephalomyelopathy, is included among the mitochondrial cytopathies (Table 1). The mitochondrial cytopathies represent disorders of mitochondrial function that result in impaired production of adenosine triphosphate in affected cells. Impaired aerobic metabolism of pyruvate results in anaerobic conversion to lactate and transamination to alanine. Most of these conditions result in myopathic weakness and fatiguability of muscles (particularly those in the limb girdles), ophthalmoplegia, peripheral neuropathy, and CNS deficits. Leigh disease typically affects infants and young children, but there may be late presentations in older children and adults. Mitochondrial deoxyribonucleic acid is maternally inherited, making the mitochondrial disorders heterogeneous and complex because of an often unequal distribution of mitochondria in daughter cells. Although most human mitochondrial disorders are either maternally inherited or sporadic, some are associated with nuclear rather than mitochondrial genes and are inherited in an autosomal dominant or recessive fashion.

Etiology

Leigh disease encompasses a group of enzyme deficiencies that have a common clinical phenotype and may therefore be more correctly referred to as Leigh syndrome. Genetic and biochemical abnormalities identified in patients with Leigh disease include pyruvate dehydrogenase deficiency, pyruvate carboxylase deficiency, and cytochrome-c oxidase deficiency.

Clinical Findings

Patients typically present during the first year of life with hypotonia, brainstem dysfunction, ophthalmoplegia, ataxia, and ptosis. The clinical course may be acute, relapsing-remitting, or slowly progressive. Elevated lactate may be present in blood and CSF.

Pathology

- Spongy degeneration associated with astroglial and microglial reaction and vascular proliferation affects the basal ganglia, brainstem, and spinal cord
- Demyelination of basal ganglia, midbrain, cerebral, and cerebellar white matter

Imaging Findings

CT

- CT is far less sensitive than MR, but low-density lesions in the putamina may be observed

MR

- T2 prolongation in the putamina bilaterally, with atrophy of the putamina over time
- Variable T2 prolongation in the caudate heads, substantia nigra, periaqueductal gray matter, thalami, and dorsomedial medulla
- Low signal on T1-WI may be observed in areas of T2 prolongation
- Mild peripheral enhancement may be seen around these areas
- Delayed myelination or diffuse demyelination may be present
- MR spectroscopy may show an elevated lactate peak

Treatment

None, except for minimizing stresses and infections that may precipitate metabolic crisis

Prognosis

Relentless progression at a variable rate

Suggested Readings

Barkovich AJ, Good WV, Koch TK, Berg BO. Mitochondrial disorders: analysis of their clinical and imaging characteristics. *AJNR* 14:1119–1137, 1993.

Kendall BE. Disorders of lysosomes, peroxisomes, and mitochondria. *AJNR* 13:621–653, 1992.

Case 96

Clinical Presentation

A 6-month-old female presents with fever and irritability. She had been noted to have delayed development as well.

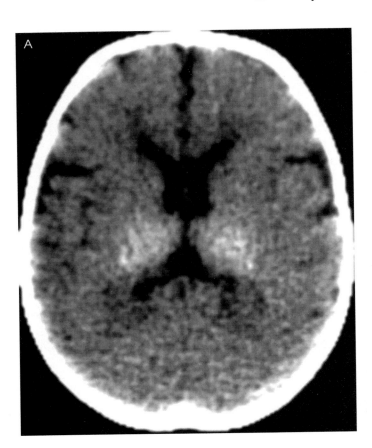
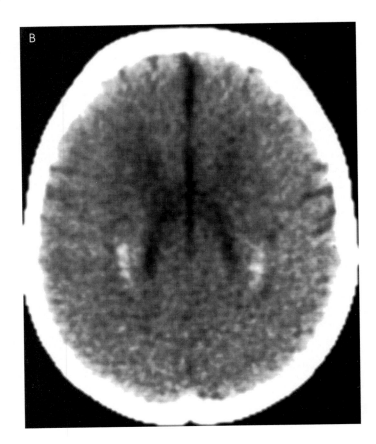

Radiologic Findings

An axial non-contrast CT scan (Fig. A) demonstrates increased attenuation in the thalami bilaterally, as well as mildly decreased attenuation in the periventricular white matter. A more superior image from the CT scan (Fig. B) demonstrates high-attenuation material in the posterior aspect of the corona radiata.

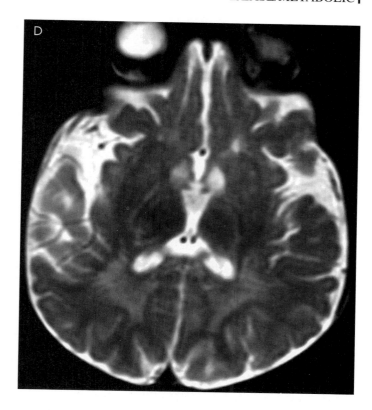

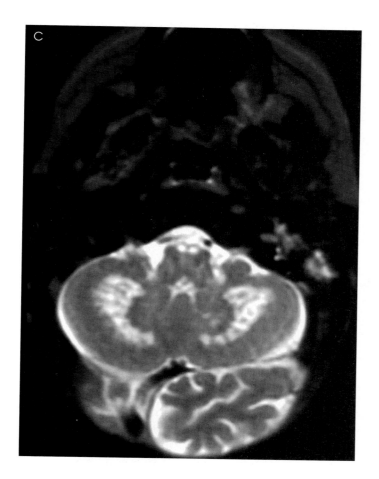

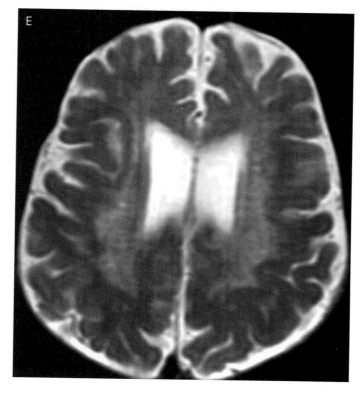

An MR scan was performed several months later. An axial T2-WI through the cerebellum (Fig. C) demonstrates abnormal high-signal intensity in the cerebellar white matter, as well as in the brainstem. A more cephalad image (Fig. D) shows abnormal T2 prolongation in the periatrial white matter. The thalami are mildly hypointense. A T2-WI at the level of the corona radiata (Fig. E) demonstrates abnormal T2 prolongation within the white matter. Note also the progressive volume loss with prominence of ventricles and sulci as compared with the earlier CT scans.

Diagnosis

Krabbe's disease (globoid cell leukodystrophy)

Differential Diagnosis

Early changes

- Include other lysosomal storage diseases such as GM1 and GM2 gangliosidoses

Late changes

- Include other inborn errors of metabolism leading to severe white matter loss and atrophy

Discussion

Background

Krabbe's disease is a lysosomal leukodystrophy that has an autosomal recessive pattern of inheritance. Lysosomes are cytoplasmic enzyme-containing vesicles that digest cellular debris. Abnormal lysosomal storage of a substance occurs when the enzyme responsible for its breakdown is absent or deficient, and the stored material interferes with normal cellular functions. In this case, the accumulation of toxic intermediate products interferes with myelin production and maintenance, and oligodendrocytes are destroyed.

Etiology

Krabbe's disease is caused by a deficiency of galactosylceramidase (galactocerebrosidase β-galactosidase), a lysosomal enzyme that normally degrades galactosylceramide, a major component of the myelin sheath, to ceramide and galactose. Accumulation of toxic metabolites leads to early destruction of oligodendroglia, while accumulation of galactosylceramide itself elicits a globoid cell reaction. The gene has been localized to chromosome 14.

Clinical Findings

Krabbe's disease typically has an acute onset between ages 3 and 6 months, with restlessness, irritability, fevers, difficulty feeding, and developmental delay. Optic atrophy and hyperacusis are also common. Over time, flaccidity and bulbar signs develop, and the disease is usually fatal within the first few years of life. Atypical and late-onset forms have been described.

Pathology

Gross

- Atrophic brain with extensive symmetric demyelination
- Both cerebrum and cerebellum are affected, but the subcortical U fibers are relatively spared

Microscopic

- Perivascular clusters of large multinucleated "globoid" cells
- Almost total loss of myelin and oligodendroglia
- Astrocytic gliosis in the white matter

Imaging Findings

CT

- Symmetric high density is seen in the thalami, caudate nuclei, and corona radiata early in the course of the disease
- Over time, progressive atrophy of white matter occurs

MR

- Nonspecific T1 and T2 prolongation is seen in the cerebral and cerebellar white matter, especially in the peritrigonal regions and corpus callosum. Subtle enhancement may rarely be observed peripherally. The thalami may show decreased T1- and/or T2-relaxation times.

Treatment

- No effective treatment is currently available
- Future prospects: bone marrow transplantation, enzyme replacement therapy

Prognosis

Generally poor, but patients with relatively mild enzyme deficiencies may have late presentation and slow deterioration

Suggested Readings

Bernardini GL, Herrera DG, Carson D, et al. Adult-onset Krabbe's disease in siblings with novel mutations in the galactocerebrosidase gene. *Ann Neurol* 41:111–114, 1997.

Ieshima A, Eda I, Matsui A, et al. Computed tomography in Krabbe's disease: comparison with neuropathology. *Neuroradiology* 25:323–327, 1983.

Sasaki M, Sakuragawa N, Takashima S, et al. MR and CT findings in Krabbe's disease. *Pediatr Neurol* 7:283–288, 1991.

Case 97

Clinical Presentation

A 10-month-old male with nystagmus and developmental delay presents for evaluation.

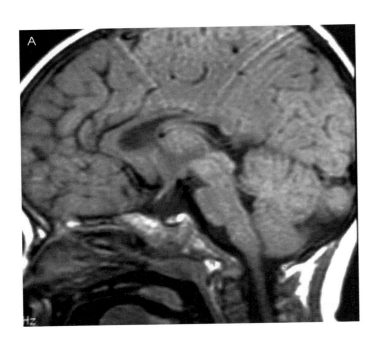

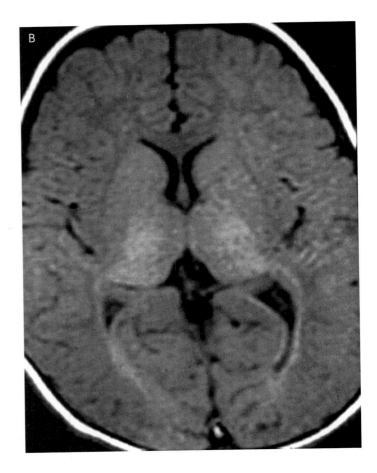

Radiologic Findings

A sagittal T1-WI (Fig. A) demonstrates a thin corpus callosum with a small splenium. The corpus callosum does not demonstrate the high signal that would be expected in an infant of 10 months. An axial T1-WI (Fig. B) at the level of the internal capsules similarly does not demonstrate the expected high signal from myelinated fibers that should be present in the internal capsules. There is slightly increased signal intensity in the thalami bilaterally as well as in the periatrial regions (corresponding to the optic radiations), but myelination is clearly deficient for the patient's age as a T1-WI should demonstrate essentially an adult pattern by the age of 10 months.

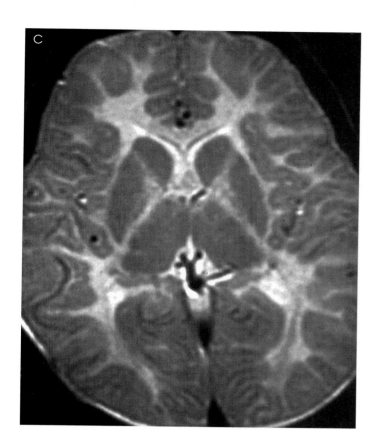

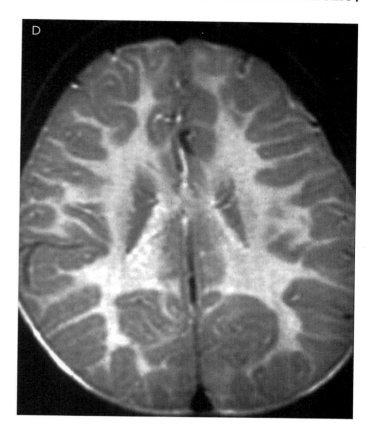

Axial T2-WIs at the level of the internal capsules (Fig. C) and the centrum semiovale (Fig. D) demonstrate diffuse hyperintensity within the white matter, consistent with a near-complete lack of normal myelination. *(Figures courtesy of Nancy Bass, M.D., San Francisco, CA.)*

Diagnosis

Pelizaeus-Merzbacher disease (PMD)

Differential Diagnosis

- Trichothiodystrophy (autosomal recessive transmission, clinical phenotype includes brittle hair)
- Cockayne's syndrome (characteristic facies, pigmentary retinopathy)

Discussion

Background

PMD is a rare dysmyelinating disorder that affects the CNS. Three basic varieties of this disorder are distinguished. Type I is the "classic" form of the disease, has onset during infancy or late infancy, and shows X-linked recessive inheritance. Type II, the "connatal" form, has its onset in utero or in the first weeks of life, progresses more rapidly than the classic form, shows total lack of myelination, generally leads to death during early childhood, and may have X-linked or autosomal recessive transmission. Type III is a transitional form that resembles the connatal type, but its course is not so rapid. Males are typically affected because

Pearls

- If some myelination is initially evident, it may slowly diminish over time.
- Dysmyelinating disorders tend to lead to symmetric, uniform white matter involvement, while demyelinating disorders are more likely to lead to patchy and asymmetric involvement.

Pitfall

- The end stage of PMD presents as diffuse atrophy and is indistinguishable on imaging from the end stage of many other leukodystrophies.

the majority of the cases are inherited in an X-linked recessive manner. However, subtle abnormalities on brain MR scans have been reported in obligate female carriers.

Etiology

The defect in the X-linked form has been shown to involve a gene encoding proteolipid protein (PLP), a crucial structural protein of myelin. This gene is located at the Xq22 position, and multiple different mutations have been associated with the PMD phenotype. Additionally, duplication of the PLP gene has been shown to be a major cause of PMD.

Clinical Findings

Consistent initial clinical features include nystagmus and inspiratory stridor. Spasticity, extrapyramidal features, and cerebellar ataxia are prominent. Other findings include developmental delay, seizures, and optic atrophy with blindness. Brainstem and somatosensory evoked potentials are useful in establishing the diagnosis by demonstrating marked disturbances of CNS nerve conduction.

Pathology

Gross

- Marked atrophy

Microscopic

- Virtually a total absence of myelin with diminished oligodendroglia
- A "tigroid" pattern may be seen where islands of myelin are separated by areas of no stainable myelin

Imaging Findings

CT

- Low density in the white matter
- Progressive white matter atrophy

MR

- Generalized lack of myelination
- On T1-WI, high-signal intensity may be seen only in the internal capsules, optic radiations, and proximal corona radiata
- The supratentorial white matter shows diffuse high signal on T2-WI
- Proton MR spectroscopy has not shown significant differences in levels of N-acetyl aspartate (NAA), creatine, and choline as compared with normal controls

Treatment

None

Prognosis

Death usually occurs in adolescence or young adulthood

Suggested Readings

Takanashi J, Sugita K, Osaka H, Ishii M, Niimi H. Proton MR spectroscopy in Pelizaeus-Merzbacher disease. *AJNR* 18: 533–535, 1997.

van der Knaap MS, Valk J. The reflection of histology in MR imaging of Pelizaeus-Merzbacher disease. *AJNR* 10:99–103, 1989.

Wang PJ, Hwu WL, Lee WT, Wang TR, Shen YZ. Duplication of the proteolipid protein gene: a possible major cause of Pelizaeus-Merzbacher disease. *Pediatr Neurol* 17:125–125, 1997.

Case 98

Clinical Presentation

A 16-month-old child with developmental delay and a seizure disorder presents with severe lethargy several days after the onset of an upper respiratory infection.

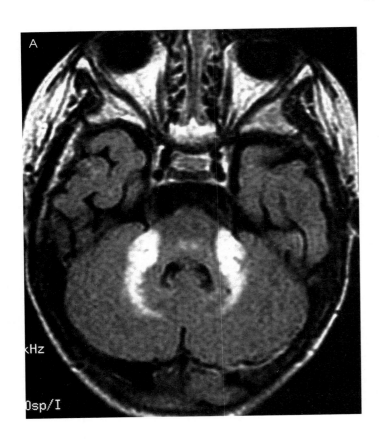

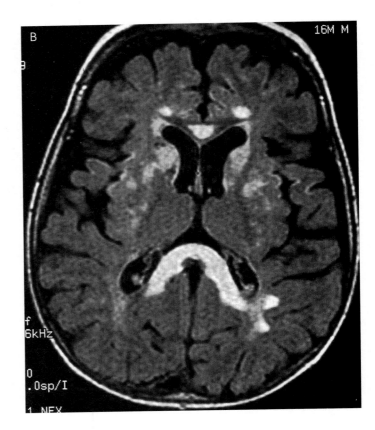

Radiologic Findings

An axial fluid-attenuated inversion recovery (FLAIR) image (Fig. A) through the posterior fossa demonstrates abnormal high signal within the middle cerebellar peduncles bilaterally. There is a suggestion of abnormal hyperintensity in the mid-pons as well. An axial FLAIR image at a more cephalad level (Fig. B) demonstrates multifocal areas of T2 prolongation in the caudate nuclei and putamina bilaterally, as well as strikingly abnormal signal in the genu and splenium of the corpus callosum.

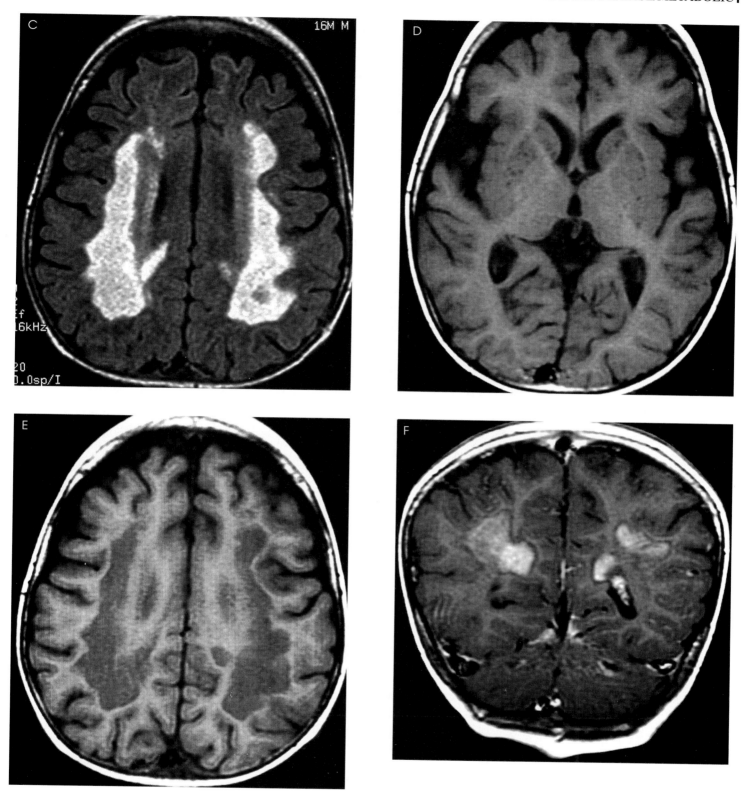

An axial FLAIR image through the hemispheric white matter (Fig. C) demonstrates extensive abnormal confluent T2 high signal in the white matter bilaterally, without significant mass effect. An axial T1-WI through the basal ganglia (Fig. D) demonstrates multiple punctate hypointensities in the caudate nuclei and putamina bilaterally. An axial T1-WI (Fig. E) through the hemispheric white matter shows abnormal hypointensity in the areas that were bright on the FLAIR image. Again, note the relative lack of mass effect. Also note that the sulci are globally prominent in this 16-month-old child. A coronal post-gadolinium T1-WI (Fig. F) demonstrates abnormal enhancement within the affected areas of white matter. The basal ganglia lesions were nonenhancing (not shown) and were felt to represent areas of more remote injury.

Diagnosis

Organic acidopathy [multiple acyl-CoA dehydrogenase deficiency (MACDD), also known as glutaric aciduria type II]

Differential Diagnosis

• Other inborn error of metabolism (diagnosis made by clinical history and laboratory analysis)
• Toxic ingestion (clinical history, laboratory data)
• Viral encephalitis (often more patchy and asymmetric, often cortical gray matter involvement, acute onset, may be febrile or have associated meningeal signs)
• Demyelinating disease such as acute disseminated encephalomyelitis (typically patchy and asymmetric, often involves subcortical U fibers, usually a monophasic illness and so would not explain areas of recent and remote injury)

Discussion

Background

The organic acidopathies constitute a diverse group of metabolic disorders that may have serious harmful effects on the CNS and may affect both gray and white matter to variable degrees. The term "organic acid" includes fatty acids and ketoacids, with the amino acidopathies generally being considered separately. Dozens of organic acidopathies have been distinguished; the specific diagnosis of any one of these disorders rests on laboratory analysis. As an example, MACDD is a disorder of mitochondrial fatty acid oxidation, a complex process that plays a major role in energy production, particularly during periods of fasting. MACDD is characterized clinically by hypoketotic or nonketotic hypoglycemia and metabolic acidosis. It is characterized biochemically by the accumulation in the urine, serum, and CSF of metabolites of compounds oxidized by the electron transfer flavoprotein system. Most organic acidopathies present during infancy, but the age at presentation and the clinical phenotype depend on the nature and severity of the underlying metabolic defect. Acute exacerbations ("crises") are commonly superimposed upon a baseline of developmental delay. In families at risk for certain organic acidemias, prenatal diagnosis can be made based on amniotic fluid levels of organic acids.

Etiology

Organic acidopathies typically show autosomal recessive inheritance. MACDD has been related to deficiency of either electron transfer flavoprotein (ETF) or an enzyme that transfers electrons to ETF, electron transfer flavoprotein-ubiquinone oxidoreductase.

Clinical Findings

Organic acidopathies typically present with either recurrent attacks of acidotic coma or progressive encephalopathy. Such episodes may be triggered by an infection, vomiting, excessive protein intake, or fasting. Developmental delay, hypotonia or hypertonia, and seizures are common. Laboratory tests show variable hypoglycemia, hyperammonemia, hypoketonemia, carnitine deficiency, and severe metabolic acidosis, often with an anion gap. These findings may be intermittent and present only during acute episodes. Evaluation of the urine consistently demonstrates elevated organic acids, with the pattern of urinary excretion related to the specific enzyme defect(s) present.

Pathophysiology

Elevated concentrations of either normal or abnormal compounds accumulate in the intra- and/or extracellular spaces, leading to neuronal and/or glial injury.

Imaging Findings

CT

- Widening of CSF spaces
- Areas of hypodensity in the deep gray nuclei and white matter

MR

- Between attacks (chronic phase), findings include widening of CSF spaces, open opercula, and punctate foci of T1 hypointensity and T2 hyperintensity in caudate and/or lentiform nuclei. Delayed myelination is frequent.
- During attack (acute phase), findings include swollen basal ganglia. White matter and cortex show areas of T1 hypointensity and T2 hyperintensity of variable severity. Contrast enhancement may be seen.

Treatment

- Avoidance of fasting
- High carbohydrate, low fat diet
- Supplementation with riboflavin and carnitine may be useful

Prognosis

Prognosis is improved by early diagnosis and prompt institution of dietary therapy

Suggested Readings

Bhala A, Willi SM, Rinaldo P, et al. Clinical and biochemical characterization of short-chain acyl-coenzyme A dehydrogenase deficiency. *J Pediatr* 126:910–915, 1995.

Brismar J, Ozand PT. CT and MR of the brain in the diagnosis of organic acidemias. Experiences from 107 patients. *Brain Dev* 16:104–124, 1994.

Stigsby B, Yarworth SM, Rahbeeni Z, et al. Neurophysiologic correlates of organic acidemias: a survey of 107 patients. *Brain Dev* 16:125–144, 1994.

Section VI

Non-Infectious
Inflammatory/Idiopathic

Case 99

Clinical Presentation

Six months prior to presentation, this 13-year-old girl developed fatigue and weight loss. She then presented with a generalized seizure and lapsed into coma for 3 days. Upon awakening, she was disoriented and inappropriate. An MR scan was obtained.

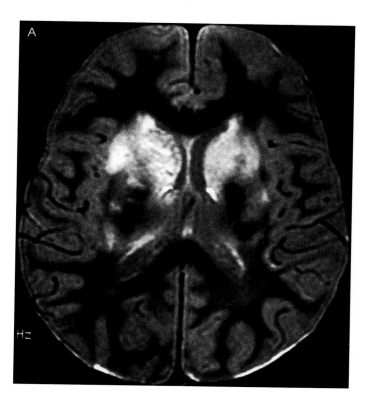

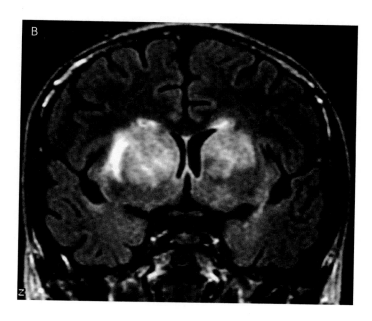

Radiologic Findings

An axial proton density-weighted image (Fig. A) and a coronal FLAIR image (Fig. B) demonstrate extensive patchy T2 prolongation involving the caudate nuclei and putamina bilaterally, as well as the internal capsules.

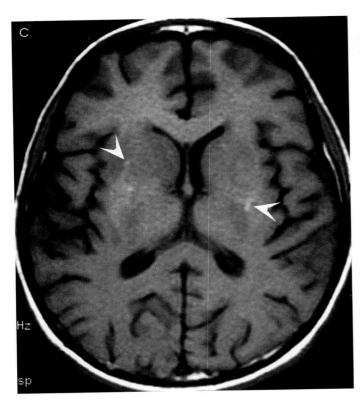

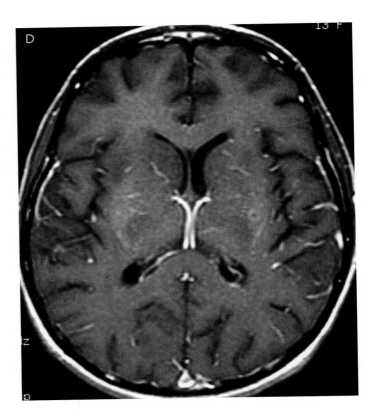

An axial T1-WI (Fig. C) shows mild hypointensity in the affected regions. There is minimal if any mass effect associated with the process. A few small foci of T1 shortening (*arrowheads*) likely represent small hemorrhages. Post-gadolinium (Fig. D), a T-1WI shows slightly prominent enhancement of the lenticulostriate vessels, but no focal areas of parenchymal enhancement are appreciated.

Diagnosis

Cerebritis secondary to systemic lupus erythematosus (SLE)

Differential Diagnosis

- Vasculitis (true vasculitis is rare in SLE, but the imaging findings may be identical)
- Encephalitis (viral infection could mimic this imaging picture)
- Acute disseminated encephalomyelitis (generally multifocal, patchy and asymmetric lesions)
- Extrapontine myelinolysis (requires an appropriate clinical context, often associated with central pontine myelinolysis)

Discussion

Background

SLE is a condition of unknown cause that has multisystem effects. It has an annual incidence of 50 to 70 cases per million, with the highest incidence in women aged 20 to 40 years. CNS involvement is frequent in patients with SLE, with a prevalence of overt neuropsychiatric symptoms ranging from 10 to 70% in multiple studies, and with the incidence of CNS involvement higher in females than in males. This wide range may be due to the fact that clinical manifestations may be transient and reversible, and that it is often difficult to distinguish a primary involvement of the CNS from secondary disturbances (iatrogenic, infectious, hypertensive, etc.). The peripheral nervous system may be affected as well.

Etiology

SLE is an autoimmune disease characterized by autoantibody production and multisystem involvement.

Clinical Findings

Clinical manifestations are remarkably heterogeneous and affect the heart, lungs, kidneys, and nervous system. Most patients present with constitutional signs, rashes, arthritis, and serositis. Central nervous system manifestations may be diffuse and include organic brain syndromes (cognitive dysfunction, dementia), psychosis, seizures, headache, and pseudotumor cerebri, or may be focal and include strokes, venous thrombosis, cranial neuropathy, and transverse myelitis.

Peripheral nervous system manifestations include peripheral neuropathy (sensory polyneuropathy, mononeuritis multiplex, Guillain-Barré syndrome), autonomic neuropathy, or myasthenia gravis.

In the appropriate clinical context, the diagnosis of SLE is supported by laboratory tests including elevated ANA (antinuclear antibody, sensitive but not specific) and anti-dsDNA (anti-double strand DNA, which is quite specific).

Pathogenetic Mechanisms of Neuropsychiatric Lupus

CNS damage in SLE may be primary or secondary. Primary mechanisms include autoantibody mediated, vaso-occlusive, and cytokine effects. Autoantibody-mediated mechanisms cause the production of antineuronal antibodies. Vaso-occlusive mechansims include immune-complex–mediated vasculitis and/or antiphospholipid antibody-associated hypercoagulability, resulting in vascular thrombosis and/or cardiac emboli. Secondary mechanisms of CNS injury include infection, hypertension, uremia, medication side effects, and electrolyte disturbances.

Pathology

• Pathologic findings are highly variable and may be normal
• Findings include parenchymal volume loss, hemorrhage, infarction, and bland vasculopathy (vascular hyalinization, perivascular inflammation, and endothelial proliferation). True vasculitis is rare.

Imaging Findings

CT

• Useful to detect parenchymal hemorrhages and large vessel infarctions
• Basal ganglia and paraventricular calcifications may be seen
• Global atrophy has been described but may be secondary to corticosteroid therapy

MR

• May be normal in patients with diffuse presentations such as organic brain syndrome, psychosis, and major depression
• Acutely ill patients may have areas of cortical and subcortical edema

- Multiple small high-signal intensity lesions may be seen in the white matter on T2-weighted sequences in the chronic phase of the disease
- Hemorrhages and large vessel infarctions may be seen

Treatment

- Depends upon the clinical presentation
- Steroids are the mainstay of therapy
- Cytotoxic/immunosuppressive agents such as cyclophosphamide, methotrexate, azathioprine, or cyclosporin A may be used
- Plasmapheresis may be employed during acute, severe flares

Prognosis

- The prognosis for CNS lupus is guarded. Although many patients with diffuse symptoms appear to recover, many are left with residual cognitive dysfunction. Status epilepticus, stroke, and coma are particularly poor prognostic signs.
- Complications of drug treatment, particularly corticosteroids, contribute significantly to long-term morbidity

Suggested Readings

Klippel JH. Systemic lupus erythematosus: demographics, prognosis, and outcome. *J Rheumatol* 24: 67–71, 1997.

Steinlin MI, Blaser SI, Gilday DL, et al. Neurologic manifestations of pediatric systemic lupus erythematosus. *Pediatr Neurol* 13:191–197, 1995.

West SG. Neuropsychiatric lupus. *Rheum Dis Clin North Am* 20:129–158, 1994.

Case 100

Clinical Presentation

A 12-year-old boy who had previously undergone biopsy of a calvarial lesion presents with ataxia and multiple cranial nerve palsies.

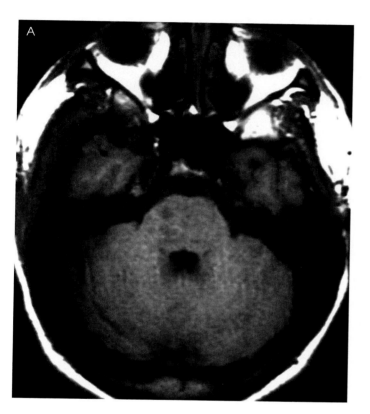

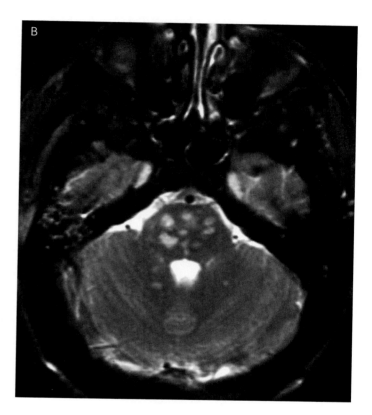

Radiologic Findings

An axial T1-WI (Fig. A) shows subtle patchy hypointensity within the pons. The right temporalis muscle is slightly thickened, related to recent biopsy. An axial T2-WI (Fig. B) demonstrates multiple rounded foci of T2 prolongation within the substance of the pons and also the anteromedial cerebellum. Fluid in the right mastoid air cells presumably is postoperative in nature.

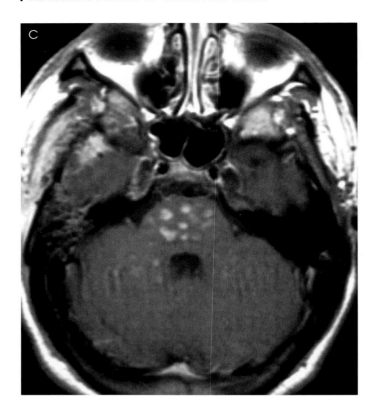

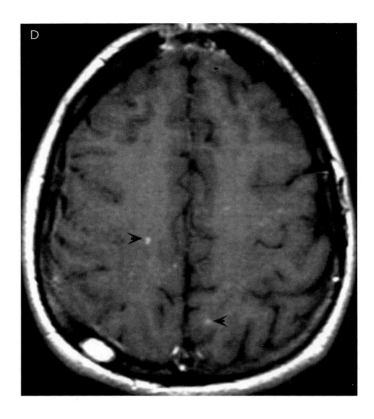

Pearls

- A sharply marginated, homogeneously enhancing lytic lesion of the calvarium or skull base in a child should raise the question of LCH.

- In patients with LCH and DI, the high signal of the posterior pituitary is typically absent.

- In some patients with dural involvement by LCH, the soft tissue masses may be strikingly hypointense on T2-WI.

Pitfalls

- In the absence of typical skeletal lesions, LCH can only be suggested as part of a differential diagnosis as there are no pathognomonic features.

- Germ cell tumors of the hypothalamus and pituitary stalk can have an appearance identical to LCH on imaging studies and occur in the same age group.

On a post-gadolinium T1-WI (Fig. C), the pontine and cerebellar lesions demonstrate homogeneous enhancement. A focus of enhancement at the anterior aspect of the right middle cranial fossa represents the recent biopsy site. A contrast-enhanced T1-WI at a more cephalad level (Fig. D) shows multiple subtle punctate foci of parenchymal enhancement (*arrowheads*), as well as an intensely enhancing lesion in the right parietal bone. Mild dural enhancement and a destructive calvarial lesion are present anteriorly.

Diagnosis

Langerhans' cell histiocytosis (LCH)

Differential Diagnosis

- Metastatic disease (the lack of a known primary and the patient's young age would argue against this)
- Infection (edema usually more prominent around lesions, patient would be expected to be sicker with disseminated CNS infection)
- Demyelinating disease (often a periventricular predominance, would not account for calvarial lesions)
- Sarcoidosis (usually adult patient, often associated with leptomeningeal and/or dural disease, bone lesions are uncommon)

Discussion

Background

LCH, formerly known as histiocytosis X, is a systemic disease with several modes of presentation ranging from the mild solitary eosinophilic granuloma of bone to

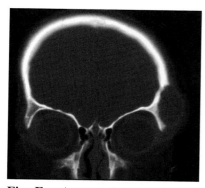

Fig. E. A coronal image from a non-contrast CT scan photographed in bone window shows a destructive lesion of the left frontal bone, with an associated soft tissue mass.

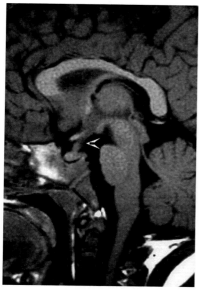

Fig. F. A sagittal T1-WI shows abnormal thickening of the pituitary stalk (*arrowhead*). Note also the absence of the posterior pituitary bright spot. Major differential considerations included LCH versus germinoma. Biopsy confirmed LCH in this 10-year-old male with diabetes insipidus.

Table 1. Organ System Involvement by LCH During the Course of Disease

Bone	80%
Skin	45%
Liver, spleen	35%
Lymphatic system	35%
Hematopoietic	30%
CNS	10-50%
Pulmonary	25%
Orbital	25%
Otologic	20%
Dental	20%

more severe forms with disseminated granulomata in bones and soft tissue. The severe forms include Hand-Schuller-Christian disease and Letterer-Siwe disease (see below). LCH typically appears during the first decade of life, with an estimated incidence of 0.05 to 0.5 cases per 100,000 children per year. Males are more commonly affected than females, and it is rare in African-Americans. CNS manifestations occur in 10 to 50% of cases and occur most frequently with multisystem disease (Table 1); only rarely do patients present initially or solely with CNS disease. Common sites of CNS disease include the skull (especially the temporal bones and orbit), the bony spinal column, and the hypothalamus and pituitary infundibulum. Less common sites include the dura, cerebral and cerebellar parenchyma, optic chiasm, and spinal cord. Rarely, LCH may present as an isolated hemispheric mass.

Etiology

The etiology is unknown. The common pathologic element in LCH is proliferation of an antigen-presenting dendritic cell of bone marrow origin. Although LCH is typically treated as a neoplasm, it is unlikely that it is a true neoplastic process; it is most likely to be due to dysfunction of the immune system.

Clinical Findings

Symptoms of CNS involvement vary with the site(s) of disease:

Diabetes insipidus is common in patients with hypothalamic/infundibular involvement. DI occurs in 5% of cases at the time of original diagnosis, and up to one third of cases on follow-up evaluation.

Calvarial lesions come to attention as a mass. Temporal bone lesions may lead to hearing loss and a chronically draining ear. Orbital lesions frequently present with proptosis.

Dural involvement may lead to headache, while the presentation of brain parenchymal lesions varies with their location. Dysmetria and ataxia are common with cerebellar involvement.

Complications

Systemic manifestations include hematopoietic, hepatic, and pulmonary dysfunction. Hand-Christian-Schuller disease (15% of LCH cases) usually affects children 1 to 5 years of age and is classically described as the triad of DI, exophthalmos, and destructive bone lesions. Letterer-Siwe disease (10% of LCH cases) is the acute disseminated form of LCH, usually occurs in patients less than

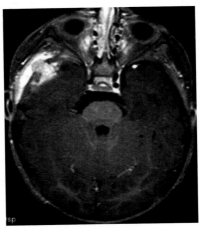

Fig. G. A post-gadolinium T1-WI with fat saturation demonstrates an enhancing lesion centered in the right greater wing of the sphenoid, with extension into the scalp soft tissues and epidural space, in a patient with known LCH.

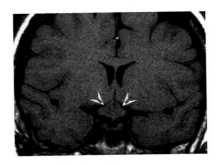

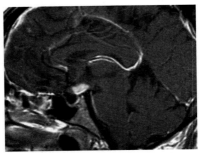

Figs. H and I. A coronal T1-WI (Fig. H) shows a mass involving the hypothalamus and optic chiasm (*arrowheads*). On a post-gadolinium T1-WI (Fig. I), this mass shows intense and homogenous enhancement. Biopsy confirmed LCH.

2 years of age, and presents with fever, anemia, thrombocytopenia, hepatosplenomegaly, and a skin rash.

Pathology

Gross

- Rubbery, soft masses

Microscopic

- CNS granulomata begin as periadventitial infiltrates around small blood vessels and are composed of Langerhans' histiocytes, microglial cells, fibrillary astrocytes, and inflammatory cells (plasma cells, leukocytes). A pathognomonic finding by electron microscopy is the presence of Birbeck granules, a unique organelle of the Langerhans cell.
- Brain parenchymal lesions may simply show demyelination and gliosis

Imaging Findings

CT

- Lytic lesions of calvarium (Fig. E) and/or temporal bones
- Significantly less sensitive to dural and parenchymal disease than is MR

MR

Findings may include:

- Infiltration of the pituitary stalk by enhancing soft tissue and absence of the posterior pituitary bright spot (Fig. F)
- Destructive lesions of calvarium and/or temporal bones (Fig. G)
- A focal mass in the hypothalamus and/or optic chiasm (Figs. H and I)
- Parenchymal lesions in the cerebral hemispheres, brainstem, and/or cerebellum (most common parenchymal site). These lesions are typically small nodules that are isointense on T1-WI, iso- or mildly hyperintense on T2-WI, and enhance post-gadolinium, although nonenhancing parenchymal lesions have also been described.
- Nodular thickening of the dura and/or leptomeninges

Treatment

- Surgery to relieve mass effect acutely or for isolated bone lesions. Some would also favor complete microsurgical excision of certain CNS lesions such as hypothalamic granulomas.
- Radiation therapy
- Chemotherapy

Prognosis

- In general, the younger the patient at presentation and the greater the extent of disease, the worse the prognosis
- Overall, estimated survival rates at 5, 10, and 15 years are 88%, 88%, and 77%, respectively, with an estimated event-free survival rate of only 30% at 15 years

Suggested Readings

Grois N, Barkovich AJ, Rosenau W, Ablin AR. Central nervous system disease associated with Langerhans cell histiocytosis. *Am J Pediatr Hematol Oncol* 15:245–254, 1993.

Maghnie M, Arico M, Villa A, et al. MR of the hypothalamic-pituitary axis in Langerhans cell histiocytosis. *AJNR* 13:1365–1371, 1992.

Poe LB, Dubowy RL, Hochhauser L, et al. Demyelinating and gliotic cerebellar lesions in Langerhans cell histiocytosis. *AJNR* 15:1921–1928, 1994.

Case 101

Clinical Presentation

A 45-year-old woman status post-bone marrow transplant has been suffering from severe mucositis, diarrhea, and malnutrition. She becomes delirious and rapidly progresses to coma.

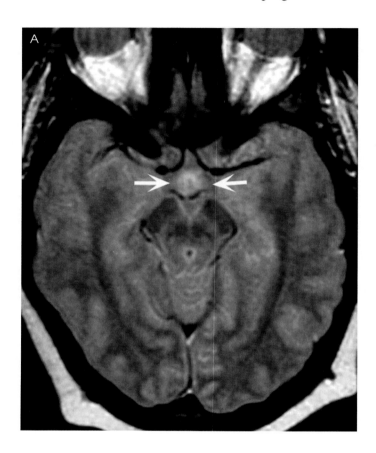
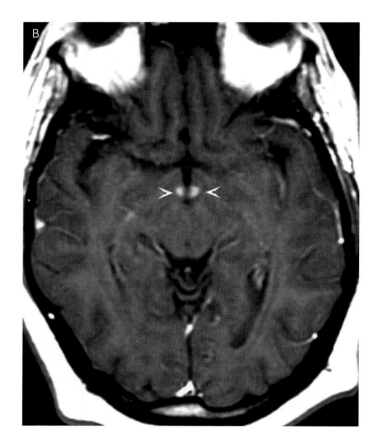

Radiologic Findings

A proton density-weighted image (Fig. A) demonstrates mild questionable hyperintensity in the region of inferior hypothalamus and mamillary bodies (*arrows*). On an axial post-gadolinium T1-WI (Fig. B), there is focal enhancement within the mamillary bodies (*arrowheads*).

Pearls

- MR is more sensitive than CT to the characteristic changes of WE and may play a critical role when the diagnosis is not suspected. In particular, contrast enhancement of the mamillary bodies is very suggestive of this diagnosis.

- The thalamic involvement usually affects the dorsal medial nuclei.

- Follow-up scans generally show improvement or resolution of lesions, although the mamillary bodies may be left severely atrophic (Fig. D)

Pitfalls

- Wernicke's syndrome is not confined to the chronic alcoholic population; other settings in which WE has been described include hyperemesis gravidarum, small bowel obstruction, anorexia nervosa, and prolonged voluntary starvation.

- This diagnosis may be missed on MR if contrast is not given.

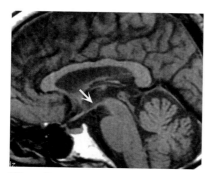

Fig. D. Sagittal T1-WI in a chronic alcoholic with a history of WE shows striking atrophy of the mamillary body (*arrow*).

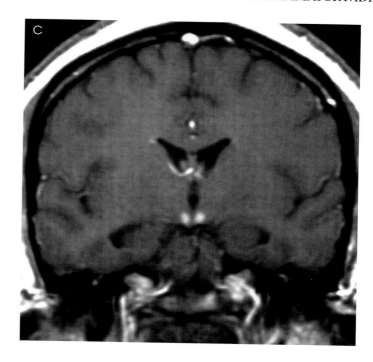

A coronal post-gadolinium T1-WI (Fig. C) shows abnormal enhancement in the inferior hypothalamus.

Diagnosis

Wernicke's encephalopathy (WE)

Differential Diagnosis

None: the symmetric and characteristic distribution of the lesions permits differentiation from other processes.

Discussion

Background

WE is caused by a severe nutritional deprivation of thiamine. It is usually observed as a neurologic complication of chronic alcoholism, but it is not confined to this population. As evidenced in this case, severe malnutrition may also lead to WE. Lesions typically occur in the mesencephalon and diencephalon, and patients experience alterations in consciousness as well as focal neurologic symptoms. The classic triad described by Wernicke included ophthalmoplegia, ataxia, and mental confusion, but this is observed in only one third of patients. Korsakoff's psychosis is an amnestic syndrome that often follows WE, emerging as the other mental symptoms of WE respond to treatment.

Etiology

WE is caused by severe thiamine (vitamin B1) deficiency.

Clinical Findings

Typical symptoms includes headache, vomiting, confusion, lethargy, and ataxia. Abducens and conjugate gaze palsies and nystagmus are also common.

Pathogenesis

The pathogenesis is poorly understood, but thiamine-deficient membranes are unable to maintain osmotic gradients, resulting in cellular swelling and damage.

Pathology

Gross

- Atrophy of mamillary bodies, vermis, and the cerebrum in the chronic phase

Microscopic

- Early: marked intracellular edema with swelling of astrocytes, oligodendrocytes, myelin sheath, and neuronal dendrites
- Late: demyelination, capillary proliferation, and astrocytic and microglial proliferation; tissue necrosis may occur
- Hemorrhage, usually petechial, is found in 20% of cases and is probably agonal as it is not usually demonstrated on imaging studies

Imaging Findings

CT

- Often normal
- May show hypodense nonenhancing lesions around the aqueduct and in the dorsal medial thalamus

MR

- Symmetric T2 prolongation may be seen in the periaqueductal gray matter, the mamillary bodies, the paraventricular regions of the thalamus and hypothalamus, and/or the floor of the fourth ventricle
- Post-gadolinium, these areas may enhance
- Hemorrhage is rarely observed on imaging studies

Treatment

- Thiamine repletion
- Magnesium is usually replaced as well

Prognosis

- Mortality is 100% in untreated WE and approximately 10% with treatment
- Most symptoms can be reversed partially or completely depending on the duration of symptoms before the institution of therapy

Suggested Readings

Doraiswamy PM, Massey EW, Enright K, Palese VJ, Lamonica D, Boyko O. Wernicke-Korsakoff syndrome caused by psychogenic food refusal: MR findings. *AJNR* 15:594–596, 1994.

Gallucci M, Bozzao A, Splendiani A, Masciocchi C, Passariello R. Wernicke encephalopathy: MR findings in five patients. *AJNR* 11:887–892, 1990.

Shogry MEC, Curnes JT. Mamillary body enhancement on MR as the only sign of acute Wernicke encephalopathy. *AJNR* 15:172–174, 1994.

Case 102

Clinical Presentation

A 25-year-old patient with longstanding partial complex seizures has recently become refractory to medical management and presents for imaging.

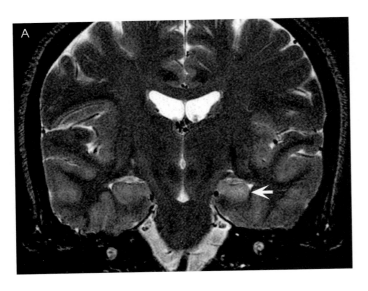

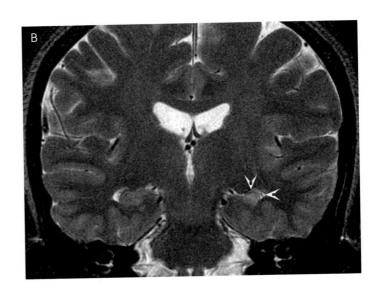

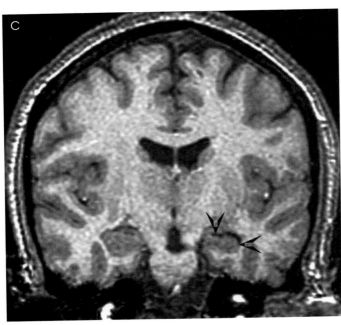

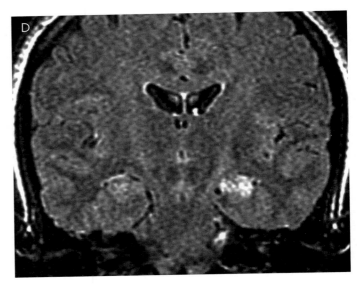

Pearls

- The imaging features of MTS are best appreciated in the coronal plane. Coronal high-resolution fast spin-echo T2-weighted images best demonstrate hippocampal signal abnormalities, while a coronal three-dimensional (3-D) T1-weighted volumetric acquisition such as 3-D SPGR is useful to demonstrate a decrease in size of the hippocampus and atrophy of collateral white matter pathways.

- The most common imaging features of MTS are high signal intensity on T2-WI (80-95%), loss of definition of internal architecture, and atrophy.

- Interictal positron emission tomography with 18F-fluorodeoxyglucose has been shown to demonstrate hypometabolism in mesial temporal sclerosis.

- Proton MR spectroscopy demonstrates relatively low N-acetyl aspartate levels in the temporal lobes of patients with MTS.

- Phosphorous MR spectroscopy shows increased pH (more alkalotic) on the affected side.

Radiologic Findings

A coronal fast spin-echo T2-WI (Fig. A) shows abnormal signal in the head of the left hippocampus (*arrow*). Slightly more posteriorly (Fig. B), another fast spin-echo T2-WI shows the body of the left hippocampus to be abnormally small and hyperintense (*arrowheads*), with poor definition of internal architecture. A thin section coronal SPGR image (Fig. C) confirms the atrophy of the left hippocampus (*arrowheads*). A coronal fluid-attenuated inversion recovery (FLAIR) image (Fig. D) nicely demonstrates striking high signal within the left hippocampus.

Diagnosis

Mesial temporal sclerosis (MTS)

Differential Diagnosis

- Infiltrating glioma of medial temporal lobe (mass effect rather than volume loss)
- Viral encephalitis (acute history, hippocampal enlargement and often enhancement)
- Post-ictal changes in hippocampus (often bilateral, expect hippocampal swelling rather than volume loss, though long-term follow-up may show changes consistent with MTS)
- Cortical dysplasia involving medial temporal lobe (often involves more than just hippocampus and amygdala, not necessarily associated with hippocampal volume loss)

Discussion

Background

Epilepsy is characterized by chronic seizures. In the United States, there are over 1 million people with epilepsy. Seizures are usually described as generalized or partial (Table 1), with the latter believed to originate focally within the brain. Partial seizures are more common, accounting for approximately 65% of all seizures. A particular subset of partial seizures is the complex partial seizure, defined as an alteration of consciousness accompanying a seizure that has focal

Table 1. Classification of Seizure Subtypes

Partial or focal seizures
    Simple partial seizures (consciousness not impaired)
    Complex partial seizures (consciousness is impaired)
        Simple partial onset followed by impaired consciousness
        Impairment of consciousness at seizure onset (rare)
        With automatisms
    Partial seizures evolving to secondary generalization

Generalized seizures of nonfocal origin (convulsive or nonconvulsive, loss of consciousness occurs at onset)
    Absence seizures
    Myoclonic seizures
    Tonic-clonic seizures
    Tonic seizures
    Atonic seizures

Unclassified seizures

Pitfalls

- Normal hippocampi appear mildly hyperintense on fast FLAIR imaging.
- MTS may be bilateral and symmetric or asymmetric in up to 20% of patients (Fig. E).
- Dual pathology (i.e., MTS and a small tumor, heterotopion, or cryptic vascular malformation) may be present, so look for additional lesions.
- A choroid fissure cyst or enlarged temporal horn may distort and compress the hippocampus, making morphological assessment more difficult.

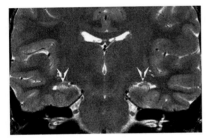

Fig. E. A coronal fast spin-echo T2-WI shows that the hippocampi (*arrowheads*) are small and hyperintense bilaterally, consistent with bilateral MTS.

onset. Approximately 70% of complex partial seizures have their origin in the temporal lobe, and a number of these patients become refractory to medical therapy. Mesial temporal sclerosis is the most common pathologic entity associated with refractory temporal lobe epilepsy, being described as the cause (or the end result) of complex partial seizures in as many as 60 to 80% of cases. Because temporal lobectomy is an effective treatment for MTS refractory to medical management, much attention has been directed at the detection of MTS in order to appropriately guide surgical resection. MTS is uncommonly detected before age 10, but most patients with MTS will have a history of early seizures.

Etiology

It is unclear whether MTS is a primary cause of seizures or a consequence of other events that then becomes a cause of seizures. It has been postulated that MTS may be related to febrile convulsions during childhood, status epilepticus, and/or complicated delivery. Presumably these situations induce metabolic disturbances in the hippocampal neurons, which disappear and are replaced by gliosis.

Clinical Findings

Partial seizures have a focal onset, and the first component is often an aura that may be visual, auditory, or olfactory. This may be followed by a period of behavioral change and altered consciousness (complex partial seizure), during which the patient may perform repetitive or stereotypical acts and is unaware of his surroundings. Secondary generalization of the seizure may occur, with tonic-clonic movements and loss of consciousness.

Pathology

Gross

- Shrunken hippocampus +/– amygdala

Microscopic

- Decrease in the number of neurons in the hippocampus, with concomitant gliosis
- In some cases, there may be loss of as few as 50 neurons in the enfolium (area CA4 of the hippocampus)
- In most cases, areas CA1 and CA3 of the hippocampus are prominently affected, while CA2 is spared until late in the process
- White matter in the ipsilateral temporal lobe may show oligodendroglial cell clusters and perivascular macrophages

Imaging Findings

CT

- Typically normal unless mesial temporal volume loss is severe

MR

- Features in approximate descending order of frequency include:
  1. High-signal intensity in the hippocampus on T2-WI
  2. Hippocampal volume loss
  3. Ipsilateral atrophy of the hippocampal collateral white matter
  4. Enlarged temporal horn (very nonspecific)

5. Reduced gray-white matter demarcation in the temporal lobe
6. Decreased temporal lobe size

- Ipsilateral atrophy of the fornix has been described with MTS, but this is relatively infrequent and is generally associated with severe hippocampal atrophy
- Ipsilateral atrophy of the mamillary body has also been described and is uncommon
- Mass effect and enhancement are not features of MTS

Treatment

- Medical management
- Surgical resection of mesial temporal structures in appropriate candidates who have medically refractory seizures

Prognosis

- Approximately two thirds of patients with medically refractory MTS become seizure-free following surgical resection. Reasons for failure include incomplete resection, bilateral MTS, "dual pathologies" overlooked on preoperative imaging, or extrahippocampal abnormalities that are not visualizable with current neuroimaging techniques.
- As many as 95% of patients with unilateral MTS by electroencephalogram and MR imaging are seizure-free after surgery

Suggested Readings

Bronen RA, Fulbright RK, Spencer DD, et al. Refractory epilepsy: comparison of MR imaging, CT, and histopathologic findings in 117 patients. *Radiology* 201:97–105, 1996.

Garcia PA, Laxer KD, Barbaro NM, Dillon WP. Prognostic value of qualitative magnetic resonance imaging of hippocampal abnormalities in patients undergoing temporal lobectomy for medically refractory seizures. *Epilepsia* 35:520–524, 1994.

Meiners LC, van Gils A, Jansen GH, et al. Temporal lobe epilepsy: the various MR appearances of histologically proven medial temporal sclerosis. *AJNR* 15:1547–1555, 1994.

Section VII

Neurodegenerative/Basal Ganglia Disorders

Case 103

Clinical Presentation

A 49-year-old male presents with lower extremity weakness. On examination he has hyperreflexia as well as fasciculations of his tongue.

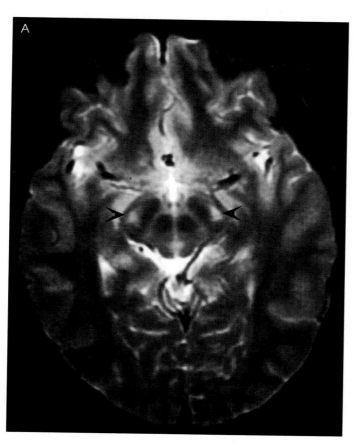

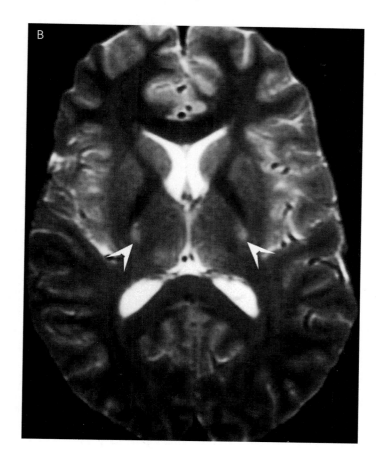

Radiologic Findings

Axial T2-WIs at the level of the cerebral peduncles (Fig. A), and internal capsules (Fig. B) show abnormal high signal intensity in the expected location of the corticospinal tracts (*arrowheads*).

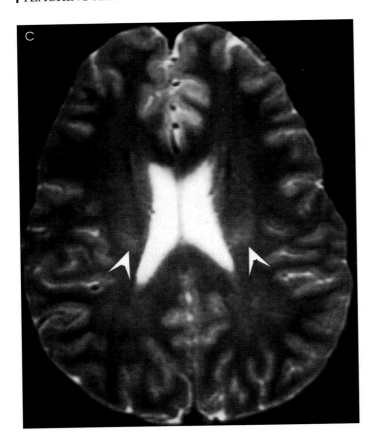

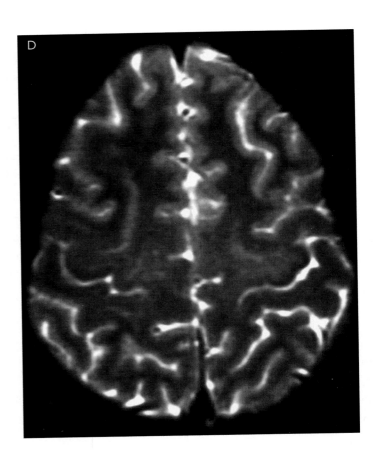

In the corona radiata (Fig. C) (*arrowheads*) and central sulcus (Fig. D) there is also abnormal T2 prolongation along the course of the corticospinal tracts (*arrowheads*). T1-WIs were normal, and no enhancement was appreciated on post-gadolinium images (not shown).

Diagnosis

Amyotrophic lateral sclerosis (ALS)

Differential Diagnosis

- HIV encephalopathy (usually involves the white matter more diffusely)
- Adrenomyeloneuropathy (often prominent involvement of the spinal cord associated with adrenal dysfunction/insufficiency)

Discussion

Background

ALS is a progressive neurodegenerative illness with a prevalence of approximately 5 cases per 100,000 people. Despite this low prevalence, it is the most common form of motor neuron disease. It is usually a sporadic disease with male predominance that typically has its onset between the ages of 50 and 70 years. Three subtypes are described: the classic form in which both upper and lower motor neurons are affected, the upper motor neuron type in which only central motor neurons are affected, and the lower motor type in which only peripheral (anterior horn) neurons are affected.

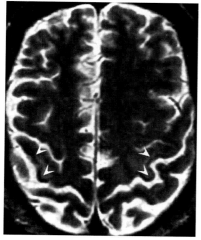

Fig E. An axial T2-WI in a patient with ALS demonstrates striking hypointensity in the motor cortex (*arrowheads*).

Etiology

The etiology is unknown. However, about 5 to 10% of cases are familial with an autosomal dominant pattern of inheritance, and 20% of these cases map to chromosome 21 at the site of the gene for superoxide dismutase, suggesting a role for free radicals in the pathogenesis of this disease.

Clinical Findings

The diagnosis of classic ALS is made by clinical and electromyographic examination. Clinically the diagnosis is established by the presence of both lower motor neuron dysfunction (weakness, wasting, fasciculation) and upper motor neuron dysfunction (hyperactive tendon reflexes, clonus, Babinski sign). Bulbar signs (dysarthria, difficulty swallowing) are also common.

Complications

Respiratory failure and recurrent aspiration are common problems as the disease progresses.

Pathology

Gross

- Usually normal, although long-surviving patients may demonstrate atrophy of the precentral gyrus

Microscopic

- Loss of cortical pyramidal and Betz cells, which is most apparent in the motor cortex
- Neuronal loss in the motor nuclei of cranial nerves, especially V, VII and XII
- Loss of neurons in the anterior horns of the spinal cord

Imaging Findings

CT

- Usually normal

MR

- The corticospinal tracts may demonstrate areas of T2 prolongation, presumably representing Wallerian degeneration, which are best seen at the level of the middle or lower internal capsule
- Low-signal intensity may be identified within the motor cortex (Fig. E)

Treatment

Supportive care

Prognosis

Relentless and progressive course, with death usually resulting from pneumonia or respiratory failure after 3 to 6 years

Suggested Readings

Cheung G, Gawal MJ, Cooper PW, Farb RI, Ang LC. Amyotrophic lateral sclerosis: correlation of clinical and MR imaging findings. *Radiology* 194:263–270, 1995.

Goodin DS, Rowley HA, Olney RK. Magnetic resonance imaging in amyotrophic lateral sclerosis. *Ann Neurol* 23:418–420, 1988.

Oba H, Araki T, Ohtomo K, et al. Amyotrophic lateral sclerosis: T2 shortening in motor cortex at MR imaging. *Radiology* 189:834–846, 1993.

Case 104

Clinical Presentation

A 70-year-old female presents with rapidly progressive memory loss and extrapyramidal symptoms.

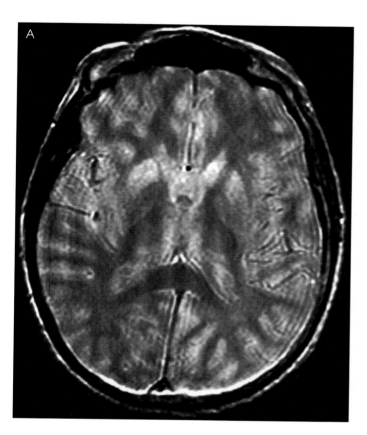

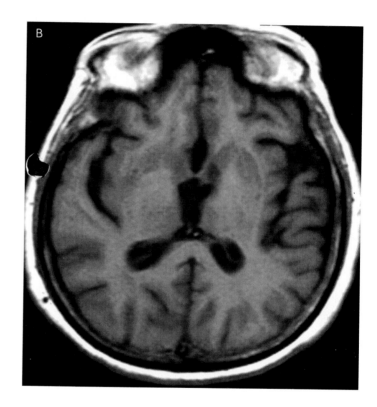

Radiologic Findings

A proton density-weighted image (Fig. A) demonstrates abnormal hyperintensity within the caudate nuclei and putamina bilaterally, as well as in the pulvinar of the thalami bilaterally. An axial T1-WI (Fig. B) shows slight hypointensity within the putamina and caudate heads bilaterally.

Diagnosis

Creutzfeldt-Jakob disease (CJD)

Differential Diagnosis

- Hypoxic-ischemic insult (often involves thalami prominently)
- Toxic exposure (appropriate history, may see globus pallidus necrosis)
- Metabolic dysfunction (metabolic errors usually present in younger patient)

- Wilson's disease (other clinical findings such as Kayser-Fleischer rings)
- Osmotic myelinolysis (pons and subcortical white matter may be affected, history of electrolyte imbalance)
- Encephalitis (associated with fever and meningeal signs, not usually limited to the deep gray nuclei)

Discussion

Background

CJD is a rare transmissible illness that usually affects older adults. Worldwide there is an annual incidence of 1 case per million persons. This disease is usually fatal within 1 year of symptom onset. Most cases are sporadic, but 10 to 15% of cases are familial. CJD has been associated with the injection of non-recombinant human growth hormone, corneal transplantation, and implantation of cerebral electrodes.

Etiology

CJD is considered a transmissible spongiform encephalopathy, and the causative agent is a transmissible infectious particle called a "prion." The human prion protein is encoded on the short arm of chromosome 20. It exists in two isoforms: a normal cellular form, and a form that differs only in physical characteristics (the protein undergoes a post-translational conformational change) and is found in prion diseases. The prion does not evoke an immune response during infection.

Clinical Findings

Patients generally present with rapidly progressive dementia. Ataxia and myoclonus, pyramidal and extrapyramidal signs, and akinetic mutism are common as well. The diagnosis may be assisted by characteristic EEG findings: periodic sharp wave complexes.

Pathology

Gross

- Severe cerebral atrophy

Microscopic

- Characteristic spongiform degeneration that involves gray matter
- Individual and clustered vacuoles in neuronal and glial processes
- Late: gross neuronal loss, marked fibrillary gliosis without inflammation

Imaging Findings

CT

- Often normal early on
- Cortical and deep gray nuclear atrophy are present in later stages

MR

- Moderate to marked T2 prolongation is present in the putamina and caudate nuclei. The thalami and globi pallidi may also be affected

- T1-WIs are usually normal except for parenchymal atrophy, although there may be mild hypointensity in the putamina and caudate nuclei. Progressive cerebral atrophy varies with the duration of disease.
- No enhancement post-gadolinium

Treatment

None

Prognosis

Poor, usually fatal within 1 year of symptom onset

Suggested Readings

Barboriak DP, Provenzale JM, Boyko OB. MR diagnosis of Creutzfeldt-Jakob disease: significance of high-signal intensity of the basal ganglia. *AJR* 162:137–140, 1994.

Finkenstaedt M, Szudra A, Zerr I, et al. MR imaging of Creutzfeldt-Jakob disease. *Radiology* 199:793–798, 1996.

Kovanen J, Erkinjuntti T, Iivanainen M, et al. Cerebral MR and CT imaging in Creutzfeldt-Jakob disease. *J Comput Assist Tomogr* 9:125–128, 1985.

Case 105

Clinical Presentation

A 19-year-old boy presents with progressive dystonia, rigidity, and choreoathetosis.

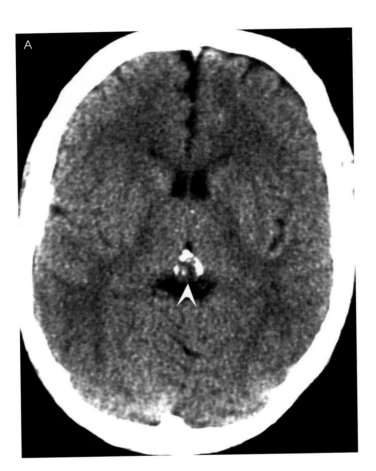

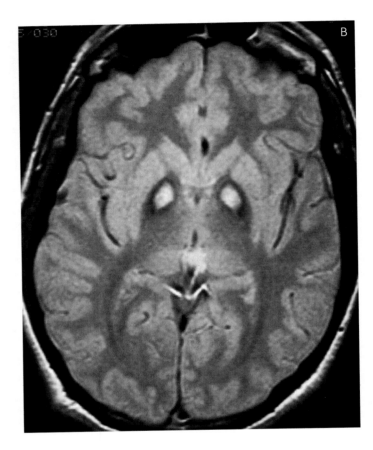

Radiologic Findings

A non-contrast CT scan (Fig. A) is unremarkable except for an incidental pineal cyst with peripheral calcification (*arrowhead*). On an axial proton density-weighted image (Fig. B) and a T2-WI (Fig. C, next page), there is striking high signal within the globi pallidi bilaterally, with surrounding low-signal intensity. This gives the so-called "eye of the tiger" appearance.

Pearl

- Characteristic MR imaging features can strongly support the diagnosis of HSD.

Pitfalls

- When the "eye of the tiger" appearance is not present, the imaging features are nonspecific because preferential deposition of iron occurs within the extrapyramidal nuclei in association with many neurodegenerative disorders.

- The "eye of the tiger" appearance may also be a transient phase which is lost as iron is progressively deposited.

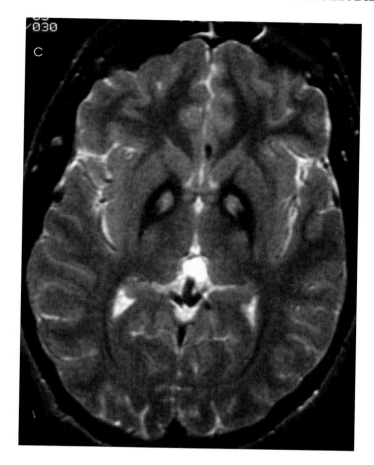

Diagnosis

Hallervorden-Spatz disease (HSD)

Differential Diagnosis

- Carbon monoxide poisoning (clinical history of exposure, often accompanying white matter disease)
- Cyanide poisoning (typically prominent involvement of the cerebellar hemispheres)
- Mineralization of the globi pallidi (CT scan shows increased density in the globi pallidi)

Discussion

Background

HSD is a rare, autosomal recessive, neurodegenerative disorder with accumulation of brain iron as a prominent finding. It typically presents in childhood or early adolescence with motor disturbances. The clinical course is relentless, with progressive dystonic and choreoathetotic movements, dysarthria, gait instability, and dementia. Systemic and CSF iron levels are normal, as are plasma levels of ferritin, transferrin, and ceruloplasmin.

Etiology

The HSD gene has been mapped to the short arm of chromosome 20, but the specific biochemical and genetic abnormalities that underlie HSD remain to be identified.

Clinical Findings

The clinical diagnosis of HSD is made if patients have all the obligatory features, two or more of the corroborative features, and none of the exclusionary features of the syndrome:

- Obligatory features: onset of extrapyramidal dysfunction (dystonia, rigidity, choreoathetosis) during first two decades of life, progressive signs and symptoms
- Corroborative features: corticospinal tract involvement, retinitis pigmentosa and/or optic atrophy, seizures, family history, basal ganglia abnormalities on MRI, and abnormal cytosomes in circulating lymphocytes and/or sea-blue histiocytes in bone marrow
- Exclusionary features: abnormalities of copper metabolism, family history of dominantly inherited movement disorders, and deficiency of β-hexosaminidase A or GM_1-galactosidase

Pathology

Gross

- Rusty brown discoloration of the globus pallidus and substantia nigra

Microscopic

- Massive nonheme iron deposits in the globus pallidus and zona reticulata of substantia nigra
- Loss of myelinated fibers, axonal swelling, and neuronal degeneration in the basal ganglia and corticospinal tracts, and sometimes the cerebellum

Imaging Findings

CT

- Often normal
- May see increased density due to dystrophic calcification in the globi pallidi

MR

- Striking low-signal intensity on T2-WI in the globi pallidi and in the zona reticularis of the substantia nigra
- In some cases, the low signal surrounds a central area of high signal, the so-called "eye of the tiger"

Treatment

None

Prognosis

Relentlessly progressive, leads to death after approximately 15 years

Suggested Readings

Casteels I, Spileers W, Swinnen T, et al. Optic atrophy as the presenting sign in Hallervorden-Spatz syndrome. *Neuropediatrics* 25:265–267, 1994.

Feliciani M, Curatolo P. Early clinical and imaging (high-field MR) diagnosis of Hallervorden-Spatz disease. *Neuroradiology* 36:247–248, 1994.

Porter-Grenn L, Silbergleit R, Mehta BA. Hallervorden-Spatz disease with bilateral involvement of globus pallidus and substantia nigra: MR demonstration. *J Comput Assist Tomogr* 17:961–963, 1993.

Case 106

Clinical Presentation

A 27-year-old man with known cirrhosis presents with worsening tremor and rigidity.

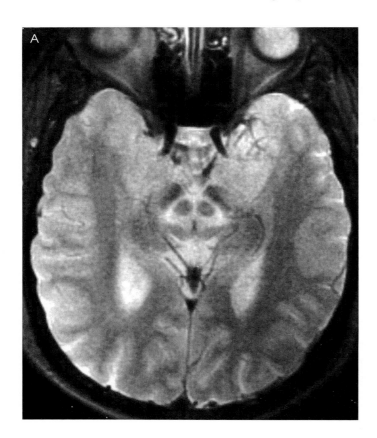
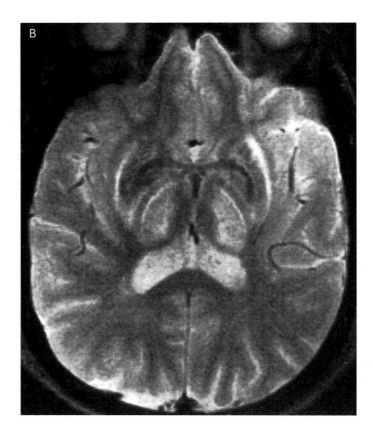

Radiologic Findings

An axial T2-WI (Fig. A) demonstrates abnormal high signal intensity within the midbrain. A more cephalad T2-WI (Fig. B) demonstrates T2 prolongation within the thalami bilaterally, as well as along the external capsules.

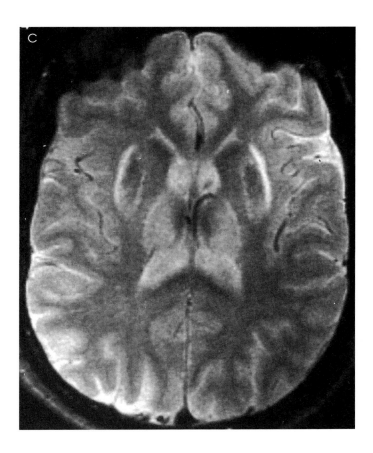

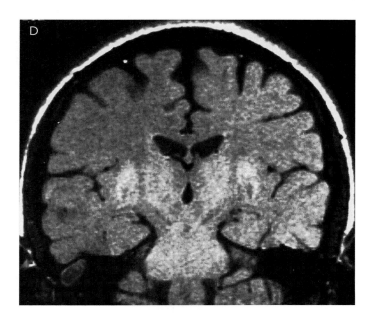

At a higher level, a T2-WI (Fig. C) again demonstrates T2 prolongation within the thalami, as well as along the internal and external capsules. The putamina and caudate nuclei appear mildly hypointense, and the ventricles and sulci are prominent for the patient's age. A coronal T1-WI (Fig. D) shows intrinsic T1 shortening within the thalami and putamina bilaterally, as well as in the brainstem.

Diagnosis

Wilson's disease (WD)

Differential Diagnosis

- Creutzfeldt-Jakob disease (older, dementia is a prominent feature, lack white matter abnormality)
- Hypoxic-ischemic insult (clinical history, may involve thalamus, often involves watershed areas)
- Toxins such as carbon monoxide (globus pallidus necrosis is frequent)
- Viral encephalitis (typically acute onset, often fever and reactive CSF)

Discussion

Background

WD is a rare, autosomal recessive disorder of copper metabolism that is also known as hepatolenticular degeneration. It is characterized by cirrhosis of the liver, basal ganglia degeneration, and corneal Kayser-Fleischer rings. This disorder is usually diagnosed in adolescents or young adults, and the diagnosis is made from clinical, biochemical, and histologic data. Supportive studies include urine copper (increased), blood ceruloplasmin (decreased), slit-lamp examination for Kayser-Fleischer rings, and liver biopsy with quantitative copper assay.

Etiology

WD is caused by an inborn error of copper metabolism that is characterized by the inability of the liver to excrete copper into bile. The defective gene product is a copper-binding ATPase. Serum ceruloplasmin levels are markedly reduced.

Clinical Findings

A movement disorder characterized by tremor and rigidity predominates if neurologic symptoms are present; however, most patients present with cirrhotic symptoms.

Pathology

Gross

• The basal ganglia appear brick-red, and the brain is atrophic

Microscopic

• The basal ganglia demonstrate neuronal loss, axonal degeneration, and large numbers of protoplasmic astrocytes
• There may also be spongy degeneration and neuronal loss involving the cortex

Imaging Findings

CT

• Often normal
• Calcifications in the globus pallidus and caudate nucleus have been observed

MR

• T2-WIs show high signal in the white matter and/or deep gray nuclei. White matter abnormalities have been described in the brainstem, cerebellum, posterior limb of internal capsule, and hemispheric white matter. Basal ganglia, thalami, and hypothalami are frequently involved.
• T1-WI may demonstrate high-signal intensity in the globus pallidus in patients with hepatic dysfunction, as well as frequent T1 shortening in the putamina
• Post-gadolinium images do not demonstrate enhancement
• Atrophy is common in the later stages of the disease

Treatment

• Medical therapy with penicillamine, zinc, trientine, and/or tetrathiomolybdate
• Liver transplantation may be indicated for fulminant disease or end-stage cirrhosis

Prognosis

• If untreated, the disease is progressive and fatal
• Most patients will do well with appropriate therapy
• Even in the presence of severe neurologic symptoms, a complete recovery may occur with aggressive therapy

Suggested Readings

King AD, Walshe JM, Kendall BE, et al. Cranial MR imaging in Wilson's disease. *AJR* 167:1579–1584, 1996.

van Hall HNV, van den Heuvel AG, Algra A, et al. Wilson disease: findings at MR imaging and CT of the brain with clinical correlation. *Radiology* 198:531–536, 1996.

van Hall HNV, van den Heuvel AG, Jansen GH, et al. Cranial MR in Wilson disease: abnormal white matter in extrapyramidal and pryamidal tracts. *AJNR* 16:2021–2027, 1995.

Case 107

Clinical Presentation

A 41-year-old man presents with increasing clumsiness, forgetfulness, and irritability.

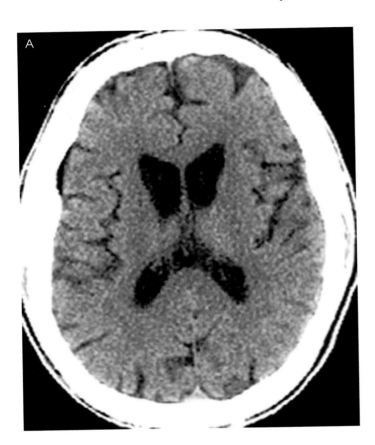

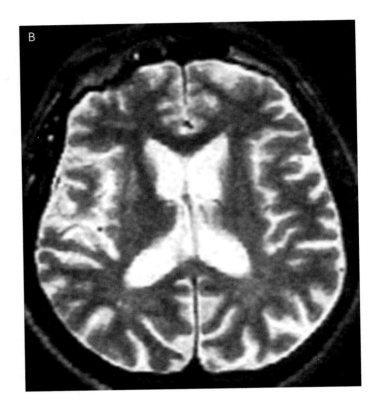

Radiologic Findings

A non-contrast CT scan (Fig. A) demonstrates enlargement of the frontal horns bilaterally due to severe atrophy of the caudate nuclei. An axial T2-WI (Fig. B) shows generalized prominence of ventricles and sulci for the patient's age, as well as T2 prolongation in the caudate nuclei and putamina.

Pearls

- Fluorodeoxyglucose (FDG)-positron emission tomography scanning may demonstrate hypometabolism in the caudate and putamen, which precedes caudate atrophy.

- The juvenile form of HD usually presents with rigidity rather than chorea. This makes the clinical diagnosis more difficult and the MR features more important to the diagnosis.

Pitfall

- Decreased rather than increased putaminal signal intensity has been reported in HD.

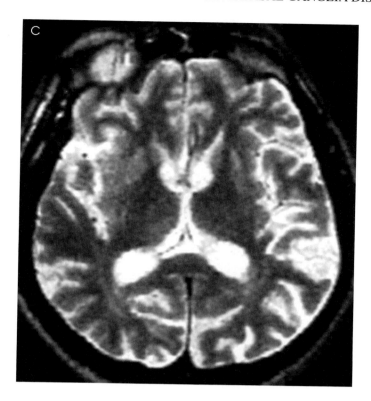

On a slightly more inferior image (Fig. C), abnormal signal affecting the caudate nuclei and putamina bilaterally is seen to better advantage.

Diagnosis

Huntington's disease (HD)

Differential Diagnosis

- Wilson's disease (lacks preferential caudate atrophy and dementia)
- Alzheimer's disease (myoclonus rather than chorea, lacks basal ganglia abnormalities)
- Pick's disease (preferential frontal atrophy, lacks basal ganglia abnormalities)
- Creutzfeldt-Jakob disease (more acute onset, usually affects older individuals, atrophy of caudate less prominent)

Discussion

Background

HD can be diagnosed without difficulty in an adult presenting with the classic clinical triad of chorea, dementia and personality disorder, and a positive family history. HD is a progressive disorder that is inherited in an autosomal dominant fashion. HD occurs worldwide and in all ethnic groups. The prevalence in the United States is approximately 4 to 8 cases per 100,000 people.

Etiology

A mutation on chromosome 4p16.3 with an expanded polyglutamine tract has been identified as the cause of HD. The HD gene is a large gene of unknown function whose product is referred to as the "huntingtin" protein. The extent of polyglutamine expansion correlates with the extent of striatal damage.

Clinical Findings

Symptoms usually appear between 35 and 40 years of age, although they may be seen as early as age 5 and as late as age 70. The onset is often insidious with clumsiness and irritability; later, overt psychotic episodes and depression may occur. Over the course of years, there is progression to striking choreiform movements and frank dementia.

Complications

Aspiration is common due to difficulties with speech and swallowing.

Pathophysiology

Disturbed energy metabolism is thought to contribute to the pathogenesis of HD. Proton MR spectroscopy shows lactate peaks in cerebral cortex that are not present in control subjects. Phosphorous MR spectroscopy shows a decrease in the muscle phosphocreatine to inorganic phosphate ratio in HD patients.

Pathology

Gross

- The brain is severely atrophic, with the caudate nuclei most severely affected

Microscopic

- The caudate and putamen show severe neuronal loss
- The cerebral cortex also shows neuronal loss, especially in layer 3

Imaging Findings

CT

- May be normal early in the course of the disease
- Over time there is parenchymal atrophy, especially involving the caudate nuclei

MR

- Cortical atrophy
- Caudate volume loss with focal enlargement of the frontal horns
- Increased signal in caudate nuclei and putamina on T2-WI

Treatment

None; however, prenatal screening is now available

Prognosis

- The disease typically runs a progressive course over 15 to 20 years
- In the setting of childhood onset, there is generally a fatal outcome within 10 years

Suggested Readings

Aylward EH, Li Q, Stine OC, et al. Longitudinal change in basal ganglia volume in patients with Huntington's disease. *Neurology* 48:394–399, 1997.

Chen JC, Hardy PA, Kucharczyk W, et al. MR of human postmortem brain tissue: correlative study between T2 and assays of iron and ferritin in Parkinson and Huntington disease. *AJNR* 14:275–281, 1993.

Koroshetz WJ, Jenkins BG, Rosen BR, Beal MF. Energy metabolism defects in Huntington's disease and effects of coenzyme Q10. *Ann Neurol* 41:160–165, 1997.

Case 108

Clinical Presentation

A 42-year-old man with a long history of dysarthria and a gait disorder presents with increasingly severe cerebellar ataxia.

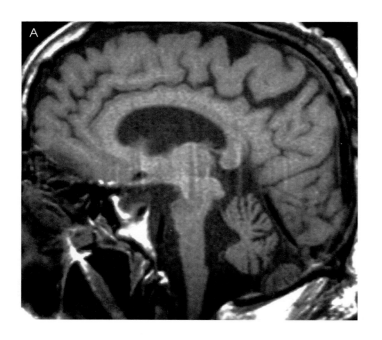

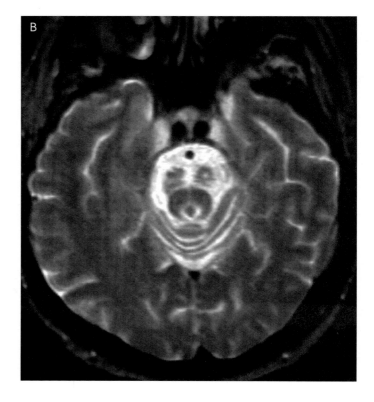

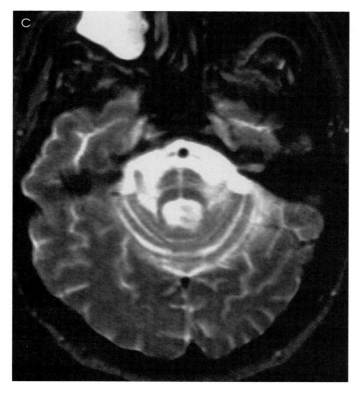

Pearls

- Mixed forms of the disease exist (multisystem atrophy, MSA), with extrapyramidal and autonomic abnormalities. In these conditions, atrophy of the putamina is typically observed, with accompanying low signal on T2-WIs.
- The pons appears flattened in OPCA.
- Alcohol-associated vermian atrophy is far more common than OPCA and usually spares the brainstem (Figs. D and E).

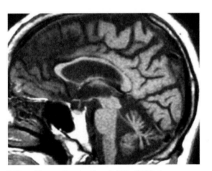

Fig. D. A sagittal T1-WI in a patient with chronic alcoholism demonstrates striking vermian atrophy, but a relatively normal appearing brainstem.

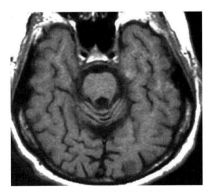

Fig. E. An axial T1-WI (same patient as Fig. D) confirms the vermian atrophy and relative preservation of the substance of the pons.

Radiologic Findings

A sagittal T1-WI (Fig. A) demonstrates marked atrophy of the cerebellar vermis, as well as atrophy of the pons and medulla. Incidental note is made of a mildly enlarged and partially empty sella. An axial T2-WI (Fig. B) confirms the atrophy of the vermis and pons. Note also T2 prolongation within the transverse pontine fibers. An axial T2-WI at a slightly lower level (Fig. C) shows enlargement of the fourth ventricle due to brainstem and cerebellar atrophy, as well as T2 prolongation within the middle cerebellar peduncles. Incidental note is made of a right maxillary retention cyst.

Diagnosis

Olivopontocerebellar atrophy (OPCA)

Differential Diagnosis

The various forms of cerebellar degeneration are difficult to distinguish without neuropathological confirmation. The differential diagnosis includes:

- Cerebello-olivary degeneration (spares brainstem except for olives)
- Cerebellar cortical degeneration (relative sparing of brainstem)
- Friedreich's ataxia (brainstem and cerebellum appear relatively normal on imaging studies)
- Alcohol-induced acquired cerebellar degeneration (preferentially affects vermis, need appropriate clinical history)

Discussion

Background

OPCA is a progressive disorder characterized by neuronal degeneration in the cerebellar cortex, pons, and inferior olives. OPCA occurs in both a sporadic and a heritable form, with both dominant and recessive forms of transmission. This disorder typically affects adults when sporadic, but may have its onset in childhood when hereditary. The primary degeneration is thought to affect the pontine nuclei, with secondary antegrade degeneration of pontocerebellar fibers and the cerebellar cortex. OPCA may be part of a larger group of disease processes referred to as "multisystem atrophy" (MSA) in which pyramidal, extrapyramidal, and autonomic symptoms occur in association with cerebellar symptoms. Most patients who present with OPCA and later develop MSA have the sporadic rather than the hereditary form of the disorder.

Etiology

OPCA is considered to represent a diagnostic grouping of a number of not-fully-characterized degenerative disorders that primarily affect posterior fossa structures. For example, carbohydrate-deficient glycoprotein syndrome type I is an autosomal recessive multisystem disorder whose manifestations include severe OPCA. Additionally, autoantibodies to the glutamate receptor subunit GluR2 have been identified in some cases of sporadic OPCA.

Clinical Findings

Progressive cerebellar ataxia is the dominant feature, usually beginning with gait disorder and dysarthria and later evolving into severe disturbances of coordination. Disturbances of extraocular movements are also common. The onset of OPCA in childhood is uncommon except in dominant pedigrees. Affected children present with gross motor developmental delay and hypotonia.

Pathology

Gross

• Atrophy of cerebellar folia, shrinkage of the brainstem, and dilatation of the fourth ventricle

Microscopic

• Myelin sheath loss and gliosis in affected regions, as well as marked reduction of Purkinje cells and granule cells in the cerebellum
• Poor or no staining for myelin in the anterior and lateral surfaces of the pons, the posterior part of the basis pontis, and the middle cerebellar peduncles
• In cases of OPCA associated with MSA, characteristic argyrophilic cytoplasmic inclusion bodies are found in oligodendroglia and neurons

Imaging Findings

CT

• Marked atrophy of the pons, vermis, and cerebellar hemispheres

MR

• Marked atrophy of the pons, vermis, and cerebellar hemispheres
• Atrophy of the medulla may also be appreciated
• T2 prolongation has been identified in structures known to degenerate in OPCA: pontine nuclei, transverse pontine fibers, cerebellar subcortical white matter, and middle cerebellar peduncles
• The pontine pyramidal tracts are spared

Treatment

Supportive care

Prognosis

Slow progression to death, usually over the course of 10 to 20 years

Suggested Readings

Kumar SD, Chand RP, Gururaj AK, Jeans WD. CT features of olivopontocerebellar atrophy in children. *Acta Radiol* 36:593–596, 1995.

Pavone L, Fiumara A, Barone R, et al. Olivopontocerebellar atrophy leading to recognition of carbohydrate-deficient glycoprotein syndrome type I. *J Neurol* 243:700–705, 1996.

Savoiardo M, Grisoli M, Girotti F, Testa D, Caraceni T. MRI in sporadic olivopontocerebellar atrophy and striatonigral degeneration. *Neurology* 48:790–791, 1997.

Case 109

Clinical Presentation

An 82-year-old man with progressive dementia presents for MR evaluation.

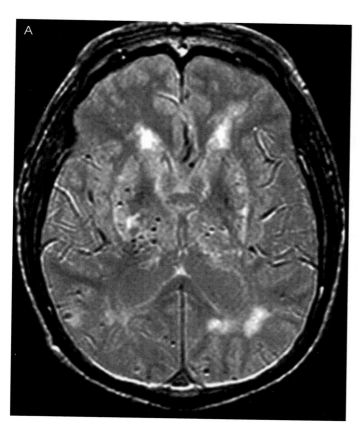

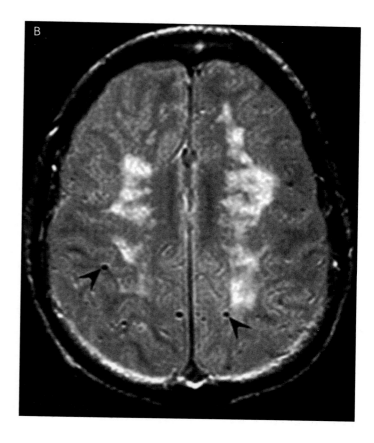

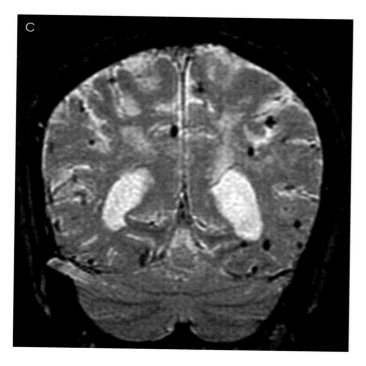

Radiologic Findings

An axial proton density-weighted image (PDWI) (Fig. A) shows patchy high signal around the ventricles, as well as multiple foci of hypointensity in the deep gray nuclei and subcortical regions. A PDWI at a slightly higher level (Fig. B) also shows patchy areas of high signal in the white matter and multiple foci of low attenuation in the subcortical regions (*arrowheads*). A coronal multiplanar gradient echo (MPGR) image (Fig. C) demonstrates to good advantage innumerable foci of hypointensity located predominantly in the peripheral subcortical regions, consistent with focal areas of hemosiderin deposition.

Diagnosis

Primary cerebral amyloid angiopathy (PCAA)

Differential Diagnosis

- Multiple cryptic vascular malformations (often familial, often occur in patients of Hispanic origin, typically present with hemorrhage at a younger age)
- Multiple parenchymal calcifications as in cysticercosis or remote tuberculosis (may need CT to distinguish)
- Chronic hypertension (punctate foci of T2 shortening or seen primarily in the basal ganglia and central pons)
- Trauma (clinical history, characteristic distribution of shearing injury)

Discussion

Background

Amyloidosis is often divided into systemic or localized forms. Systemic amyloidosis may be further subdivided into primary amyloidosis, amyloid associated with multiple myeloma or chronic infectious/inflammatory processes, amyloidosis associated with chronic hemodialysis, and other uncommon amyloid syndromes. Localized amyloidosis includes tumorlike deposits of amyloid in isolated organs without evidence of systemic involvement, and cerebral amyloidosis. PCAA is a subset of cerebral amyloidosis characterized by deposition of amyloid material in the walls of cerebral and leptomeningeal vessels. Other cerebral amyloidoses include Alzheimer's disease, Down's syndrome, and the Dutch and Icelandic-type familial cerebrovascular amyloidoses.

Etiology

The cause is uncertain, but may be related to a substitution of glutamine for glutamic acid at position 22 of the amyloid beta protein.

Clinical Findings

PCAA is associated with spontaneous intraparenchymal hemorrhage in elderly, normotensive patients. Amyloid deposits may also encroach on the vascular lumen, producing chronic cerebral ischemia and dementia. The frequency of PCAA in the elderly is high, with estimates ranging from 10% in the seventh decade to 60% in the tenth decade in unselected autopsy series.

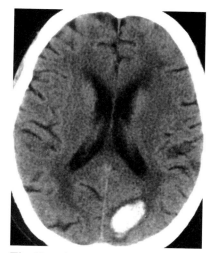

Fig. D. A non-contrast CT scan in an 82-year-old woman demonstrates a left parietal subcortical hematoma.

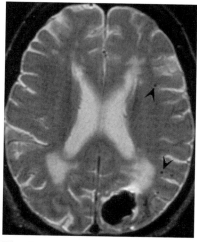

Fig. E. A corresponding axial T2-WI from an MR scan (same patient as Fig. D) demonstrates the parenchymal hematoma as well as deep white matter ischemic changes and multiple punctate foci of hypointensity (*arrowheads*) consistent with amyloid angiopathy.

Complications

PCAA is associated with an increased risk of hemorrhage in the setting of chronic anticoagulation. These patients are also at increased risk of hemorrhage during neurosurgical procedures.

Pathology

Gross

- Multiple punctate foci of hemosiderin staining, particularly near the cortical surface of the parietal and occipital lobes, although any region including the basal ganglia, brainstem, and cerebellum may be affected
- Frank hematoma formation may be observed

Microscopic

- Deposition of amyloid beta protein in arterial, arteriolar, and capillary walls of cortical and leptomeningeal vessels
- Characteristic staining of amyloid deposits with Congo red dye and birefringence under a polarized microscope

Imaging Findings

CT

- May demonstrate a frank parenchymal hematoma, which is typically lobar (Figs. D and E)

MR

- Multiple cerebral cortical and subcortical punctate foci of low-signal intensity on T2-WIs or gradient-echo images due to hemosiderin deposition
- Basal ganglia, brainstem, and cerebellum may also be affected
- No enhancement, and no abnormal flow voids are seen

Treatment

- Surgical evacuation of hematoma if necessary
- Avoid anticoagulation if possible

Prognosis

It is estimated that 40 to 70% of patients with PCAA as proven by autopsy will have died from a cerebral hemorrhage

Suggested Readings

Awasthi D, Voorhies RM, Eick J, Mitchell WT. Cerebral amyloid angiopathy presenting as multiple intracranial lesions on magnetic resonance imaging. *J Neurosurg* 75:458–460, 1991.

Greenberg SM, Vonsattel JPG, Stakes JW, Gruber M, Finkelstein SP. The clinical spectrum of cerebral amyloid angiopathy: presentations without lobar hemorrhage. *Neurology* 43:2073–2079, 1993.

Opeskin K. Cerebral amyloid angiopathy: a review. *Am J Forensic Med Path* 17:248–254, 1996.

Section VIII

Trauma

Case 110

Clinical Presentation

A 25-year-old man is status-post motor vehicle accident. He was unconscious at the scene of the accident, then regained consciousness in the ambulance. In the emergency room, his level of consciousness started to decline, and an emergent CT scan was obtained.

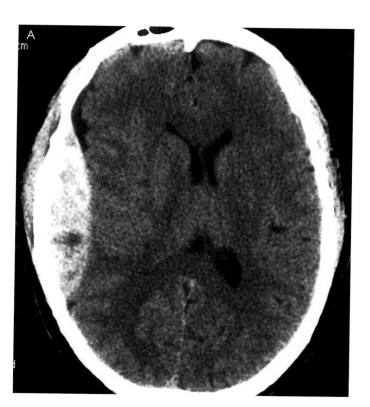 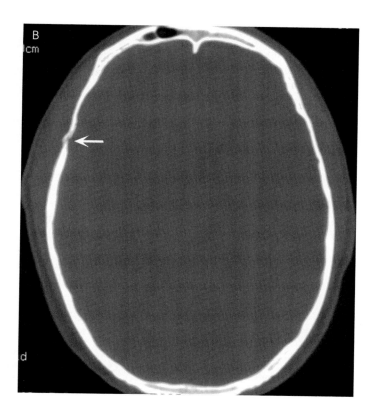

Radiologic Findings

A non-contrast CT scan (Fig. A) demonstrates a somewhat heterogeneous, hyperdense, lentiform extra-axial mass consistent with hematoma over the right posterior frontal region. The underlying brain parenchyma is displaced and compressed, and there is a moderate degree of right-to-left midline shift (subfalcial herniation). A hematoma of the right temporalis muscle is present, confirming this area to be the impact or "coup" site. An image at the same level photographed in bone window (Fig. B) demonstrates slight buckling of the skull at the level of the groove for the middle meningeal artery, consistent with a skull fracture (*arrow*).

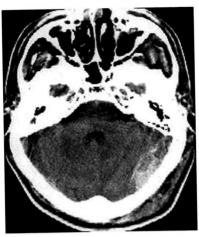

Fig. C. A non-contrast CT scan demonstrates a left occipital sub-galeal hematoma. An underlying hyperdense, lentiform collection in the left posterior fossa is most consistent with a venous epidural hematoma.

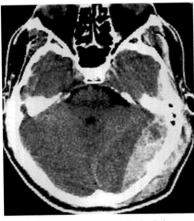

Fig. D. A more cephalad image (same patient as Fig. C) shows the venous epidural hematoma extending into the supratentorial compartment.

Diagnosis

Epidural hematoma (EDH)

Differential Diagnosis

Subdural hematoma (usually crescentic, holohemispheric; typically contrecoup)

Discussion

Background

Under normal conditions, the epidural space is a potential space as the outer layer of the dura forms the periosteum of the inner table of the skull. In the setting of trauma, the dura may be forcefully stripped from the skull, creating an epidural space that fills with blood from damaged arteries or veins. EDHs usually do not cross suture lines as the periosteum is tightly bound to the calvarium at sutures, thus EDHs typically assume a lentiform configuration. Arterial extravasation may be of sufficient pressure that the epidural collection rapidly enlarges, stopping only when intracranial pressure becomes greater than arterial pressure or when thrombosis of the damaged vessel supervenes. The most common location for an EDH is over the temporoparietal convexity, as the thin temporal squamosa easily fractures and causes damage to the partially embedded middle meningeal artery.

Etiology

EDHs are of arterial origin in approximately 90% of cases and of venous origin in approximately 10% of cases. EDHs usually occur at the coup site, and an accompanying skull fracture is seen in about 90% of cases. Arterial EDHs most commonly arise from injury to the middle meningeal artery, while venous EDHs are typically due to injury to the transverse sinuses (Figs. C and D), the superior sagittal sinus, or the sphenoparietal sinus.

Clinical Findings

The "classic" presentation of an EDH, occurring in only 30% of cases, is a brief period of unconsciousness at the moment of trauma followed by a lucid interval. Consciousness then rapidly declines as the EDH enlarges.

In general, the presentation of EDH depends on the nature of any associated brain injuries, the size and rapidity of growth of the collection, the location of the collection, and the pressure within the collection. Decompression of the EDH into the subgaleal or subarachnoid space, or diploic or meningeal veins, may alter the pressure within the collection.

Complications

Rapid enlargement results in subfalcial and uncal herniation.

Imaging Findings

CT

- Classically a biconvex hyperdense collection bounded by cranial sutures and associated with a skull fracture
- May be heterogeneous or atypical if active bleeding is occurring

Pearls

- EDHs may enlarge in a delayed manner, so repeat scanning is indicated if there is clinical decline.

- Axial CT is the imaging study of choice except for EDHs near the vertex related to injury to the superior sagittal sinus. In these cases, coronal CT scanning or MR may be very useful.

- Vertex EDHs may cross the sagittal suture as the periosteum is not tightly invested in this location because of the presence of the dural sinus.

- Common locations for venous EDHs include the posterior fossa (injury to transverse sinus), convexity (injury to superior sagittal sinus), and temporal tip (injury to sphenoparietal sinus). MR imaging and MR venography may be helpful in assessing the patency of an injured sinus.

Pitfalls

- Arterial EDHs may cross a suture line if sutural diastasis has occurred.

- EDHs are relatively uncommon in children because of a compliant calvarium.

- If an EDH occurs in a child, it may not be associated with a skull fracture.

MR

- A biconvex extra-axial collection is present
- The displaced dura may be directly visualized on MR as a thin, dark line along the medial margin of the collection
- The signal characteristics vary with the age of the blood

Treatment

- Arterial EDHs are usually surgically evacuated unless very small and the patient is stable
- Venous EDHs are generally observed

Prognosis

- Depends on extent of associated brain injuries
- Rapid evacuation of an isolated EDH generally has an excellent prognosis

Suggested Readings

Gean AD. Extra-axial collections. In *Imaging of Head Trauma*. New York, Raven Press, 1994.

Guha A, Perrin RG, Grossman H, Smyth HS. Vertex epidural hematomas. *Neurosurgery* 25:824–828, 1989.

Knuckey NW, Gelbard S, Epstein MH. The management of "asymptomatic" epidural hematomas. A prospective study. *J Neurosurg* 70:392–396, 1989.

Case 111

Clinical Presentation

A 65-year-old male who was mildly confused after a fall in the shower was brought to the emergency room by his family.

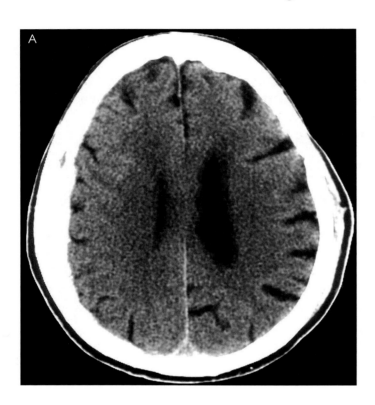

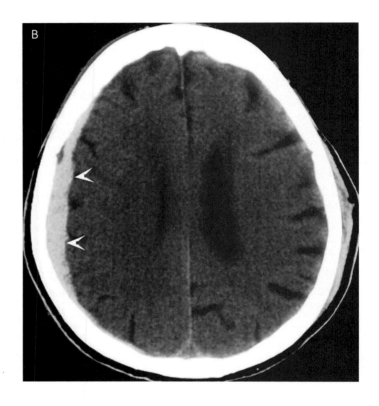

Pearls

- SDHs typically occur at the contre-coup location, 180 degrees opposite the site of initial impact.

- All trauma CT scans should be viewed with wide window settings to avoid missing a small subdural collection obscured by the calvarium.

Radiologic Findings

A non-contrast CT scan photographed with brain windows (Fig. A) demonstrates a left frontal subgaleal hematoma. Right-sided sulci are effaced compared with the left, and the right lateral ventricle is smaller than the left, but on this image it is difficult to define a collection next to the dense calvarium. An image photographed with subdural windows (Fig. B) clearly demonstrates a hyperdense crescentic right-sided holohemispheric extra-axial collection (*arrowheads*), which is exerting mild mass effect on the underlying brain.

Diagnosis

Subdural hematoma (SDH)

Differential Diagnosis

- Epidural hematoma (usually confined by sutures, usually associated with fracture)
- Subdural hygroma (should be CSF density)

Discussion

Background

The subdural space is considered to represent a potential space located between the inner layer of the dura mater (the so-called meningeal layer) and the arachnoid membrane. Bridging cortical veins heading from the brain surface to the dural venous sinuses traverse the subdural space. In the setting of head trauma where the brain is subjected to shear-strain forces, these veins may be torn. An SDH results. Being of venous origin, SDHs accumulate until the intracranial pressure rises above the level of venous pressure. The majority of these collections are located over the cerebral convexity, although they may occur along the falx or over the tentorium (Figs. C and D). Posterior fossa SDHs are uncommon except in neonates.

Clinical Findings

SDHs may present *acutely*, at the time of trauma, with symptoms related to mass effect from the collection itself or associated brain injuries. An isolated SDH is termed a *simple* SDH. SDHs may also present in a *chronic* phase, with multiple hemorrhages into a pre-existent collection. This is more common in elderly patients, who may present with progressive dementia.

Evolution

SDHs have traditionally been divided into three stages: acute (<1 week), subacute (1 to 3 weeks), and chronic (>3 weeks).

Imaging Findings

Acute SDH

CT

- Typically a homogeneous hyperdense crescentic mass lying over the cerebral convexity
- Some acute SDHs may appear atypical (i.e., heterogeneous), demonstrating areas of low attenuation thought to be related to active bleeding, serum extrusion during the early phase of clot retraction, and/or an associated arachnoid tear with admixture of CSF into the SDH. Atypical SDHs may also demonstrate a convex inner margin, simulating epidural hematoma.

MR

- The presence of deoxyhemoglobin generally renders the collection isointense on T1-WI and hypointense on T2-WI
- Toward the end of the first week, conversion to methemoglobin begins to shorten T1

Subacute SDH

CT

- Approximately 70% will be isodense to brain parenchyma by 3 weeks
- An isodense SDH can be recognized by abnormal separation of the gray-white junction from the inner table of the skull, distortion or effacement of the ven-

---

Pitfalls

- CT scan may be relatively insensitive to an isodense SDH. Note that even acute SDHs may be isodense in the setting of severe anemia or rapid scanning before clot formation.

- A remote SDH may lead to dural thickening and enhancement, which is usually unilateral.

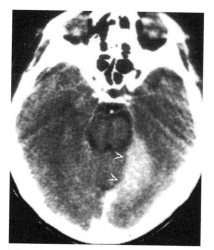

Fig. C. A non-contrast CT scan demonstrates asymmetric density along the left tentorium. Note the sharp medial margin (*arrowheads*) indicating its supratentorial location.

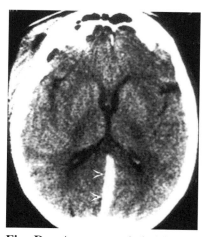

Fig. D. A more cephalad image (same patient as Fig. C) demonstrates a right frontal subgaleal hematoma and a left interhemispheric SDH (*arrowheads*) along the posterior falx.

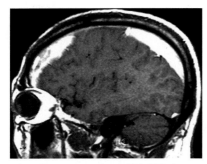

Fig. E. A sagittal T1-WI in an elderly patient with progressive confusion shows lentiform areas of T1 shortening overlying the frontal and parietal convexities.

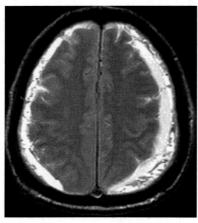

Fig. F. An axial proton density-weighted image (same patient as Fig. E) demonstrates bilateral holo-hemispheric heterogeneous subdural collections with multiple internal septations. These findings are consistent with bilateral chronic SDHs.

tricular system, inward displacement of cortical veins, effacement of sulci on the affected side, and the presence of midline shift without an identifiable mass lesion

MR

- The collection is hyperintense on T1-WI due to the presence of methemoglobin
- On T2-WI, intensity is variable depending on the location of the methemoglobin (intracellular or extracellular)

Chronic SDH

CT

- The typical chronic SDH appears as a well-defined low-attenuation collection containing multiple internal septations and fluid-fluid levels
- In the absence of rebleeding, a chronic SDH may appear as a homogeneously hypodense collection
- Note that most small acute SDHs are medically managed (rather than surgically evacuated), resolve completely, and do not evolve to the chronic phase

MR

- Variably homogeneous or heterogeneous depending on rehemorrhage
- Signal intensity varies with the stage of evolution of the blood (Figs. E and F)

Treatment

- Surgical evacuation if indicated by the patient's neurologic status
- Small collections in a stable patient may be observed

Prognosis

- Varies with accompanying injuries, with an overall mortality of 50 to 90%
- Favorable prognostic features include early surgery, young patient age, Glasgow Coma Scale score >5, and the presence of a lucid interval

Suggested Readings

Boyko OB, Cooper DF, Grossman CB. Contrast-enhanced CT of acute isodense SDH. *AJNR* 12:341–343, 1991.

Fobben ES, Grossman RI, Atlas SW, Hackney DB, Goldberg HI, Zimmerman RA, Bilaniuk LT. MR characteristics of subdural hematomas and hygromas at 1.5 T. *AJNR* 10:687–693, 1989.

Gean AD. Extra-axial collections. In *Imaging of Head Trauma*. New York, Raven Press, 1994.

Case 112

Clinical Presentation

A 45-year-old man status post-motor vehicle accident has a Glasgow Coma Scale score of 8 when he is initially seen in the emergency room, and a CT scan of the head is obtained.

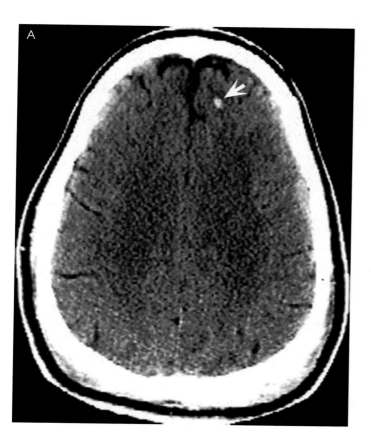 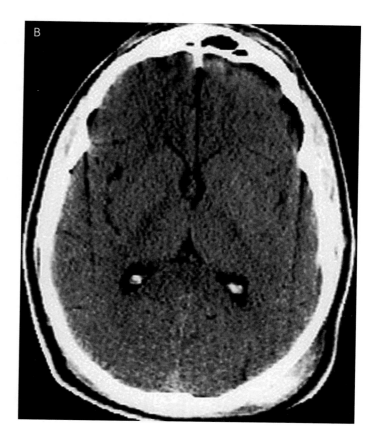

Radiologic Findings

An axial image through the high convexity (Fig. A) demonstrates biparietal subgaleal hematomas. A high-density focus is noted in the left frontal subcortical white matter (*arrow*), with a small zone of surrounding edema. A more inferior image (Fig. B) again shows evidence of scalp injury. No areas of hemorrhage are identified, but the splenium of the corpus callosum appears mildly enlarged and hypodense.

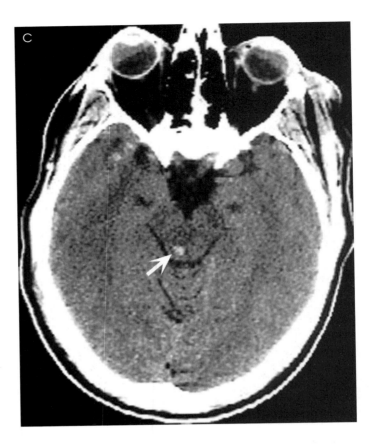

An image through the brainstem (Fig. C) shows a focus of high density in the dorsal midbrain (*arrow*). Several focal areas of high density are also noted in the right anterior temporal lobe.

Diagnosis

Diffuse axonal injury (DAI)

Differential Diagnosis

In trauma setting:

• Essentially none

In nontrauma setting:

• Multiple cryptic vascular malformations
• Amyloid angiopathy with multiple hemorrhages
• Septic emboli with hemorrhages

Discussion

Background

Primary mechanical injury to the brain occurs through two major mechanisms: direct injury due to skull distortion and gross brain motion, and indirect injury due to shear-strain forces that develop in tissues because of differential movements of one portion of the brain with respect to another portion. These forces are greatest at the junction of tissues of different density and rigidity, such as the gray-white junction. White matter shearing injury, usually termed "DAI," is common in severe head trauma and tends to occur in three major anatomic areas: the lobar white matter, the corpus callosum, and the dorsolateral aspect of the upper brainstem. These areas tend to be involved successively as the severity of the traumatic insult increases.

Clinical Findings

Patients with DAI have classically been described as presenting with severe impairment of consciousness from the moment of trauma. It is increasingly recognized that there is a spectrum of shearing injury. In the long term, mildly affected patients may be asymptomatic while severely affected patients may remain in a vegetative state.

Pathology

Gross

- Multiple small focal lesions, often hemorrhagic, are identified in the peripheral white matter, corpus callosum and brainstem

Microscopic

- Injury is always more extensive than is visible on imaging studies or grossly
- Acute: axonal retraction balls, perivascular hemorrhages
- Chronic: astrogliosis, endothelial proliferation, accumulation of hemosiderin-laden macrophages

Imaging Findings

CT

- Relatively insensitive: lesions are visible only if large or hemorrhagic

MR

Cerebral hemispheres

- Typically small, ovoid lesions that are bright on T2-WI and spare the overlying cortex
- Low signal on T2-WI and/or high signal on T1-WI sequences may be seen if the lesion is hemorrhagic
- The parasagittal frontal lobes and periventricular region of temporal lobes are most commonly involved

Corpus callosum

- Callosal lesions typically affect the posterior body and splenium (70%)

Brainstem

- Lesions typically occur in the dorsolateral midbrain and upper pons
- Lesions of DAI are hemorrhagic approximately 20% of the time

Treatment

None—supportive care and rehabilitation

Prognosis

Varies with extent of injury, but patients may suffer severe cognitive impairment and amnesia

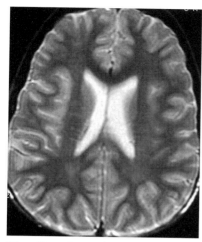

Fig. D. An axial T2-WI in a 6-year-old boy who remains cognitively impaired several months following a motor vehicle accident is unremarkable.

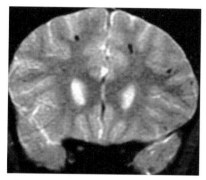

Fig. E. A coronal gradient-echo image (same patient as Fig. D) shows multiple foci of hypointensity at the gray-white junction consistent with shear hemorrhages.

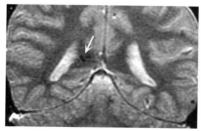

Fig. F. A more posterior gradient-echo image (same patient as Figs. D and E) shows injury to the splenium of the corpus callosum (*arrow*), as well as the left temporal lobe.

Suggested Readings

Gentry LR. Imaging of closed head injury. *Radiology* 191:1–17, 1994.

Gentry LR, Godersky JC, Thompson B. MR imaging of head trauma: review of the distribution and radiopathologic features of traumatic lesions. *AJNR* 9:101–110, 1988.

Gentry LR, Thompson B, Godersky JC. Traumatic brainstem injury: MR imaging. *Radiology* 171:177–187, 1989.

Case 113

Clinical Presentation

A young man was admitted following a motor vehicle accident. Several days after admission he underwent MR scanning to fully characterize his injuries.

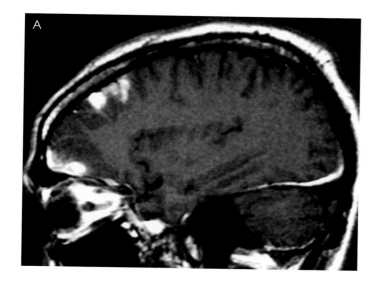

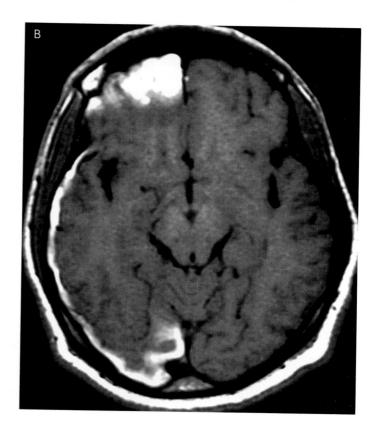

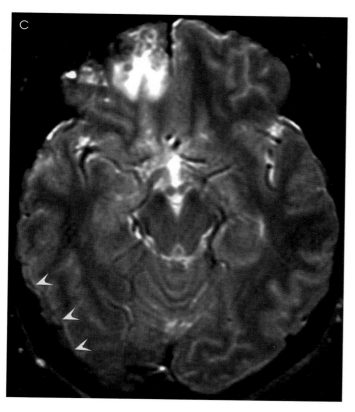

Radiologic Findings

A sagittal T1-WI (Fig. A) demonstrates areas of intrinsic T1 shortening involving the anteroinferior frontal lobe as well as the superior frontal lobe, consistent with cortical contusions. In addition, a subdural hematoma is noted layering around the occipital and temporal lobes. An axial T1-WI (Fig. B) similarly demonstrates the hemorrhagic contusion of the right frontal cortex, as well as the temporo-occipital subdural hematoma. An axial T2-WI (Fig. C) demonstrates mixed high- and low-signal intensity within the cortical contusion, consistent with evolving blood products. Surrounding vasogenic edema is present. Note how subtle the right temporo-occipital collection is on the T2-WI (*arrowheads*).

Diagnosis

Traumatic parenchymal contusions

Differential Diagnosis

Essentially none—the location and appearance are pathognomonic. If there is no history of trauma given, this history should be sought, and the scalp should be carefully inspected (on physical examination and imaging) for signs of trauma.

Discussion

Background

The cerebral contusion is the most common primary traumatic intra-axial lesion. Contusions classically occur in areas of the brain that directly contact and slide over irregular surfaces of the inner skull in the setting of trauma. Typical locations include the anteroinferior frontal lobes, anterior temporal lobes, and inferior temporal lobes. The bony structures contacted are the orbital roof, sphenoid wing, and petrous ridges. Contusions of the occipital lobes and cerebellum are uncommon because the inner aspect of the occipital bone is very smooth. By definition, contusions involve primarily the superficial gray matter of the brain, with relative sparing of the underlying white matter.

Clinical Findings

Headache and confusion are common. The clinical picture will often be dominated by associated traumatic injuries such as an epidural hematoma or diffuse axonal injury.

Complications

Significant edema and hemorrhage due to cerebral contusion may cause brain herniation, usually descending transalar herniation from frontal lobe mass effect or uncal herniation from temporal lobe mass effect. Delayed hemorrhage into an area of contused parenchyma, usually occurring within 24 to 48 hours of trauma, may result in a dramatic clinical decline.

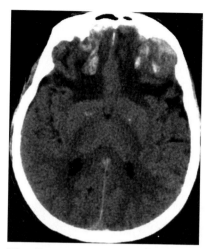

Fig. D. A non-contrast CT scan demonstrates hemorrhagic contusions of the frontal lobes bilaterally, with associated vasogenic edema.

Pathology

Gross

- Acute: edema, petechial hemorrhage; microhemorrhages may coalesce into a focal hematoma
- Chronic: volume loss, hemosiderin staining

Microscopic

- Acute: edema, capillary disruption, petechial hemorrhage, areas of focal necrosis
- Chronic: demyelination, gliosis, cyst forrmation, hemosiderin staining

Imaging Findings

CT

- Ill-defined area of low attenuation
- May be admixed with petechial hemorrhage or frank hematoma (Fig. D)

MR

- Ill-defined regions of T1 and T2 prolongation involving superficial surfaces of brain
- Hemorrhage is common, and the MR appearance varies with the stage of evolution of the blood products
- Ill-defined enhancement may be present in the resolving phase due to disruption of the blood-brain barrier and capsule formation around hematoma

Treatment

Surgical evacuation of hematoma due to contusion may be necessary

Prognosis

Varies with size and extent of contusion itself, as well as the presence of associated injuries

Suggested Readings

Gean AD. *Imaging of Head Trauma*. New York Raven Press, 1994, pp.150–187.

Gentry LR, Godersky JC, Thompson B. MR imaging of head trauma: review of the distribution and radiopathologic features of traumatic lesions. *AJNR* 9:101–110, 1988.

Gentry LR. Imaging of closed head injury. *Radiology* 191:1–17, 1994.

Case 114

Clinical Presentation

A 22-month-old male is brought to the emergency room because of apnea and lethargy. The patient's mother comments that he had fallen off a bed several hours earlier.

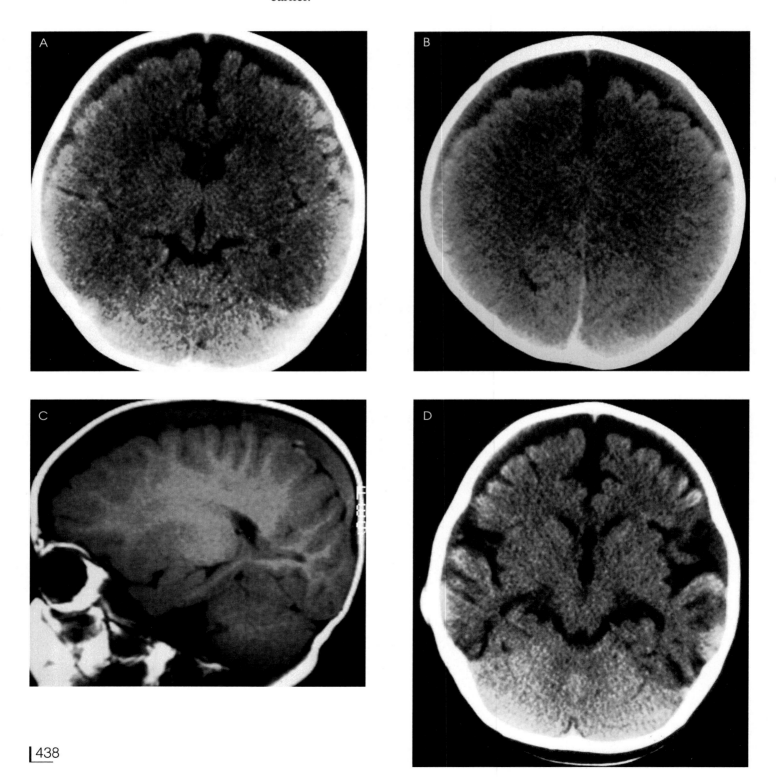

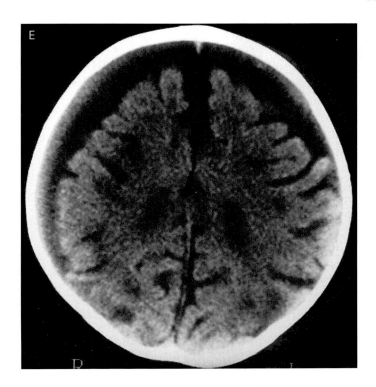

Pearls

- CT scanning is often useful in the acute setting to assess for surgical lesions, but MR is better able to support a suspected diagnosis of abuse given its ability to detect subdural hematomas of varying ages and diffuse axonal injury. Gradient-echo imaging should be done to increase sensitivity for shear hemorrhages.

- Skull films are still occasionally useful in the evaluation of suspected child abuse, as fractures on both sides of the midline are very strong evidence for abuse.

- Intrafalcial hematomas may be observed due to microtears within the relatively vascular pediatric falx.

- Evaluate the orbits carefully as retinal hemorrhages may sometimes be visible on imaging studies.

Pitfalls

- Children with enlarged extra-axial spaces are at increased risk of subdural bleeding in the setting of minimal accidental trauma. Predisposing conditions include benign enlargement of the subdural spaces and Menke's kinky hair syndrome.

- Children with osteogenesis imperfecta are at increased risk of fracture in the setting of minimal accidental trauma.

Radiologic Findings

A non-contrast head CT (Fig. A) shows bifrontal extra-axial collections that appear isodense to CSF. On a more cephalad image (Fig. B), the bifrontal extra-axial collections are again seen. Because of streak artifact underlying the calvarium, it is difficult to determine whether they are truly subdural collections or prominent subarachnoid spaces. Note that this patient is too old for so-called benign enlargement of the subarachnoid spaces. Additionally, there is subtle hyperdensity along the posterior falx, representing an acute interhemispheric subdural hematoma. On a sagittal T1-WI (Fig. C) from an MR scan that was obtained to assess the extra-axial collections, a large holohemispheric subdural collection can be seen. The presence of subdural collections of varying age is a characteristic of child abuse. A CT scan obtained 3 weeks after the original study shows striking parenchymal volume loss, with global prominence of ventricles and sulci (Figs. D and E). (*Figures courtesy of Alisa D. Gean, M.D., San Francisco, CA.*)

Diagnosis

Non-accidental trauma (child abuse)

Differential Diagnosis

- Subdural hematoma secondary to accidental trauma
- Subdural hematoma in the setting of a predisposing condition such as: benign enlargement of the subarachnoid spaces (usually in patients <18 months of age), blood dyscrasia, and meningitis with subdural effusions (CSF intensity unless complicated)

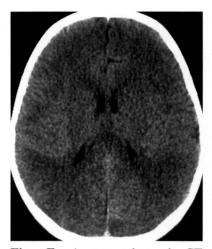

Fig. F. A non-enhanced CT shows loss of distinction of the deep gray nuclei as well as bifrontal and biparieto-occipital loss of cortical gray-white differentiation in a young child who had been strangled.

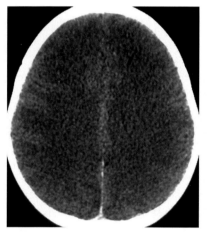

Fig. G. A CT scan at a higher level (same patient as Fig. F) shows diffuse sulcal effacement as well as abnormal hypodensity of cortex and white matter.

Discussion

Background

It is estimated that there are 3000 deaths per year in the United States due to non-accidental injury and that at least 10% of children with mental retardation and cerebral palsy have been damaged by abuse. Most cases of child abuse occur in children under 2 years of age. In these children, non-accidental injury accounts for ≥80% of deaths from head trauma. Clinically, a marked discrepancy between the explanation of how an injury occurred and the extent of the observed lesions should raise the question of abuse.

Clinical Findings

The presentation is highly variable. Abused children are commonly irritable or abnormally subdued, and may have episodes of vomiting or cyanosis. These children may present with seizures, focal neurologic signs, or coma related to parenchymal damage and intracranial hematomas. Any child suspected of being a victim of abuse should have a careful ophthalmologic examination to look for retinal hemorrhages because many authorities believe that the finding of retinal hemorrhages in a child with a head injury suggests a nonaccidental cause. Children under the age of 2 years often have no external signs of trauma.

Complications

Complications of abuse vary with the mechanism of injury. Strangulation or suffocation may lead to cerebral infarction and global hypoxic/ischemic damage. Shaking may lead to a characteristic syndrome of retinal hemorrhages, subdural and/or subarachnoid hemorrhage, cerebral edema, diffuse axonal injury, and cerebral contusion with little or no evidence of external trauma. Direct impact may lead to skull fractures, extra-axial hematomas, and cerebral contusions.

Imaging Findings

Findings are dependent on the mechanism and severity of trauma and include:

CT

- Skull fractures in approximately 65% of abused children with head injury
- Epidural, subdural, and parenchymal hematomas
- Traumatic subarachnoid and intraventricular hemorrhage
- Diffuse anoxic injury with cerebral edema and loss of gray-white distinction (Figs. F and G) may lead to the "reversal sign" or "white cerebellum sign"

MR

- More sensitive to shear hemorrhages, small extra-axial collections and small cortical contusions than CT
- May demonstrate posttraumatic infarction or hypoxic/ischemic injury to the cerebral cortex and deep gray nuclei (Fig. H)

Treatment

- Surgical therapy for mass lesions as needed
- Removal of the child from the abusive environment

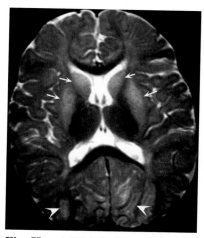

Fig. H. A T2-WI shows high signal in the caudate nuclei and putamina (*arrows*) in an infant who had been smothered. Note also the subtle T2 prolongation in the cortex, best seen in the occipital lobes (*arrowheads*).

Prognosis

Nearly half of all abuse cases lead to physical disfigurement, permanent neurologic or psychologic deficits, or death

Suggested Readings

Hart BL, Dudley MH, Zumwalt RE. Postmortem cranial MRI and autopsy correlation in suspected child abuse. *Am J Forensic Med Path* 17:217–224, 1996.

Harwood-Nash DC. Abuse to the pediatric central nervous system. *AJNR* 13:569–575, 1992.

Zimmerman RA, Bilaniuk LT. Pediatric head trauma. *Neuroimag Clin North Am* 4:349–366, 1994.

Section IX

Phakomatoses

Case 115

Clinical Presentation

A 7-year-old boy with inguinal freckling noted on routine exam is referred for MR imaging.

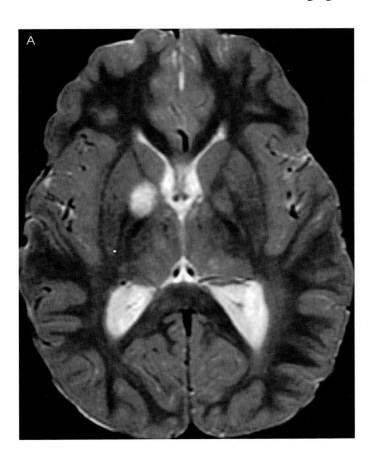

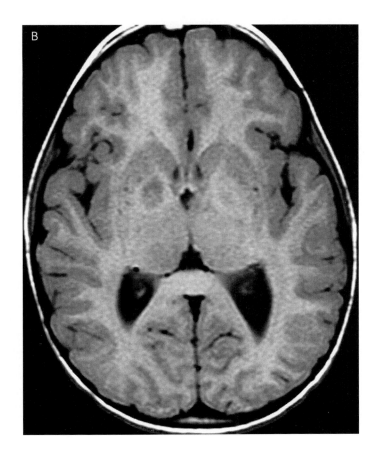

Radiologic Findings

A rounded focus of increased signal intensity on a T2-WI (Fig. A) and decreased signal on a T1-WI (Fig. B) is seen in the right globus pallidus. More subtle ill-defined areas of T2 prolongation are seen in the left globus pallidus and in the thalami (Fig. A).

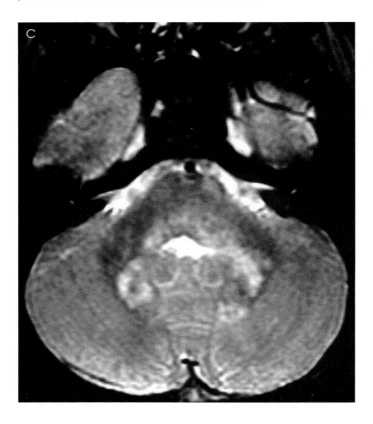

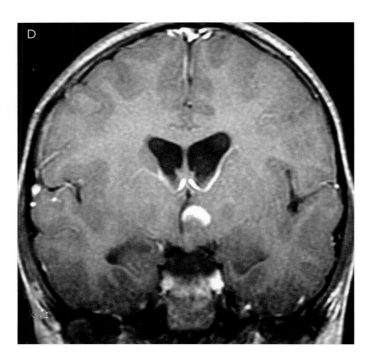

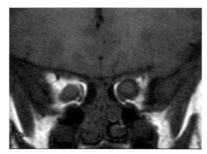

Fig. E. A coronal T1-WI in a patient with NF1 demonstrates bilateral marked enlargement of the optic nerves, as well as dilatation of the left optic sheath, consistent with bilateral ON gliomas.

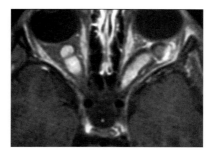

Fig. F. An axial post-gadolinium T1-WI with fat saturation (same patient as Fig. E) demonstrates homogeneous enhancement of the enlarged optic nerves.

An axial T2-WI (Fig. C) through the posterior fossa demonstrates ill-defined T2 prolongation in the white matter of the middle cerebellar peduncles and dorsal pons, as well as in the dentate nuclei. A coronal post-gadolinium T1-WI (Fig. D) shows an enhancing mass in the left hypothalamus consistent with a hypothalamic glioma. However, no enhancement was identified in any of the other areas of T2 prolongation.

Diagnosis

Neurofibromatosis Type 1 (NF1)

Differential Diagnosis

None for this characteristic constellation of findings

Discussion

Background

NF1 is the most common neurocutaneous disorder, with an incidence of approximately 1 per 3,000 births. The disorder is autosomal dominant with 50% of cases representing spontaneous mutations. The common lesions encountered in patients with NF1 include cutaneous cafe au lait spots, peripheral nerve neurofibromas, and optic nerve gliomas (Figs. E and F). Additional often-seen abnormalities include "Lisch" nodules (iris hamartomas), seen in >90% of patients; intertriginous (i.e., axillary and inguinal) freckling; vascular dysplasias; bony abnormalities (i.e., "ribbon ribs"); macrocephaly; dysplasia of the greater and lesser wing of

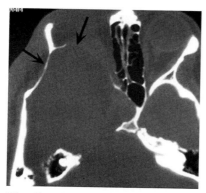

Fig. G. An axial non-contrast CT scan in a different patient with NF1 shows enlargement of the middle cranial fossa and focal thinning and deficiency of the right sphenoid wing (*arrows*), consistent with sphenoid wing dysplasia.

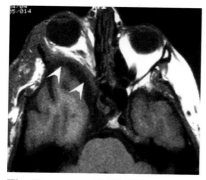

Fig. H. An axial T1-WI (same patient as Fig. G) through the same level of the sphenoid bone reveals herniation of the anterior temporal lobe into the right orbit (*arrowheads*). Additionally, a plexiform neurofibroma infiltrates and thickens the skin lateral to the right eye.

the sphenoid bone (Figs. G and H); pseudoarthrosis, thinning, and bowing of the long bones; scoliosis; dural ectasia and associated enlargement of neural foramina; and lateral thoracic meningoceles.

NF1 is also associated with some malignancies including astrocytomas, malignant nerve sheath tumors, Wilms' tumor, rhabdomyosarcoma, leukemia, melanoma, and medullary thyroid carcinoma. There is also an association with pheochromocytoma.

Etiology

The gene for NF1 has been isolated to chromosome 17. The gene product, neurofibromin, is thought to function as a growth suppressor.

Clinical Findings

The age at presentation is quite variable, as are the penetrance and expressivity of this disorder. The cafe au lait spots are usually the first manifestation of the disease and can be seen in the first year of life. Cutaneous neurofibromas begin to appear in later childhood and can develop throughout the patient's life. Approximately 15% of patients will develop CNS manifestations of NF1. Some of the symptoms encountered in these patients include diminished vision or blindness in patients with optic nerve gliomas, mental retardation (9.7%), seizures (7.3%), and precocious puberty (4.8%).

Pathology

- Neurofibroma: Schwann cells, neurons, and acellular matrix; unencapsulated
- Optic glioma: usually a low-grade astrocytoma
- "Hamartomas" of NF1: myelin vacuolization
- Parenchymal glioma: usually low or intermediate grade tumors

Imaging Findings

Only intracranial manifestations will be considered here.

CT

- Fusiform enlargement of optic nerve(s), optic tract(s), and/or optic chiasm in cases of optic pathway glioma
- Parenchymal mass representing astrocytoma
- Sphenoid wing dysplasia may be present and is usually associated with plexiform neurofibroma and buphthalmos

MR

- Optic nerve glioma: abnormal enlargement of the optic nerve(s), chiasm, and/or optic tract(s) with increased signal on T2-WI and mild to moderate contrast enhancement
- Nonenhancing foci of T2 prolongation within the deep gray nuclei and the white matter, thought to represent areas of myelin vacuolization. These are most common in the globi pallidi, followed by the cerebellum and brainstem, internal capsules, centrum semiovale, and corpus callosum. T1 signal characteristics are variable.
- Parenchymal tumors (usually astrocytomas) have a predilection for the thalami and basal ganglia and typically present as T2 prolonging mass lesions with variable post-gadolinium enhancement. Brainstem gliomas are relatively common as well.

Pearls

- Foci of T2 prolongation in the globi pallidi may be accompanied by T1 shortening that is thought to represent paramagnetic metals, remyelination, and/or calcification.

- Both the T1 and the T2 signal abnormalities evolve over time and typically resolve by adulthood.

- Brainstem gliomas (BSGs) in patients with NF1 have a more indolent course and better prognosis than isolated BSGs, and may not require aggressive therapy.

- Patients with optic nerve tumors have a higher incidence of brain tumors.

Pitfall

- Enhancing hypothalamic masses may spontaneously resolve for reasons that are unclear. Therefore, unless mass effect from the lesions is causing symptoms, conservative therapy is warranted.

Treatment

- Surgery and/or radiation therapy as needed for malignancy
- Surgery may be required for disfiguring plexiform neurofibromas

Prognosis

- Varies with expression of disease and presence or absence of malignancy
- Many patients have a normal life span

Suggested Readings

Bognanno JR, Edwards MK, Lee TA, et al. Cranial MR imaging in neurofibromatosis. *AJR* 151:381–388, 1988.

DiPaolo DP, Zimmerman RA, Rorke LB, Zackai EH, Bilaniuk LT, Yachnis AT. Neurofibromatosis type 1: pathologic substrate of high-signal-intensity foci in the brain. *Radiology* 195:721–724, 1995.

Terada H, Barkovich AJ, Edwards MSB, Ciricillo SF. Evolution of high-intensity basal ganglia lesions on T1-weighted MR in neurofibromatosis type 1. *AJNR* 17:755–760, 1996.

Case 116

Clinical Presentation

A 29-year-old male presents with gradually progressive right-sided hearing loss. He has a history of surgery for left-sided hearing loss. The patient's mother went deaf at an early age.

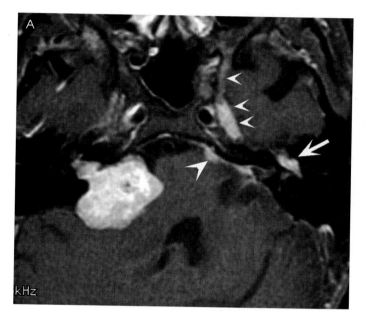

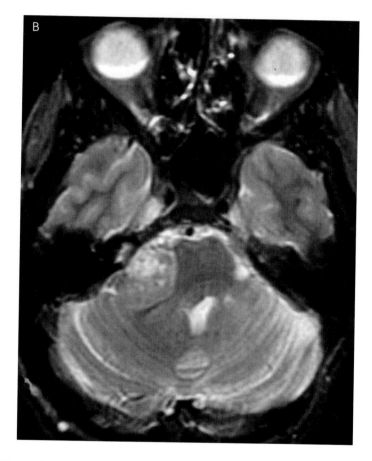

Radiologic Findings

An axial post-gadolinium T1-WI with fat saturation (Fig. A) demonstrates an enhancing mass in the right cerebellopontine angle and right internal auditory canal consistent with an acoustic neuroma (vestibular schwannoma). There is a smaller enhancing mass involving the left facial nerve canal (*arrow*) most consistent with a facial nerve schwannoma, and postoperative enhancement is seen in the left internal auditory canal related to prior resection of a left-sided acoustic neuroma. An ovoid focus of enhancement anterior to the left internal auditory canal (*large arrowhead*) most likely represents a small meningioma. In addition, an enhancing mass is present in Meckel's cave on the left, with enhancement extending anteriorly along foramen rotundum (*arrowheads*), most consistent with a trigeminal schwannoma. On an axial T2-WI (Fig. B), the right cerebellopontine angle mass is noted to be somewhat heterogenous in signal intensity. There is significant mass effect on the adjacent cerebellum and pons.

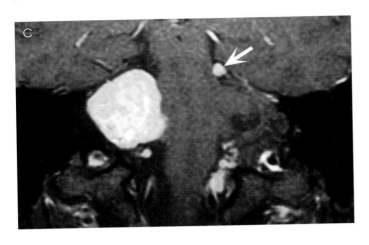

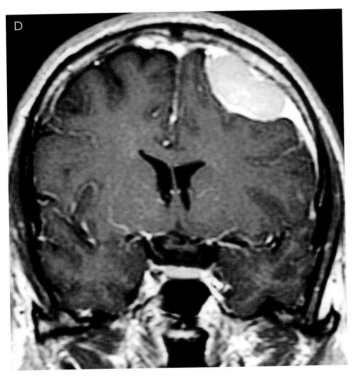

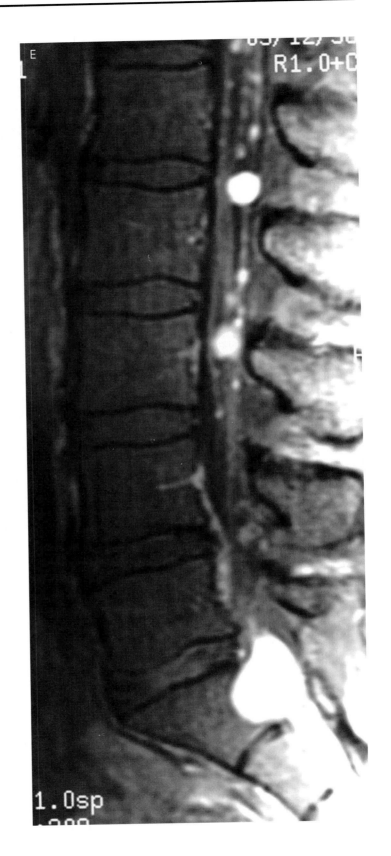

On a coronal post-gadolinium T1-WI with fat saturation (Fig. C), in addition to the large right-sided acoustic neuroma, there is abnormal enlargement and enhancement of the left fourth cranial nerve (*arrow*) secondary to a trochlear nerve schwannoma. A coronal post-gadolinium T1-WI (Fig. D) reveals a large enhancing extra-axial mass overlying the left frontal convexity, consistent with meningioma. A sagittal post-gadolinium T1-WI of the lumbar spine (Fig. E) demonstrates multiple abnormal enhancing nodules studding the surface of the cauda equina, most consistent with multiple schwannomas.

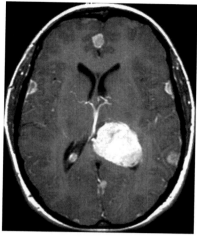

Fig. F. An axial post-gadolinium T1-WI through the brain in a different patient with NF2 reveals multiple meningiomas, including a large intraventricular meningioma in the atrium of the left lateral ventricle.

Table 1. NF1 versus NF2

Characteristic	NF1	NF2
Incidence	1 per 3000	1 per 20,000-50,000
Location of gene	Chromosome 17	Chromosome 22
Skin lesions	Multiple	Few
Intracranial lesions	Astrocytomas, "hamartomas"	Bilateral vestibular schwannomas, other cranial nerve schwannomas, meningiomas
Orbital findings	Optic gliomas, Lisch nodules	Cataracts, optic nerve sheath meningiomas, epiretinal membranes

Diagnosis

Neurofibromatosis Type 2 (NF2) with vestibular schwannoma, facial nerve schwannoma, trigeminal schwannoma, multiple spinal schwannomas, and meningioma

Differential Diagnosis

None: this is a pathognomonic appearance

Discussion

Background

The hallmark of NF2 is bilateral acoustic neuromas (vestibular schwannomas), which typically come to attention in the third or fourth decade of life. Unlike NF1, in which glial tumors predominate, the tumors associated with NF2 generally arise from Schwann and meningothelial cells (Table 1). Schwannomas of the cranial and spinal nerves are the most common tumors, followed by meningiomas (which are frequently multiple, Fig. F). Vestibular schwannomas are the most common schwannomas, followed by trigeminal schwannomas. Ependymomas also occur with increased frequency in NF2 and usually arise within the spinal cord. Ocular abnormalities are common in NF2 and include early onset cataracts (both posterior subcapsular and cortical), retinal hamartomas, and epiretinal membranes.

Etiology

NF2 is inherited as an autosomal dominant trait with nearly 100% penetrance and has been linked to a genetic defect on the long arm of chromosome 22. The protein product of the NF2 gene is called schwannomin or merlin, and it is thought to function as a tumor suppressor.

Clinical Findings

Patients usually present with hearing loss in the second to fourth decades, but there is heterogeneity with regard to clinical course, age at onset, and the presence of other cranial and spinal tumors. Some patients present as late as the seventh or eighth decades. Other presenting symptoms include tinnitus, skin tumors, neck or back pain, and ocular complaints.

Complications

Hemorrhage into a vestibular schwannoma may result in sudden hearing loss or acute hydrocephalus. Spine tumors may compress the spinal cord and present with myelopathy.

Imaging Findings

Schwannomas

- Usually round or ovoid extra-axial masses
- Iso- to mildly hypodense on non-contrast CT scan unless cystic or hemorrhagic
- Iso- to hypointense compared to brain parenchyma on T1-WI
- Iso- to hyperintense to brain parenchyma on T2-WI. As these lesions are typically hypointense compared with CSF, they stand out clearly against the bright CSF in the internal auditory canals and basal cisterns.
- Fairly intense, homogeneous enhancement postcontrast is typically seen, although areas of cystic change or hemorrhage may lead to heterogeneous enhancement
- Large lesions may cause brainstem compression and/or hydrocephalus

Meningiomas

- Dural-based extra-axial masses, often with an associated dural tail
- Typically isodense to brain on nonenhanced CT scan and isointense to gray matter on T1- and T2-WIs
- Usually enhance intensely and homogeneously
- Frequently calcified

Treatment

- Observation with serial MR examinations may be indicated as many schwannomas will only slowly progress over time
- Surgical resection of symptomatic, accessible lesions
- Gamma knife radiosurgery is an option for treatment of vestibular schwannomas in appropriate cases

Prognosis

Variable as both mild and severe phenotypes exist

Suggested Readings

Aoki S, Barkovich AJ, Nishimura K, et al. Neurofibromatosis types 1 and 2: cranial MR findings. *Radiology* 172:527–534, 1989.

Mautner VF, Lindenau M, Baser ME, et al. The neuroimaging and clinical spectrum of neurofibromatosis 2. *Neurosurgery* 38:880–886, 1996.

Pont MS, Elster AD. Lesions of skin and brain: modern imaging of the neurocutaneous syndromes. *AJR* 158:1193–1203, 1992.

Case 117

Clinical Presentation

A 16-month-old female with medically refractory seizures presents for evaluation.

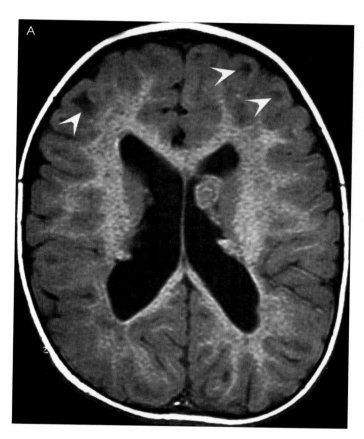
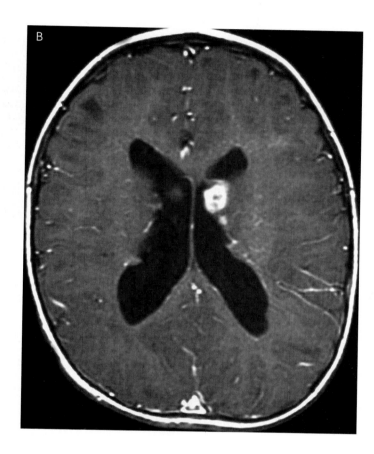

Radiologic Findings

An axial T1-WI through the level of the lateral ventricles (Fig. A) demonstrates multiple subependymal nodules isointense to white matter along the ventricular surface. In addition, several broad gyri are noted in the frontal lobes bilaterally (*arrowheads*), with hypointensity of the subcortical white matter. After administration of gadolinium (Fig. B), a T1-WI shows variable contrast enhancement of these subependymal nodules, with the largest nodule enhancing intensely.

Pearls

- The fluid-attenuated inversion recovery sequence is superior to standard spin-echo sequences in detecting subtle cortical and subcortical lesions.

- The classic clinical triad occurs in only approximately 50% of patients, so imaging findings are key to the diagnosis of TS, especially in infancy.

Pitfalls

- Subependymal nodules should not be mistaken for periventricular nodular heterotopia. Subependymal nodules are isointense to mature white matter on T1-WI, while nodular heterotopia are isointense to gray matter on all sequences.

- Subependymal nodules are rarely calcified in the newborn.

- Subependymal nodules may appear bright on T1-WI compared to unmyelinated white matter in the neonate. These should not be mistaken for subependymal hemorrhages.

- A gyral pattern of cortical calcification, which can mimic Sturge-Weber syndrome, may occasionally be seen in TS.

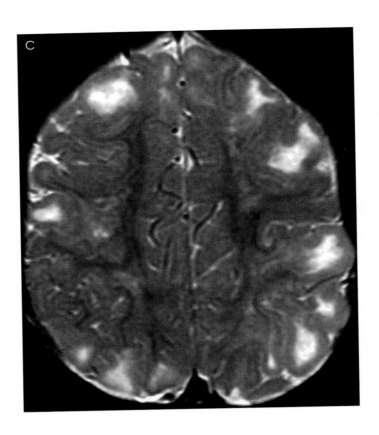

An axial T2-WI (Fig. C) demonstrates multiple areas of abnormal hyperintensity in the subcortical white matter, with associated expansion of the overlying gyri.

Diagnosis

Tuberous sclerosis (TS) (Bourneville's disease)

Differential Diagnosis

None

Discussion

Background

TS is a neurocutaneous disorder with an estimated prevalence of 1 per 20,000. It is inherited in an autosomal dominant manner in 20 to 50% of cases, with the rest resulting from spontaneous mutations. Clinically, the classic triad of TS includes mental retardation, seizures, and adenoma sebaceum, although not all patients manifest these features. A plethora of organ systems is involved in TS, and associated findings include CNS subependymal and cortical hamartomas, white matter lesions, giant cell astrocytomas of the foramen of Monro, cutaneous lesions (facial angiofibromas, shagreen patches, ash leaf spots, and subungual fibromas), retinal hamartomas, renal angiomyolipomas and cysts, interstitial lung disease, and cardiac rhabdomyomas.

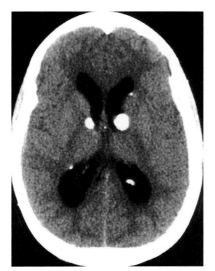

Fig. D. A non-contrast CT of the brain in an adult with TS reveals densely calcified subependymal nodules.

Etiology

Two separate genes have been identified that are mutated or deleted in patients with TS. TSC1 is at 9q34, and TSC2 is at 16p13.3. The TSC2 gene codes for a protein called tuberin, which may be involved in regulation of cell proliferation.

Clinical Findings

Myoclonic seizures beginning in infancy or early childhood are the presenting symptom in 80% of cases. Some neonates may present with congestive heart failure due to cardiac rhabdomyomas. Mental retardation is present in 45 to 82% of affected individuals. The severity and probability of mental retardation correlate with the number of subependymal tubers and early age of seizure onset.

Pathogenesis

Intracranial manifestations are thought to be secondary to a dysplasia of stem cells in the germinal zone. This results in disorganized and dysplastic collections of cells extending from the subependymal region to the cortex. Thus, the cortical brain lesions can be thought of as transmantle cortical dysplasias.

Pathology

Gross

- Broad flat gyri represent cortical tubers; these may be calcified, may show central depressions, and are usually firm to palpation

Microscopic

- Cortical hamartomas ("tubers") are small nodular lesions that expand involved gyri and are composed of giant cells with varying degrees of neuronal and astrocytic differentiation, and abnormal, deficient myelin sheaths
- White matter lesions are composed of bizarre, heterotopic giant cells ("balloon cells") and associated hypomyelination
- Subependymal nodules are hamartomatous lesions that are frequently calcified
- Subependymal giant cell astrocytomas are located at or near the foramen of Monro and enlarge over time while remaining histologically benign

Imaging Findings

Subependymal nodules

CT

- Slightly hyperdense nodules which line the ventricular surface
- Usually calcified (Fig. D), though rarely in the first year of life

MR

- In the neonate, subependymal nodules appear hyperintense on T1-WI and proton density-weighted imaging and relatively hypointense on T2-WI
- As the brain myelinates, these lesions become more isointense with white matter on T1-WI and hypointense to white matter on T2-WI
- Gradient-echo images (T2*) enhance visualization of the calcified nodules due to magnetic susceptibility effects
- These lesions demonstrate variable enhancement, and the degree of enhancement has no apparent clinical significance

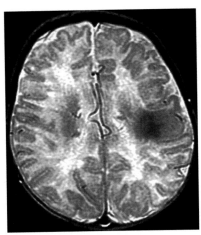

Fig. E. A proton density-weighted image in a 3-month-old girl with seizures demonstrates T2 shortening in a large left frontal lobe cortical tuber. This lesion will gradually become hyperintense relative to white matter as the brain myelinates.

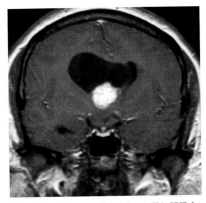

Fig. F. Post-gadolinium T1-WI in a different patient with TS and increasing headaches shows a giant cell astrocytoma arising in the region of the foramen of Monro and obstructive hydrocephalus.

Cortical tubers

CT

- Low attenuation areas in slightly expanded gyri
- Become isodense to normal cortex in older children and adults
- May calcify (by age 10, 50% of patients demonstrate calcifed cortical hamartomas)

MR

- Like their subependymal counterparts, the cortical hamartomas change in appearance as the brain myelinates; they are initially hyperintense on T1-WI and hypointense on T2-WI (Fig. E), but as myelination occurs, a reversal of this pattern occurs

White matter lesions

CT

- Relatively insensitive to white matter lesions

MR

- Hyperintense linear bands in cerebrum and cerebellum
- In infants, these bands are hypointense to unmyelinated white matter on T2-WI, becoming hyperintense to white matter in older children and adults

Giant cell atrocytomas

CT and MR

- Located at or near the foramen of Monro (Fig. F)
- Exhibit growth on serial imaging studies
- Intense enhancement post-contrast is typical

Treatment

- Medical management of seizure activity
- Surgical resection of dominant seizure foci in selected cases
- Surgical resection of giant cell astrocytomas as necessary
- Screening and appropriate intervention for cardiac and renal tumors

Prognosis

Varies with the severity of expression of the disease

Suggested Readings

Curatolo P. Neurological manifestations of tuberous sclerosis complex. *Childs Nerv Syst* 12:515–521, 1996.

Menor F, Marti-Bonmati L, Mulas F, et al. Neuroimaging in tuberous sclerosis: a clinico-radiological evaluation in pediatric patients. *Pediatr Radiol* 22:485–489, 1992.

Shepherd CW, Houser OW, Gomez MR. MR findings in tuberous sclerosis complex and correlation with seizure development and mental impairment. *AJNR* 16:149–155, 1995.

Case 118

Clinical Presentation

A 48-year-old man with ataxia presents for MR imaging of the brain and spine.

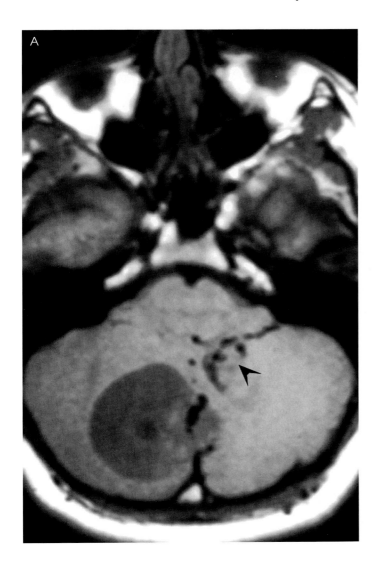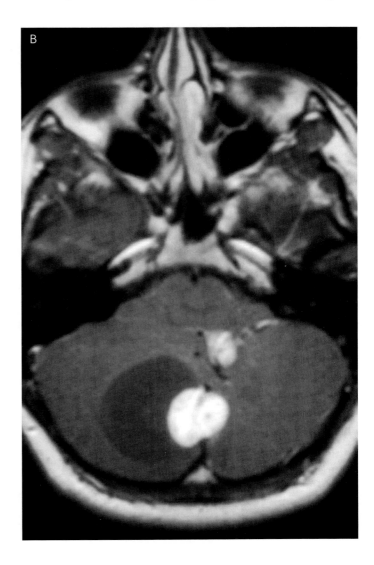

Radiologic Findings

An axial T1-WI of the cerebellum (Fig. A) demonstrates a well-circumscribed low-attenuation mass associated with serpiginous low-signal intensity structures consistent with flow voids. There is a suggestion of a second isointense mass more anteriorly (*arrowhead*). A post-gadolinium T1-WI (Fig. B) demonstrates intense enhancement of a mural nodule along the margin of a large cyst in the right cerebellar hemisphere. In addition, a second enhancing mass is identified more anteriorly.

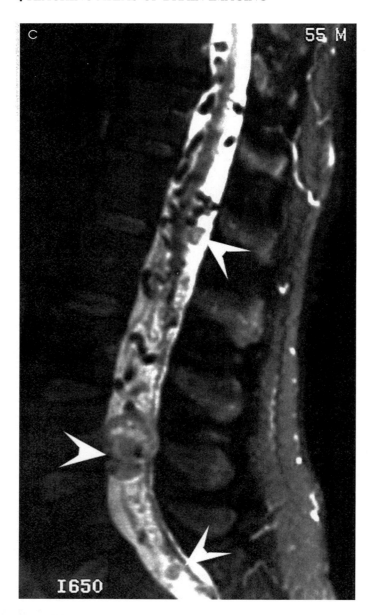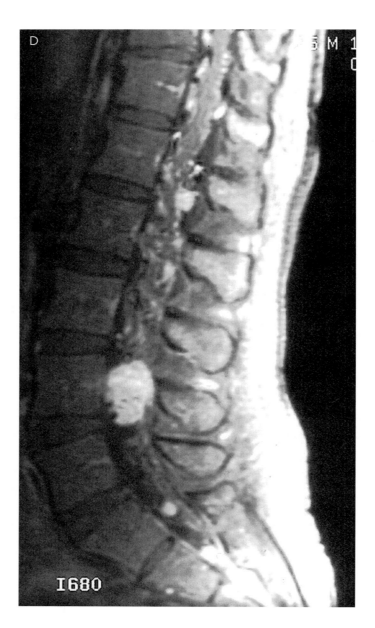

A sagittal fast spin-echo T2-WI of the lumbar spine (Fig. C) reveals strikingly prominent flow voids within the spinal canal, as well as several soft tissue masses (*arrowheads*). A post-gadolinium T1-WI with fat saturation of the lumbar spine (Fig. D) demonstrates innumerable enhancing nodules, as well as prominent flow voids.

Diagnosis

von Hippel-Lindau (VHL) disease

Differential Diagnosis (of cerebellar lesion)

- Juvenile pilocytic astrocytoma (usually not associated with enlarged vessels)
- Cystic medulloblastoma (uncommon, typically a younger patient)
- Cystic metastasis (usually not associated with enlarged vessels, often significant surrounding edema)
- Arachnoid cyst (no enhancement, no nodularity)

Discussion

Background

VHL disease is an autosomal dominant neurocutaneous syndrome with ~90% penetrance. It has a prevalence of approximately 1 per 40,000 people and is characterized by hemangioblastomas of the cerebellum (75%), spinal cord (13%), and medulla (5%), as well as rarely the supratentorial brain (1.5%); retinal angiomas; renal cell carcinoma; pheochromocytoma; angiomas of liver and kidney; cysts of the pancreas, kidney, and liver; papillary cystadenoma of the epididymis; and endolymphatic sac tumors. Relatively few patients exhibit all the manifestations of VHL disease, and approximately 50% of patients will have only one manifestation of the disease.

Etiology

The VHL gene is located on the short arm of chromosome 3 and is thought to encode a tumor suppressor gene.

Clinical Findings

Patients usually present in adulthood. Initial symptoms are often visual and related to retinal angiomas, with a mean age of onset of 25 years. Symptoms from cerebellar hemangioblastomas generally present somewhat later and include headaches, disequilibrium, and/or nausea and vomiting. A clinical diagnosis of VHL requires a family history of VHL and one CNS hemangioblastoma or visceral lesion. In the absence of familial history, either two or more hemangioblastomas or one hemangioblastoma, and one characteristic visceral lesion are required for diagnosis.

Pathology

Gross

• Hemangioblastomas usually consist of a cyst and an associated mural nodule, but they may be solid in 20 to 30% of cases

Microscopic

• A vascular lesion that contains channels lined by cuboidal epithelium interspersed with nests of foamy stromal cells and pericytes
• Mast cells are often present

Imaging Findings

CT

• Low-density cystic mass in posterior fossa
• Isodense mural nodule that intensely enhances postcontrast

MRI

• Cyst may be isointense to CSF or proteinaceous (hyperintense on T1, variable hyper- or hypointensity on T2)
• The mural nodule strongly enhances and usually abuts a pial surface

- Prominent flow voids are generally present in and adjacent to the solid portions of the hemangioblastoma

Angiography

- Vascular nodule in posterior fossa with intense tumor blush
- Supply to the tumor(s) is typically from superior cerebellar, anterior inferior cerebellar or posterior inferior cerebellar arteries, but may be from internal carotid artery and/or external carotid artery branches

Treatment

- Surgical removal of symptomatic lesions
- External beam radiation or radiosurgical ablation may be helpful for multiple or inaccessible lesions

Prognosis

- Median age of death is 49 years; 53% of deaths are due to complications of cerebellar hemangioblastoma, 32% are due to metastatic renal cell carcinoma
- It is important to screen asymptomatic family members for the disease. Screening tools include urinary catecholamines, ophthalmologic exam, MRI of the brain and spine, and abdominal CT ultrasound.
- Purely solid lesions have a worse prognosis than mixed cystic and solid hemangioblastomas

Suggested Readings

Choyke PL, Glenn GM, Walther MM, Patronas NJ, Linehan WM, Zbar B. von Hippel-Lindau disease: genetic, clinical and imaging features. *Radiology* 194:629–642, 1995.

Filling-Katz MR, Choyke PL, Oldfield E, et al. Central nervous system involvement in von Hippel-Lindau disease. *Neurology* 41:41–46, 1991.

Neumann HPH, Eggert HR, Scheremet R, et al. Central nervous system lesions in von Hippel-Lindau syndrome. *J Neurol Neurosurg Psychiatry* 55:898–901, 1992.

Case 119

Clinical Presentation

A 6-year-old female with a long history of seizures has a port-wine nevus on the right side of her face.

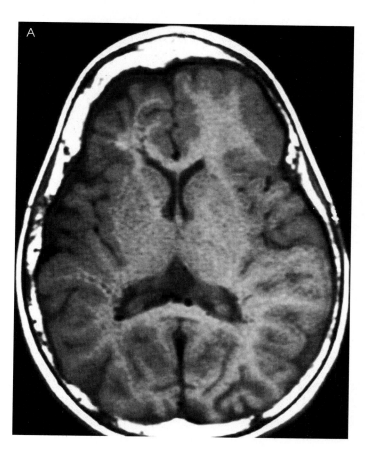

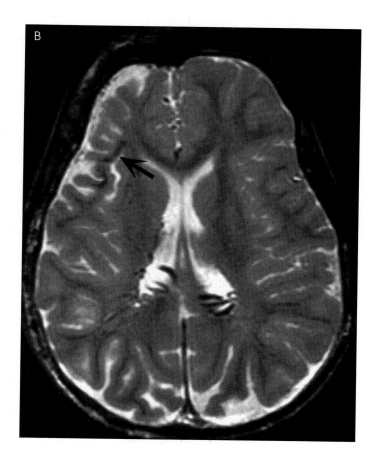

Radiologic Findings

An axial T1-WI (Fig. A) demonstrates volume loss in the right frontal lobe with associated enlargement of the diploic space of the right hemicalvarium, especially the right frontal region. An axial T2-WI (Fig. B) reveals low signal in the parenchyma of the right frontal lobe (arrow) as well as multiple abnormally prominent flow voids along the ependymal surfaces of the atria of the lateral ventricles.

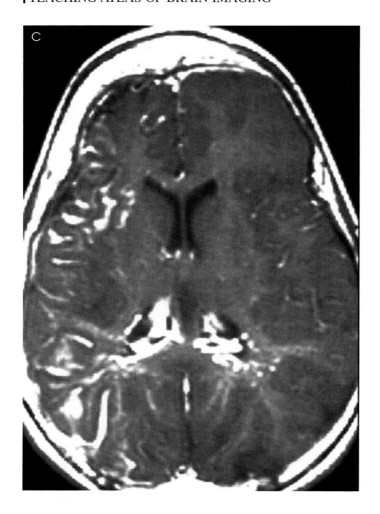

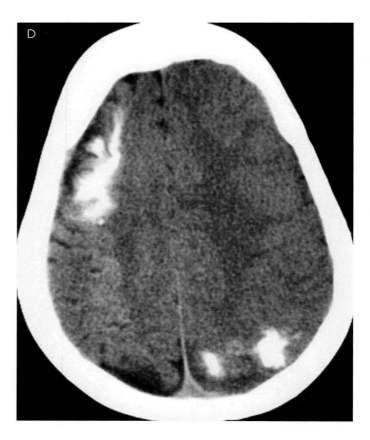

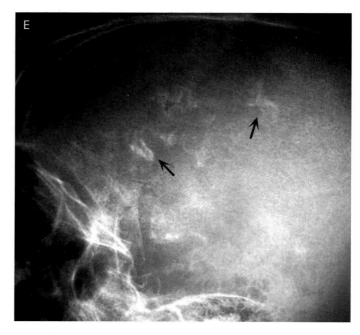

Following gadolinium administration, a T1-WI shows extensive leptomeningeal enhancement over the surface of the right cerebral hemisphere and deep in multiple sulci (Fig. C). There is also prominent enhancement of the subependymal draining vessels. An axial non-contrast CT in this patient (Fig. D) demonstrates abnormal calcification in the cortex of the right frontal lobe, as well as the left parietal lobe. On a lateral plain film of the skull (Fig. E), gyriform "tram-track" calicification can be appreciated (*arrows*).

Diagnosis

Sturge-Weber syndrome

Differential Diagnosis

None: this is a pathognomonic appearance.

Discussion

Background

Sturge-Weber syndrome is a rare neurocutaneous syndrome that includes a facial port-wine stain and associated leptomeningeal angiomatosis. It is generally considered nonhereditary, but familial cases have been reported. The facial angioma usually occurs in the distribution of the first and second divisions of the trigeminal nerve; it is typically unilateral, but may be bilateral. The angiomatous malformation often involves the choroid of the eye as well. Ten percent of children with facial port-wine stains are at risk for leptomeningeal angiomatosis.

Etiology

The gene locus has not yet been mapped. Embryologically, a lack of development of cortical veins is thought to play a role in the development of the leptomeningeal angioma.

Clinical Findings

The "classic clinical triad" includes mental retardation, seizures, and a port-wine facial nevus. Seizures often begin in the first year of life. They are the initial presenting feature in 80% of patients and are often intractable. Hemiparesis is also present. Glaucoma or buphthalmos occurs on the affected side in up to 40% of patients.

Pathology

Gross

- A lack of superficial cortical veins leads to imparied venous drainage, resulting in hemostasis and eventually ischemic injury to the brain

Microscopic

- The meningeal angioma is usually confined to the pia mater and consists of a tangle of small venous channels
- Cortical calcifications occur subjacent to the meningeal angioma, but are usually not present in the first year or two of life. They are most common in the parieto-occipital region but may occur throughout the hemisphere and may be bilateral.

Imaging Findings

CT

- Gyral or "tram-track" cortical calcifications (absent in very young patients) occur most commonly over the posterior hemispheres

- Underlying cortical atrophy
- Enlargement of skull, diploic space, subarachnoid space, sinuses, and mastoid air cells ipsilateral to the port-wine stain
- Contrast-enhanced scan may reveal diffuse staining of the involved cerebral cortex and intense leptomeningeal enhancement if performed prior to the development of cortical calcifications

MR

- Ipsilateral parenchymal atrophy and compensatory skull thickening and sinus enlargement as described above
- Marked gadolinium enhancement in areas of leptomeningeal angiomatosis
- Enlargement of the ipsilateral choroid plexus secondary to angiomatous involvement
- T2 shortening in the white matter underlying the angiomatous malformation, usually seen in infants and possibly due to ischemia. In later life, areas of T2 shortening are usually secondary to calcification.
- Enlargement of deep venous structures ipsilateral to the meningeal angioma

Treatment

- Medical therapy for seizure activity and glaucoma
- In cases of intractable seizures, surgical resection (occasionally hemispherectomy) may be required

Prognosis

Early development of intractable seizures associated with hemiparesis and bilateral involvement are poor prognostic signs

Suggested Readings

Braffman B, Naidich TP. The phakomatoses: part II. Von Hippel-Lindau disease, Sturge-Weber syndrome, and less common conditions. *Neuroimag Clin North Am* 4:325–348, 1994.

Oakes J. The natural history of patients with the Sturge-Weber syndrome. *Pediatr Neurosurg* 18:287–290, 1992.

Wasenko JJ, Rosenbloom SA, Duchesneau PM, et al. The Sturge-Weber syndrome: comparison of MR and CT characteristics. *AJNR* 11:131–134, 1990.

Case 120

Clinical Presentation

A 3-year-old child with a giant congenital scalp nevus presents for evaluation.

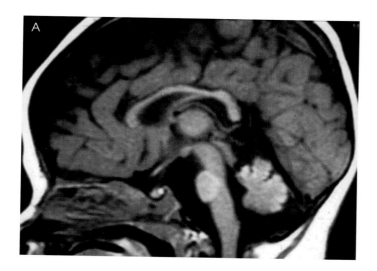

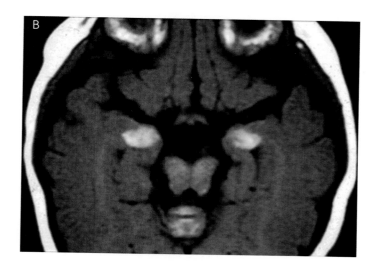

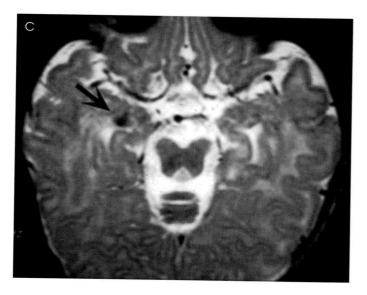

Radiologic Findings

A sagittal T1-WI (Fig. A) demonstrates abnormal T1 shortening involving the surface of the pons and the superior and posterior vermis. There is associated pontine and cerebellar hypogenesis. An axial T1-WI (Fig. B) reveals T1 shortening in the mesial temporal lobes bilaterally. An axial T2-WI (Fig. C) shows a focus of T2 shortening in the right mesial temporal lobe (*arrow*).

Diagnosis

Neurocutaneous melanosis

Differential Diagnosis

None: this is a pathognomonic appearance in a child with a large cutaneous melanotic nevus.

Discussion

Background

Neurocutaneous melanosis is a rare, nonfamilial congenital syndrome that consists of large melanocytic nevi and benign or malignant melanotic lesions of the CNS. Over 100 cases have been reported, and criteria for diagnosis include large or multiple (three or more) congenital nevi in association with CNS melanoma or meningeal melanosis (note that a "large" nevus is defined as having a diameter equal to or larger than 20 cm in an adult, 9 cm in the scalp of infant, and/or 6 cm on the body of an infant), no cutaneous melanoma except in patients where the examined CNS lesions are histologically benign, and no CNS melanoma except in patients where the examined cutaneous lesions are histologically benign (i.e., the CNS lesion cannot be a metastasis from another source).

Etiology

Neurocutaneous melanosis is thought to represent an embryonal neuroectodermal dysplasia, possibly due to a disorder of migration of melanocyte precursors or abnormal expression of melanin-producing genes within the skin and leptomeninges.

Clinical Findings

Most patients are asymptomatic. Those with symptoms may demonstrate seizures, signs of increased intracranial pressure, cranial nerve palsies, hemiparesis, and psychiatric disturbances/mental retardation.

Pathology

Gross

- The leptomeninges may appear abnormally dark

Microscopic

- Basilar meninges show nodularity and a markedly increased number of melanocytes
- Leptomeningeal melanocytes can infiltrate neural tissue via perforating vessels

Imaging Findings

CT

- Usually normal unless there has been malignant transformation

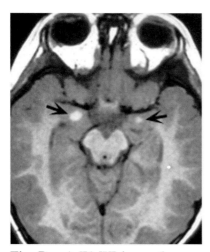

Fig. D. A T1-WI in another patient with neurocutaneous melanosis demonstrates abnormal T1 shortening in the mesial temporal lobes (*arrows*).

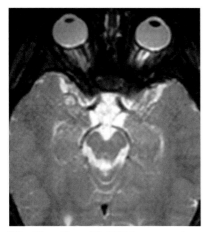

Fig. E. On a T2-WI (same patient as Fig. D), no definite signal abnormality is seen in the mesial temporal lobes.

MR

- Foci of T1 shortening are present within the pia mater as well as the parenchyma, involving predominently the cerebellum and anterior paramedian temporal lobes (especially the amygdala). The pons and colliculi may be involved as well.
- T2 shortening is usually absent or mild (Figs. D and E)
- The leptomeninges of the brain (convexities, basal cisterns, posterior fossa) and/or spine (posterior aspect) occasionally enhance post-gadolinium

Treatment

- Ventricular shunting in patients with hydrocephalus (must be careful to prevent seeding of potential CNS melanoma into the peritoneal cavity)
- Resection of malignant melanoma if mass effect is present

Prognosis

Poor if melanoma develops

Suggested Readings

Barkovich AJ, Frieden IJ, Williams ML. MR of neurocutaneous melanosis. *AJNR* 15:859–867, 1994.

Byrd SE, Darling CF, Tomita T, et al. MR imaging of symptomatic neurocutaneous melanosis in children. *Pediatr Radiol* 27:39–44, 1997.

Demirci A, Kawamura Y, Gordon S, et al. MR of parenchymal neurocutaneous melanosis. *AJNR* 16:603–606, 1995.

Section X

Congenital Malformations/Syndromes

A.   Supratentorial

Case 121

Clinical Presentation

A child is referred for MR imaging because of mild developmental delay.

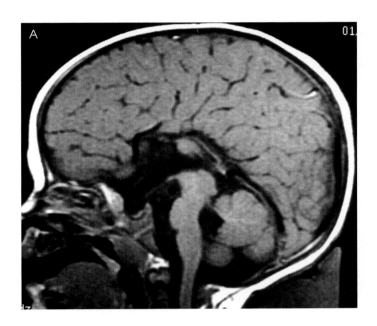

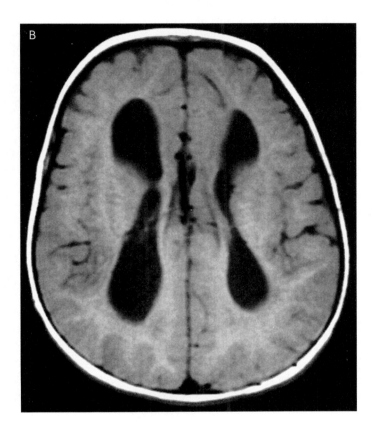

Radiologic Findings

A sagittal T1-WI (Fig. A) demonstrates absence of the corpus callosum. Sulci radiate to the third ventricle because of the lack of formation of the cingulate sulcus. An axial T1-WI (Fig. B) demonstrates mild ventriculomegaly and a parallel configuration to the lateral ventricles.

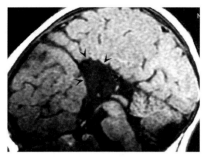

Fig. C. A sagittal T1-WI demonstrates absence of the corpus callosum and extension of the superior third ventricle into the interhemispheric fissure (*arrowheads*).

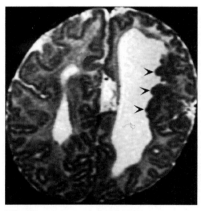

Fig. D. An axial T2-WI (same patient as Fig. C) demonstrates multiple nodules isointense to gray matter consistent with subependymal heterotopia along the surface of the left lateral ventricle (*arrowheads*). The overlying cortex of the left frontal lobe is also abnormal, with a pattern consistent with polymicrogyria. This female infant had typical clinical and imaging findings of Aicardi syndrome.

Diagnosis

Agenesis of the corpus callosum

Differential Diagnosis

None: this is a pathognomonic appearance

Discussion

Background

Callosal dysgenesis may be considered in three distinct categories: callosal agenesis, hypogenesis, and hypoplasia. In callosal agenesis, the corpus callosum is completely absent. In callosal hypogenesis, the corpus callosum is variably formed. Callosal hypoplasia refers to a corpus callosum that is completely formed but focally or generally small in size; this usually occurs in the setting of cerebral cortical dysgenesis, with poor development and/or abnormal myelination of crossing callosal fibers. Characteristic features of agenesis or hypogenesis of the corpus callosum include the presence of Probst bundles, representing the uncrossed callosal fibers running parallel to the interhemispheric fissure in the medial walls of the lateral ventricles; colpocephaly, abnormal dilatation of the ventricular atria and occipital horns; and a high-riding third ventricle opening into the interhemispheric fissure or an interhemispheric "cyst."

Etiology/Embryology

Formation of the corpus callosum begins with formation of the massa commissuralis between the lamina reuniens in the dorsal aspect of the lamina terminalis at 10 to 12 weeks' fetal gestation. If this structure fails to form, then callosal fibers cannot decussate. Once the induction bed develops, it must then be maintained normally, or interruption of callosal development will occur. It is generally accepted that the corpus callosum forms in an overall anterior to posterior manner, although in fact the posterior aspect of the genu forms first, followed by the body, the anterior genu, the splenium, and finally the rostrum. Therefore, the anterior callosum is typically present in cases of callosal hypogenesis although it may be malformed and the rostrum is typically absent. The first callosal axons cross at the level of the foramen of Monro. By 20 weeks' gestation, the corpus callosum assumes a form similar to an adult as the rostrum forms.

Clinical Findings

Patients with isolated callosal agenesis are typically asymptomatic, with cognitive abnormalities detected only with sophisticated neuropsychiatric testing. Symptoms are usually related to associated conditions (see below) that may lead to developmental delay, mental retardation, and/or seizures. Hydrocephalus may result if a loculation related to the interhemispheric cyst enlarges and compresses the ventricular system.

Associated Conditions

Conditions that have a high incidence of associated callosal agenesis or hypogenesis include Dandy-Walker malformation, Chiari II malformation, septo-optic dysplasia, and anomalies of neural migration. Aicardi's syndrome (Figs. C and D) is

Pearls

- MR with its multiplanar capability is much more sensitive to callosal anomalies than is CT; mild hypogenesis may be easily missed on an axial CT scan.

- A congenital lipoma may be associated with a hypogenetic corpus callosum, as the presence of this tissue interferes with normal callosal development.

- Colpocephaly likely results from absence of the compact fibers of the callosal splenium, which allows the ventricular atria and occipital horns to expand into the soft white matter surrounding them while the basal ganglia maintain the shape of the ventricles more anteriorly.

Pitfalls

- The unmyelinated neonatal corpus callosum may normally be quite thin.

- Callosal dysgenesis may be atypical; in holoprosencephaly an isolated splenium may be present, while in some patients with complete callosal agenesis a prominent hippocampal commissure may mimic a callosal splenium.

a syndrome defined by the diagnostic tetrad of infantile spasms, chorioretinal lacunae, mental retardation, and agenesis of the corpus callosum. It is seen only in females and is transmitted as an X-linked dominant trait with male lethality.

Imaging Findings

Characteristic findings of agenesis of the corpus callosum are generally better appreciated on MR than on CT and include:

- Absence of all portions of the corpus callosum
- Parallel configuration of the lateral ventricles
- The longitudinal bundles of Probst lie lateral to the cingulate gyri and invaginate the medial borders of the lateral ventricles, giving them a characteristic lateral convexity. The bundles of Probst represent the axons that would normally cross the corpus callosum and are best seen in the coronal plane.
- The third ventricle is located higher than normal and is continuous with the interhemispheric fissure
- The cingulate gyri are everted, and the cingulate sulcus does not form; this results in radiation of the medial hemispheric sulci into the third ventricle, best seen on midline sagittal images
- Colpocephaly (dilatation of the trigones and occipital horns of the lateral ventricles) is frequent

Treatment

- Management of associated hydrocephalus
- Management of associated syndromic complications

Prognosis

Excellent for isolated callosal agenesis—if associated with a syndrome, the prognosis is usually determined by the associated syndrome

Suggested Readings

Barkovich AJ. Apparent atypical callosal dysgenesis: analysis of MR findings in six cases and their relationship to holoprosencephaly. *AJNR* 11:333–339, 1990.

Curnes JT, Laster DW, Koubek TD, et al. MRI of corpus callosum syndromes. *AJNR* 7:617–622, 1986.

Kier EL, Truwit CL. The normal and abnormal genu of the corpus callosum: an evolutionary, embryologic, anatomic, and MR analysis. *AJNR* 17:1631–1641, 1996.

Case 122

Clinical Presentation

A 1-day-old female is referred for MR evaluation of the brain because of midline facial anomalies.

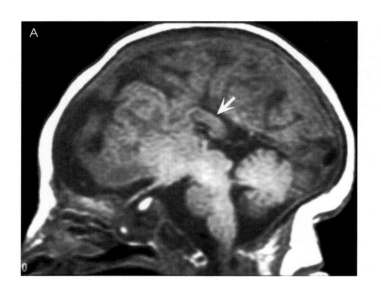

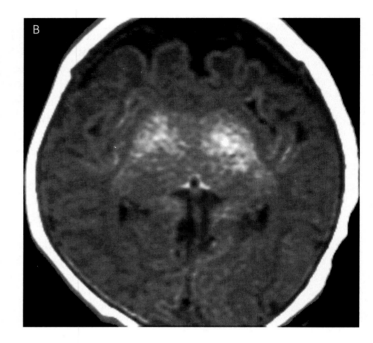

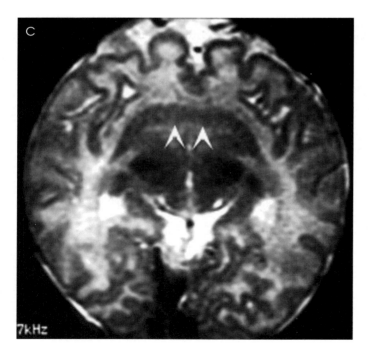

Radiologic Findings

A sagittal T1-WI (Fig. A) demonstrates an abnormal corpus callosum, with formation of the splenium (*arrow*) but absence of the body and genu. An axial

Pearls

- HP is the only condition in which the anterior corpus callosum is malformed in the presence of a normal-appearing posterior corpus callosum.

- The septum pellucidum is absent in all forms of HP, and patients with mild lobar HP may also be classified as having septo-optic dysplasia.

Pitfalls

- The face may be normal even with alobar HP, as the severity of the brain malformation does not necessarily predict the severity of facial anomalies.

- The subtypes of HP represent a continuum rather than discrete categories; therefore, classification of a given patient may be difficult.

- Midline interhemispheric fusion in the presence of nearly normal anterior and posterior interhemispheric fissures has been described and is considered a variant of HP.

T1-WI image (Fig. B) shows fusion of the thalami, absence of the anterior falx and continuity of white matter tracts across the midline. An axial T2-WI (Fig. C) also demonstrates lack of an interhemispheric fissure anteriorly. The anterior commissure (*arrowheads*) is strikingly prominent.

Diagnosis

Holoprosencephaly (HP), semilobar

Differential Diagnosis

Of semilobar HP:

- Lobar HP (see discussion below)

Of alobar HP:

- Hydranencephaly (destruction of cerebral hemispheres in part or in total, thalami may be normal, no facial anomalies)
- Hydrocephalus, severe (thin cortical mantle usually identifiable, septum pellucidum may be very thin but is present)
- Agenesis/hypogenesis of the corpus callosum (if any callosum has formed, it should be the anterior aspect not the posterior aspect; lacks fusion of thalami)

Discussion

Background

HP results from failure of the normal cleavage of the prosencephalon or forebrain into two discrete hemispheres. The failure of cleavage is of variable extent and results in a spectrum of abnormalities that ranges from minimal fusion of the basal forebrain to complete fusion of the hemispheres and a single horseshoe-shaped monoventricle. Patients with HP are divided into three subgroups (lobar, semilobar, and alobar) (Table 1) of increasingly severe malformation, but this disorder should be thought of as a continuum rather than strict divisions. The corpus callosum is always anomalous. The corpus callosum is completely absent in severe forms and partially formed in less severe forms. Typically, the posterior portion of the corpus callosum is formed, and the anterior portion is absent. In contrast, the anterior corpus callosum is normal and the posterior portion is malformed in callosal anomalies outside the HP spectrum. Facial anomalies are also common and typically manifest as hypoplasia of the central face.

Etiology

A failure of cleavage of the embryonic forebrain into discrete hemispheres leads to HP. As complete cleavage occurs over 1 to 5 months of gestation, the time at which this process is disturbed defines the spectrum of anomalies seen in HP. Chromosomal anomalies are found in approximately 40% of cases of HP, most commonly trisomy 13. Familial cases have also been reported.

Clinical Findings

Alobar and semilobar HP may be detected by prenatal sonography. Midline facial anomalies such as cleft lip and/or palate and nasal anomalies that are detected at

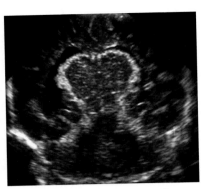

Fig. D. A coronal image from a transfontanel neonatal sonogram demonstrates fusion of the thalami.

Table 1. Features of Subtypes of Holoprosencephaly

Alobar
  Microcephaly
  Interhemispheric fissure is absent
  Falx cerebri is absent
  Septum pellucidum is absent
  Corpus callosum is absent
  Olfactory bulbs and tracts are absent
  Fusion of gray and white matter across midline
  Thalami and basal ganglia are fused
  Large dorsal cyst in continuity with a monoventricle may be present
  Cortical sulci are not well formed
  Migration anomalies are common
  Azygous anterior cerebral artery
Semilobar
  Posterior aspect of interhemispheric fissure is formed
  Falx cerebri is partially present
  Monoventricle shows some differentiation into two components
  Rudimentary temporal horns may be present
  Partial thalamic cleavage gives rise to a small third ventricle
  The posterior aspect of the corpus callosum may be formed
  Septum pellucidum, olfactory bulbs, and olfactory tracts are absent
Lobar
  Interhemispheric fissure is well formed except in basal frontal region
  Falx may be deficient anteriorly or normal
  Lateral ventricles assume a normal or near-normal shape
  Anterior aspect of the corpus callosum is deficient
  Septum pellucidum is absent
  Fusion of the cingulate gyri may be observed

birth often lead to screening examination of the brain, commonly with transfontanel sonography (Fig. D) followed by MR. Other facial features associated with HP include hypotelorism, a single midline incisor, and formation of a midline proboscis (a rudimentary soft tissue structure resembling a nose but associated with abnormal formation of the nasal passages). Neonates with alobar or semilobar HP are hypotonic and have poor neonatal reflexes, and as infants they are developmentally delayed and typically have seizures.

Imaging Findings

The imaging findings vary with the severity of the malformation. MR is more sensitive than CT in evaluating:

- Formation of the interhemispheric fissure (absent to nearly complete)
- Presence of the falx cerebri (absent to nearly normal)
- Fusion of the thalami and basal ganglia (variable in extent)
- Continuity of gray and white matter across the midline
- Variable ventricular differentiation (ranges from a horseshoe-shaped monoventricle to nearly normal morphology)
- Absence of the septum pellucidum
- Callosal anomalies (vary from absent to partly formed posteriorly to nearly normal)

Treatment

- Supportive care
- Chromosomal analysis is important to genetic counseling

Prognosis

- The severity of the malformation is inversely correlated with the length of survival
- Children with lobar HP may have normal or nearly normal long-term survival, while children with alobar HP often die in the neonatal period or infancy

Suggested Readings

Castillo M, Bouldin TW, Scatliff JH, Suzuki K. Alobar holoprosencephaly. *AJNR* 14:1151–1156, 1993.

Croen LA, Shaw GM, Lammer EJ. Holoprosencephaly: epidemiologic and clinical characteristics of a California population. *Am J Med Genet* 64:465–472, 1996.

Oba H, Barkovich AJ. Holoprosencephaly: an analysis of callosal formation and its relation to development of the interhemispheric fissure. *AJNR* 16:453–460, 1995.

Case 123

Clinical Presentation

A 10-year-old boy with poor visual acuity presents following a seizure.

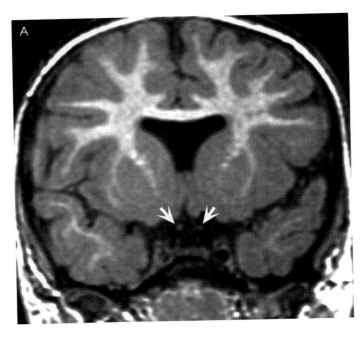

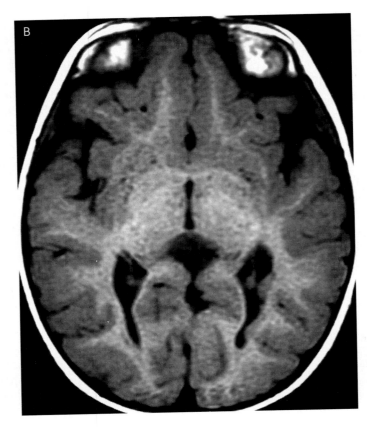

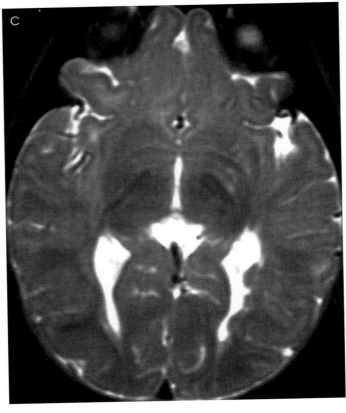

Radiologic Findings

A coronal image from a volumetric T1-weighted gradient-echo sequence (Fig. A) demonstrates absence of the septum pellucidum and hypoplasia of the optic nerves (*arrows*). Axial T1-WI (Fig. B) and T2-WI (Fig. C) demonstrate nodules along the surface of the left lateral ventricle that are isointense to gray matter, diagnostic of subependymal heterotopia.

Diagnosis

Septo-optic dysplasia

Differential Diagnosis

• Holoprosencephaly, lobar (may be indistinguishable [see below], but typically the interhemispheric fissure is abnormal, the falx is partly deficient, and callosal anomalies are present)
• Severe, longstanding hydrocephalus with pressure necrosis of the septum pellucidum and optic nerve atrophy (clinical history, evidence of severe hydrocephalus)
• Isolated septal deficiency (rare, need to search for associated anomalies)

Discussion

Background

Septo-optic dysplasia, also known as de Morsier's syndrome, consists of hypoplasia or aplasia of the septum pellucidum and hypoplasia of the optic nerves. Septo-optic dysplasia is more common in females than in males. This syndrome is heterogeneous and is likely the end result of a number of different abnormalities, including genetic abnormalities and in utero ischemic injuries. Several subgroups of patients with septo-optic dysplasia have been identified. One group has a high incidence of schizencephaly and gray matter heterotopia in association with partial absence of the septum pellucidum and hypothalamic dysfunction. A second group may actually represent a mild form of lobar holoprosencephaly, as hypoplasia of the anterior falx cerebri and the genu of the corpus callosum have been described. A third subset includes patients with an ectopic posterior pituitary.

Etiology

Multiple causes are likely. The vascular vulnerability of the components affected in the syndrome and a decreased maternal age effect similar to that of other abnormalities with presumed vascular origins suggest a vascular disruption sequence possibly involving the proximal trunk of the anterior cerebral artery. However, familial cases in a highly consanguineous pedigree support a heritable basis for at least some forms of this syndrome.

Clinical Findings

Visual findings include decreased visual acuity and nystagmus, but vision may be normal. Hypothalamic-pituitary dysfunction leading to growth retardation is present in two thirds of patients.

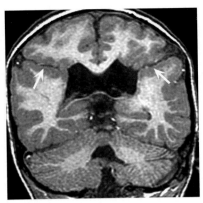

Fig. D. A coronal SPGR image demonstrates absence of the septum pellucidum, as well as bilateral gray matter-lined clefts (*white arrows*) consistent with bilateral schizencephaly.

Imaging Findings

CT

- Absent septum pellucidum
- Optic canals may be small
- Thinning of the optic nerves may be observed

MR

- Hypoplasia or complete absence of the septum pellucidum
- Boxlike frontal horns, often with inferior pointing
- Hypoplasia of the optic nerves is visible in approximately 50% of cases
- Hypoplasia of the optic chiasm and hypothalamus may lead to dilatation of the anterior recesses of the third ventricle
- Associated schizencephaly (Fig. D), polymicrogyria, and/or gray matter heterotopia may be seen
- The fornices are present but low in location, typically attaching to the postero-inferior aspect of the splenium of the corpus callosum

Treatment

- Management of associated problems such as seizures in association with schizencephaly
- Hormone replacement if pituitary dysfunction is present

Prognosis

- Varies with severity of associated malformations
- Children with septo-optic dysplasia and hypocortisolism are at risk of sudden death in the setting of febrile illness

Suggested Readings

Barkovich AJ, Fram EK, Norman D. Septo-optic dysplasia: MR imaging. *Radiology* 171:189–192, 1989.

Barkovich AJ, Norman D. Absence of the septum pellucidum: a useful sign in the diagnosis of congenital brain malformations. *AJNR* 9:1107–1114, 1988.

Fitz CR. Holoprosencephaly and septo-optic dysplasia. *Neuroimag Clin North Am* 4:263–281, 1994.

Case 124

Clinical Presentation

A 5-year-old child with severe cognitive and motor retardation presents for imaging evaluation.

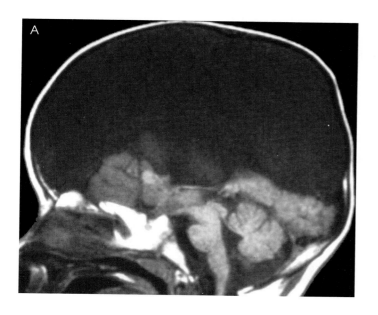
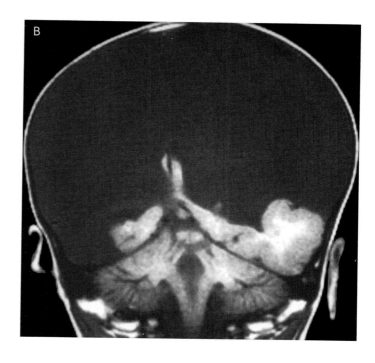

Radiologic Findings

A sagittal T1-WI (Fig. A) demonstrates fluid filling most of the cranium in the expected location of the cerebral hemispheres, with only portions of frontal and occipital lobes present. The posterior fossa is unremarkable, though the upper cervical spinal cord appears thinned. A coronal T1-WI (Fig. B) shows residual portions of the temporal lobes bilaterally.

Diagnosis

Hydranencephaly

Differential Diagnosis

- Severe hydrocephalus (thin cortical mantle usually present)
- Alobar holoprosencephaly (absent falx, fused thalami, monoventricle)
- Multicystic encephalomalacia (irregular septations between fluid-filled spaces)

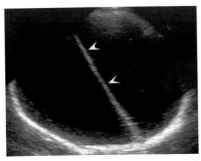

Fig. C. An image from a prenatal ultrasound demonstrates absence of the cerebral hemispheres bilaterally. Artifactual echos are present on the inner aspect of the calvarium, but no cortical mantle is seen. Note the presence of the falx cerebri (*arrowheads*). *(Case courtesy of Ruth B. Goldstein, M.D., San Francisco, CA.)*

Pearls

• Posterior circulation structures may be affected in cases where the posterior cerebral artery originates from the internal carotid artery.

• The immature human brain tends to undergo dissolution and cavitation, while older brains undergo gliosis and scarring.

Pitfalls

• Hydranencephaly may be confused with severe hydrocephalus (Fig. D), so look for the presence of a thinned cortical mantle in hydrocephalus.

• Hydranencephaly may be confused with holoprosencephaly. Remember that the anterior falx is deficient in cases of semilobar or alobar holoprosencephaly but is typically present in hydranencephaly.

Discussion

Background

Hydranencephaly is characterized by destruction of the cerebral hemispheres and replacement by a thin membranous sac filled with CSF and necrotic debris. This destruction is thought to result from occlusion of both supraclinoid internal carotid arteries, with or without concomitant encephalitis, during the second trimester of gestation. A normal falx is usually present and posterior fossa structures are typically well developed. The thin sac is considered to represent the intact leptomeninges along with remnants of cortex and white matter. Hydranencephaly is relatively more common among babies born to young mothers, and disorders related to prenatal vascular disruptions have been observed to show a decreased maternal age effect.

Etiology

The exact cause of hydranencephaly is unknown, but it is thought to result from bialteral in utero disruption of the anterior circulation. The striking loss of brain substance (dissolution and cavitation) is reproducible experimentally when bilateral injuries to the carotid arteries are induced early in the second trimester.

Clinical Findings

Hydranencephaly is easily diagnosed at prenatal sonography (Fig. C). If undetected prenatally, hydranencephaly presents in infancy with irritability, infantile spasms, and retarded motor development.

Imaging Findings

Similar findings are present on ultrasound, CT, and MR:

• Absence of the cerebral hemispheres with preservation of parts of the inferomedial aspects of the frontal and temporal lobes
• The falx cerebri is usually present
• Relative preservation of the thalami and cerebellum
• The brainstem is usually atrophic

Treatment

• Supportive care
• CSF diversion may be indicated in cases of progressive macrocephaly due to superimposed hydrocephalus

Prognosis

Death in infancy is common

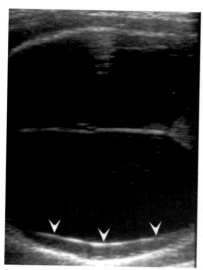

Fig. D. An image from a prenatal ultrasound in a patient with severe hydrocephalus secondary to aqueductal stenosis demonstrates marked enlargement of the lateral ventricles. The falx is present in the midline. Note the presence of a severely compressed cortical mantle (*arrowheads*). (*Case courtesy of Ruth B. Goldstein, M.D., San Francisco, CA.*)

Suggested Readings

Lubinsky MS, Adkins W, Kaveggia EG. Decreased maternal age with hydranencephaly. *Am J Med Genet* 69:232–234, 1997.

Raybaud C. Destructive lesions of the brain. *Neuroradiology* 25:265–291, 1983.

Wintour EM, Lewitt M, McFarlane A, et al. Experimental hydranencephaly in the ovine fetus. *Acta Neuropath* 91:537–544, 1996.

Case 125

Clinical Presentation

At birth, a neonate is noted to have a large mass emanating from the posterior skull.

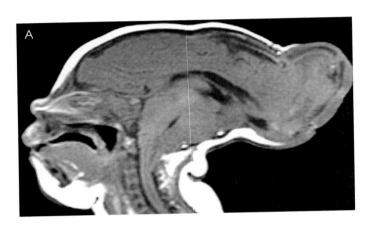

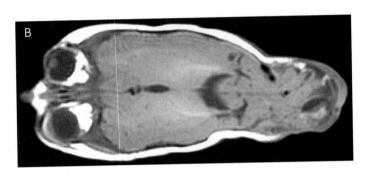

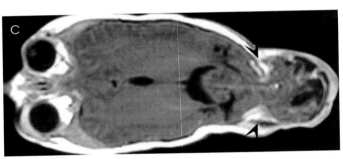

Radiologic Findings

A sagittal T1-WI (Fig. A) demonstrates herniation of brain and meninges through a large parieto-occipital bony defect. The corpus callosum is very thin and poorly seen. Note also cerebellar tonsillar herniation through the foramen magnum, consistent with a Chiari I malformation. An axial T1-WI (Fig. B) demonstrates striking dolichocephaly. The mass of herniated brain tissue has areas that appear cystic, consistent with gliosis and encephalomalacia. The mass is covered by a thickened membrane, but it is not covered by normal skin or subcutaneous fat. An axial post-gadolinium T1-WI (Fig. C) demonstrates enhancement of dural venous structures (*arrowheads*), which have partly herniated through the large bony defect.

Diagnosis

Occipital cephalocele

Differential Diagnosis

None: this is a pathognomonic appearance

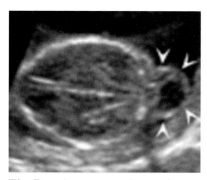

Fig. D. A transverse image from a prenatal ultrasound demonstrates herniation of brain, CSF, and leptomeninges through a defect in the occipital bone (*arrowheads*). Typical meningoencephalocele. *(Case courtesy of Ruth B. Goldstein, M.D., San Francisco, CA.)*

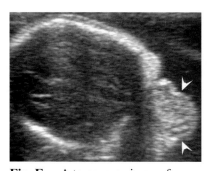

Fig. E. A transverse image from a prenatal ultrasound demonstrates a solid echogenic mass protruding through a defect in the occipital bone, consistent with a solid cephalocele (*arrowheads*). *(Case courtesy of Ruth B. Goldstein, M.D., San Francisco, CA.)*

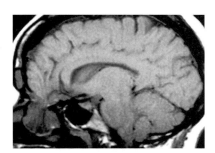

Fig. F. A sagittal T1-WI in a 23-year-old woman with chronic nasal stuffiness demonstrates herniation of brain and meninges through a defect in the floor of the anterior cranial fossa.

Discussion

Background

A cephalocele is a congenital defect in the cranium and dura with extracranial herniation of intracranial structures. The incidence of cephaloceles is approximately 1.9 per 10,000 births. Cephaloceles are described by the site of the cranial defect through which the herniation occurs. In the United States, 66 to 89% of cephaloceles affect the occipital region. Four subtypes of cephalocele are recognized:

1. Cranial meningocele: protruding structures consist solely of leptomeninges and CSF
2. Cranial gliocele: protruding structures consist solely of a glial-lined cyst containing CSF
3. Cranial meningoencephalocele: protruding structures include brain, CSF, and leptomeninges
4. Atretic cephalocele: a forme fruste of a cephalocele that usually contains no cerebral tissue but may include neural remnants. It is characterized by a skull defect in association with a flat or nodular lesion and often a hairless patch in the midline. Typical locations are near the vertex (parietal form) or cephalic to the external occipital protruberance (occipital form).

Etiology

Occipital cephaloceles are related to neural tube defects. Approximately 7% of children with occipital cephaloceles have a concurrent myelomeningocele. The majority of cases are of sporadic occurrence, and their cause is unknown. In the laboratory, cephaloceles have been related to exposure to radiation, excess vitamin A, and folic acid antagonists.

Clinical Findings

Cephaloceles may be detected at prenatal ultrasonography (Figs. D and E). Cephaloceles that are not identified prenatally typically present at birth, although basal cephaloceles may remain clinically occult for many years (Figs. F and G).

Associated Findings

Associated findings include hydrocephalus and agenesis or hypogenesis of the corpus callosum. The anterior commissure, septum pellucidum, and fornices are absent in 80% of cases. The vermis and cerebellar hemispheres may be malformed or absent, and the Dandy-Walker malformation occurs in approximately 17% of occipital cephaloceles. The Meckel-Gruber syndrome is an autosomal recessive condition that is associated with occipital encephalocele (in 80% of cases), along with holoprosencephaly, orofacial clefting, retinal dysplasia, polydactyly, and polycystic kidneys.

Pathology

Gross

- Vary tremendously in size, shape, and extent of skin cover
- May be broad-based or pedunculated

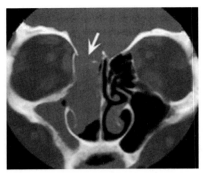

Fig. G. A coronal CT scan (same patient as Fig. F) demonstrates a bony defect in the roof of the ethmoid (*arrow*).

Pearls

• Most cephaloceles occur as isolated anomalies, unassociated with syndromes, though other midline defects such as cleft palate and tracheoesophageal fistulas have been observed.

• The so-called "Chiari III" malformation consists of an occipitocervical cephalocele, with herniation of posterior fossa contents (cerebellum, possibly brainstem) through a posterior spina bifida at the C1-2 level. This condition is very rare.

Pitfall

• An ethmoidal cephalocele may be misdiagnosed as a nasal polyp on a screening sinus CT scan. Look carefully for a bony defect in the floor of the anterior cranial fossa to rule out cephalocele.

Microscopic

• Cephaloceles typically contain disorganized neural and glial tissue

Imaging Findings

CT

• Focal skull defect
• Sac containing variable amounts of brain and CSF

MR

• Focal defect in the calvarium
• Herniation of portions of the cerebral hemisphere(s) through the bony defect, often asymmetrically
• The residual intracranial content is rotated, elongated, and shows progressive constriction toward the hernia orifice
• Herniating tissues may show evidence of ischemia/infarction, with increased signal intensity on T2-WI
• Hydrocephalus is common

Treatment

• Small lesions may be observed, as they may disappear following ventricular shunting or closure of an associated myelomeningocele
• Larger lesions are generally resected to improve cosmesis and patient management, as well as to protect the child from ulceration of the sac with subsequent hemorrhage or infection

Prognosis

• In older series, 50% of patients died, and 76% of survivors were mentally retarded. More recently, mortality has been reduced to the 20 to 30% range.
• Prognosis depends heavily on the site, size, and contents of the cephalocele, as well as the presence of any associated brain malformations

Suggested Readings

Martinez-Lage JF, Poza M, Sola J, et al. The child with a cephalocele: etiology, neuroimaging, and outcome. *Childs Nerv Syst* 12:540–550, 1996.

Naidich TP, Altman NR, Braffman BH, McLone DG, Zimmerman RA. Cephaloceles and related malformations. *AJNR* 13:655–690, 1992.

Section X

Congenital Malformations/Syndromes

B. Infratentorial

Case 126

Clinical Presentation

A 5-year-old male has a history of occipital headaches that increase during exertion and crying.

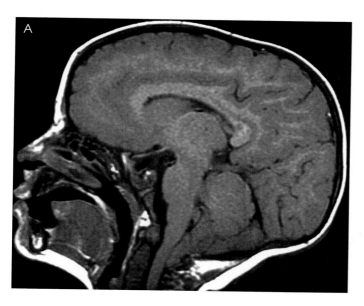

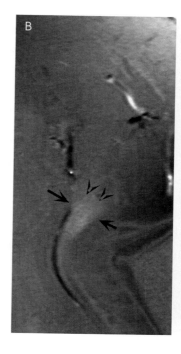

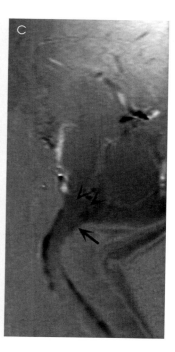

Radiologic Findings

A sagittal T1-WI (Fig. A) demonstrates descent of the cerebellar tonsils through the foramen magnum and absence of CSF within the cisterna magna. The tonsils appear pointed and extend to the level of C2-3. Sagittal cine phase-contrast images (Figs. B and C) with the flow-sensitive gradient in the superior-inferior direction were obtained. By convention, high-signal intensity is associated with superior-to-inferior motion; low signal is associated with inferior-to-superior motion. These two images, at the same slice location, were obtained at different points in the cardiac cycle. Figure B was obtained during systole and demonstrates absence of normal CSF flow at the foramen magnum (*arrows*) and foramen of Magendie. The high-signal intensity of the cerebellar tonsils indicates abnormal downward tonsillar motion (*arrowheads*). Figure C, obtained during diastole, demonstrates abnormal reduced signal intensity of the cerebellar tonsils indicating upward movement (*arrowheads*), as well as absence of CSF flow within both the posterior and the anterior aspects of the spinal subarachnoid space (*arrow*).

Pearls

- MR is much more sensitive than CT to the diagnosis of Chiari I malformation because of imaging in the sagittal plane and the lack of beam-hardening artifact.

- Alterations in CSF flow dynamics may contribute to symptoms and to syrinx formation in patients with Chiari I malformation. Cine phase-contrast MR studies directly assess the flow of CSF at the foramen magnum and may help predict which patients will benefit from posterior fossa decompression.

Pitfalls

- Intracranial CSF hypotension is not uncommonly mistaken for a Chiari I malformation.

- In children under 15 years of age, the tonsils may normally extend 6 mm below the foramen magnum.

- Tonsillar descent may be easily overlooked on axial CT studies.

Diagnosis

Chiari I malformation

Differential Diagnosis

- Intracranial hypotension (diffuse dural enhancement, prominence of dural venous sinuses)
- Tonsillar herniation due elevated intracranial pressure or posterior fossa mass (signs of downward herniation or a mass lesion, effacement of dural sinuses)

Discussion

Background

The Chiari I malformation consists of an abnormal caudal extension of the cerebellar tonsils below the foramen magnum. The true incidence of this abnormality is difficult to determine because many patients have mild or no symptoms. The foramen magnum is defined by a line drawn from the basion to the opisthion, and normally the cerebellar tonsils lie above this line. Tonsillar ectopia of 5 mm or less is not thought to be clinically significant, while tonsillar ectopia of greater than 5 mm is often clinically significant. The Chiari I malformation is usually isolated but can be seen in association with other anomalies that result in a small posterior fossa such as multiple craniosynostosis syndromes.

Etiology

The cause of the Chiari I malformation is uncertain, but most hypotheses implicate a primarily small and shallow posterior fossa due to a dysplastic or underdeveloped occipital bone that cannot accommodate the normal volume of cerebellar tissue. In some patients, the tonsillar descent may be due to in utero hydrocephalus, with the tonsils retaining the low-lying position and pointed configuration they had when myelination occurred, despite resolution of the hydrocephalus.

Clinical Findings

Patients are usually asymptomatic until late childhood or early adult life. Common presenting signs and symptoms include headache (often occipital); worsening of headache or neck pain with neck flexion or extension, coughing, or the Valsalva maneuver; weakness in the extremities (upper>lower); unsteadiness and dysequilibrium; and nystagmus (50%). Less common symptoms include cranial neuropathies (trigeminal neuralgia most common) and otoneurologic findings.

Imaging Findings

CT

- Cerebellar tonsillar tissue surrounds the medulla and upper cervical spinal cord, extending below the foramen magnum on axial images
- Craniovertebral junction anomalies may be present

MR

- Sagittal images demonstrate caudally-displaced cerebellar tonsils that extend at least 5 mm below the forman magnum
- The tonsils are often pointed ("peglike")
- Syringohydromyelia may be present in 20 to 40% of cases, most commonly in the cervical spinal cord

Treatment

- The decision to operate largely depends on clinical findings (severity of symptoms), as well as the presence of a syrinx
- Potential surgical interventions include decompression of the foramen magnum, with or without upper cervical laminectomy, and shunting of the associated syringomyelia (advocated by some when the cavity size is 35% the diameter of the cord)

Prognosis

There are few reports of the natural history of Chiari I malformation. Symptoms are usually progressive and relate to brainstem compression or untreated syringomyelia. Some patients may have extended periods of relatively few complaints. Overall, 65% of those symptomatic patients who undergo surgical intervention have total or partial relief of symptoms, although up to 30% of these patients may have recurrent symptoms at a later time.

Suggested Readings

Bhadelia RA, Bogdan AR, Wolpert SM, Lev S, Appignani BA, Heilman CB. Cerebrospinal fluid flow waveforms: analysis in patients with Chiari I malformation by means of gated phase-contrast MR imaging velocity measurements. *Radiology* 196:195–202, 1995.

Bindal AK, Dunsker SB, Tew JM. Chiari I malformation: classification and management. *Neurosurgery* 37:1069–1074, 1995.

Elster AD, Chen MYM. Chiari I malformations: clinical and radiologic reappraisal. *Radiology* 183:347–353, 1992.

Case 127

Clinical Presentation

A 7-week-old male with a history of myelomeningocele presents for cranial MR evaluation.

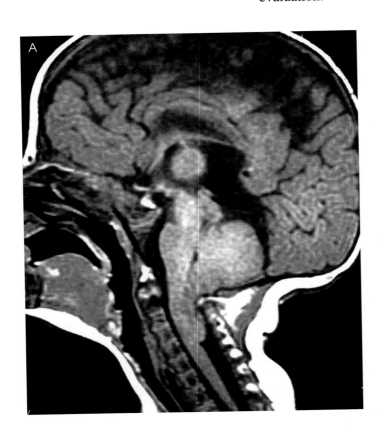

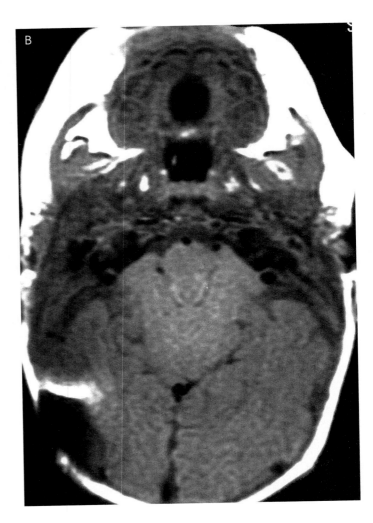

Radiologic Findings

A sagittal T1-WI (Fig. A) demonstrates descent of the cerebellar vermis through the foramen magnum, a cervicomedullary kink, low-lying brainstem and fourth ventricle, and enlargement of the massa intermedia. The corpus callosum is also poorly formed, with a deficient splenium. An axial T1-WI (Fig. B) demonstrates "towering" of the vermis through the tentorial incisura secondary to the small posterior fossa.

Pearls

- CT is often used to monitor ventricular size, especially after ventriculoperitoneal shunt placement, but MR is superior to CT for evaluation of the craniocervial junction and for assessment of subtle anomalies of the corpus callosum or gray matter heterotopia.

- Progression of neurologic deficit in a patient with the Chiari II malformation should prompt an evaluation to exclude hydrocephalus, syringohydromyelia, other spinal cord malformations such as diastematomyelia, or tethered cord.

Pitfall

- The fourth ventricle is low in position and narrowed in its anteroposterior dimension in a Chiari II malformation. Therefore, a "normal-sized" fourth ventricle in a Chiari II patient may indicate hydrocephalus.

Diagnosis

Chiari II malformation

Differential Diagnosis

None: this is a pathognomonic appearance

Discussion

Background

The Chiari II malformation (sometimes referred to as the Arnold-Chiari malformation) includes a constellation of abnormalities that predominately affect the hindbrain. The most significant features include inferior displacement of the cerebellum, brainstem, and fourth ventricle; a small posterior fossa; narrowing of the fourth ventricle; and a kink between the medulla and upper cervical spinal cord. In severe cases, the cerebellum may wrap anterolaterally around the brainstem. Virtually all of these patients present at birth because of an associated myelomeningocele which is most commonly lumbosacral. After repair of the myelomeningocele, most of these patients will develop hydrocephalus and require CSF shunting.

Etiology

Several theories have been proposed as to the cause of the Chiari II malformation and the associated myelomeningocele. The most likely etiology is a failure of expression of certain molecules required for both the closure of the neural tube and the development of the cerebral ventricles. This failure of ventricular development is thought to prevent the normal growth of the posterior fossa. The small posterior fossa may in turn lead to the observed hindbrain anomalies.

Clinical Findings

Patients usually present with a myelomeningocele that requires surgery immediately after birth. At the present time, many affected individuals will have had their condition diagnosed prenatally because of screening for maternal serum alpha-fetoprotein, a marker of neural tube defects, and prenatal sonography. Some patients will develop signs and symptoms referable to herniation of their hindbrain, with lower cranial nerve dysfunction, upper extremity weakness, opisthotonus, and/or spasticity.

Imaging Findings

CT

- Hydrocephalus is frequent
- Scalloping of the petrous bones and dorsal clivus
- Large foramen magnum
- Tectal "beaking" (posterior pointing)
- So-called "Luckenschadel" or lacunar skull, which largely resolves by 6 months of age

MR

- Small posterior fossa

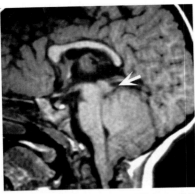

Fig. C. A sagittal T1-WI in a different patient demonstrates tectal beaking (*arrow*), as well as other features of the Chiari II malformation including descent of the cerebellar vermis through the foramen magnum and callosal dysgenesis.

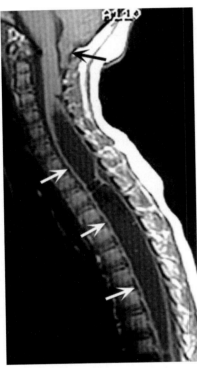

Fig. D. A sagittal T1-WI in another patient with the Chiari II malformation demonstrates syringohydromyelia (*white arrows*). The cerebellum is abnormally positioned below the level of the foramen magnum (*black arrow*). The fourth ventricle is narrow and inferiorly displaced.

- Caudal displacement of the inferior cerebellar vermis through a widened foramen magnum and cephalad displacement of the upper vermis through an enlarged tentorial incisura
- Varying degrees of dysgenesis of the corpus callosum
- Tectal "beaking" (Fig. C) with fusion of the colliculi
- Kinking or buckling at the cervicomedullary junction, often with associated syringohydromyelia (Fig. D)
- Hydocephalus is present in approximately 90%
- Interdigitation of paramedian gyri due to either absence or fenestration of the falx cerebri
- Large massa intermedia
- Less common findings include gray matter heterotopia and aqueductal stenosis

Treatment

- Closure of the myelomeningocele
- Ventriculoperitoneal shunt placement as indicated for hydrocephalus

Prognosis

Varies with the level of the myelomeningocele and the severity of associated anomalies such as agenesis of the corpus callosum

Suggested Readings

El Gammal T, Mark EK, Brooks BS. MR imaging of Chiari II malformation. *AJR* 150:163–170, 1988.

McLone DG, Knepper PA. The cause of Chiari II malformation: a unified theory. *Pediatr Neurosci* 15:1–12, 1989.

Wolpert SM, Anderson M, Scott RM, et al. Chiari II malformation: MR imaging evaluation. *AJR* 149:1033–1042, 1987.

Case 128

Clinical Presentation

A 2-year-old child presents with large head circumference and prominence of the occipital region.

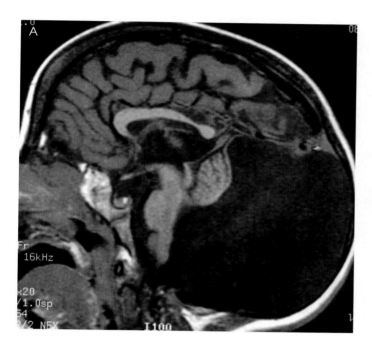

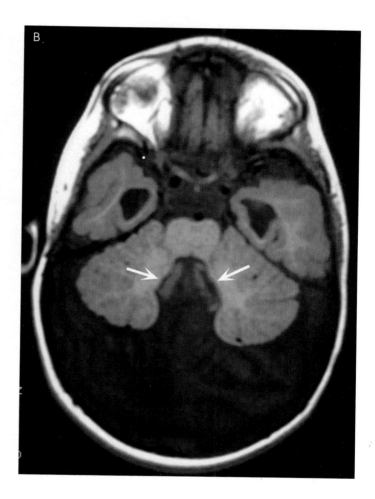

Radiologic Findings

A midline sagittal T1-WI (Fig. A) demonstrates a large posterior fossa cyst communicating with the fourth ventricle, rotating and elevating the cerebellar vermis, and remodeling the calvarium. An axial T1-WI (Fig. B) through the cerebellar hemispheres shows a large CSF-intensity fluid collection that expands the posterior fossa and communicates in the midline with the fourth ventricle (*arrows*). The cerebellar hemispheres are hypoplastic.

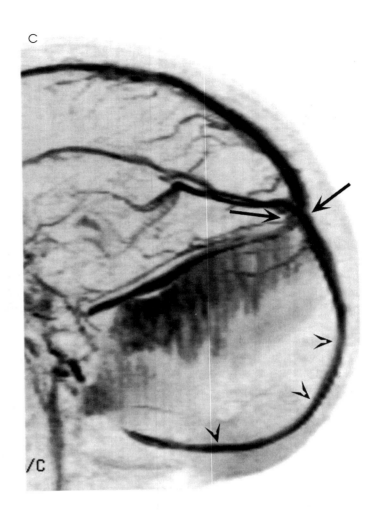

An MR venogram (Fig. C, sagittal projection) shows that the torcular Herophili (*arrows*) is elevated and a large occipital sinus (*arrowheads*) is present.

Diagnosis

Dandy-Walker malformation (DWM)

Differential Diagnosis

- Cerebellar agenesis/aplasia (absence of cerebellar hemispheres)
- Cerebellar hypogenesis/hypoplasia (rudimentary cerebellar hemispheres, the brainstem often small, the posterior fossa not enlarged)
- Posterior fossa arachnoid cyst (exerts mass effect on cerebellum, cerebellum itself is normally formed)
- Mega cisterna magna (midline location, cerebellum is normally formed, posterior fossa is not enlarged, normal vessels typically traverse the mega cisterna magna)

Discussion

Background

The typical DWM is characterized by complete or partial agenesis of the cerebellar vermis, cystic dilatation of the fourth ventricle, and enlargement of the posterior fossa with upward displacement of the transverse sinuses, tentorium, and torcular Herophili. The DWM, Dandy-Walker variant, and mega cisterna magna may represent a continuum of developmental anomalies of the posterior fossa and are best described under the broader category of Dandy-Walker complex. The DWM occurs in approximately 1 per 30,000 births and accounts for 14% of cystic posterior fossa malformations.

Etiology

The DWM likely results from interference with the normal migration of either the Purkinje cells from the germinal matrix in the roof of the fourth ventricle or the young neurons from the rhombic lips. An insult to the fourth ventricle with maldevelopment of the outlet foramina of Magendie and Luschka may also play a role in the development of the DWM. The DWM is associated with a number of genetic syndromes including Meckel-Gruber syndrome, Warburg's syndrome, Aicardi's syndrome, neurocutaneous syndromes (neurocutaneous melanosis, PHACE syndrome, posterior fossa malformations, hemangiomas, arterial anomalies, coarctation of the aorta and cardiac defects, and eye abnormalities), and diverse chromosomal abnormalities.

Clinical Findings

The classic presentation of DWM is with macrocephaly, developmental delay, and seizures, but all three are present in the minority of cases. The majority of patients present with hydrocephalus, which occurs in more than 80% of patients and usually presents by 3 months of age. Some patients may remain asymptomatic into adulthood when they may present with headache and/or cerebellar signs.

Complications

Approximately 15% of patients with DWM have severe intellectual delay and spastic cerebral palsy. DWM may be complicated by sudden death, which is thought to be related to vascular compromise. Associated anomalies of the CNS are present in approximately 68% of cases and include agenesis or hypogenesis of the corpus callosum (~20%), gray matter heterotopia, polymicrogyria, agyria, and schizencephaly.

Pathology

Gross

- Marked expansion of the posterior fossa
- Hypoplasia of cerebellar hemispheres
- Aplasia (~25% of cases) or hypoplasia of the vermis
- Grossly normal cerebellar lobular pattern
- The fourth ventricular outlet foramina of Luschka and Magendie are inconsistently patent in patients with DWM
- The brainstem may appear small

Microscopic

- Disorganization and heterotopia of the cerebellar cortex may be present
- Brainstem nuclei may be dysplastic

- The thin wall of the Dandy-Walker cyst is composed of three layers:
  1. An inner ependymal layer continuous with the lining of the anterior fourth ventricle
  2. An intermediate layer of stretched neuroglial tissue that would have formed portions of the vermis and hemispheres
  3. An outer pial layer continuous with the pia of the cerebellar hemispheres

Imaging Findings

Findings are similar on CT and MR, although better defined on MR

- Enlargement of the posterior fossa with elevation of the tentorium and "torcular-lambdoid inversion" (the torcular is higher than the confluence of the lambdoid sutures)
- Vermian hypogenesis or agenesis
- The inferior vermis, if present, is often rotated posterosuperiorly
- A posterior fossa "cyst" representing an enlarged fourth ventricle is present, occupying most of the enlarged posterior fossa

Treatment

CSF diversion if necessary

Prognosis

- The majority of patients with isolated DWM do well with CSF diversion
- Approximately 40% of patients have normal intellect and little or no motor deficit
- DWMs that occur as part of developmental or genetic syndromes have a worse prognosis for intellectual and motor functioning

Suggested Readings

Altman NR, Naidich TP, Braffman BH. Posterior fossa malformations. *AJNR* 13:691–724, 1992.

Barkovich AJ, Kjos BO, Norman D, Edwards MSB. Revised classification of posterior fossa cysts and cystlike malformations based on the results of multiplanar MR imaging. *AJNR* 10:977–988, 1989.

Frieden IJ, Reese V, Cohen D. PHACE syndrome. The association of posterior fossa brain malformations, hemangiomas, arterial anomalies, coarctation of the aorta and cardiac defects, and eye abnormalities. *Arch Dermatol* 132:307–311, 1996.

Kalidasan V, Carroll T, Allcutt D, Fitzgerald RJ. The Dandy-Walker syndrome–a 10-year experience of its management and outcome. *Eur J Pediatr Surg* 5:16–18, 1995.

Case 129

Clinical Presentation

An 18-year-old male complains of gradually progressive headache and ataxia.

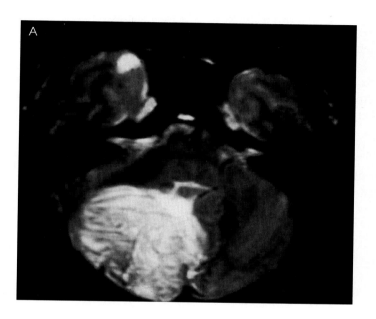
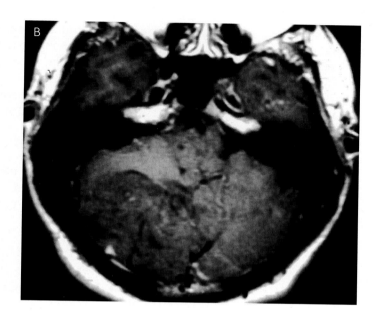

Radiologic Findings

An axial T2-WI (Fig. A) demonstrates a large mass in the right cerebellar hemisphere. The lesion is mostly hyperintense, with bands of isointensity running through it. No enhancement is observed after contrast administration (Fig. B). Note that there is mild mass effect on the inferior fourth ventricle and medulla.

Diagnosis

Lhermitte-Duclos disease (LDD)

Differential Diagnosis

- Cerebellar astrocytoma (lacks characteristic striated appearance and usually enhances)
- Cerebellar infarction or ischemia (follows a vascular territory, usually acute onset of symptoms)

Discussion

Background

LDD was first described in 1920. The disease has various synonyms including dysplastic gangliocytoma of the cerebellum and granular cell hypertrophy. It is a rare disorder, with approximately 100 cases reported in the literature. Controversy exists over whether LDD is a neoplastic or hamartomatous process (see below). LDD is generally sporadic, although familial cases and an association with Cowden disease (an autosomal dominant phakomatosis characterized by multiple hamartomas) have been described.

Etiology

It is unclear whether LDD is dysplastic, hamartomatous, or neoplastic in origin. Some have suggested that LDD represents a developmental hypertrophy of the inner granular cell layer of the cerebellum. Others favor a hamartomatous origin because immunohistochemical studies demonstrate a heterogeneous cellular composition, the lesion exhibits slow growth and no malignant potential, and LDD is associated with Cowden disease (a disorder characterized by development of a wide variety of hamartomatous lesions in various organs). Regrowth of the lesion following partial resection has been described and supports a neoplastic origin.

Clinical Findings

Patients usually present as young adults (mean age of 34 years). Common presenting signs and symptoms include ataxia, headache, and hydrocephalus. Associated abnormalities include megalencephaly, hydromyelia, and heterotopia.

Pathology

Gross

• Mixture of normal and pale, enlarged cerebellar folia

Microscopic

• Hypertrophy of the granular cell neurons, hypermyelination of the molecular layer, Purkinje cell loss, and demyelination of white matter within affected folia
• Mitosis, necrosis, and neovascularity are not observed

Imaging Findings

CT

• Low-density cerebellar mass, which may contain calcifications
• No enhancement post-contrast
• Thinning of the ipsilateral occipital bone may be seen

MR

• Large, typically nonenhancing mass located in the cerebellar hemisphere with occasional involvement of the vermis and/or cerebellar peduncle
• Striated pattern of hypointensity on T1-WI and hyperintensity on T2-WI alternating with isointense bands of tissue
• Enlarged cerebellar folia

Treatment

Surgical resection, especially in cases of brainstem compression

Prognosis

• The natural history of LDD is not well known

- Poor outcome in the past may reflect inadequate management of obstructive hydrocephalus
- Regrowth of the lesion following resection has been reported, so careful follow-up is advisable

Suggested Readings

Kulkantrakorn K, Awwad EE, Levy B, et al. MRI in Lhermitte-Duclos disease. *Neurology* 48:725–731, 1997.

Meltzer CC, Smirniotopoulos JG, Jones RV. The striated cerebellum: an MR imaging sign in Lhermitte-Duclos disease (dysplastic gangliocytoma). *Radiology* 194:699–703, 1995.

Smith RR, Grossman RI, Goldberg HI, Hackney DB, Bilaniuk LT, Zimmerman RA. MR imaging of Lhermitte-Dulos disease: a case report. *AJNR* 10:187–189, 1989.

Section XI

Malformations of Cortical Development

Case 130

Clinical Presentation

A 7-year-old hemiparetic, mentally retarded boy with a chronic seizure disorder presents for MR evaluation.

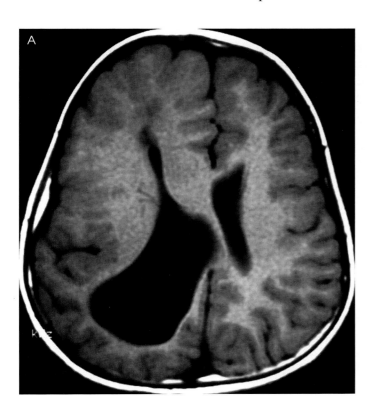

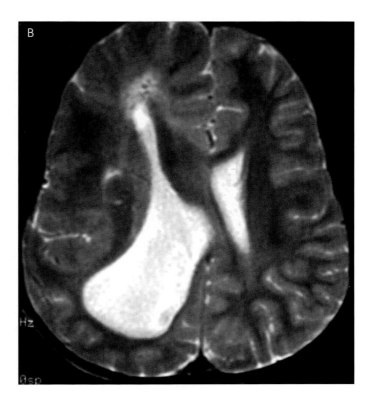

Radiologic Findings

An axial T1-WI (Fig. A) shows overall enlargement of the right cerebral hemisphere as compared with the left. The gyri of the right hemisphere appear somewhat broadened as compared with the left hemisphere, consistent with areas of pachygyria. The posterior aspect of the right lateral ventricle is abnormally enlarged, and the right frontal horn has an abnormally straight contour. Hypointensity is noted in the right frontal white matter. On a T2-WI (Fig. B), the right frontal white matter appears abnormally hyperintense. Marked asymmetry of the cerebral hemispheres is again appreciated.

Diagnosis

Hemimegalencephaly

Differential Diagnosis

- Sturge-Weber syndrome (the small hemisphere is the abnormal one, with marked enhancement of a leptomeningeal angioma, and cortical calcification)

- Ischemic hemiatrophy (the small hemisphere may show areas of gliosis or frank infarction, while the larger hemisphere appears normal)
- Unilateral polymicrogyria (lacks characteristic abnormal ventricular morphology that is seen with hemimegalencephaly, and the affected hemisphere is usually of normal size)

Discussion

Background

Hemimegalencephaly, also known as unilateral megalencephaly, is a disorder of neuronal and glial proliferation that results in enlargement of all or part of a cerebral hemisphere. Neuronal migration defects occur in the affected hemisphere, with areas of polymicrogyria, pachygyria, and heterotopia commonly observed. Hemimegalencephaly may occur in isolation, but it has also been described in association with the linear sebaceous nevus syndrome, neurofibromatosis Type I, hypomelanosis of Ito, and Klippel-Trénaunay-Weber syndrome. Males and females are equally affected.

Etiology

Hemimegalencephaly is a heterogeneous disorder, probably with many different causes. The etiology is as yet unknown.

Clinical Findings

Patients usually present in infancy with macrocephaly and intractable seizures. Contralateral hemiparesis and mental retardation may manifest in childhood. Hemihypertrophy of all or part of the ipsilateral body may be observed. Findings of an associated syndrome such as neurofibromatosis Type I may be present.

Pathology

Gross

- Enlargement of the affected cerebral hemisphere
- The brain surface may show pachygyria or polymicrogyria

Microscopic

- Nerve cells are larger and less densely packed than in the normal side of the brain, and the number of glial cells is increased
- Areas of polymicrogyria, neuronal heterotopia, and pachygyria occur
- White matter may show areas of gliosis

Imaging Findings

Many appearances have been described. Common findings include:

CT

- Enlargement of all or part of a cerebral hemisphere
- Enlargement of the ipsilateral ventricle in over half of cases
- White matter volume may be increased or decreased, and may show areas of low attenuation
- Cortical calcification is occasionally observed

MR

- Enlargement of at least one lobe of a cerebral hemisphere
- Enlargement of the ipsilateral ventriclular atrium and straightening of the frontal horn is present in more than 50% of cases
- The hemisphere may show areas of agyria, pachygyria, and/or polymicrogyria
- White matter frequently shows areas of abnormal hyperintensity on T2-WIs

Angiography

- Usually unremarkable, though arteriovenous shunting in the affected hemisphere has been described

Treatment

- Medical management of seizures
- Surgical treatment (anatomical or functional hemispherectomy, or corpus callosotomy) of intractable epilepsy may be indicated

Prognosis

Hemispherectomy may result in seizure control and neurologic improvement

Suggested Readings

Barkovich AJ, Chuang SH. Unilateral megalencephaly: correlation of MR imaging and pathologic characteristics. *AJNR* 11:523–531, 1990.

Mathis JM, Barr JD, Albright AL, Horton JA. Hemimegalencephaly and intractable epilepsy treated with embolic hemispherectomy. *AJNR* 16:1076–1079, 1995.

Wolpert SM, Cohen A, Libenson MH. Hemimegalencephaly: a longitudinal MR study. *AJNR* 15:1479–1482, 1994.

Case 131

Clinical Presentation

A 26-year-old male with a history of seizures presents for evaluation.

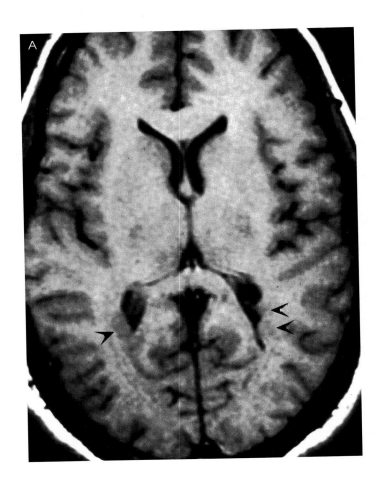 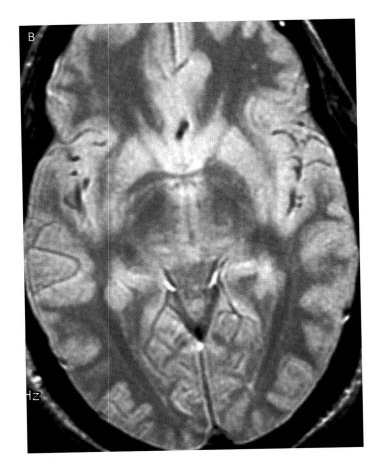

Radiologic Findings

An axial T1-WI demonstrates subtle nodular foci of tissue in the subependymal region of the trigones of the lateral ventricles bilaterally, which are isointense to gray matter (Fig. A, *arrowheads*).

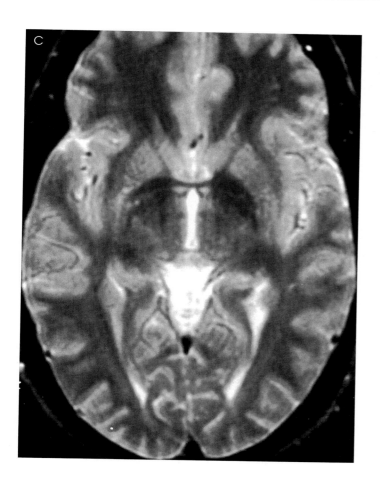

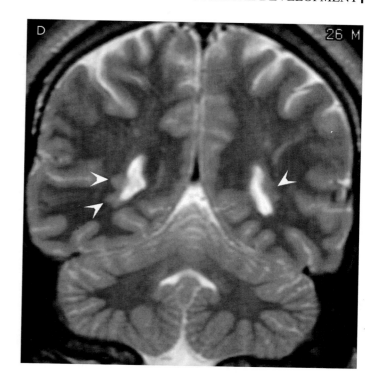

On an axial proton density-weighted image (Fig. B) and a T2-WI (Fig. C), these nodular foci remain isointense to gray matter. A coronal fast spin-echo T2-WI (Fig. D) demonstrates these subependymal nodular lesions to better advantage (*arrowheads*).

Diagnosis

Subependymal nodular heterotopia (SENH)

Differential Diagnosis

- Subependymal nodules of tuberous sclerosis (TS) (often calcified, not isointense to gray matter on all sequences, may enhance; other findings of TS such as cortical tubers typically present)
- Subependymal spread of neoplasm (typically enhancing, may have hydrocephalus, patients usually have a history of known neoplasm)

Discussion

Background

Heterotopia are malformations that result from abnormal radial neuronal migration and consist of gray matter in abnormal locations. They may be subcortical and/or subependymal in location, depending when interference with normal mi-

- Subcortical heterotopia typically extend from the cortical surface to the ventricular surface (Fig. E).

Pitfalls

- Periventricular nodular heterotopia may be very subtle and require careful attention to imaging technique and interpretation. A thin-section volumetric sequence such as a three-dimensional T1-weighted gradient echo sequence may be very useful in detecting subtle periventricular nodules (Fig. F).
- Coronal sequences are also useful to reveal heterotopia along the inferior aspect of the temporal horns of the lateral ventricles.

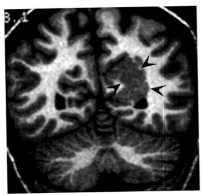

Fig. E. A 1.5-mm section from a volumetric T1-weighted gradient echo acquisition in a young woman with refractory seizures and visual complaints demonstrates an irregular mass of heterotopic gray matter (*arrowheads*) extending from the cortex to the ventricular surface. This is consistent with a subcortical heterotopia.

gration occurred. The cases of subependymal or periventricular nodular heterotopia may be further subdivided into those that are sporadic and those that are X-linked. Patients with periventricular nodular heterotopia may have concomitant brain anomalies such as cerebellar hypoplasia and callosal maldevelopment. The periventricular nodules may be diffuse, focal, or multifocal; bilateral and symmetrical; or asymmetric with a posterior predominance. A female predominance is noted in most series, suggesting that there may be some degree of prenatal lethality in males.

Etiology

The exact mechanism of migration arrest is uncertain. Direct injury (genetic, vascular, environmental) to the radial glial fibers that guide neurons in their migration has been postulated. Alternatively, the radial glial cells or migrating neurons may fail to express certain surface molecules which guide migration. It is also possible that the periventricular heterotopia are a manifestation of a failure of programmed cell death (apoptosis) of collections of neuroblasts within the periventricular germinal matrix.

Clinical Findings

Patients may be asymptomatic, with periventricular nodular heterotopia discovered during investigation of unrelated symptoms. Seizures are the most common presenting symptom and are usually partial. The age of seizure development is variable, ranging from infancy to young adulthood. Intelligence may be normal, or mild retardation may be present. Spasticity, hemiparesis, and/or hemisensory deficits may be present, but these are variable and are more common with subcortical heterotopia than with periventricular nodular heterotopia.

Pathology

Gross

- Nodules of normal-appearing gray matter up to 2 cm in size line the ventricular surface

Microscopic

- Normal-appearing neurons and astrocytes

Imaging Findings

CT

- May appear normal in subtle cases
- Nodular irregularity of gray matter attenuation may be seen along the ventricular surface

MR

- Nodular lesions in the subependymal region of the lateral ventricles with signal intensity equal to gray matter on all sequences
- The number of heterotopic nodules may vary widely, from a few small nodules to a thick layer of nodules
- When focal or multifocal, the trigones and occipital horns are most frequently involved
- White matter is typically normal in signal and quantity

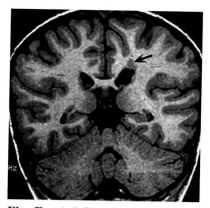

Fig. F. A 1.5-mm section from a volumetric T1-weighted gradient echo acquisition in a different patient demonstrates a single sub-ependymal heterotopic focus (*arrow*). This abnormality was missed on other sequences.

Treatment

- Medical management of seizures
- Surgery may have a role in treating relatively localized subcortical heterotopia

Prognosis

Lifespan is generally normal

Suggested Readings

Barkovich AJ, Kjos BO. Gray matter heterotopias: MR characteristics and correlation with developmental and neurologic manifestations. *Radiology* 182:493–499, 1992.

Dubeau F, Tampieri D, Lee N, et al. Periventricular and subcortical nodular heterotopia: a study of 33 patients. *Brain* 118:1273–1287, 1995.

Raymond AA, Fish DR, Stevens JM, Sisodiya SM, Alsanjari N, Shorvon SD. Subependymal heterotopia: a distinct neuronal migration disorder associated with epilepsy. *J Neurol Neurosurg Psych* 57:1195–1202, 1994.

Case 132

Clinical Presentation

A 35-year-old woman with long-standing epilepsy undergoes MR imaging after her son is diagnosed with lissencephaly.

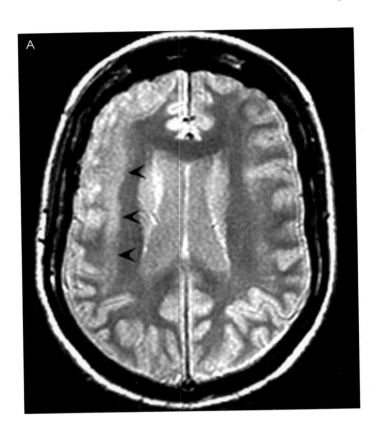

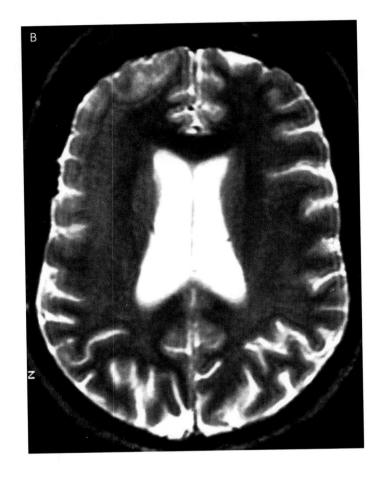

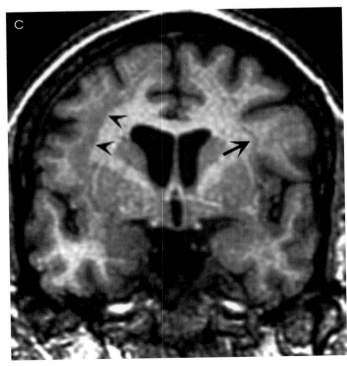

Pearls

- The typical band heterotopia is symmetrical and encompasses most of the brain circumference, but it may be partial and asymmetrical. When partial, the frontal lobes are involved.

- Fluorodeoxyglucose (FDG)-positron emission tomography scanning shows glucose uptake in the band that is similar to overlying cortex.

Pitfalls

- When bilateral and symmetric, the band heterotopia can be missed if one simply examines the imaging study for any asymmetry.

- The neurologic exam is frequently normal in patients with band heterotopia.

Radiologic Findings

A proton density-weighted image (Fig. A) demonstrates a right frontal subcortical band of tissue that is isointense to gray matter (*arrowheads*). On an axial T2-WI (Fig. B), the band of tissue remains isointense to gray matter. A coronal thin-section T1-weighted gradient echo image (Fig. C) clearly demonstrates a 5- to 10-mm-thick subcortical band of tissue, which remains isointense to gray matter on all sequences (*arrowheads*). In this patient, the band is partial and involves mainly the right frontal lobe, although a subtle band is seen on the left as well (*arrow*).

Diagnosis

Band heterotopia

Differential Diagnosis

- The appearance is essentially pathognomonic
- A leukodystrophy may on occasion mimic band heterotopia, but the areas of abnormal white matter will not be isointense to gray matter on all sequences

Discussion

Background

Band heterotopia or "double cortex" is a brain malformation that is considered to result from a premature arrest of neuronal migration. Neuroblasts migrate from the subependymal periventricular germinal matrix to the cortex between the 8th and 20th weeks of gestation, guided by radial glial fibers. Band heterotopia results from migrational arrest that is typically widespread but may be more focal. The typical appearance of band heterotopia is of bilateral and symmetric ribbons of gray matter located between the cortex and the ventricular walls and separated from both by layers of white matter. This disorder affects females significantly more often than males, and males with the same genetic mutation (see below) have lissencephaly. Band heterotopia typically presents with developmental delay and a seizure disorder that becomes progressively more complex as patients age. Associated brain anomalies include ventriculomegaly, T2 prolongation in the white matter, and cerebellar vermian hypoplasia.

Etiology

Although most cases of band heterotopia are sporadic, sex-linked dominant inheritance has been shown in some cases. Affected women may have daughters with band heterotopia and/or sons with lissencephaly. An abnormality at Xq22.3 is associated with X-linked lissencephaly in males and subcortical band heterotopia in females.

Clinical Findings

Patients may present in the neonatal period, childhood, or adolescence, with a mean age at presentation of 5 years. Typical presenting symptoms include seizures, delayed motor development, and delayed speech development. The types of seizures vary and include complex partial, focal motor, atonic, primarily or secondarily generalized, or any combination of the above. Patients presenting in infancy may have infantile spasms.

Pathology

Gross

- Complete or incomplete subcortical band of gray matter

Microscopic

- The band contains large, well-differentiated ganglion cells without lamination
- The overlying cortex has a normal six-layered configuration

Imaging Findings

CT

- May demonstrate a subcortical band of tissue that is isodense to gray matter

MR

- A subcortical "band" of tissue that is isointense to gray matter on all sequences is present
- The band is variable in thickness, ranging from 2 to 12 mm
- The band is also variable in location, sometimes forming a complete continuous band around the entire cerebrum. When it is partial, the frontal lobes are typically involved.
- The heterotopic band has sharp borders at the interface with white matter and does not follow the gyral pattern of the overlying cortex
- Overlying cerebral cortical abnormalities are common and range from mildly shallow sulci to very shallow sulci
- The thickness of cortex external to the band is typically normal or slightly decreased

Treatment

- Medical management of seizures
- Genetic counseling of affecting females

Prognosis

- The clinical course of band heterotopia is highly variable
- Patients with early seizure onset, more severe overlying cerebral cortical abnormalities, and greater ventricular enlargement have significantly worse prognoses for normal intelligence and neurologic development

Suggested Readings

Barkovich AJ, Guerrini R, Battaglia G, et al. Band heterotopia: correlation of outcome with magnetic resonance imaging parameters. *Ann Neurol* 36:609–617, 1994.

Barkovich AJ, Jackson DE Jr, Boyer RS. Band heterotopias: a newly recognized neuronal migration anomaly. *Radiology* 171:455–458, 1989.

Ono J, Mano T, Andermann E, et al. Band heterotopia or double cortex in a male: bridging structures suggest abnormality of the radial glial guide system. *Neurology* 48:1701–1703, 1997.

Case 133

Clinical Presentation

A 7-month-old male with developmental delay and infantile spasms presents for MR imaging.

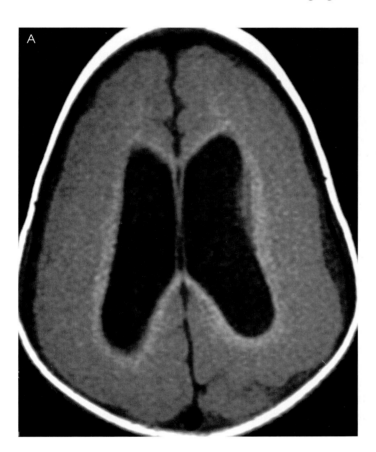 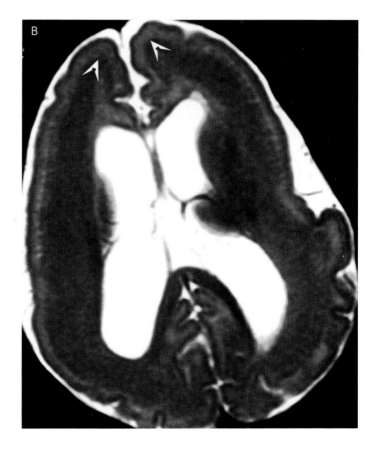

Radiologic Findings

An axial T1-WI (Fig. A) shows a strikingly smooth brain surface without normal sulcal or gyral formation. The ventricles are mildly enlarged as well. On an axial T2-WI (Fig. B), the abnormally smooth brain surface is again appreciated, although a few relatively normal appearing sulci and gyri are identified in the medial occipital lobes bilaterally. On this T2-WI, a thin outer layer of cortex is separated from a thick inner layer of gray matter by a thin layer of white matter (*arrowheads*).

Diagnosis

Classical (Type I) lissencephaly

Pearls

- Classical lissencephaly specifically excludes polymicrogyria, diffuse or focal heterotopia, and severe congenital microcephaly with head circumference at birth ≥4 standard deviations below the mean ("microlissencephaly").

- In cases of Type I lissencephaly, it may be useful for purposes of counseling to obtain an MR of the maternal brain in order to look for subcortical band heterotopia if chromosome 17p13.3 is normal.

Pitfalls

- Congenital CMV infection may result in abnormal neuronal migration, but clues to CMV infection include parenchymal calcifications, lack of an inner cortical layer, areas of polymicrogyria, and involvement of other organ systems.

Differential Diagnosis

- Cobblestone (Type 2) lissencephaly (irregular interface between cortex and white matter, typically associated with congenital muscular dystrophy)
- Partial lissencephaly (spares a portion of the brain)
- Microlissencephaly (profound microcephaly is expected)

Discussion

Background

Lissencephaly, or "smooth brain," denotes a severe disorder of abnormal neuronal migration in which there are no or few cerebral gyri and sulci. However, other causes of "smooth brain" exist and include congenital cytomegalovirus (CMV) infection, diffuse polymicrogyria of other causes, and smooth brain secondary to premature exhaustion or destruction of the germinal matrix. Lissencephaly is subdivided into two main types (Table 1), Type 1 or classical lissencephaly, and Type 2 or cobblestone lissencephaly. Type 1 lissencephaly is also known as the agyria-pachygyria spectrum and is characterized by a markedly thickened cerebral cortex with four coarse histological layers. The cerebral surface is largely smooth, but more normal gyral development may be seen in the orbitofrontal and inferior temporal regions, and the hippocampi. The normally myelinated white matter is very thin, the gray-to-white matter ratio is inverted, and there are no gray-white interdigitations. Associated anomalies such as hypogenesis of the corpus callosum and cardiac anomalies are frequent.

Etiology

Classical lissencephaly has been linked to abnormalities of chromosome 17 and the X chromosome. Large deletions in chromosome 17p13.3 are associated with Miller-Dieker syndrome (see below) and smaller deletions with cases of isolated lissencephaly. The abnormality on the X chromosome has been linked to Xq21.3-q24. The deficient gene product(s) is as yet unknown but may function as a receptor for a diffusible directional signal, a cell adhesion molecule, or a transcription factor regulating genes required for neuronal migration.

Clinical Findings

Patients with Type I lissencephaly are typically severely mentally retarded and have seizure disorders that are often medically refractory. The severity of the clini-

Table 1. Type I vs. Type 2 Lissencephaly

Classical (Type I) lissencephaly (smooth interface between gray and white matter)
    1. Chromosome 17-linked
        a. Miller-Dieker syndrome
        b. Isolated lissencephaly
    2. X-linked
        a. X-linked lissencephaly (males)
        b. Subcortical band heterotopia (females)
Cobblestone (Type 2) lissencephaly (irregular interface between gray and white matter)
    1. Fukuyama type congenital muscular dystrophy
    2. Walker-Warburg syndrome
    3. Muscle-eye-brain disease

cal syndrome correlates with the severity of the lissencephaly. Characteristic facial anomalies are associated with the Miller-Dieker syndrome, which includes midface hypoplasia, micrognathia, a short nose with upturned nares, and a small jaw, along with Type I lissencephaly.

Pathology

Gross

- Mild microcephaly
- Agyria and/or pachygyria with failure of opercularization
- Markedly thickened cortex
- The claustrum and extreme capsule are typically absent
- Ventricular dilatation is present

Microscopic

- Four coarse layers of cortex are present: a molecular layer, an outer cellular layer, a sparsely cellular layer, and a thick inner cellular layer
- Severe hypoplasia of the pyramidal tracts and the brainstem is common

Imaging Findings

CT

- Absent or decreased surface convolutions and underdeveloped opercula lead to a "figure-of-eight" configuration on axial images

MR

- Better defines areas of pachygyria or more normal gyral formation than does CT
- The cortex appears as a thin outer layer and a thicker inner layer separated by a layer of normal-appearing white matter
- Associated findings include callosal anomalies and ventricular dilatation

Treatment

- Medical management of seizures
- Surgery is generally not indicated because of the diffuse nature of the malformation

Prognosis

Patients typically die in childhood or adolescence, often due to pneumonia or sepsis

Suggested Readings

Barkovich AJ, Kuzniecky RI, Dobyns WB, Jackson GD, Becker LE, Evrard P. A classification scheme for malformations of cortical development. *Neuropediatrics* 27:59–63, 1996.

Kuchelmeister K, Bergmann M, Gullotta F. Neuropathology of lissencephalies. *Childs Nerv Syst* 9:394–399, 1993.

Ross ME, Allen KM, Srivastava AK, et al. Linkage and physical mapping of X-linked lissencephaly/SBH (XLIS): a gene causing neuronal migration defects in human brain. *Hum Molec Genet* 6:555–562, 1997.

Case 134

Clinical Presentation

A 4-year-old male who had had a mild left hemiparesis since birth presents with increasingly frequent staring spells that are thought to represent seizures. His prenatal history was notable for maternal hyperthyroidism and hypertension.

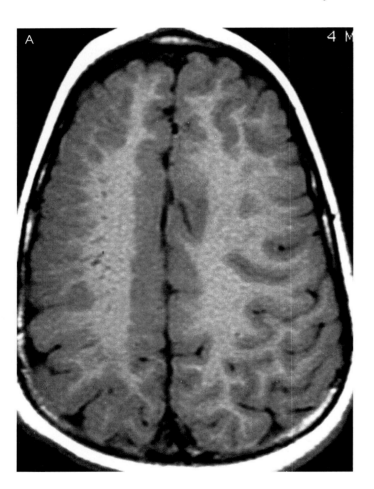

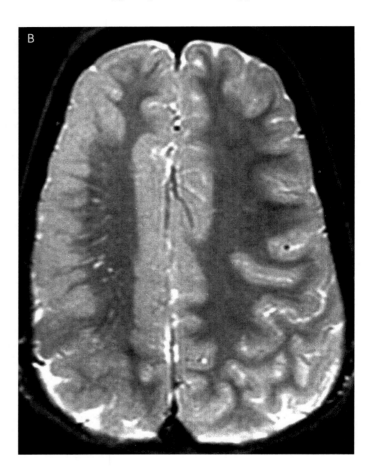

Radiologic Findings

An axial T1-WI (Fig. A) demonstrates an abnormal gyral pattern involving the right frontal lobe. Focal linear and rounded hypointensities in the subjacent white matter represent dilated perivascular spaces. A T2-WI (Fig. B) confirms the abnormal gyral pattern. The abnormal cortex is isointense with normal cortex on both T1- and T2-WIs.

Pearls

- High-resolution volumetric gradient-echo scanning with thin partitions increases the sensitivity of detection of small focal areas of PMG.

- Interictal fluorodeoxyglucose (FDG)-positron emission tomography scanning may be useful to localize areas of hypometabolism for further study with high-resolution MR imaging techniques.

- Ictal HMPAO-SPECT scanning may detect areas of hyperperfusion.

Pitfalls

- Focal areas of PMG can be easily missed on CT or on an MR with thick sections. It is therefore critical to obtain thin sections (3 mm or less) with high signal-to-noise ratio.

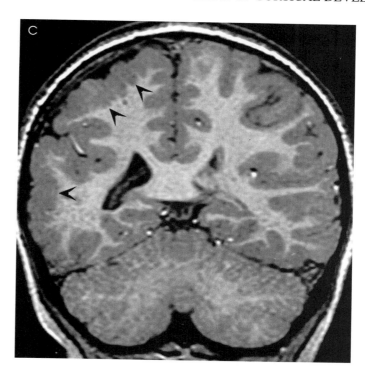

A coronal image from a T1-weighted volumetric acquisition (Fig. C) better demonstrates the somewhat irregular and bumpy inner and outer surfaces of the abnormal cortex, a finding which is present in both right frontal and right temporal lobes (*arrowheads*).

Diagnosis

Polymicrogyria (PMG)

Differential Diagnosis

- Pachygyria (broad flat gyri, could be confused with polymicrogyria on thick-section images or images with poor resolution)
- Schizencephaly (associated with a parenchymal cleft)
- Ulegyria (small gyri secondary to perinatal ischemia)
- Stenogyria (abnormal gyri secondary to congenital hydrocephalus)

Discussion

Background

PMG literally means "too many small gyri" and is characterized grossly by numerous abnormally small convolutions on the brain surface. Sulci may be shallow or may be obliterated by fusion of the molecular layer. Because neurons reach the cortex normally but then distribute and organize abnormally, polymicrogyria is classified as a malformation of cortical organization. PMG may be focal, multifocal, or generalized. Any region of the brain may be affected.

Etiology

PMG results from cortical injury during the period of cortical organization. In humans, toxic and ischemic insults during the early to middle portion of the second trimester have been linked to PMG, although causality cannot be unequivocally established. Congential cytomegalovirus infection is an important cause of PMG. Genetic syndromes may also result in PMG.

Clinical Findings

The age at presentation and the severity of the clinical syndrome depend on the extent of the malformation, but patients typically present with seizures and developmental delay. Motor dysfunction is variably present depending on the location of the lesion.

Pathology

Gross

- Multiple abnormally small convolutions are typically seen over the surface of the brain, although the brain surface may appear smooth if there is fusion across microsulci

Microscopic

- Two major variants are described that are indistinguishable on imaging studies:
  1. *Unlayered PMG* (associated with injury during early second trimester, 12 to 17 weeks): this is characterized by poorly laminated cortex in which layers are not distinctly evident
  2. *Layered PMG* (associated with later injury, 18 to 24 weeks gestation): in this case, the cortex is laminated but contains only four layers instead of the normal six

Imaging Findings

CT

- An irregular, bumpy cortical surface may be seen, but PMG often mimics pachygyria on CT
- Calcification is evident in less than 5% of cases not associated with congenital cytomegalovirus
- CT may appear normal if the areas of involvement are small

MR

- MR may detect an irregular bumpy inner and outer cortical surface consistent with PMG
- The abnormal cortex is isointense to normal cortex on all sequences in most cases, although it may rarely be calcified
- The subjacent white matter may demonstrate high signal intensity on T2-WIs in approximately 20% of cases
- Anomalous vessels may overlay regions of dysplastic cortex and are more common when there is an infolding of dysplastic cortex

Treatment

- Medical management of seizures
- Surgical treatment of intractable seizures is an option if imaging findings and electroencephalogram findings are concordant and localized

Prognosis

Varies with the extent of cortical involvement

Suggested Readings

Barkovich AJ, Kuzniecky RI, Dobyns WB, Jackson GD, Becker LE, Evrard P. A classification scheme for malformations of cortical development. *Neuropediatrics* 27:59–63, 1996.

Barkovich AJ, Lindan CE. Congenital cytomegalovirus infection of the brain: imaging analysis and embryologic considerations. *AJNR* 15:703–715, 1994.

Thompson JE, Castillo M, Thomas D, Smith MM, Mukherji SK. Radiologic-pathologic correlation: polymicrogyria. *AJNR* 18:307–312, 1997.

Case 135

Clinical Presentation

A 31-year-old woman with mild spastic quadriparesis and mild intellectual impairment presents for evaluation.

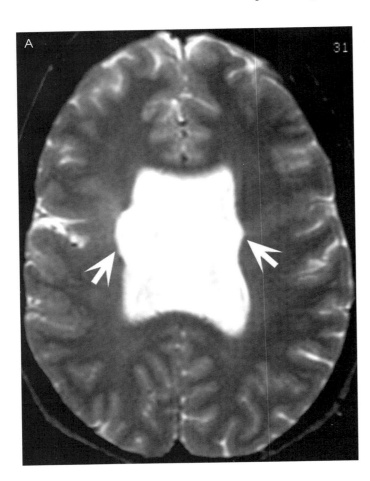

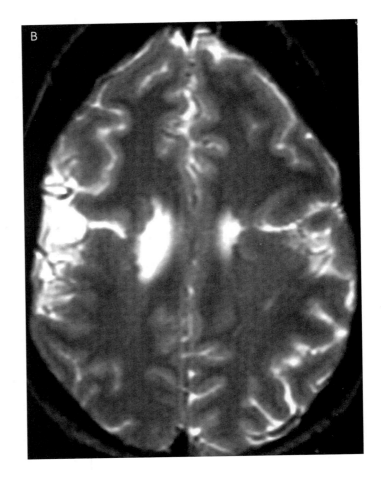

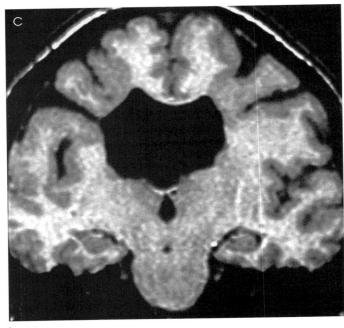

Radiologic Findings

An axial T2-WI (Fig. A) shows a focal outpouching along the lateral surface of each lateral ventricle (*arrows*). There is a suggestion of a faint linear area with gray matter signal intensity extending from the outpouching to the brain surface. A T2-WI at a slightly higher level (Fig. B) shows a narrow cleft of CSF signal intensity extending from the brain surface toward the margin of the lateral ventricle. The signal intensity of brain alongside the cleft is equivalent to gray matter. A coronal image from a volumetric T1-weighted gradient echo sequence (Fig. C) more clearly demonstrates the bilateral clefts lined with dysplastic-appearing gray matter. On this particular image, the communication of the right-sided cleft with the ventricle is clearly delineated. Note also the absence of the septum pellucidum.

Diagnosis

Bilateral small open-lip schizencephalies

Differential Diagnosis

Porencephalic cyst (secondary to a destructive process, lined by gliotic white matter rather than dysplastic gray matter)

Discussion

Background

Schizencephaly is defined as a gray matter-lined cleft that extends from the pial surface to the ventricle, with the subarachnoid space in continuity with ventricular CSF. By definition, the ependymal lining of the ventricle contacts the pial covering of the brain surface. The clefts are classified as unilateral or bilateral, large or small, and open- or closed-lip. Closed-lip clefts have their gray matter-lined walls in apposition at one or more points in more than one plane, while in open-lip schizencephaly, the walls are separated. Clefts may be located in any area of the brain but are most common in the frontal and frontoparietal regions. Patients may present at any age depending on the severity of impairment.

Etiology/Pathogenesis

Schizencephaly is an uncommon disorder of cerebral cortical development that likely results from an insult in the early second trimester that damages the full thickness of the developing cerebral hemisphere. The insult may be sporadic and related to external factors (infection, ischemia). In some cases, familial occurrence has been documented, suggesting a genetic cause. This hypothesis has been furthered by the discovery of functional mutations in the EMX2 homeobox gene in a family with schizencephaly. The EMX2 gene is the human counterpart of a mouse gene that is expressed in proliferating neuroblasts during development of the cerebral cortex.

Clinical Findings

Presenting findings vary with the size and location of the lesion and include seizures, hydrocephalus, developmental delay, language impairment, and motor dysfunction (hypotonia, hemiparesis, quadriparesis). Hemiparesis and motor delay are the common presenting features in patients with closed-lip schizencephaly, while patients with open-lip schizencephaly typically present with hydrocephalus or seizures.

Pathology

Gross

- A gray matter-lined cleft extends from the ventricle through the full thickness of the hemisphere

Microscopic

- Variably-sized areas of polymicrogyria are present in the cortex lining and surrounding the clefts

Imaging Findings

CT

- Open-lip defects: cleft extending from brain surface to ventricle
- Closed-lip defects: often difficult to detect

MR

- In open-lip defects, the cleft extends from brain surface to ventricle and is lined by irregular polymicrogyric gray matter
- In closed-lip defects, a "dimple" sought along the ventricular surface

Treatment

- Medical management of seizures with anticonvulsant therapy
- In cases of medically refractory seizures, there may be a role for surgical treatment such as subpial resection of the dysplastic cortex surrounding the cleft

Prognosis

- Varies with size, location, and uni- or bilaterality of process
- In general, patients with small unilateral lesions have an excellent prognosis, while those with large and/or bilateral lesions often have significant motor and intellectual impairment

Suggested Readings

Barkovich AJ, Kjos BO. Schizencephaly: correlation of clinical findings with MR characteristics. *AJNR* 13:85–94, 1992.

Maehara T, Shimizu H, Nakayama H, Oda M, Arai N. Surgical treatment of epilepsy from schizencephaly with fused lips. *Surg Neurol* 48:507–510, 1997.

Packard AM, Miller VS, Delgado MR. Schizencephaly: correlations of clinical and radiologic features. *Neurology* 48:1527–1434, 1997.

Case 136

Clinical Presentation

A 10-year-old female has a history of medically refractory seizures. An electro-encephalogram (EEG) has localized the seizure focus to the left frontal lobe, and a surface coil MR examination is performed.

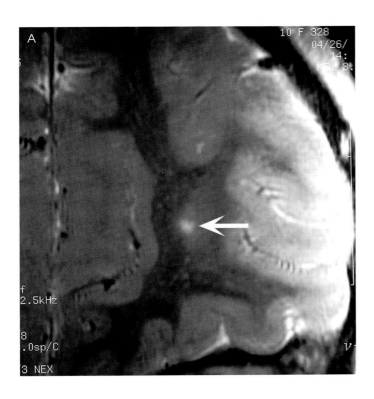

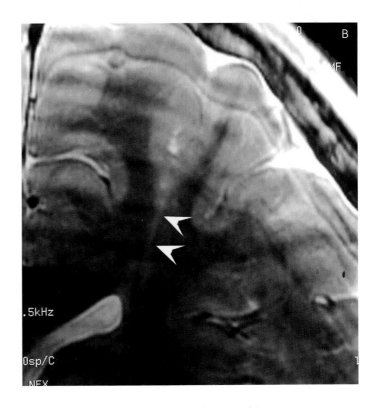

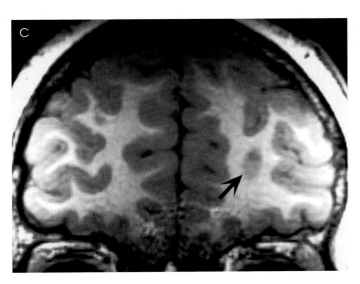

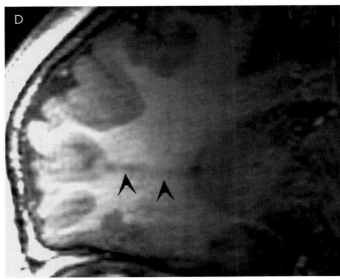

Radiologic Findings

A coronal fast spin-echo T2-WI (Fig. A) demonstrates a focus of high signal in the left frontal subcortical white matter (*arrow*). On a more posterior coronal fast spin-echo T2-WI (Fig. B), a linear area of hyperintensity is seen to extend from the cortical surface toward the left frontal horn (*arrowheads*). A coronal T1-weighted gradient echo image (Fig. C) demonstrates subtle blurring and decreased signal intensity in the focally abnormal left frontal cortex (*arrow*). A sagittal reformation from the same acquisition (Fig. D) also demonstrates the abnormal linear signal extending from the right frontal cortex to the ventricular surface (*arrowheads*). (*Case courtesy of P. Ellen Grant, M.D., Boston, MA.*)

Diagnosis

Focal transmantle cortical dysplasia, surgically confirmed

Differential Diagnosis

- Encephalomalacia/glial scarring (volume loss, may have clinical history of an insult such as trauma or infection)
- Primary glial neoplasm (mass effect, growth over time)
- Solitary cortical tuber (gyral expansion, predominantly subcortical signal abnormality, no blurring of gray-white distinction, other manifestations of tuberous sclerosis)
- Polymicrogyria (irregular, small, disorganized gyri)

Discussion

Background

Malformations of cortical development can be considered in three broad categories: abnormalities of cellular proliferation in the germinal zone, abnormalities of cellular migration to the developing cerebral cortex, and abnormalities of cellular organization within the cortex. Within this classification scheme, focal cortical dysplasia (FCD) may be considered a result of abnormal neuronal and glial proliferation if it is associated with balloon cells (transmantle dysplasia, see below), or as a result of abnormal cortical organization if balloon cells are not present. Focal cortical dysplasia was initially described in 1971 by Taylor and colleagues and has come to be recognized as an important cause of epilepsy. FCD is characterized by abnormal neurons and glial cells arranged abnormally in focal areas of the cerebral cortex. Patients with focal cortical dysplasia typically present with seizures during infancy or childhood, but may also present in young adulthood. FCD is most common in the temporal lobe, followed by the frontal and occipital lobes.

Clinical Findings

Patients present with infantile spasms or medically refractory epilepsy with seizures that are typically complex partial, complex partial with secondary generalization, or complex and simple partial. Patients may also have developmental delay, hemiparesis, and/or hypotonia.

Pathology

Gross

- Often normal to palpation
- Not associated with major abnormalities of gyration
- A slightly thickened cortical ribbon or an indistinct junction between cortex and white matter may be recognized

Microscopic

- A spectrum of changes may be seen ranging from mild disruption of cortical lamination without apparent giant neurons to the most severe form in which cortical dyslamination and bizarre giant (balloon) cells are present. Balloon cells are large cells with pale eosinophilic glassy cytoplasm and eccentric nuclei, which resemble cells seen in cortical tubers.
- White matter may demonstrate a decrease in the number of myelinated fibers, reactive gliosis, and ectopic neurons

Imaging Findings

CT

- Usually normal

MR

- Blurring of the gray matter-white matter junction may be observed on T1- and/or T2-WIs
- White matter and deep layers of the cortex may show abnormal T2 prolongation, which is often best visualized on proton density or fluid-attenuated inversion recovery (FLAIR) images
- In transmantle dysplasia, the abnormal signal may be observed to extend from the cortex toward the ventricular surface in a linear fashion
- Variable presence of a thick cortex
- Abnormal sulcal orientation
- Focal enlargement of the overlying subarachnoid space or adjacent ventricle may be seen

Treatment

- Medical management of epilepsy
- Surgical resection of the epileptogenic focus is indicated in those with medically refractory seizures, provided that the focus can be localized and is accessible to surgical removal

Prognosis

In medically refractory cases, surgical outcome is excellent if single focal concordant abnormalities are identified with MRI and EEG.

Suggested Readings

Barkovich AJ, Kuzniecky RI, Bollen AW, Grant PE. Focal transmantle dysplasia: a specific malformation of cortical development. *Neurology* 49:1148–1152, 1997.

Grant PE, Barkovich AJ, Wald LL, Dillon WP, Laxer KD, Vigneron DB. High-resolution surface-coil MR of cortical lesions in medically-refractory epilepsy: a prospective study. *AJNR* 18:291–301, 1997.

Taylor D, Falconer M, Bruton C, Corsellis J. Focal dysplasia of the cerebral cortex in epilepsy. *J Neurol Neurosurg Psychiatr* 34:369–387, 1971.

Section XII

Cranial Nerves

The twelve cranial nerves mediate motor and sensory functions for the head and neck, including innervation of both voluntary and involuntary muscles and reception of both general and special sensory information. Of note, the first two cranial nerves are actually evaginations of the brain itself and represent white matter tracts rather than true cranial nerves. Cranial nerve functions can be divided into six categories (Table 1).

Table 1. Subcategories of Cranial Nerve Function

Category	Function
Somatic motor	Innervates muscles derived from somites
Branchial motor	Innervates muscles derived from the branchial arches
Visceral motor	Innervates glands and smooth muscle
General sensory	Receives touch, pain, temperature, pressure, vibration, and proprioceptive information
Special sensory	Receives olfactory, visual, auditory, taste, and balance information
Visceral sensory	Receives sensory information from viscera

When imaging a patient with cranial nerve dysfunction, it is essential to cover the entire course of the nerve in order not to overlook pathology. In some cases, clinical findings can help to limit the area that needs to be imaged, but often clinical history will not be adequate to make this determination. In general, the nerve should be covered from its brainstem nucleus to the end-organ level. This will include the cranial nerve nucleus, the cisternal or subarachnoid segment of the nerve, the cavernous or foraminal segment of the nerve (depending on its course), and the extracranial portion of the nerve. If symptoms suggest a possible supranuclear origin for cranial nerve dysfunction (i.e., a "central" facial palsy versus a "peripheral" facial palsy), the whole brain should be studied. Certain visual symptoms may also warrant a study of the brain rather than a study targeted to the optic nerves. General pathologies at various levels are summarized in Table 2.

Table 2. General Categories of Pathology Affecting Cranial Nerves

Level of Pathology	Types of Pathology
Brainstem	Ischemia/infarction
	Demyelinating disease
	Neoplasm
	Trauma (shear injury or contusion)
	Hemorrhage/vascular malformation
	Infection (encephalitis, abscess)

(continued)

Level of Pathology	Types of Pathology
Cisternal	Vascular (aneurysm, compressive vascular loop)
	Neoplasm (neural tumor, compressive mass, leptomeningeal spread of tumor)
	Infection (basilar meningitis, viral neuritis)
	Ischemic (microvascular infarction of nerve)
	Miscellaneous (brain herniation with neural compression, sarcoidosis)
Cavernous (III, IV, V1, V2, VI)	Neoplasm (sellar, paracavernous)
	Vascular (aneurysm, fistula, dissection)
	Inflammation (pseudotumor)
	Infection (cavernous sinus thrombophlebitis)
Orbital (II, III, IV, V1, V2, VI)	Neoplasm
	Trauma
	Inflammation (i.e., viral neuritis)
	Infection
Internal auditory canal (VII, VIII)	Neoplasm (schwannoma, hemangioma)
	Trauma (temporal bone fracture)
	Inflammation (neuritis)
	Infection (skull base osteomyelitis)
Foraminal (V3, IX, X, XI, XII)	Neoplasm (schwannoma, meningioma, paraganglioma, perineural spread of disease, bony tumors)
	Vascular (dissection, pseudoaneurysm
	Infection (skull base osteomyelitis)
	Trauma (skull base fracture)
Extracranial	Neoplasm (schwannoma, squamous cell carcinoma, lymphoma, perineural tumor)
	Inflammation (abscess)
	Trauma

Also note that the proximity of certain cranial nerves to one another may result in multiple cranial nerves being affected by a single pathologic process. This provides useful clinical localizing information and can give advance information to the radiologist about where to focus an imaging study.

Suggested Readings

Harnsberger HR. Handbook of Head and Neck Imaging. St. Louis, Mosby, 1995.

Kelly WM, guest editor. Cranial neuropathy. *Neuroimag Clin North Am* 3:1993.

Waxman SG, de Groot J. Correlative Neuroanatomy, 22nd ed. Stanford, Connecticut, Appleton and Lange, 1995.

Wilson-Pauwels L, Akesson EJ, Stewart PA. Cranial Nerves: Anatomy and Clinical Comments. Toronto, B.C. Decker Inc, 1988.

Cranial Nerve I

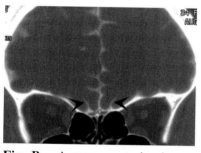

Fig. A. A coronal image from a CT cisternogram demonstrates the normal olfactory bulbs (*arrows*) lying below the frontal lobes and above the cribriform plate.

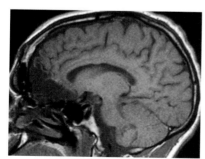

Fig. B. A more posterior image from the CT cisternogram demonstrates normal, well-defined olfactory sulci (*arrowheads*). The olfactory tracts are seen inferior to the frontal lobes.

Function

The first cranial nerve (CN I), the olfactory nerve, has only a special sensory function, subserving the sense of smell.

Anatomy

The olfactory system is specialized for the detection and processing of molecules called odorants. Odorants interact with olfactory receptor cells in the olfactory epithelium. The olfactory epithelium is located in the roof of the nasal cavity and contains three cell types: olfactory receptor neurons, sustentacular or supporting cells, and basal cells (which give rise to new receptor cells). The olfactory receptor cell is a bipolar neuron whose function is to detect odorants and transmit sensory information to the olfactory bulb. Peripheral processes of these primary sensory neurons act as sensory receptors and transmit sensation via bundles of central processes which traverse the cribriform plate of the ethmoid bone. The olfactory bulbs lie just above the cribriform plate and below the frontal lobe (Fig. A). Within the olfactory bulbs, the primary sensory neurons synapse with the secondary sensory neurons, and the axons of the secondary sensory neurons then travel posteriorly in the olfactory tracts. The olfactory tract divides into medial, lateral, and intermediate olfactory striae, which then project to the anterior perforated substance and the olfactory centers in the medial temporal lobe. Normally, prominent olfactory sulci should be seen in the frontal lobes (Fig. B).

Pathology

Anosmia is most commonly either idiopathic or due to sinonasal inflammatory disease (rhinitis, sinusitis, sinonasal polyposis). The olfactory pathways themselves are most commonly compromised by trauma (Figs. C and D) or surgery, mass lesions of the anterior cranial fossa, and mass lesions of the upper nasal cavity. The olfactory system may be congenitally deficient as in Kallmann's syndrome (Fig. E).

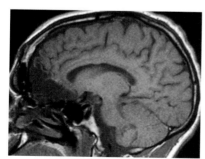

Fig. C. A sagittal T1-WI in a patient with a history of head trauma and post-traumatic anosmia demonstrates cystic encephalomalacia of the frontal lobe.

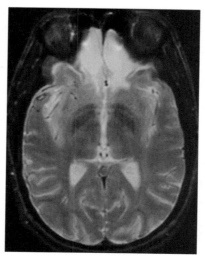

Fig. D. An axial T2-WI in the patient from Figure C shows the classic bifrontal changes of post-traumatic encephalomalacia.

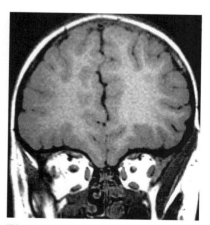

Fig. E. A coronal T1-WI in an eight-year-old boy with congenital anosmia and hypogonadism (Kallmann's syndrome) demonstrates absence of the olfactory sulci bilaterally (compare with Figure B).

531

Case 137

Clinical Presentation

A 47-year-old woman with 6 months of nasal stuffiness and anosmia presents for evaluation.

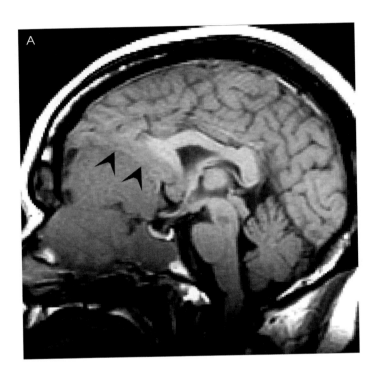

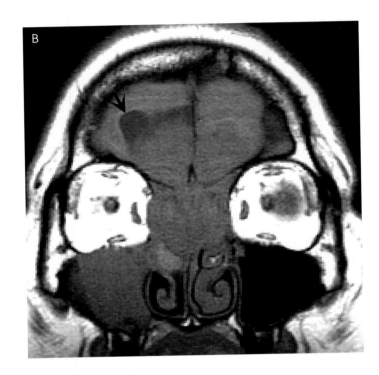

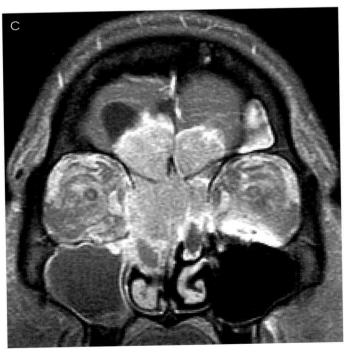

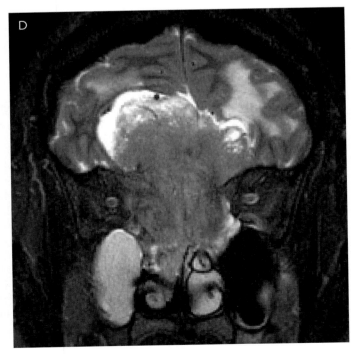

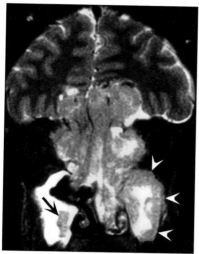

Fig. E. A coronal fast spin-echo T2-WI with fat saturation in a patient with sinonasal undifferentiated carcinoma demonstrates an extensive intermediate-signal intensity mass involving the anterior cranial fossa, nasal cavity and ethmoid air cells, and medial orbits. The mass also extends along the mucosal surface of the left maxillary sinus (*arrowheads*). Central inter- mediate-intensity material in the right maxillary sinus represents inspissated secretions (*arrow*).

Radiologic Findings

A sagittal T1-WI (Fig. A) demonstrates a large lobulated soft tissue mass filling the anterior and superior aspect of the nasal cavity and ethmoid air cells, with extension into the anterior cranial fossa. The sphenoid sinus is obstructed and filled with fluid. There is mass effect on the frontal lobe (*arrowheads*) and the genu of the corpus callosum. A coronal T1-WI (Fig. B) demonstrates the lobulated soft tissue mass extending from the sinonasal cavity into the anterior cranial fossa. There is extension into the medial aspect of the right orbit. The right maxillary sinus is obstructed and filled with fluid. A peripheral cyst is present along the margin of the intracranial mass (*arrow*). Following administration of gadolinium, a coronal T1-WI (Fig. C) demonstrates moderately intense and homogeneous enhancement of the soft tissue mass. Note the lack of enhancement of the intracranial cyst, as well as the lack of enhancement of the material within the maxillary sinus, confirming that this represents obstructed secretions rather than tumor extension. A coronal fast spin-echo T2-WI (Fig. D) demonstrates that the mass is of relatively homogeneous intermediate signal intensity, while the peripheral cyst has high-signal intensity. In addition to the peripheral intracranial cyst, note the reactive vasogenic edema in the compressed frontal lobes bilaterally.

Diagnosis

Olfactory neuroblastoma (esthesioneuroblastoma)

Differential Diagnosis

- Meningioma (more of a broad dural base, often a "dural tail")
- Primary paranasal sinus tumors, including squamous cell carcinoma (often more infiltrative, less lobulated, lacks peripheral cysts); sinonasal undifferentiated carcinoma [SNUC; may be indistinguishable except by electron microscopy, but often more extensive, aggressive, and destructive, (Fig. E)], and malignant minor salivary gland tumor (may be indistinguishable, but often more infiltrative rather than lobulated)
- Lymphoma (may be indistinguishable, but lacks peripheral cysts)

Discussion

Olfactory neuroblastoma, also known as esthesioneuroblastoma, is an uncommon tumor that arises from the basal neural cell of the olfactory mucosa at the level of the cribriform plate. Therefore, it typically presents as a superior nasal fossa tumors. Symptoms are quite nonspecific (patients have often had many months of nasal stuffiness, epistaxis, and headache), so these tumors are generally large at the time of presentation. Gross intracranial spread occurs in approximately 30% of cases, but microscopic involvement of the dura overlying the cribriform plate is the rule, as would be expected based on the site of origin of the lesion. This tumor is composed of small round cells and is typically of intermediate signal on both T1- and T2-WIs. Post-gadolinium, there is generally intense and relatively homogeneous enhancement. Cystic areas at the margins of the intracranial tumor component have been described, and it has been suggested that this is a relatively specific sign of esthesioneuroblastoma. These cysts demonstrate variable enhancement of their margins, and it is not always clear whether they are part of the tumor itself, or reactive or secondary arachnoid loculations. These tumors are generally treated with a combination of surgery (anterior skull base resection) and radiation therapy, with chemotherapy in some cases as well. The overall reported cure rate for esthesioneuroblastoma is approximately 70%, though small tumors with limited intracranial extension have cure rates in the 85 to 90% range. Cervical lymph node and distant metastases may occur but are relatively uncommon.

Case 138

Clinical Presentation

A 33-year-old man with a known systemic illness presents with mild headache and multiple cranial neuropathies.

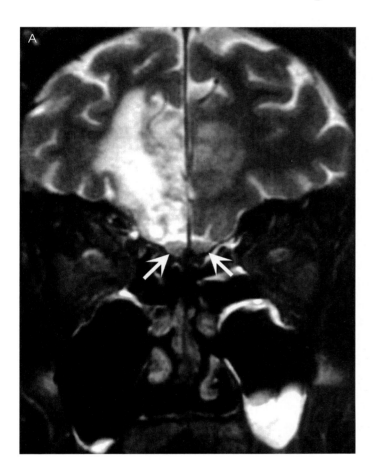

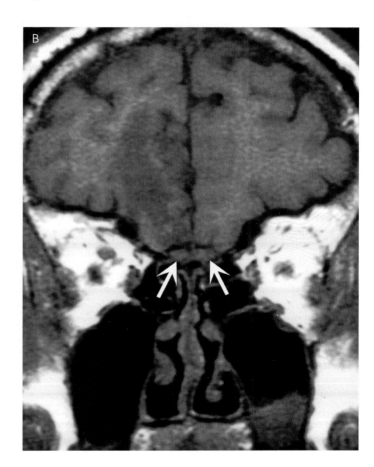

Radiologic Findings

A coronal fast spin-echo T2-WI with fat saturation (Fig. A) demonstrates abnormal high signal in the subcortical white matter of the right frontal lobe. In addition, the right frontal cortex shows abnormal high signal. More subtle high signal is noted in the left medial frontal lobe. In addition, note that the olfactory nerves are strikingly enlarged bilaterally (*arrows*). A coronal T1-WI (Fig. B) demonstrates abnormal hypointensity in the right frontal parenchyma. The abnormally enlarged olfactory nerves are seen to be isointense to normal parenchyma (*arrows*).

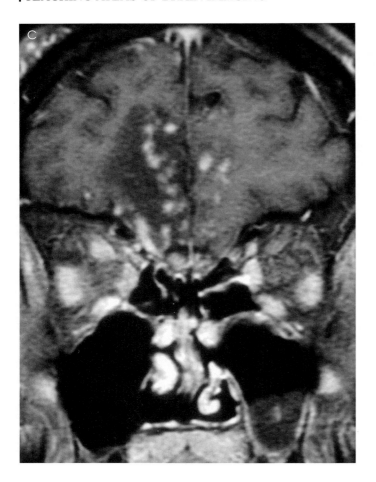

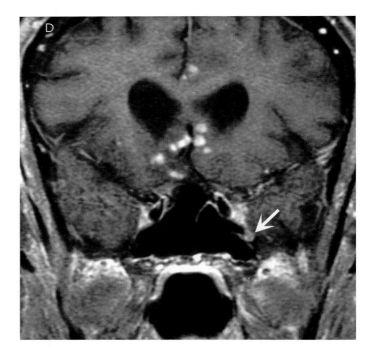

Following administration of gadolinium, a coronal T1-WI with fat saturation (Fig. C) demonstrates multiple nodular areas of enhancement involving the periphery of the frontal lobes bilaterally. The abnormally enlarged olfactory nerves show intense enhancement. Note, incidentally, that the right extraocular muscles are slightly enlarged as compared with the left, and there is mild stranding and enhancement of the right intraconal fat as compared with the left. A more posterior coronal post-gadolinium T1-WI with fat saturation (Fig. D) demonstrates additional foci of parenchymal enhancement as well as abnormal enlargement and enhancement of the second division of the trigeminal nerve (*arrow*) as it traverses the left foramen rotundum.

Diagnosis

Neurosarcoidosis

Differential Diagnosis

- Lymphoma (pattern of brain parenchymal enhancement is atypical)
- Tuberculosis (generally expect a basilar meningitis in the context of multiple cranial neuropathies)
- Lyme disease (frequently involves cranial nerves; brain involvement is more typically patchy white matter disease, with variable enhancement)

Discussion

Involvement of the nervous system is uncommon in sarcoidosis, with only 5% of patients developing symptomatic CNS disease. Cranial nerve involvement is, however, the most common manifestation of neurosarcoidosis. The facial nerve is affected most frequently, followed by the optic, abducens, and vestibulocochlear nerves. Optic nerve involvement may mimic optic nerve meningioma, as the sheath is typically involved. The remaining cranial nerves are involved far less frequently, and even if involved radiographically, may not be clinically sympathetic. Additional CNS manifestations include periventricular white matter lesions, dural and leptomeningeal involvement, and parenchymal enhancing mass lesions (which are often peripheral and may be related to extension of disease along perivascular spaces). Peripheral nerves are involved in 15% of patients with neurosarcoidosis. Cranial and peripheral nerve involvement with sarcoidosis generally responds well to steroid therapy. In general, the diagnosis of neurosarcoidosis is made by demonstrating the presence of sarcoidosis in other organ systems, the absence of another explanation for CNS disease, and a response to steroid therapy. Biopsy may be performed if the diagnosis cannot be established by other means.

Suggested Readings

Salvage DR, Spencer JA, Batchelor AG, MacLennan KA. Sarcoid involvement of the supraorbital nerve: MR and histologic findings. *AJNR* 18:1785–1787; 1997. (Case 138)

Som PM, Lidov M, Brandwein M, Catalano P, Biller HF. Sinonasal esthesioneuroblastoma with intracranial extension: marginal tumor cysts as a diagnostic MR finding. *AJNR* 15:1259–1262; 1994. (Case 137)

Cranial Nerve II

Function

The second cranial nerve (CN II), also known as the optic nerve, is purely a special sensory nerve, conveying visual information from the retina to the brain. CN II is formally considered to be part of the diencephalon, and it differs from the other cranial nerves in that its fascicles are coated with central nervous system myelin, not peripheral nervous system myelin.

Anatomy

The primary sensory neurons in the visual pathway are the bipolar cells, which are located in the retina and receive information from the rods and cones. Information is passed from the bipolar cells to ganglion cells in the anterior layers of the retina. Ganglion cell axons converge toward the optic disc, then turn posteriorly and exit the globe as the optic nerve. The optic nerves exit the orbit via the optic canals (Fig. A), course in the suprasellar cistern (Fig. B), and then join to form the optic chiasm (Fig. C). At the chiasm, the axons from the nasal halves of the retinas cross in the midline, and the optic tracts are formed (Fig. D). Because of this crossing, information from the right half of the visual field from both eyes is carried in the left optic tract, while information from the left half of the visual field in both eyes is carried in the right tract. The tracts continue posteriorly to the superior colliculus and lateral geniculate body of the thalamus, where synapse occurs. The optic radiations then course to the visual cortex in the occipital lobes.

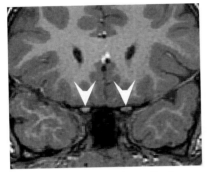

Fig. A. A coronal spoiled gradient-recalled (SPGR) image demonstrates the optic nerves in the optic canals (*arrowheads*).

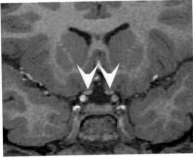

Fig. B. A more posterior image demonstrates the optic nerves (*arrowheads*) traversing the suprasellar cistern and converging toward each other.

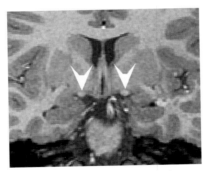

Fig. D. A more posterior image demonstrates the optic tracts (*arrowheads*) diverging from the chiasm.

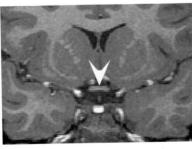

Fig. C. A more posterior image demonstrates the optic chiasm (*arrowhead*) in the suprasellar cistern.

Pathology

The orbital segment of the optic nerve may be affected by neoplastic, infectious/inflammatory, and traumatic lesions. Within the optic canal, the optic nerve may be damaged by trauma and impingement of bony fragments. The subarachnoid segment of the optic nerve is most commonly affected by neoplastic or inflamma-

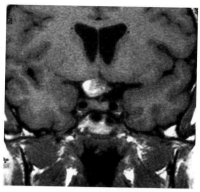

Fig. E. A coronal T1-WI in a 25-year-old male with sudden headache and bitemporal visual field defect demonstrates smoothly marginated enlargement and intrinsic T1 shortening involving the mid and right sides of the optic chiasm.

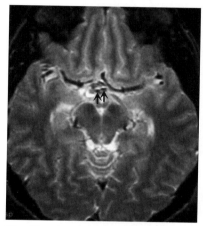

Fig. F. An axial T2-WI in the patient in Figure E demonstrates areas of mixed high and low signal within the chiasmal lesion as well as two fluid- fluid levels indicative of hemorrhage (*arrows*). At surgery, a cavernous malformation of the chiasm and associated hematoma were identified.

tory processes. The optic chiasm may be affected by intrinsic lesions or by extrinsic compression, most frequently in the setting of pituitary macroadenomas or other compressive sellar/suprasellar masses. The optic tracts and intracerebral segments of the visual pathways are most frequently affected by neoplastic and ischemic processes. When there is injury to the prechiasmal visual pathway, partial or complete monocular vision loss results. A lesion at the level of the chiasm classically produces bitemporal hemianopia (Figs. E and F) or heteronymous field defects (i.e., parts of both visual fields are affected). Injury posterior to the chiasm results in homonymous hemianopia (i.e., visual field defect restricted to a single side). These clinical-anatomic correlations are summarized in Table 1.

Table 1. Clinical/Anatomic Correlation of Optic Pathway Lesions

Level of Injury	Clinical Correlate
Optic nerve	Ipsilateral loss of vision
Optic chiasm	
Damage to one side	Nasal hemianopia of ipsilateral eye due to damage to noncrossing fibers
Damage to center	Bitemporal hemianopia
Optic tract	Contralateral homonymous hemianopia
Brain parenchyma	
Temporal lobe	Contralateral homonymous hemianopia or superior quadrantanopia, depending on the extent of damage to the optic radiation
Parietal lobe	Contralateral homonymous inferior quadrantanopia
Occipital lobe	Massive damage: contralateral homonymous hemianopia (variable macular sparing)
	Limited damage: contralateral superior or inferior homonymous quadrantanopia

Shibuya M, Baskaya MK, Saito K, et al. Cavernous malformations of the optic chiasm. *Acta Neurochir (Wien)* 136:29-36, 1995.

Case 139

Clinical Presentation

A 44-year-old female presented with abrupt onset of blurred vision in the left eye.

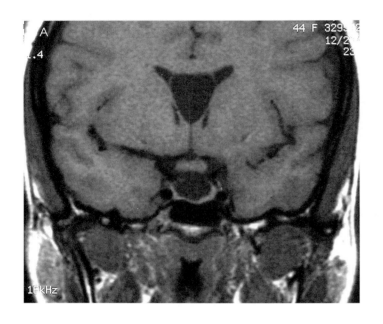

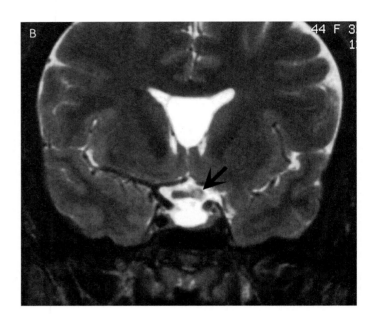

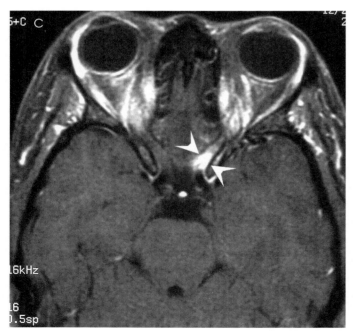

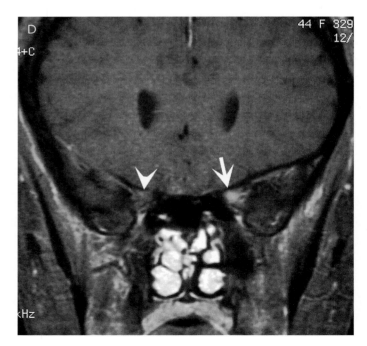

Radiologic Findings

A coronal T1-WI (Fig. A) shows questionable prominence of the optic chiasm. Incidental note is made of an enlarged, partially empty sella, as well as a cavum septum pellucidum. A coronal fast spin-echo T2-WI (Fig. B) demonstrates enlargement and T2 prolongation within the left anterior aspect of the optic chiasm (*arrow*). An axial post-gadolinium T1-WI with fat saturation (Fig. C) demonstrates intense focal enhancement of the intracanalicular segment of the left optic nerve (*arrowheads*). A coronal post-gadolinium T1-WI with fat saturation (Fig. D) confirms the abnormal enhancement in the left optic nerve (*arrow*). Note the normal right optic nerve for comparison (*arrowhead*).

Diagnosis

Optic neuritis

Differential Diagnosis

- Optic glioma (more common in children, often associated with neurofibromatosis type 1 (NF1), symptoms generally not abrupt in onset)
- Optic nerve sheath meningioma (involves sheath around optic nerve rather than the nerve itself)

Discussion

Optic neuritis usually presents with decreased visual acuity or visual field defects occurring over hours to days. It is most commonly idiopathic or related to multiple sclerosis. Approximately 50% of patients with optic neuritis go on to develop multiple sclerosis, and in fact it is useful to screen the brain with MR in patients with optic neuritis in order to look for clinically silent demyelinating plaques. Other causes of optic neuritis include infection (viral, tuberculous, or syphilitic), sarcoidosis, radiation therapy and vasculitis. MR imaging of optic neuritis may be normal or may show T2 prolongation and post-gadolinium enhancement of the involved nerve(s). In rare cases, the optic nerve will be enlarged.

Case 140

Clinical Presentation

A 17-year-old girl with NF1 complains of visual changes.

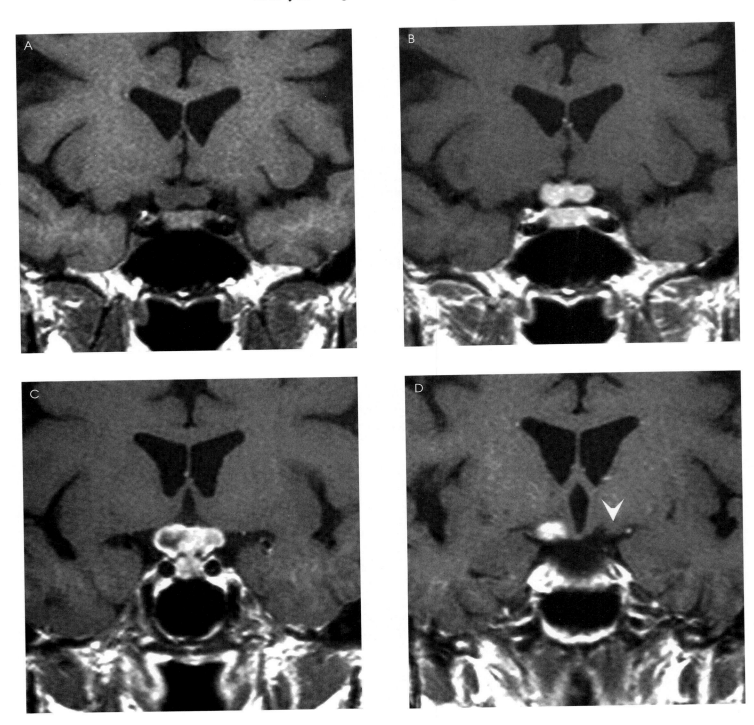

Radiologic Findings

A coronal T1-WI (Fig. A) demonstrates abnormal enlargement and hypointensity of the optic chiasm. Post-gadolinium, a coronal T1-WI at the same level (Fig. B) demonstrates intense and homogeneous enhancement of the chiasm. A slightly more anterior postgadolinium coronal T1-WI (Fig. C) demonstrates a more globular chiasmal lesion, with areas of irregular hypointensity representing cyst formation or necrosis. A somewhat more posterior coronal post-gadolinium T1-WI (Fig. D) demonstrates abnormal enhancement extending along the right optic tract. Note the normal left optic tract (*arrowhead*) for comparison.

Diagnosis

Chiasmal glioma

Differential Diagnosis

- Craniopharyngioma (tends to displace chiasm rather than enlarge it, frequently calcified, often cystic)
- Lymphoma (more likely to involve periphery of nerves in the context of lymphomatous meningitis, typically homogeneous enhancement in the non-HIV population)
- Tuberculosis (may involve the optic chiasm, but generally in the setting of a basal meningitis with diffuse leptomeningeal enhancement and multiple cranial neuropathies)

Discussion

Astrocytomas of the visual pathways may involve the optic nerves, optic chiasm, hypothalamus, optic tracts, and temporal lobes. These lesions generally present during the first decade of life and together represent 5% of all primary CNS tumors of childhood. Most patients present with visual difficulties, although endocrine dysfunction and headache are frequent, particularly when the tumors are large. These lesions are associated with NF1 and may be incidentally detected on screening examinations. Chiasmal glioma patients have associated NF1 in 15 to 25% of cases. These lesions are almost always low grade gliomas, with approximately 75% representing juvenile pilocytic astrocytomas (grade I) and 25% representing low grade fibrillary astrocytomas (grade II). On CT, these lesions are usually hypodense compared with gray matter, and cyst formation and calcification are rare. On MR, the tumors are typically iso- to hypointense on T1-WIs and hyperintense on T2-WIs. Moderate enhancement is usually present, although nonenhancing cystic regions are not infrequent. Extension of tumor beyond the visual axis may occur, with infiltration of the thalamus, frontal and temporal lobes, and basal ganglia. Treatment includes various combinations of surgery, radiation, chemotherapy, and expectant management (usually in patients with NF1), depending on the age of the patient, although most patients are treated with radiation therapy. Overall prognosis is difficult to assess, but 5-year survival is 85 to 90%. Of note, children under 5 years of age at the time of diagnosis have a much poorer prognosis for survival and also for long-term severe disability.

Case 141

Clinical Presentation

A 75-year-old female presents with abrupt onset of a left homonymous superior quadrantanopia.

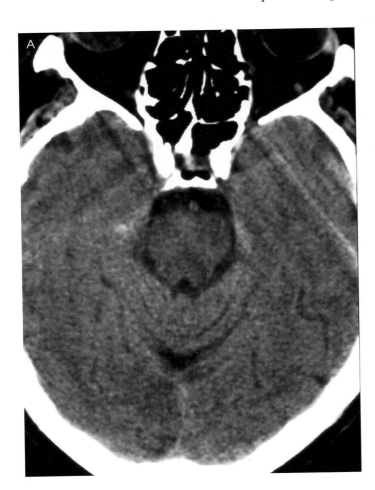

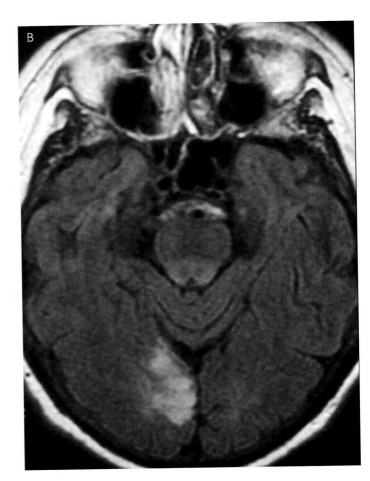

Radiologic Findings

An axial image from a non-contrast head CT (Fig. A) demonstrates subtle hypointensity in the right medial occipital lobe. An axial fluid-attenuated inversion recovery (FLAIR) image (Fig. B) confirms the lesion, showing striking high signal in the anteroinferior aspect of the right medial occipital lobe.

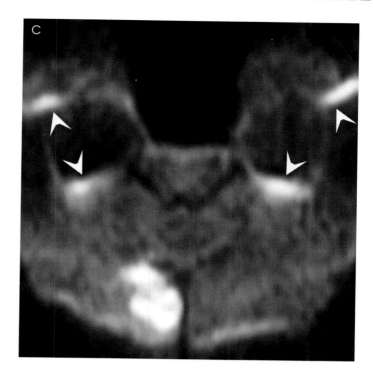

A diffusion-weighted image (Fig. C) demonstrates high signal in the right medial occipital lobe, consistent with reduced diffusion. More anterior areas of symmetric high-signal intensity (*arrowheads*) are related to susceptibility artifact arising from the bones of the skull base.

Diagnosis

Occipital lobe infarction

Differential Diagnosis

- Occipital lobe tumor (symptoms often more slowly progressive, evidence of a parenchymal mass lesion, diffusion is not reduced)
- Occipital lobe hemorrhage (evidence of hematoma on imaging, may see evidence of an underlying vascular malformation)

Discussion

Homonymous visual field defects result from retrochiasmal lesions. The retrochiasmal pathways include the optic tract, lateral geniculate body (where synapse occurs), optic radiations through the parietal and temporal lobes, and the visual (medial occipital) cortex. Unilateral posterior cerebral artery (PCA) infarction most commonly results in isolated hemianopia, although there may be associated alexia or color anomia. The superior portion of the visual field projects to the inferior occipital cortex, while the inferior portion of the visual field projects to the superior occipital cortex. Therefore, a partial or branch occlusion of the PCA may lead to an isolated superior or inferior defect in the visual field. Depending on the extent of infarction, an entire half of the visual field may be affected, or only a single quadrant, as in this case. Note that occipital lobe lesions generally result in macular sparing.

Suggested Readings

Balcer LJ. Optic nerve disorders. *Curr Opin Ophthalmol* 8:3–8, 1997. (Case 139)

Gray LG, Galetta SL, Schatz NJ. Vertical and horizontal meridian sparing in occipital lobe homonymous hemianopias. *Neurology* 50:1170–1173, 1998. (Case 141)

Medlock MD, Madsen JR, Barnes PD, et al. Optic chiasm astrocytomas of childhood. *Pediatr Neurosurg* 27:121–136, 1997. (Case 140)

Cranial Nerve III

Function

The third cranial nerve (CN III), also known as the oculomotor nerve, has both somatic and visceral motor functions. The somatic motor component innervates four of the six extraocular muscles, including the superior, medial, and inferior rectus muscles and the inferior oblique muscle. It also supplies the levator palpebrae superioris, which elevates the upper eyelid. The visceral motor component provides parasympathetic supply to the constrictor pupillae and ciliary muscles. Therefore, a lesion that interrupts the parasympathetic fibers of CN III will lead to pupillary dilatation (mydriasis).

Anatomy

The motor nucleus of CN III is located in the midbrain at the level of the superior colliculus, near midline and just ventral to the cerebral aqueduct. The visceral motor (Edinger-Westphal) nucleus lies dorsal to the motor nucleus. The fibers from both nuclei course ventrally through the midbrain, traverse the red nucleus, and emerge in the interpeduncular fossa where they combine to form CN III. CN III then passes between the posterior cerebral and superior cerebellar arteries (Figs. A and B) and enters the lateral wall of the cavernous sinus (Fig. C). It enters the orbit via the superior orbital fissure, passes through the tendinous ring at the orbital apex, and splits into superior and inferior divisions. Parasympathetic fibers separate from the inferior division and terminate in the ciliary ganglion.

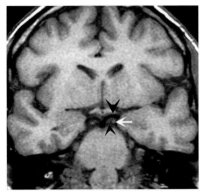

Fig. A. A coronal T1-WI demonstrates CN III (*white arrow*) passing between the left posterior cerebral artery (*large arrowhead*) and the superior cerebellar artery (*small arrowhead*). (Courtesy of Alisa D. Gean, M.D., San Francisco, CA)

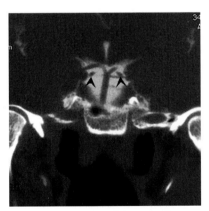

Fig. B. A coronal image from a CT cisternogram similarly demonstrates CN III (*arrowheads*) passing between the posterior cerebral and the superior cerebellar arteries.

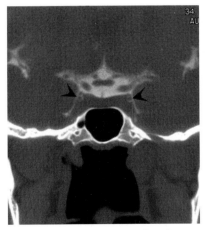

Fig. C. A more anterior image from the CT cisternogram demonstrates CN III (*arrowheads*) entering the superolateral aspect of the lateral wall of the cavernous sinus.

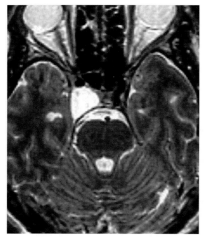

Fig. D. A 23-year-old female with diplopia is noted to have dysfunction of the right third and fourth cranial nerves, as well as numbness in the distribution of V1 on the right. An axial fast spin-echo T2-WI demonstrates a strikingly hyperintense, smoothly marginated mass lesion in the right cavernous sinus, displacing the right cavernous carotid artery anteriorly.

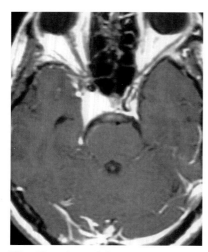

Fig. E. An axial post-gadolinium T1-WI (same patient as Fig. D) demonstrates diffuse, homogeneous, intense enhancement of the mass. Differential considerations included meningioma and schwannoma, but an extra-axial cavernous hemangioma was diagnosed at surgery.

Pathology

Third cranial nerve palsies may be categorized as isolated or complex. The main causes of an isolated CN III palsy in an adult include ischemia, aneurysm, trauma with uncal herniation, and neoplasm. Microvascular ischemic neuropathy, which usually affects patients with severe diabetes and/or hypertension, tends to produce a pupil-sparing third nerve palsy, as the pupillary fibers run along the outside of the nerve and are often spared from ischemic injury. This is in distinction from third nerve palsies due to compressive lesions (i.e., aneurysm, uncal herniation), as these lesions compress the peripheral fibers and result in mydriasis ("blown pupil"). Patients with pupil-sparing third nerve palsies present with strabismus, diplopia, and ptosis. Complex lesions involving CN III are usually due to brainstem pathologies that involve multiple tracts, meningeal pathologies that affect multiple cranial nerves, or skull base pathologies that affect multiple adjacent cranial nerves. Brainstem lesions are often associated with a contralateral hemiparesis due to involvement of the nearby corticospinal tracts. Lesions of the cavernous sinus, superior orbital fissure, and/or orbital apex often result in multiple cranial nerve palsies with involvement of cranial nerves III, IV, V1, V2, and VI in various combinations depending on the exact location of the lesion (Figs. D and E).

Suggested Readings

Bianchi-Marzoli S, Brancato R. Third, fourth, and sixth cranial nerve palsies. *Curr Opin Ophthalmol* 8:45–51, 1997.

Meyer FB, Lombardi D, Scheithauer B, Nichols DA. Extra-axial cavernous hemangiomas involving the dural sinuses. *J Neurosurg* 73:187–192, 1990.

Case 142

Clinical Presentation

A 23-year-old woman with the acute onset of a pupil-involving left CN III palsy presents for evaluation.

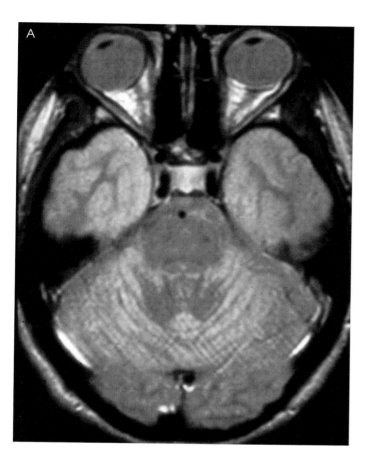

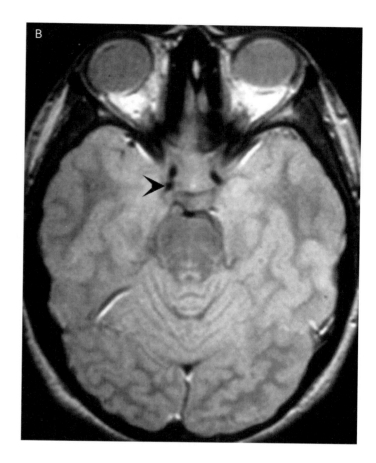

Radiologic Findings

An axial PD-WI (Fig. A) at the level of the cavernous sinuses shows symmetric-appearing cavernous carotid arteries. No mass of the cavernous sinus is appreciated. A more cephalad axial PD-WI (Fig. B) demonstrates an abnormal rounded hypointensity arising from the posterior aspect of the right supraclinoid carotid artery (*arrowhead*).

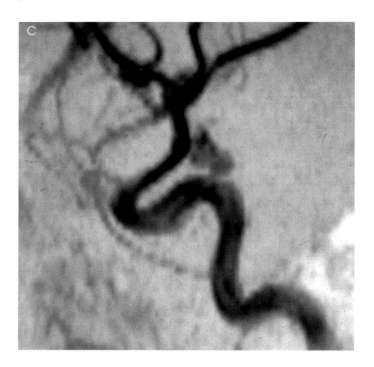

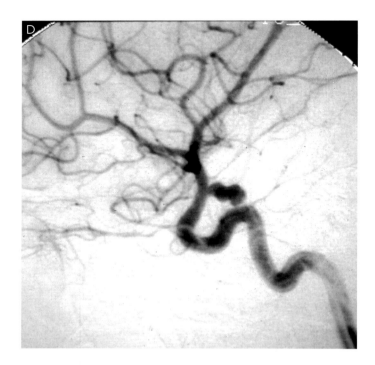

A sagitally oriented maximum intensity projection image from an intracranial MR angiogram (MRA) (Fig. C) demonstrates an abnormal bilobed structure showing flow-related enhancement arising from the dorsal aspect of the supraclinoid carotid artery. A lateral view from a cerebral angiogram obtained during injection of the right internal carotid artery (Fig. D) confirms a bilobed enhancing mass consistent with a saccular aneurysm arising at the level of the left posterior communicating artery.

Diagnosis

Aneurysm of the right posterior communicating artery

Differential Diagnosis

- None in this case
- Differential diagnosis of this clinical presentation:
  - Ischemic third nerve palsy (usually spares the pupil)
  - Cisternal mass lesion such as schwannoma or epidermoid (unlikely to cause acute symptoms, mass visible on MRI)
  - Meningitis (often causes enhancement of leptomeninges, particularly with tuberculosis, fungus, sarcoid, or lymphoma/carcinoma; often causes multiple cranial neuropathies)

Discussion

Because of their proximity to CNs III, IV, and VI, unruptured aneurysms of the circle of Willis are often associated with abnormal eye movements, and 20 to 30% of all third nerve palsies are due to aneurysms. As many as 90% of patients with posterior communicating artery (Pcomm) aneurysms who eventually develop subarachnoid hemorrhage have clinical features of an oculomotor paresis prior to rupture. Because CN III passes between the posterior cerebral artery and the superior cerebellar artery and is closely related to the posterior communicating artery, it is easily compressed by aneurysms in this region. Complete third nerve palsy results in a "down and out" eye, complete ptosis, and a dilated and unreactive pupil. Pain is a prominent feature of many aneurysmal third nerve palsies, but patients generally do not complain of double vision because the affected eye is obscured by the ptotic eyelid. An isolated third cranial nerve palsy with pupillary involvement indicates a Pcomm aneurysm until proven otherwise. In patients under the age of 50 years, emergent neuroimaging should be performed. In patients over the age of 50 years, microvascular infarction is an important confounder when the pupil is involved, as it is in 20 to 30% of cases. In these cases, patients may also require emergent neuroimaging to exclude the possibility of aneurysm. CT or preferably MR imaging is done to exclude other compressive lesions, and in some cases, CT angiography (CTA) or MR angiography (MRA) may directly demonstrate an aneurysm. Conventional arteriography is indicated in patients in whom other compressive lesions have been excluded in order to identify a small aneurysm that may have been missed with CTA or MRA, or to better define an identified aneurysm prior to treatment.

Case 143

Clinical Presentation

A 45-year-old man previously treated for nasopharyngeal carcinoma presents with diplopia.

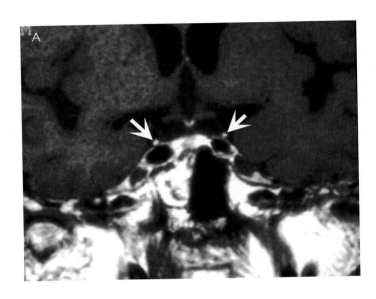

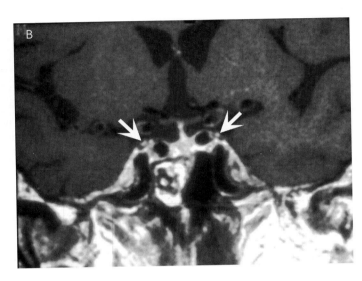

Radiologic Findings

A coronal postgadolinium T1-WI (Fig. A) demonstrates abnormal enhancement of the distal cisternal aspect of CN III bilaterally (*arrows*). A more anterior coronal postgadolinium T1-WI (Fig. B) demonstrates the abnormally enhancing third nerves entering the superolateral aspect of the lateral wall of the cavernous sinus (*arrows*).

Diagnosis

Radiation injury of CN III

Differential Diagnosis

- Perineural spread of tumor (relatively rare along CN III, nerves are often enlarged, unlikely to be bilaterally symmetric)
- Leptomeningeal metastases (nerves often enlarged, multiple cranial nerves often involved, positive CSF cytology in many cases)

Discussion

Therapeutic radiation has a number of effects on the nervous system, including diffuse white matter injury, focal necrosis, cranial and peripheral neuropathy, and radiation-induced neoplasia. The optic nerve is the most sensitive to radiation injury, with other cranial nerves involved significantly less often. It is suspected that pre-existing cranial nerve dysfunction may make the nerve more vulnerable to radiation injury. Cranial nerve injury generally does not occur with radiation doses of <60 Gy, and there is typically a latent period of 6 months to several years between the treatment and the onset of symptoms. The pathophysiology is presumed related to vascular damage and fibrosis, although direct nerve injury likely also plays a role. On MR imaging, in the acute phase (i.e., when a patient first presents with symptoms), the nerve is normal to slightly enlarged, may show high-signal intensity on T2-WIs, and may show postgadolinium enhancement. In the chronic phase, the nerve may atrophy and enhancement generally resolves.

Case 144

Clinical Presentation

An elderly male presents with acute onset of diplopia and ataxia. Examination demonstrates a left CN III palsy.

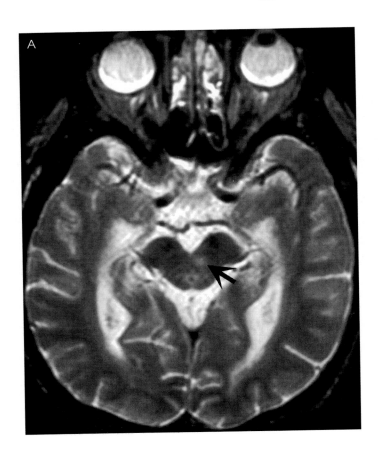

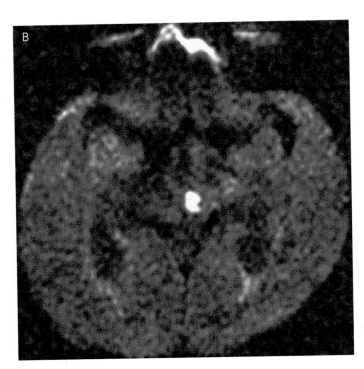

Radiologic Findings

An axial T2-WI (Fig. A) demonstrates a focal area of T2 prolongation in the left midbrain (*arrow*), along the posteromedial aspect of the left red nucleus. An axial diffusion-weighted image (Fig. B) shows striking high signal in this area, consistent with reduced diffusion.

Diagnosis

Brainstem infarction (Claude's syndrome)

Differential Diagnosis

- Acute demyelinating plaque (unusual in elderly male, would not expect reduced diffusion)

- Brainstem tumor (gradually progressive rather than acute symptoms, evidence of a mass lesion)
- Brainstem hemorrhage (evidence of blood products on imaging)

Discussion

As mentioned previously, a complex neuropathy involving CN III can be localized to the brainstem when the dysfunction occurs in conjunction with involvement of other brainstem nuclei and/or tracts. The third cranial nerve nucleus lies immediately dorsal to the red nucleus, and its fibers traverse the red nucleus and cerebral peduncle on its way to its exit point at the interpeduncular fossa. Claude's syndrome (ipsilateral third nerve palsy, contralateral hemitremor, and ataxia) is secondary to a lesion involving the red nucleus and third nerve fascicle. Weber's syndrome (ipsilateral third nerve palsy and contralateral hemiparesis) is due to a lesion involving the cerebral peduncle and third nerve fascicle. Benedikt's syndrome represents a combination of these two syndromes and is due to a larger lesion. Infarction and neoplasm are the most frequent pathologies associated with these syndromes. In this case, infarction is likely due to occlusion of a small perforating vessel arising from the distal basilar artery or the left posterior cerebral artery. The diffusion-weighted image is very useful in confirming the presence of acute infarction.

Suggested Readings

Kasner SE, Liu GT, Galetta SL. Neuro-ophthalmologic aspects of aneurysms. *Neuroim Clin N Am* 7:679–692, 1997. (Case 142)

Urie MM, Fullerton B, Tatsuzaki H, et al. A dose response analysis of injury to cranial nerves and/or nuclei following proton beam radiation therapy. *Int J Radiat Oncol Biol Phys* 23:27–39, 1992. (Case 143)

Cranial Nerve IV

Function

The fourth cranial nerve (CN IV), also known as the trochlear nerve, is a somatic motor nerve that innervates only the superior oblique muscle. Contraction of this muscle results in inward rotation and downward and lateral movement of the globe.

Anatomy

The trochlear nucleus is located in the tegmentum of the midbrain at the level of the inferior colliculus. Axons leaving the nucleus course dorsally, decussate in the superior medullary velum, and exit the dorsal brainstem. The nerve then curves around the midbrain in the ambient cistern, adjacent to the free edge of the tentorium, and emerges between the posterior cerebral and superior cerebellar arteries with CN III. CN IV continues anteriorly in the lateral wall of the cavernous sinus, below CN III, and enters the orbit through the superior orbital fissure. CN IV is the smallest of the cranial nerves and has the longest intracranial course. It is also the only cranial nerve in which all the lower motor neurons axons decussate, and it is the only cranial nerve to exit from the dorsal aspect of the brainstem.

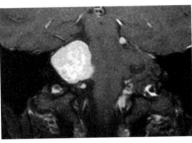

Fig. A. An axial post-gadolinium T1-WI with fat saturation in a 25-year-old man demonstrates a rounded, well-circumscribed, homogeneously enhancing extra-axial mass in the left ambient cistern.

Fig. B. A coronal post-gadolinium T1-WI with fat saturation (same patient as Fig. A) shows the perimesencephalic mass as well as a right cerebellopontine angle mass representing a known vestibular schwannoma in this patient with known neurofibromatosis type II and multiple schwannomas. The left-sided lesion is presumed to represent a schwannoma of CN IV.

Pathology

CN IV is uncommonly affected in isolation, although this may occur in the setting of trauma, as CN IV is vulnerable to injury based on its location between the dorsal brainstem and the tentorium cerebelli. The nucleus may also be injured in the setting of shear injury to the dorsolateral brainstem. The cisternal, cavernous, and foraminal segments of the nerve may be affected by any of the pathologies that affect cranial nerve III, such as uncal herniation, posterior communicating artery or cavernous carotid artery aneurysm, or other compressive mass lesions. Schwannomas of CN IV are rare except in the context of neurofibromatosis type II (Figs. A and B). Leptomeningeal and cavernous sinus processes may also lead to CN IV palsy, generally in association with palsies of other upper cranial nerves.

Suggested Readings

Santoreneos S, Hanieh A, Jorgensen RE. Trochlear nerve schwannomas occurring in patients without neurofibromatosis: case report and review of the literature. *Neurosurgery* 41:282–287, 1997.

Case 145

Clinical Presentation

A 35-year-old man presents with a complaint of retro-orbital pain and diplopia. On examination, a fourth cranial nerve palsy is evident.

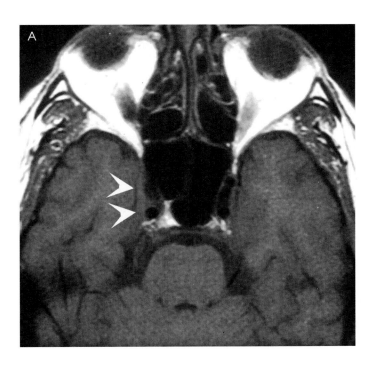

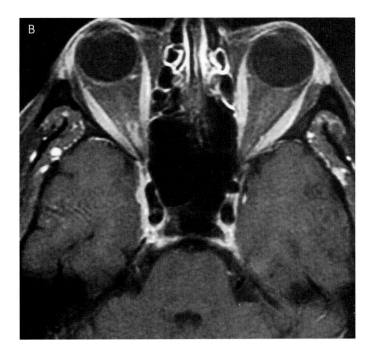

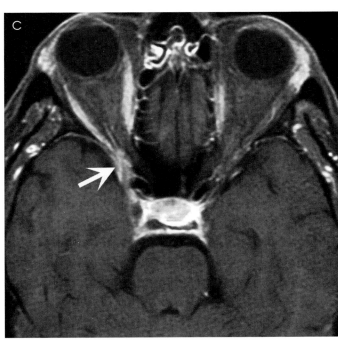

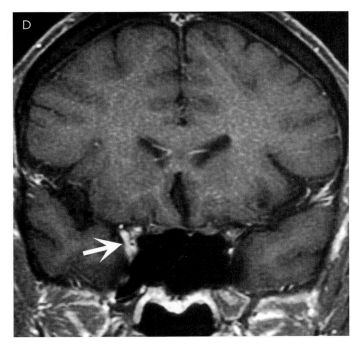

Radiologic Findings

An axial T1-WI (Fig. A) demonstrates asymmetric thickening of the right lateral wall of the cavernous sinus (*arrowheads*) as compared with the left. Post-gadolinium, an axial T1-WI with fat saturation (Fig. B) confirms abnormal soft tissue along the right lateral aspect of the right cavernous sinus, which shows intense and homogeneous enhancement. A somewhat more cephalad axial post-gadolinium T1-WI with fat saturation (Fig. C) demonstrates that the enhancing, infiltrative soft tissue extends to the right superior orbital fissure (*arrow*). A coronal post-gadolinium T1-WI with fat saturation (Fig. D) confirms the abnormal soft tissue at the level of the right superior orbital fissure (*arrow*). On a T2-WI (not shown) the asymmetric soft tissue was intermediate in signal intensity.

Diagnosis

Pseudotumor of the cavernous sinus (Tolosa-Hunt syndrome)

Differential Diagnosis

- Perineural spread of neoplasm, including lymphoma (could have an identical imaging appearance, but typically does not cause pain)
- Sarcoidosis (systemic manifestations of the disease will generally be present, but if isolated may have an identical appearance)
- Metastatic disease (could have an identical appearance, but typically occurs in an older patient with a known primary lesion)

Discussion

The Tolosa-Hunt syndrome (THS) refers to painful ophthalmoplegia secondary to idiopathic granulomatous inflammation of the cavernous sinus or the superior orbital fissure that is steroid-responsive. Two criteria must be satisfied for this diagnosis. The first is anatomic and requires that the neurologic deficits be confined to structures in the cavernous sinus, superior orbital fissure, or orbital apex. The second is clinical and requires steady periorbital or retro-orbital pain that usually precedes but may occur concomitant with the onset of ophthalmoplegia. The symptoms are often relapsing and remitting and may last for days to weeks. CT and MR typically demonstrate asymmetric enlargement of the cavernous sinus and/or abnormal soft tissue mass or infiltration of the orbital apex. Enhancement of the abnormal soft tissue is typically present. If conventional or MR angiography is performed, it may demonstrate segmental narrowing of the cavernous carotid artery. A short course of steroids usually results in dramatic relief of pain and resolution of cranial nerve dysfunction. The imaging findings of THS may be identical to sarcoidosis and lymphoma, although these entities will not typically present with painful ophthalmoplegia. If a trial of steroids is unsuccessful, or if a patient has progressive neurological deficit or relapsing disease, a biopsy may be necessary to firmly establish a tissue diagnosis.

Case 146

Clinical Presentation

A young man injured in a high-speed motor vehicle accident is noted to have outward rotation of the right eye.

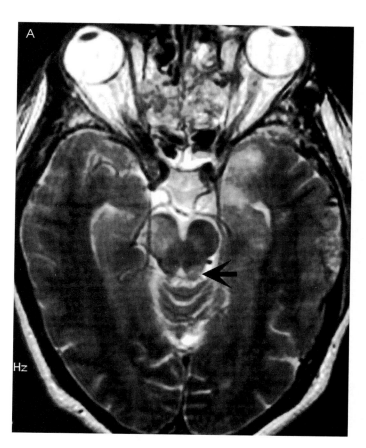

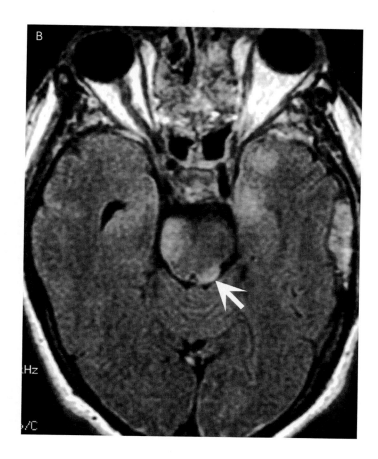

Radiologic Findings

An axial fast spin-echo T2-WI (Fig. A) demonstrates abnormal high-signal intensity in the left inferior colliculus (*arrow*). In addition, high-signal intensity secondary to parenchymal contusion is present in the right cerebral peduncle and the left anteromedial temporal lobe. A small extra-axial collection is also present along the lateral aspect of the left temporal lobe. An axial fluid-attenuated inversion recovery (FLAIR) image (Fig. B) confirms the abnormal high signal in the left inferior colliculus (*arrow*), as well as the other lesions.

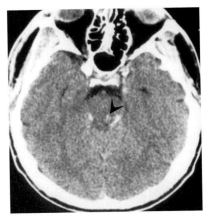

Fig. C. A non-enhanced CT (NECT) in a patient who was hit by a car while crossing the street demonstrates high density consistent with shear hemorrhage in the left dorsolateral brainstem (*arrowhead*), as well as post-traumatic subarachnoid hemorrhage in the ambient cisterns bilaterally. A fourth nerve palsy was evident on exam.

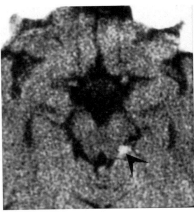

Fig. D. A NECT scan in a patient who fell from a ladder and later complained of headache and diplopia demonstrates isolated post-traumatic subarachnoid hemorrhage in the left ambient cistern (*arrowhead*). Clinical examination demonstrated an isolated palsy of CN IV.

Diagnosis

Traumatic CN IV palsy

Differential Diagnosis

None in this clinical setting

Discussion

Trauma is the most common identifiable cause of an acquired unilateral or bilateral fourth nerve palsy. The palsy may result from injury to the brainstem that affects the fourth cranial nerve nucleus, from stretching of the nerve, and/or from compression of the nerve against the tentorium. In some cases, the nerve may be avulsed from the dorsal brainstem. In general, a traumatic fourth cranial nerve palsy occurs in the setting of a severe head injury, but the fourth cranial nerve may also be injured by minor trauma. Evidence of dorsolateral brainstem shear injury should be sought on CT (Fig. C) or MR in this setting. Even the presence of isolated post-traumatic subarachnoid hemorrhage within the quadrigeminal plate cistern should raise concern about a traumatic injury to the fourth cranial nerve (Fig. D).

Suggested Readings

Kwan ESK, Wolpert SM, Hedges TR III, Laucella M. Tolosa-Hunt syndrome revisited: not necessarily a diagnosis of exclusion. *AJNR* 8:1067–1072, 1987. (Case 145)

Lavin PJM, Troost BT. Traumatic fourth nerve palsy. *Arch Neurol* 41:679–680, 1984. (Case 146)

Cranial Nerve V

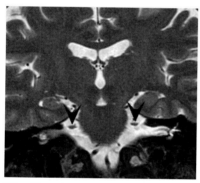

Fig. A. An axial fast spin-echo T2-WI demonstrates the trigeminal nerves exiting the lateral pons, traversing the prepontine cistern, and entering Meckel's cave (*arrowheads*), where they then ramify.

Fig. B. A coronal fast spin-echo T2-WI demonstrates the cisternal segments of the trigeminal nerves (*arrowheads*) on either side of the pons, just above the level of the internal auditory canal.

Function

The fifth cranial nerve (CN V), also known as the trigeminal nerve, has both sensory and motor functions. The branchial motor component of CN V innervates the muscles of mastication (masseter, temporalis, medial and lateral pterygoid muscles), the mylohyoid muscle, the anterior belly of the digastric muscle, the tensor tympani, and the tensor veli palatini muscles. The general sensory component receives sensory input from the skin of the face and temporal region, the mucous membranes of the sinonasal and oral cavities, the anterior two-thirds of the tongue, the conjunctiva, part of the external aspect of the tympanic membrane, from the meninges of the anterior and middle cranial fossae.

Anatomy

CN V is the largest cranial nerve and has multiple brainstem nuclei. The motor nucleus of CN V is located in the mid-pons. There are three sensory nuclei: the mesencephalic nucleus (located in the midbrain, subserves proprioception), the pontine trigeminal nucleus (located in pons, primarily subserves touch), and the spinal nucleus (extends from the pons into the upper spinal cord, subserves primarily pain and temperature). The fifth cranial nerve emerges from the lateral aspect of the pons as a large sensory root and a smaller motor root. Both pass anteriorly in the lateral pontine cistern (Figs. A and B) to enter Meckel's cave, a CSF-filled space defined by dural reflections in which the gasserian ganglion (sensory ganglion of CN V) is located. Beyond the ganglion, the nerve divides into three major divisions known as the ophthalmic (V1), maxillary (V2), and mandibular (V3) divisions. V1 and V2 then travel anteriorly in the lateral wall of the cavernous sinus. V1 continues anterosuperiorly to exit the skull via the superior orbital fissure with CNs III, IV, and VI. V2 continues anteroinferiorly to exit the skull via foramen rotundum. It then enters the pterygopalatine fossa and ramifies. V3 does not traverse the cavernous sinus but rather exits the skull inferiorly via foramen ovale, in conjunction with the motor root of CN V. These unite just below the skull base to form the mandibular nerve, which traverses the masticator space.

Once extracranial, the divisions of the trigeminal nerve branch extensively, and only the major divisions will be described. The major divisions of V1 include the lacrimal, frontal, and nasociliary branches. They carry general sensory information from the forehead, ethmoid and frontal sinuses, orbit, cornea and conjunctiva. The major divisions of V2 include the zygomatic, infraorbital, pterygopalatine, and meningeal branches. They carry sensory information from the maxilla and overlying skin, the skin of the zygomaticotemporal region, nasal cavity, palate, nasopharynx, and meninges of the anterior and middle cranial fossa. The major divisions of V3 include the lingual, inferior alveolar, buccal, auriculotemporal and meningeal. These nerves carry general sensory information from the anterior two-thirds of the tongue, the entire lower jaw, the buccal region, and the skin overlying the chin and jaw. The motor fibers of V3 are named by the muscles they innervate.

Pathology

The brainstem nuclei and cisternal segments may be affected by any of the lesions mentioned in Table 2 of the introduction to this section. The divisions of CN V may be individually affected by anatomically localizable processes, so good clinical history can help to focus the imaging evaluation of CN V. V1 and V2 may be affected by lesions of the cavernous sinus. V1 may be affected in combination with CNs III, IV and VI at the level of the superior orbital fissure or orbital apex. V2 may be affected by pathology that affects foramen rotundum and the pterygopalatine fossa. V3 is affected by lesions involving the foramen ovale or the masticator space. Each division may be individually affected by lesions arising from the skin or mucosal surfaces innervated by that division. Symptoms and signs of CN V dysfunction include loss of sensation of one or more sensory modalities of the nerve, impaired hearing from paralysis of the tensor tympani muscle, paralysis of the muscles of mastication with deviation of the mandible to the affected side, and loss of corneal and jaw jerk reflexes.

Suggested Readings

Majoie CBLM, Verbeeten B, Dol JA, Peeters FLM. Trigeminal neuropathy: evaluation with MR imaging. *Radiographics* 15:795–811, 1995.

Case 147

Clinical Presentation

A 42-year-old previously healthy female presented with left facial numbness, as well as bilateral lower extremity numbness, weakness and urinary retention. A lumbar puncture revealed elevated protein and elevated white blood cells, with 98% lymphocytes.

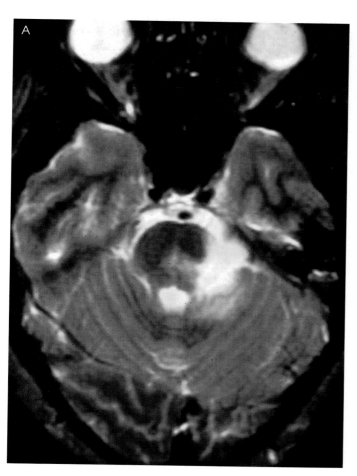

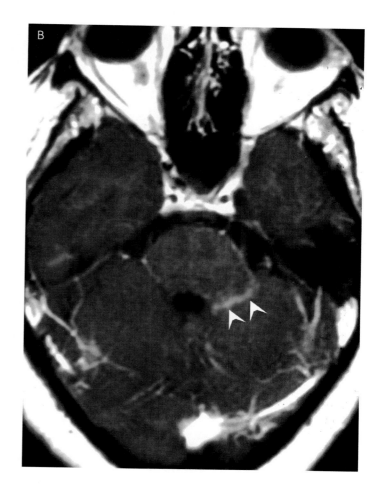

Radiologic Findings

An axial T2-WI (Fig. A) demonstrates abnormal T2 prolongation involving the left lateral pons and superior aspect of the left middle cerebellar peduncle. Post-gadolinium, an axial T1-WI (Fig. B) demonstrates an irregular, asymmetric "front" of enhancement (*arrowheads*) along the dorsolateral margin of the legion.

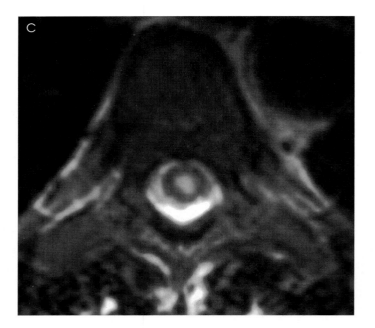

An axial fast spin-echo T2-WI through the midthoracic spine (Fig. C) demonstrates abnormal T2 prolongation within the central aspect of the thoracic spinal cord.

Diagnosis

Acute disseminated encephalomyelitis (ADEM)

Differential Diagnosis

- Multiple sclerosis (first presentation may be indistinguishable from ADEM clinically and by imaging)
- Viral encephalomyelitis (patient often febrile, may have meningeal signs)
- Lymphoma (typically a more homogeneous pattern of enhancement)
- Infiltrating glioma (the enhancement pattern and central cord abnormality would be very atypical)

Discussion

ADEM is an uncommon immune-mediated demyelinating condition affecting the CNS. It is temporally associated with viral infections and vaccinations, but may occur in the absence of a known precipitant. ADEM typically has a monophasic course. Patient presentation is variable depending on the sites and extent of parenchymal involvement, and ranges from focal sensory and motor changes to obtundation and frank coma. Children are affected more often than adults. ADEM typically responds well to high-dose steroids, although some patients are left with residual neurologic deficits, and some patients will die during the acute phase of the disease. MR imaging demonstrates multiple areas of high-signal intensity on T2-WIs in the subcortical and deep white matter, as well as the deep gray nuclei. Infratentorial and spinal cord lesions are variably present. Gadolinium enhancement is variable and may be ringlike, arclike, homogeneous, or absent. Following appropriate treatment, resolution of lesions is often complete.

Case 148

Clinical Presentation

A 31-year-old woman presents with left cheek numbness of one week's duration. The remainder of her evaluation is unremarkable. Several days later she develops multiple left buccal vesicles.

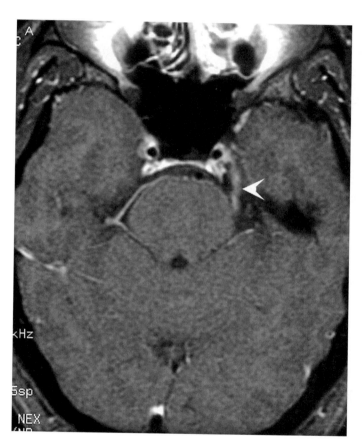

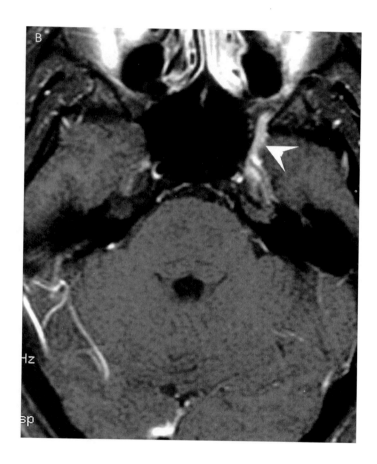

Radiologic Findings

An axial post-gadolinium T1-WI with fat saturation (Fig. A) demonstrates abnormal enhancement of the cisternal segment of the left trigeminal nerve (*arrowhead*). A more inferior axial post-gadolinium T1-WI with fat saturation (Fig. B) demonstrates abnormal enhancement in the region of the left trigeminal ganglion, with extension of abnormal enhancement along the left V2 branch in foramen rotundum (*arrowhead*).

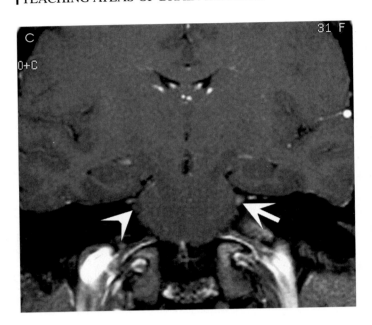

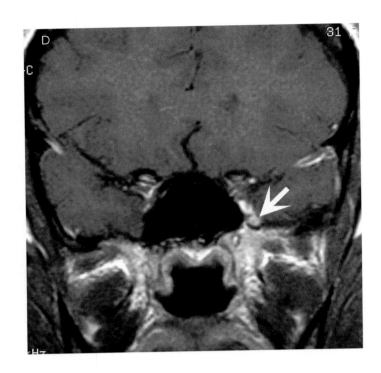

A coronal post-gadolinium T1-WI with fat saturation (Fig. C) similarly demonstrates abnormal enhancement of the left cisternal segment of CN V (*arrow*). The normal right fifth nerve is shown for comparison (*arrowhead*). More anteriorly, a coronal post-gadolinium T1-WI with fat saturation (Fig. D) demonstrates abnormal enlargement and enhancement of the second division of the left trigeminal nerve within foramen rotundum (*arrow*).

Diagnosis

Herpetic neuritis

Differential Diagnosis

- Other viral neuritides (likely indistinguishable)
- Postradiation neuritis (clinical history)
- Perineural spread of tumor (patient typically has a history of head and neck cancer)
- Sarcoidosis (usually systemic evidence of disease, but isolated CNS involvement may be indistinguishable initially from a viral process)

Discussion

Herpes simplex type 1 is the most commonly identified etiologic agent of viral neuritis. After a primary exposure, the virus lies latent within the trigeminal ganglion but may reactivate under conditions of stress or relative immunosuppression (i.e. steroid use). Antegrade spread of virus via the distal branches of the sensory divisions of the trigeminal nerve results in painful ulcers. Retrograde spread into the brainstem causing a viral rhombencephalitis has been described but is rare. Symptoms generally resolve within weeks to months, and treatment with acyclovir may help to speed resolution. Pre-gadolinium MR imaging is usually normal in the acute phase, while post-gadolinium images may demonstrate intense enhancement of the trigeminal nerve, its ganglion, and/or its main divisions. If the brainstem is involved, abnormal T2 prolongation and postgadolinium enhancement may be present. Follow-up MR after resolution of symptoms is typically normal.

Case 149

Clinical Presentation

A 45-year-old man presents with gradually progressive numbness of the right face, as well as headache, diplopia and right-sided hearing loss.

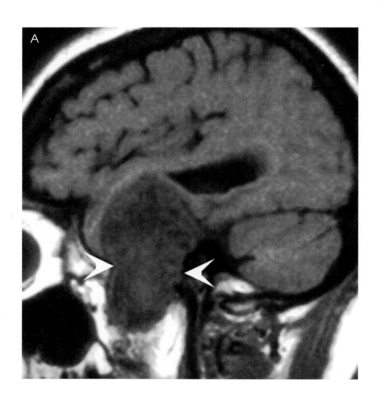
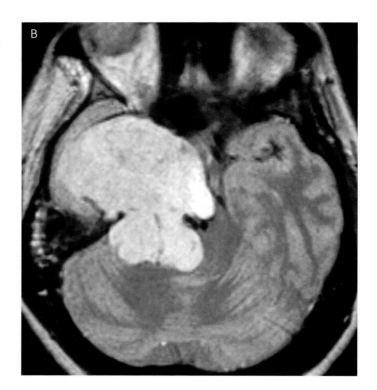

Radiologic Findings

A sagittal T1-WI (Fig. A) demonstrates a well-circumscribed mass that is mildly hypointense to brain parenchyma extending from the right middle cranial fossa through a widened foramen ovale (*arrowheads*) into the infratemporal fossa. The mass is clearly extra-axial, as evidenced by its sharp margination from adjacent brain parenchyma and the fact that it is displacing brain away from it rather than infiltrating and expanding the brain. On an axial PD-WI (Fig. B), the mass is seen to be hyperintense to brain parenchyma. The mass is displacing and compressing the right temporal lobe, pons, and cerebellum. Fluid is present within right mastoid air cells, presumably related to eustachian tube dysfunction.

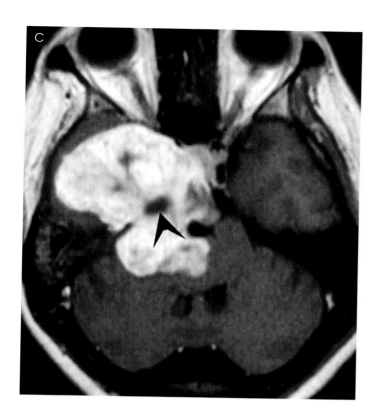
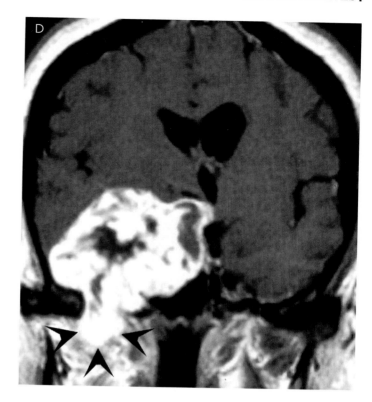

Post-gadolinium, an axial T1-WI (Fig. C) and a coronal T1-WI (Fig. D) demonstrate moderately intense enhancement of the mass. The mass is somewhat heterogeneous, with areas of irregular hypointensity and probable cyst formation (Fig. C, *arrowhead*). Note that the mass has a bilobed configuration, dumbbelling through a widened right foramen ovale with a component in the infratemporal fossa (Fig. D, *arrowheads*).

Diagnosis

Schwannoma of CN V

Differential Diagnosis

- Meningioma (broad dural base, often a "dural tail," isointense to brain parenchyma on T2-WIs, intense and homogeneous enhancement post-gadolinium)
- Lipoma (fat signal intensity, evidence of chemical shift artifact)
- Epidermoid cyst (similar to CSF signal intensity on T1- and T2-weighted sequences, nonenhancing)

Discussion

Trigeminal schwannomas account for about 0.2% of all intracranial tumors and 2 to 3% of intracranial schwannomas. Patients typically present with sensory disturbances such as numbness, hypesthesia, hypalgesia, and/or a diminished or absent corneal reflex. Weakness of the muscles of mastication or facial pain is less common. Trigeminal schwannomas may arise along any segment of the nerve, but the majority develop at the level of the trigeminal ganglion. They may then extend posteriorly into the posterior fossa or anteriorly through the skull base foramina, and they often have a "dumbbell" configuration. Trigeminal schwannomas are typically smoothly marginated, round, or ovoid masses that are isointense to brain on T1-WIs and hyperintense on T2-WIs. Enhancement is typically intense and homogeneous, although inhomogeneity may result from cystic degeneration or hemorrhage. Surgical resection is the treatment of choice, and when removed completely, these lesions have little tendency to recur.

Case 150

Clinical Presentation

A 65-year-old man presents with progressive left facial numbness and difficulty chewing. His medical history is notable for prior local excision of an invasive squamous cell carcinoma of the left face.

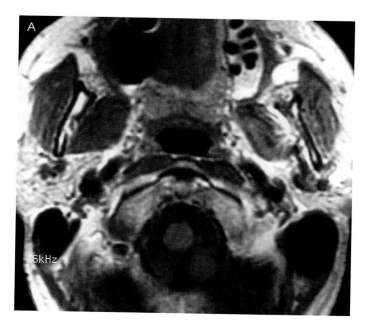

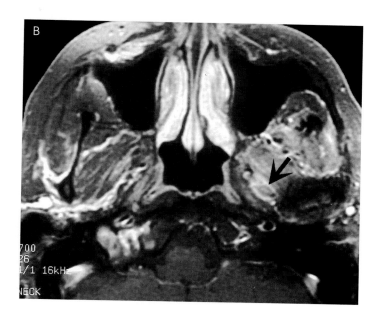

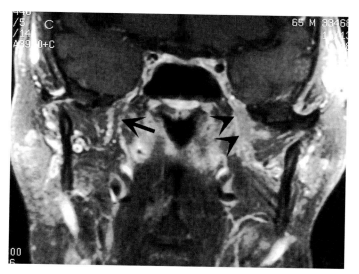

Radiologic Findings

An axial T1-WI (Fig. A) demonstrates atrophy of the left medial pterygoid and masseter muscles as compared with the right side. A more cephalad axial post-gadolinium T1-WI with fat saturation (Fig. B) demonstrates abnormal enhancement of the left muscles of mastication. In addition, there is enlargement of the third division of the left trigeminal nerve at the level of foramen ovale (*arrow*). A coronal post-gadolinium T1-WI with fat saturation (Fig. C) demonstrates abnormal enlargement and enhancement of the left third division of the fifth cranial nerve as it passes through foramen ovale and into the masticator space (*arrowheads*). The normal nerve is seen on the right (*arrow*).

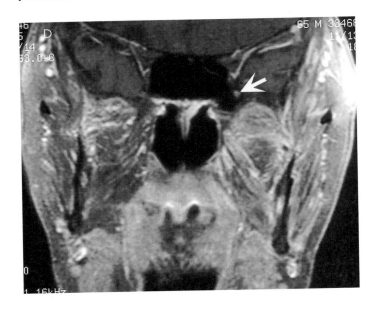

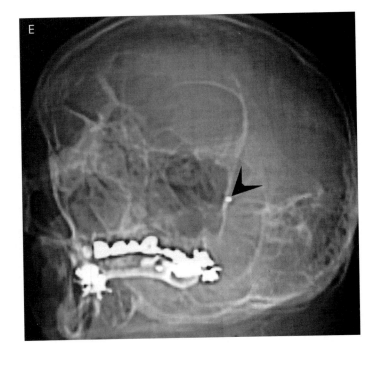

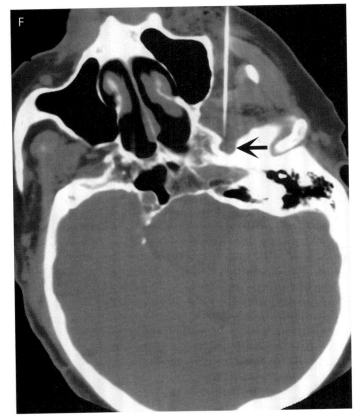

A more anterior post-gadolinium coronal T1-WI with fat saturation (Fig. D) demonstrates abnormal enhancement of the left muscles of mastication as well as abnormal enhancement of the left second division of the trigeminal nerve as it passes through foramen rotundum (*arrow*). A digital scout radiograph from a CT scan (Fig. E) was obtained in preparation for percutaneous fine needle aspiration of the abnormal tissue. Note that the patient's head is slightly extended and rotated away from the side of the lesion. A metallic marker (*arrowhead*) indicates the approximate position of foramen ovale. An axial CT image obtained during the biopsy procedure (Fig. F) demonstrates a thin needle advancing toward the left foramen ovale (*arrow*).

Diagnosis

Perineural spread of squamous cell carcinoma

Differential Diagnosis

- Lymphoma (may infiltrate multiple cranial nerves, but often a more rapid course and less likely to cause chronic denervation changes)

- Sarcoid (often known systemic disease, more often presents in younger patients, unlikely to cause chronic denervation changes)

Discussion

Perineural spread of tumor is a form of metastatic disease in which tumor disseminates along the endoneurium or perineurium of a cranial nerve, most commonly along branches of the fifth and seventh cranial nerves. Clinical evidence of perineural disease is often lacking, as patients may be asymptomatic early in the course of disease. Perineural spread most commonly occurs with adenoid cystic carcinoma and squamous cell carcinoma, but has also been described with mucoepidermoid carcinoma, basal cell carcinoma, and melanoma, among others. CT changes occur relatively late and include foraminal widening or destruction. Contrast-enhanced MR is far more sensitive to perineural spread of disease, with findings including enlargement and abnormal enhancement of nerves, obliteration of fat planes at foraminal apertures, abnormal soft tissue in Meckel's cave, cavernous sinus enlargement, and evidence of denervation change in the muscles of mastication. Early denervation changes include high signal on T2-WIs and post-gadolinium enhancement. As denervation becomes chronic, there is loss of muscle bulk and fatty infiltration.

Suggested Readings

Caldemeyer KS, Mathews VP, Righi PD, Smith RR. Imaging features and clinical significance of perineural spread or extension of head and neck tumors. *Radiographics* 18:97–110, 1998. (Case 150)

Mader I, Stock KW, Ettlin T, Probst A. Acute disseminated encephalomyelitis: MR and CT features. *AJNR* 17:104–109, 1996. (Case 147)

Samii M, Migliori M, Tatagiba M, Babu R. Surgical treatment of trigeminal schwannomas. *J Neurosurg* 82:711–718, 1995. (Case 149)

Tien RD, Dillon WP. Herpes trigeminal neuritis and rhombencephalitis on Gd-DTPA-enhanced MR imaging. *AJNR* 11:413–414, 1990. (Case 148)

Cranial Nerve VI

Function

The sixth cranial nerve (CN VI), also known as the abducens nerve, provides somatic motor innervation to the lateral rectus muscle of the eye. Because individual eye muscles must be precisely coordinated in order to change or maintain visual fixation, the nuclei of cranial nerves III, IV, and VI are controlled by higher centers in the brainstem and cerebral cortex. CN VI causes contraction of the lateral rectus muscle, which results in outward movement (abduction) of the eye.

Anatomy

The nucleus of CN VI is located in the pontine tegmentum, close to the midline and ventral to the fourth ventricle. Axons course ventrally through the pons and exit the ventral brainstem at the pontomedullary junction (Fig. A). CN VI then runs anteriorly, superiorly, and laterally in the subarachnoid space to pierce the dura at the level of the petrous apex, where it enters Dorello's canal (Fig. B). It then traverses the cavernous sinus, passing lateral to the internal carotid artery and medial to CNs III, IV, V1, and V2. The nerve accesses the orbit via the superior orbital fissure.

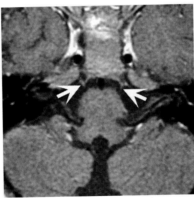

Fig. A. An axial post-gadolinium T1-WI with fat saturation demonstrates the sixth cranial nerves bilaterally (*arrows*) exiting from the ventral brainstem at the pontomedullary junction and coursing through the ventral subarachnoid space.

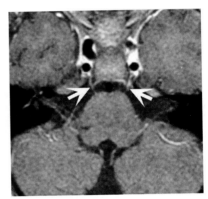

Fig. B. A more cephalad image demonstrates the sixth cranial nerves bilaterally (*arrows*) traversing the petrous apex and heading toward the cavernous sinuses.

Pathology

A sixth cranial nerve palsy may result from a lesion at any point along its course, including compressive lesions of the fourth ventricle, intrinsic brainstem pathology, cisternal/subarachnoid disease, cavernous sinus masses, or orbital apex processes. Because of the close relationship between the nuclei of CNs VI and VII (see CN VII section), these nerves are often affected together by brainstem processes. The subarachnoid segment of the nerve is vulnerable to traumatic injury and leptomeningeal processes. Where the nerve crosses the petrous ridge, it may be affected by inflammatory, expansile, or destructive processes of the petrous apex (Figs. C and D), or may be compressed in the setting of elevated intracranial pressure. More distally, CN VI is vulnerable to processes involving the cavernous sinus, superior orbital fissure and orbital apex, often in conjunction with CNs III, IV, and VI.

Suggested Readings

Brodkey JA, Robertson JH, Shea JJ III, Gardner G. Cholesterol granuloma of the petrous apex: combined neurosurgical and otological management. *J Neurosurg* 85:625–633, 1996.

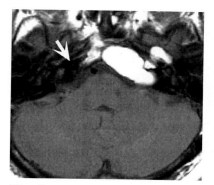

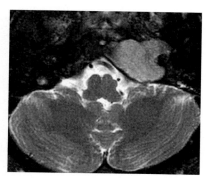

Fig. C. A patient with a history of chronic headaches presents with diplopia and a left sixth nerve palsy is diagnosed. An axial T1-WI demonstrates a strikingly hyperintense, expansile legion of the left petrous apex, with smooth remodeling of the left side of the clivus. The normally pneumatized right petrous apex is indicated for comparison (*arrow*).

Fig. D. An axial T2-WI (same patient as Fig. C) demonstrates that the lesion is of intermediate to high signal intensity. At surgery, thick "chocolate-like" fluid was drained from the lesion, diagnostic of cholesterol granuloma.

Case 151

Clinical Presentation

A young man with 1 week of fever and neck stiffness develops right CN VI and CN VII palsies.

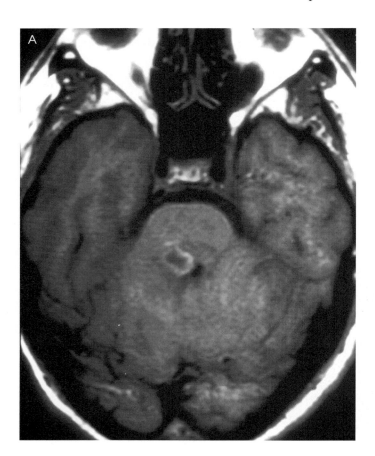
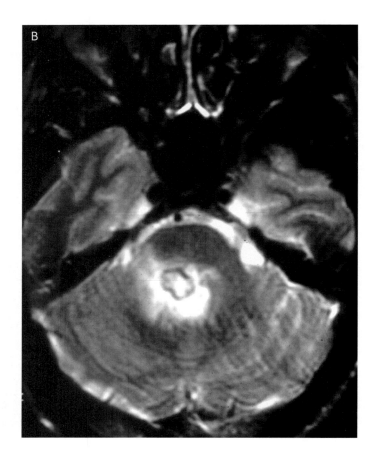

Radiologic Findings

An axial T1-WI (Fig. A) demonstrates a mass in the right dorsal pons. The lesion shows a peripheral rim of intrinsic T1 shortening. On a T2-WI (Fig. B), the lesion shows central hyperintensity and a peripheral rim of hypointensity, as well as surrounding edema.

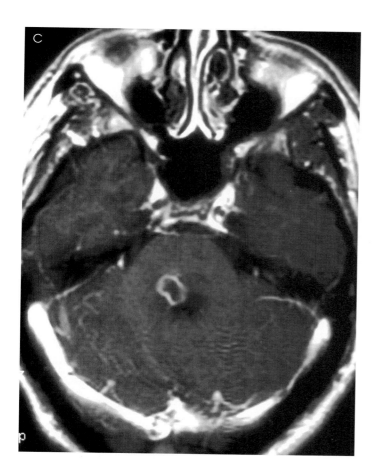

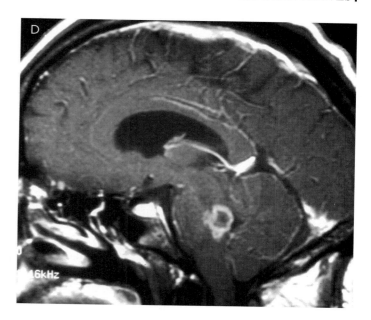

Post-gadolinium, an axial T1-WI (Fig. C) demonstrates enhancement of the thin, somewhat irregular, peripheral rim. A sagittal post-gadolinium T1-WI (Fig. D) shows the peripherally enhancing lesion in the dorsal pons, as well as possibly a small "daughter" lesion at the inferior aspect of the mass. In addition, there is slightly prominent surface enhancement overlying vermian folia, suggesting a possible associated leptomeningeal process.

Diagnosis

Brainstem abscess and meningitis. A specific organism was not isolated. The patient was treated with broad spectrum antibiotics and improved over the course of a few weeks.

Differential Diagnosis

- Brainstem glioma (often a longer duration of symptoms, typically a diffuse infiltrative lesion)
- Brainstem encephalitis (often more extensive brainstem involvement, with variable enhancement that is typically more diffuse and mild than is seen in this case)
- Metastatic lesion (usually an older patient with a known primary lesion, lacks intrinsic peripheral T1 shortening though may show evidence of hemorrhage)
- Multiple sclerosis (typically a relapsing and remitting clinical course, evidence of periventricular plaques and callosal lesions)

Discussion

Intracerebral abscesses are uncommon, with an incidence of 0.13 cases per 100,000 persons. Within this population, solitary brainstem abscesses account for 0.5 to 6% of cases, and the pons is most commonly affected. Most cases are caused by *Streptococcus* and *Staphylococcus* species and result from hematogenous seeding, often in the context of severe dental disease, but in many cases no source is identified. *Mycobacterium tuberculosis* is also a common cause of brainstem abscess, particularly in regions where pulmonary disease is prevalent. Many patients will have symptoms of an accompanying meningitis, and brainstem abscess will be identified when cranial neuropathy and/or long tract signs develop. MR is the study of choice and may demonstrate typical features of a parenchymal abscess: a rounded mass with surrounding edema and a rim that shows both T1 and T2 shortening as well as intense post-gadolinium enhancement. Because of the relatively inaccessibility of these lesions, they are often managed with antibiotics alone. In the case of a large, refractory, or enlarging lesion, however, stereotactic aspiration is useful to relieve local mass effect and arrive at a specific diagnosis.

Case 152

Clinical Presentation

A 36-year-old woman who had been diagnosed with a congenital unilateral left sixth cranial nerve palsy underwent MR imaging.

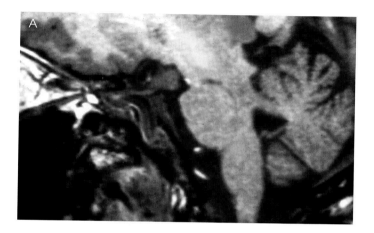 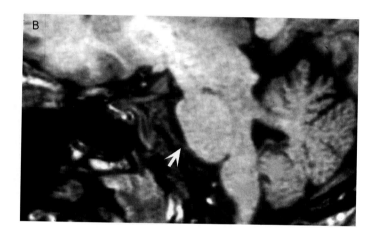

Radiologic Findings

A sagittal spoiled gradient-recalled acquisition image (Fig. A) obtained by reformatting a volumetric axial acquisition shows no evidence of a left sixth cranial nerve in its expected position in the prepontine cistern. The normal right sixth cranial nerve is shown for comparison as it ascends in the right prepontine cistern (*arrow*, Fig. B).

Diagnosis

Duane's syndrome

Differential Diagnosis

None: This is a pathognomonic appearance.

Discussion

Duane's syndrome consists of a congenital unilateral horizontal abduction deficit accompanied by retraction of the globe on attempted adduction. Pathologic studies have demonstrated two anatomic abnormalities in patients with this syndrome: absence of the abducens nerve and anomalous innervation of the affected lateral rectus muscle by a branch of the ipsilateral third cranial nerve. The left eye is more commonly affected than the right, and the syndrome is more common in females. Some patients are benefited by surgery, and indications for surgical intervention include a noticeable horizontal deviation of the globe, an abnormal head position, marked retraction on adduction, and a cosmetically unacceptable upshoot or downshoot in adduction.

Suggested Readings

Fulgham JR, Wijdicks EFM, Wright AJ. Cure of a solitary brainstem abscess with antibiotic therapy: case report. *Neurology* 46:1451–1454, 1996. (Case 151)

Parsa CF, Grant PE, Dillon WP, Du Lac S, Hoyt WF. Absence of the abducens nerve in Duane syndrome verified by magnetic resonance imaging. *Am J Ophthalmol* 125:399–401, 1998. (Case 152)

Cranial Nerve VII

Function

The seventh cranial nerve (CN VII), also known as the facial nerve, has both sensory and motor components. The branchial motor component innervates the muscles of facial expression (buccinator, platysma, frontalis, occipitalis, orbicularis oculi, and orbicularis oris muscles), the stapedius, the stylohyoid, and the posterior belly of the digastric muscle. The visceral motor component stimulates the lacrimal, submandibular, and sublingual glands, as well as the mucous membranes of the nose and palate. The general sensory component supplies a small area of skin on the concha of the auricle and behind the ear. The visceral sensory component receives taste sensation from the anterior two-thirds of the tongue and the palate.

Anatomy

The motor nucleus of CN VII is located in the dorsal pons, and the superior salivary (or lacrimal) nucleus lies adjacent to it. The superior aspect of the nucleus solitarius (shared with CNs IX and X) subserves taste. The fibers of CN VII leave the nuclei, course dorsally toward the floor of the fourth ventricle, and loop around the nucleus of CN VI. This creates a slight bulge in the floor of the fourth ventricle known as the facial colliculus. The fibers then emerge on the ventrolateral aspect of the brainstem and traverse the lateral subarachnoid space of the cerebellopontine angle (CPA). CN VII, along with CN VIII, enters the internal auditory canal (IAC) and travels in the anterosuperior aspect of the IAC.

At the fundus of the IAC, CN VII turns anteriorly and enters the narrow fallopian canal, which houses the labyrinthine segment of the nerve (Fig. A). The nerve makes a turn (anterior genu) at the level of the geniculate ganglion, where the greater superficial petrosal nerve (GSPN) takes off (Fig. B). The GSPN innervates the lacrimal gland and mucous glands in the nasal and oral cavities. The tympanic segment of the nerve then continues posteriorly in a bony canal that lies inferior to the horizontal semicircular canal (Figs. C and D). The facial nerve makes a posterior genu and gives off the nerve to the stapedius muscle, which functions in dampening loud sounds. The nerve descends further in the mastoid segment of the facial canal (Figs. E and F), gives off the chorda tympani branch (which innervates the submandibular and sublingual glands and also receives taste sensation from the anterior two-thirds of the tongue and the palate), and eventually exits the temporal bone at the level of the stylomastoid foramen to enter the parotid gland.

Pathology

CN VII may be affected at multiple points along its course. One important clinical point is whether a patient has a central or a peripheral facial palsy. As the upper muscles of facial expression receive bilateral input from higher cortical centers, they will be spared by an upper motor neuron lesion (central facial palsy) but will be affected by a lesion at the nuclear level or below (peripheral facial palsy). If both CN VI and CN VII are affected, this suggests a brainstem lesion.

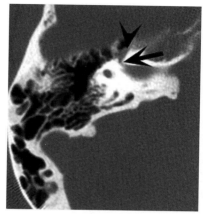

Fig. A. The bony anatomy of the facial nerve canal is illustrated in the following six images from a CT scan of the right temporal bone. In this image, the bony fallopian canal (*arrow*) is seen arising from the anterosuperior aspect of the IAC, heading toward the anterior genu (*arrowhead*).

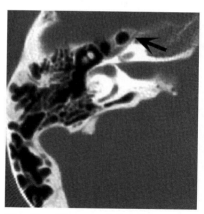

Fig. B. The canal for the greater superficial petrosal nerve (*arrow*) arises at the level of the geniculate ganglion.

If both CN VII and CN VIII are affected, this suggests a lesion of the CPA or IAC. If CN VII is affected in isolation, this suggests a lesion more peripherally in the temporal bone or in the parotid gland. Common pathologies that affect CN VII include Bell's palsy, cholesteatoma of the middle ear and mastoid, hemangioma of the temporal bone, schwannoma of CN VII, and parotid malignancy.

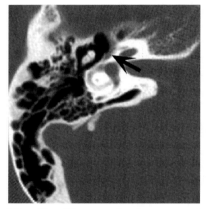

Fig. C. The proximal aspect of the canal for the tympanic segment of the facial nerve (*arrow*) is seen coursing posteriorly from the anterior genu.

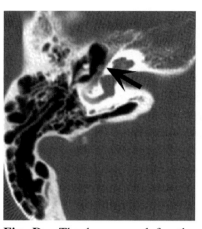

Fig. D. The bony canal for the tympanic segment of the nerve continues posteriorly (*arrow*) and passes under the lateral semicircular canal.

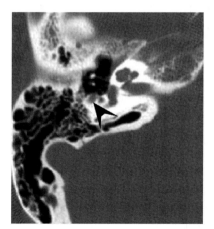

Fig. E. The nerve makes a posterior genu and continues inferiorly in the descending mastoid segment of the bony canal (*arrowhead*).

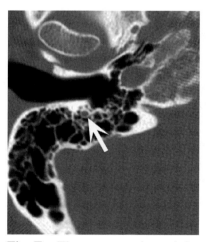

Fig. F. The nerve continues inferiorly in the mastoid (*arrow*), posterior to the bony wall of the external auditory canal.

Case 153

Clinical Presentation

A young woman has the onset of complete left-sided facial palsy over a 24-hour period.

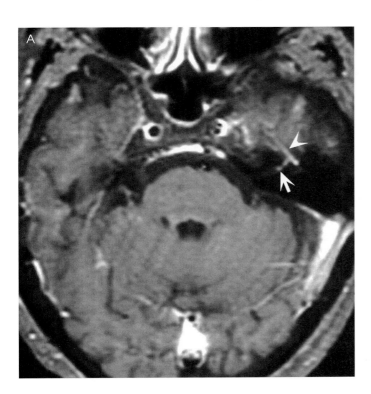
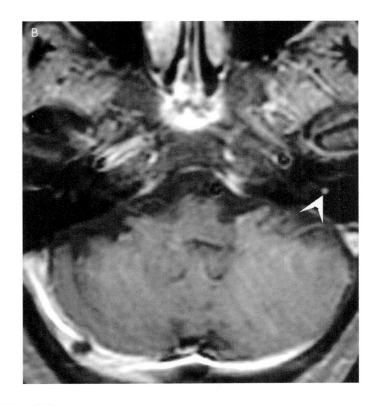

Radiologic Findings

An axial post-gadolinium T1-WI with fat saturation (Fig. A) demonstrates abnormal enhancement along the course of the left facial nerve, including the distal intracanalicular segment (*arrow*), the labyrinthine segment, the region of the geniculate ganglion, and the greater superficial pertrosal nerve (*arrowhead*). A more inferior axial post-gadolinium T1-WI with fat saturation (Fig. B) demonstrates intense enhancement of the descending mastoid segment of the left facial nerve (*arrowhead*). There is no evidence of abnormal enhancement on the right side.

Diagnosis

Bell's palsy

Differential Diagnosis

- Trauma to facial nerve (history, evidence of temporal bone fracture)
- Herpes zoster oticus (severe lancinating pain, vesicles on tympanic membrane and along ear canal)

- Retrograde spread of parotid neoplasm (usually a gradually progressive facial palsy)

Discussion

The most common causes of unilateral complete facial paralysis include Bell's palsy, trauma, and herpes zoster oticus (Ramsay Hunt syndrome). Other less common causes of facial paralysis include multiple sclerosis, Lyme disease, and neoplasm. Bell's palsy accounts for 60 to 75% of all cases of facial paralysis. As Bell's palsy is defined as facial paralysis of unknown origin, it is in effect a diagnosis of exclusion. Etiologic theories have included genetic, metabolic, autoimmune, vascular, and infectious causes. Many investigators have claimed evidence for a viral etiology (particularly herpes simplex), and treatment often includes both systemic corticosteroids and antiviral agents. About 85% of patients regain some facial movement within 3 weeks of the onset of paresis, and the remaining 15% begin to improve within 3 to 6 months. Most patients have a complete recovery, but 10 to 15% will have residual weakness. Imaging is generally not required for a diagnosis of Bell's palsy. Imaging studies are indicated if the palsy is atypical (gradual in onset or no improvement within 6 months) or recurrent.

Case 154

Clinical Presentation

An elderly patient complains of involuntary, paroxysmal, painless left facial spasms.

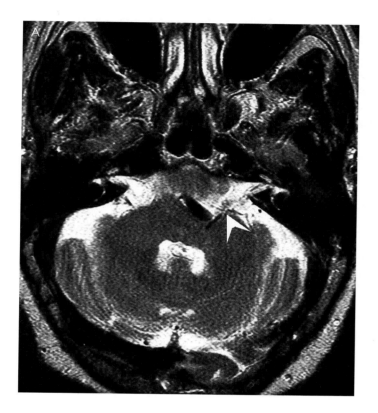

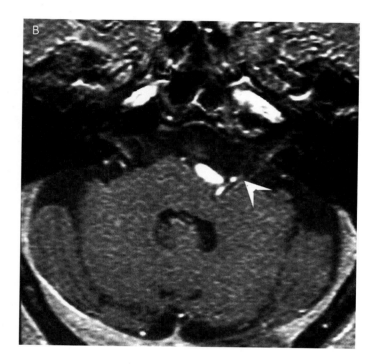

Radiologic Findings

An axial thin-section fast spin-echo T2-WI (Fig. A) demonstrates marked distortion of the left ventral and ventrolateral pons by a tortuous, ectatic vertebral artery. In addition, a prominent anterior inferior cerebellar artery (AICA) is noted at the level of the root exit zone of the left seventh cranial nerve (*arrowhead*). An axial partition image from an intracranial MR angiogram (Fig. B) similarly demonstrates the marked compression of the pons and left CPA by the tortuous, ectatic vertebral artery, and the AICA at the level of the root exit zone of the left seventh cranial nerve (*arrowhead*).

Diagnosis

Hemifacial spasm due to vascular compression

Differential Diagnosis

None: This is a pathognomonic appearance.

Discussion

Hemifacial spasm results from unilateral hyperactive dysfunction of the facial nerve. The syndrome is characterized by the onset of mild and intermittent spasms in the orbicularis oculi muscle that gradually progress in severity and frequency and spread downward to include all the muscles of facial expression. Most cases result from vascular compression at the root exit zone of the facial nerve, with responsible vessels including the AICA, the posterior inferior cerebellar artery, the vertebral artery, the basilar artery, or basal veins in descending order of frequency. Criteria for neurovascular compression include that the compressive vessel(s) should run at right angles to the nerve, should contact the root exit zone, and should deform the proximal nerve. Surgical microvascular decompression leads to relief of symptoms in 60 to 90% of cases and is widely performed. Imaging is useful to exclude other causes of hemifacial spasm such as brainstem pathology or a cisternal neoplasm. In many cases, the offending vessel can be identified using conventional MR sequences or with high-resolution three-dimensional imaging sequences.

Case 155

Clinical Presentation

A 56-year-old man with a progressive facial palsy over the course of a year presents for evaluation.

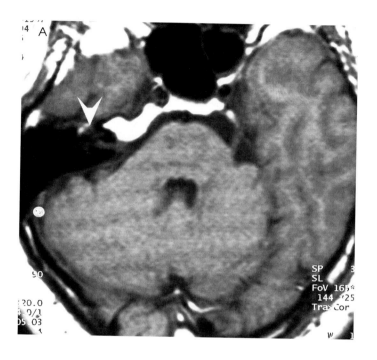

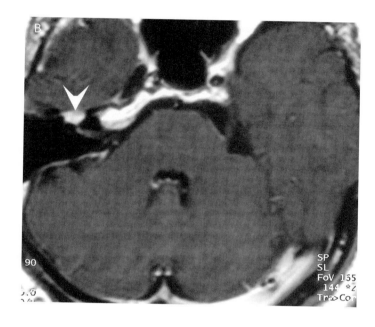

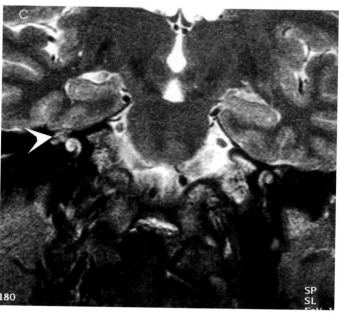

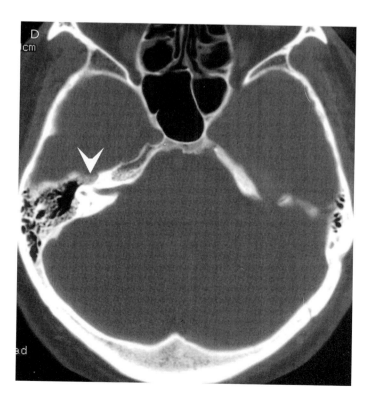

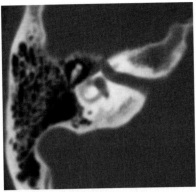

Fig. E. Axial image from a temporal bone CT scan in a 45-year-old woman with long-standing facial palsy demonstrates smooth, tubular enlargement of the fallopian canal and proximal tympanic segment of the facial canal. This facial nerve schwannoma was confirmed surgically.

Radiologic Findings

An axial T1-WI (Fig. A) suggests slightly prominent soft tissue at the level of the right geniculate ganglion (*arrowhead*). Post-gadolinium, an axial T1-WI (Fig. B) demonstrates intense, homogeneous enhancement of the geniculate region mass (*arrowhead*). A coronal fast spin-echo T2-WI (Fig. C) shows that the mass (*arrowhead*) is hyperintense to white matter and isointense to gray matter. The bone window from an axial CT scan (Fig. D) demonstrates a somewhat irregularly marginated lesion at the level of the right geniculate ganglion (*arrowhead*). Slightly increased density within the lesion is related to residual bone spicules and/or calcification within the lesion.

Diagnosis

Hemangioma of the facial canal

Differential Diagnosis

- Facial nerve schwannoma (smooth, often tubular enlargement of facial canal (Fig. E))
- Meningioma of facial nerve canal (very rare, may induce a hyperostotic response)
- Bell's palsy (acute presentation, lacks a soft tissue mass, no bone changes)

Discussion

Hemangiomas of the temporal bone are relatively rare lesions that may occur in the CPA, the IAC, or the facial canal near the geniculate ganglion. They are not true neoplasms but rather are hamartomatous lesions that represent mesodermal rests of vasoformative tissue. Neovascular enlargement occurs by canalization of hyperplastic solid masses of endothelial cells, and these lesions produce symptoms as a result of neural compression. Geniculate-region hemangiomas arise from the perigeniculate capillary plexus and present with progressive facial weakness. They are typically small lesions (< 1 cm) that have irregular and indistinct margins with bone on CT scans ("honeycomb bone"), and often intratumoral bone spicules and calcifications. Enhancement is characteristically intense and relatively homogeneous, and these lesions are generally intermediate to bright on T2-WIs.

Case 156

Clinical Presentation

An elderly man with a remote history of a parotid gland adenoid cystic carcinoma presents with facial palsy and hearing loss.

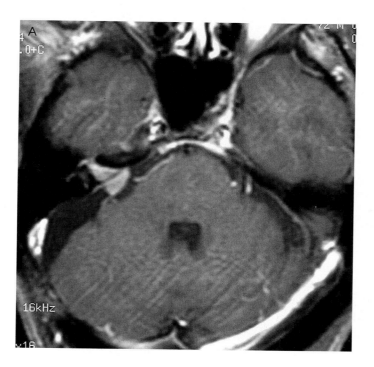
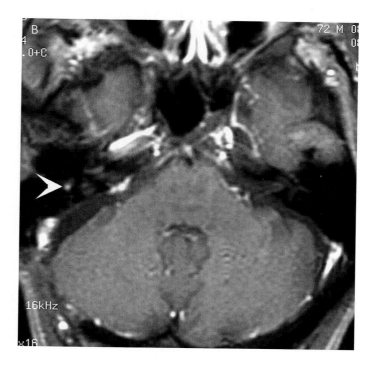

Radiologic Findings

An axial post-gadolinium T1-WI with fat saturation (Fig. A) demonstrates an enhancing soft tissue mass filling the right internal auditory canal, with a component extending into the right CPA. A more inferior axial post-gadolinium T1-WI with fat saturation (Fig. B) demonstrates abnormal enhancement along the descending mastoid segment of the right facial nerve (*arrowhead*).

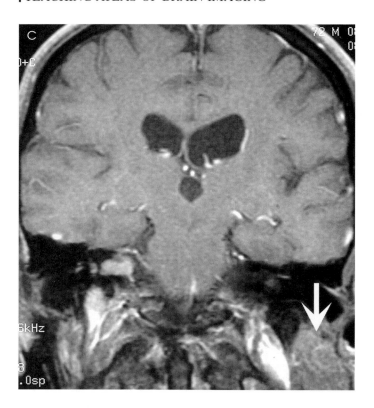

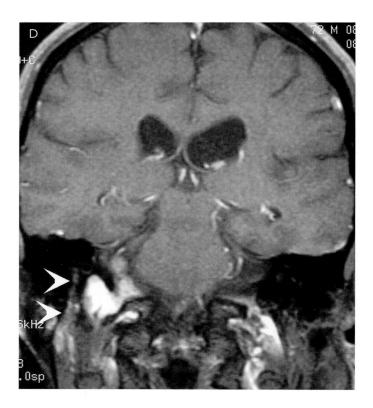

A coronal post-gadolinium T1-WI with fat saturation (Fig. C) again demonstrates the abnormally enhancing soft tissue mass filling the right IAC and extending into the CPA. In addition, enhancing soft tissue is seen within the right labyrinth. The right parotid gland is surgically absent. Note the normal parotid gland on the left (*arrow*). A slightly more posterior coronal post-gadolinium T1-WI with fat saturation (Fig. D) demonstrates abnormal enlargement and enhancement of the descending mastoid segment of the right facial nerve (*arrowheads*).

Diagnosis

Perineural spread of tumor along CN VII

Differential Diagnosis

- Vestibular schwannoma (enhancement should not extend into the facial canal)
- Facial nerve schwannoma (tubular enlargement of facial nerve canal, patients often asymptomatic until the lesion becomes very large)
- Meningioma (unusual to fill entire IAC unless large, and enhancement should not extend into the facial canal)
- CSF spread of tumor (often involves IACs bilaterally, would not expect enhancement to extend into the facial canal)
- Bell's palsy (uniform enhancement of CN VII that does not extend proximal to the distal IAC, no mass is present)

Discussion

Perineural spread of disease along the facial nerve is usually secondary to retrograde spread of parotid malignancy. This may be present at the time of initial presentation or may occur in the setting of residual or recurrent disease and represents direct extension from the primary site along branches of the facial nerve. Tumor may also reach the facial nerve from the fifth cranial nerve via the greater superficial petrosal nerve (GSPN), a branch of the facial nerve that breaks away at the level of the geniculate ganglion and courses anteromedially to exit the superior surface of the temporal bone via the facial hiatus. The GSPN passes under Meckel's cave as it heads toward foramen lacerum, at which point it joins the deep petrosal nerve to form the vidian nerve. As the GSPN passes by Meckel's cave, it may be involved by tumor that has affected the trigeminal nerve, and this tumor may extend back along the GSPN to the facial canal and IAC.

Suggested Readings

Du C, Korogi Y, Nagahiro S, et al. Hemifacial spasm: three-dimensional MR images in the evaluation of neurovascular compression. *Radiology* 197:227–231, 1995. (Case 154)

Ginsberg LE, De Monte F, Gillenwater AM. Greater superficial petrosal nerve: anatomy and MR findings in perineural tumor spread. *AJNR* 17:389–393, 1996. (Case 156)

Shelton C, Brackmann DE, Lo WWM, Carberry JN. Intratemporal facial nerve hemangiomas. *Otolaryngol Head Neck Surg* 104:116–121, 1991. (Case 155)

Engstrom M, Abdsaleh S, Ahlstrom H, et al. Serial gadolinium-enhanced magnetic resonance imaging and assessment of facial nerve function in Bell's palsy. *Otolaryngol Head Neck Surg* 117:559–566, 1997. (Case 153)

Cranial Nerve VIII

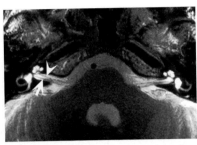

Fig. A. Axial high-resolution fast spin-echo T2-WI of the IACs demonstrates the cochlear (*arrowhead*) and inferior vestibular nerves (*arrow*) bilaterally. This image was obtained with surface coils and shows shading of intensity across the image from peripheral to central.

Function

The eighth cranial nerve (CN VIII), also known as the vestibulocochlear nerve, is a purely sensory nerve. It carries auditory information from the cochlea and balance information from the semicircular canals.

Anatomy

The peripheral processes of the primary sensory neurons of CN VIII receive input from sensory receptors in the cochlea and vestibular apparatus. The cell bodies of these neurons reside in the spiral and vestibular ganglia, respectively, and their central processes form CN VIII. CN VIII traverses the internal auditory canal (IAC) and cerebellopontine angle (CPA) (Fig. A), then enters the brainstem at the lateral aspect of the pontomedullary junction. The vestibular nuclear complex is located in the floor of the fourth ventricle. These nuclei contribute fibers to the medial longitudinal fasciculus (MLF), which terminates bilaterally in the nuclei of CNs III, IV, and VI. The MLF's primary function is maintaining orientation in space, and by coordinating extraocular muscle function with vestibular function, it allows the eyes to maintain fixation on an object while the head is moving. The dorsal and ventral cochlear nuclei are located lateral to the vestibular complex. From the cochlear nuclei, fibers decussate and ascend in the contralateral lateral lemniscus to reach the inferior colliculus, the medial geniculate body of the thalamus, and eventually the superior temporal gyrus where the conscious perception of sound occurs.

Pathology

Lesions of the auditory component of CN VIII may lead to tinnitus (ringing in the ear) and eventually deafness. Lesions of the vestibular component result in vertigo, nausea, and balance problems. If both CN VII and CN VIII are affected, a lesion can be localized to the CPA and/or IAC. Large brainstem lesions may affect multiple cranial nerves, as may large lesions of the CPA. The most common pathology of CN VIII is the vestibular schwannoma (commonly referred to as an "acoustic neuroma").

Case 157

Clinical Presentation

A 56-year-old man is evaluated for gradually progressive sensorineural hearing loss.

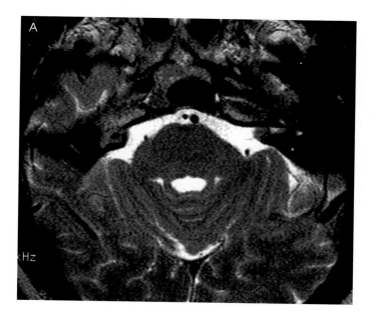

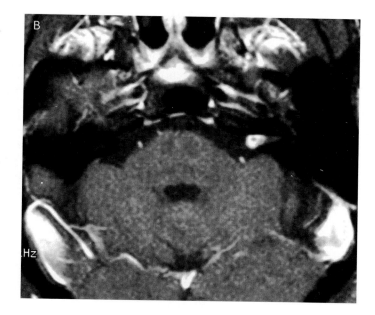

Radiologic Findings

An axial fast spin-echo T2-WI with fat saturation (Fig. A) demonstrates a well-circumscribed, rounded mass in the proximal aspect of the left IAC. The mass is hypointense to CSF and isointense to brain parenchyma. Following administration of gadolinium, an axial T1-WI with fat saturation (Fig. B) demonstrates intense, homogeneous enhancement of the left intracanalicular mass.

Diagnosis

Vestibular schwannoma

Differential Diagnosis

- Meningioma (rare to be entirely intracanalicular)
- Facial nerve schwannoma (rare compared with vestibular schwannoma, often extends into facial nerve canal)
- CSF spread of tumor (less masslike, tends to involve both internal auditory canals, usually occurs in the context of known primary malignancy)

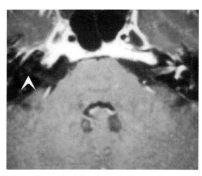

Fig. C. A 45-year-old woman has sudden onset of left-sided hearing loss, as well as ataxia and vertigo. An axial post-gadolinium T1-WI demonstrates diffuse enhancement in the left internal auditory canal, cochlea, and vestibule. The right inner ear structures show no evidence of abnormal enhancement (*arrowhead*).

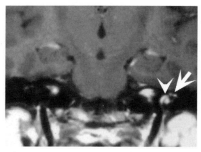

Fig. D. A post-gadolinium coronal T1-WI (same patient as in Figure B) demonstrates intense enhancement of the left cochlea (*arrowhead*). The facial nerve (*arrow*) also demonstrates asymmetric enhancement, though the patient had no symptoms referable to the left facial nerve. She was diagnosed presumptively with viral labyrinthitis, and a follow-up scan three months later when she was asymptomatic showed resolution of abnormal enhancement.

• Viral neuritis (less masslike, often causes abrupt onset of symptoms such as vertigo and hearing loss; see Figs. C and D)

Discussion

Vestibular schwannomas, still commonly referred to as acoustic neuromas, are benign nerve sheath tumors that usually arise from the vestibular portion of the eighth cranial nerve. They represent 8% of all primary intracranial neoplasms and 60 to 90% of tumors of the CPA and IAC. Small intracanalicular lesions usually result in hearing loss, tinnitus, and/or vertigo. As the lesion grows and extends into the CPA, auditory symptoms worsen, and headache may occur due to localized dural irritation. As the tumor enlarges further, trigeminal and/or facial nerve symptoms may also occur, although facial nerve symptoms are quite rare. With further growth and brainstem compression, hydrocephalus may ensue. On MR imaging, lesions are typically iso- or mildly hypointense compared with brain parenchyma on T1-WIs, unless focal hemorrhage has occurred. Lesions are hypointense to CSF and iso- or hyperintense to brain parenchyma on T2-WIs. Most lesions enhance intensely and homogeneously post-gadolinium, but areas of non-enhancement may be due to cystic degeneration. MR is the study of choice for the diagnosis of vestibular schwannoma. Although many lesions can be detected using thin-section high-resolution fast spin-echo T2-weighted imaging, administration of gadolinium is often helpful in demonstrating small lesions and other pathologies that may be confused clinically with vestibular schwannoma.

Case 158

Clinical Presentation

A 57-year-old man complains of 1 month of tinnitus and hearing loss.

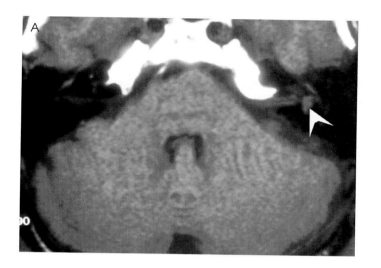

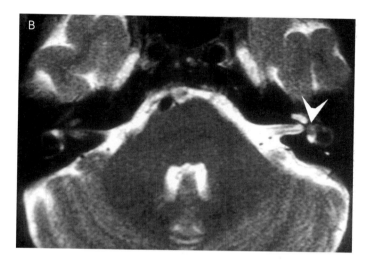

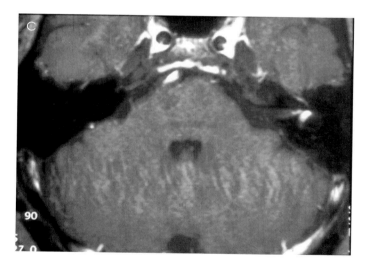

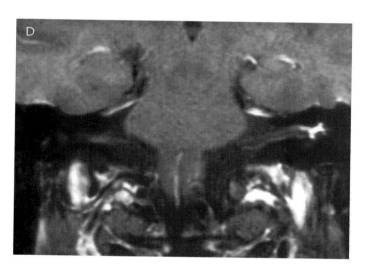

Radiologic Findings

An axial T1-WI (Fig. A) demonstrates a questionable soft tissue mass in the left vestibule (*arrowhead*). On an axial fast spin-echo T2-WI with fat saturation (Fig. B), the mass is identified within the left vestibule (*arrowhead*) and is hypointense to CSF. Post-gadolinium, an axial T1-WI with fat saturation (Fig. C) demonstrates intense abnormal enhancement in the left vestibule, as well as the fundus of the IAC. A coronal post-gadolinium T1-WI with fat saturation (Fig. D) confirms the presence of an enhancing lesion involving the left vestibule, proximal semicircular canals, and fundus of the left IAC. A follow-up MR examination 6 months later (*not shown*) showed progressive enlargement of the lesion, and the patient was taken to the operating room.

Diagnosis

Intralabyrinthine vestibular schwannoma

Differential Diagnosis

Viral labyrinthitis (acute onset of symptoms, should resolve over weeks to months, may be associated with hemorrhage)

Discussion

Primary intralabyrinthine schwannomas arise from the Schwann cells surrounding the peripheral fibers of the cochlear nerve within the turns of the cochlea or the peripheral vestibular nerve fibers innervating the vestibule or semicircular canals. They are very rare compared with the more typical schwannoma arising in the IAC and are often associated with neurofibromatosis type 2. Like the more common schwannomas of the IAC, intralabyrinthine schwannomas are encapsulated and slow growing. These lesions appear as hypointense masses compared to CSF on thin-section, high-resolution fast spin-echo T2-WIs and show homogeneous enhancement post-gadolinium. In some cases, the lesion may grow and extend throughout the labyrinth, rather than causing focal expansion and remodeling of a portion of the bony labyrinth. These lesions may rarely extend to the middle ear. The true incidence of these lesions is unknown as diagnosis is often presumptive because surgery would destroy remaining hearing in patients who still have useful hearing.

Suggested Readings

Mafee MF. MR imaging of intralabyrinthine schwannoma, labyrinthitis, and other labyrinthine pathology. *Otolaryngol Clin N Am* 28:407–430, 1995. (Case 158)

Mulkens TH, Parizel PM, Martin JJ, et al. Acoustic schwannoma: MR findings in 84 tumors. *AJR* 160:395–398, 1993. (Case 157)

O'Keefe LJ, Camilleri AE, Gillespie JE, et al. Primary tumors of the vestibule and inner ear. *J Laryngol Otol* 111:709–714, 1997. (Case 158)

Seltzer S, Mark AS. Contrast enhancement of the labyrinth on MR scans in patients with sudden hearing loss and vertigo: evidence of labyrinthine disease. *AJNR* 12:13–16, 1991. (Case 157)

Cranial Nerve IX

Function

The ninth cranial nerve (CN IX), the glossopharyngeal nerve, has both motor and sensory functions divided among five major components. The branchial motor component innervates the stylopharyngeus muscle, which elevates the pharynx during swallowing and speech. The visceral motor component stimulates secretion from the parotid gland. The visceral sensory component carries information from the carotid body and carotid sinus. The special sensory component subserves taste from the posterior one-third of the tongue. Finally, the general sensory component provides general sensory information from the posterior one-third of the tongue, the skin of the external ear, and the internal surface of the tympanic membrane.

Anatomy

Within the brainstem, the functions of CN IX are mediated by a group of nuclei, some of which also serve CNs X and V. These include the nucleus ambiguus, nucleus solitarius, and the spinal nucleus of CN V. The inferior salivatory nucleus mediates function of the parotid gland. CN IX emerges from the medulla as a series of rootlets that exit the groove between the olive and the inferior cerebellar peduncle. The rootlets converge to form the trunk of CN IX, which then traverses the jugular foramen, usually in the more anterior pars nervosa. The tympanic branch (parasympathetic supply to the parotid gland via the lesser petrosal nerve, as well as sensation to the middle ear and bony eustachian tube) is given off in the jugular foramen, and the superior and inferior glossopharyngeal ganglia are located in the foramen. Below the jugular foramen, CN IX travels in the carotid sheath with CNs X and XI before branching into multiple components and traveling to its target organs.

Pathology

Because of the close association among CNs IX, X, and XI in the brainstem, jugular foramen, and upper carotid sheath, it is rare to find an isolated lesion of CN IX. The integrity of CN IX is best assessed by testing the gag reflex. The general sensory component of CN XI mediates this response, and damage to CN IX leads to an absent gag reflex. Any lesion of the lower brainstem, jugular foramen, or carotid space may lead to dysfunction of CN IX. More common pathologies include medullary infarction, schwannomas of lower cranial nerves, and paragangliomas.

Case 159

Clinical Presentation

An elderly woman presents with brief attacks of lancinating pain that begin in the throat and radiate down the side of the neck from in front of the ear to the back of the lower jaw.

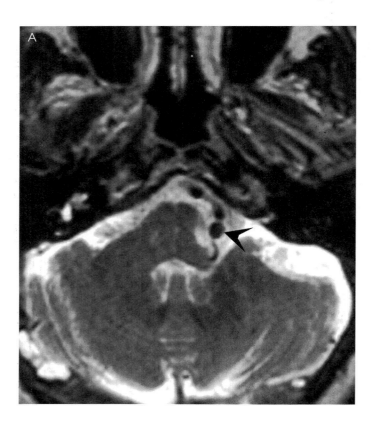
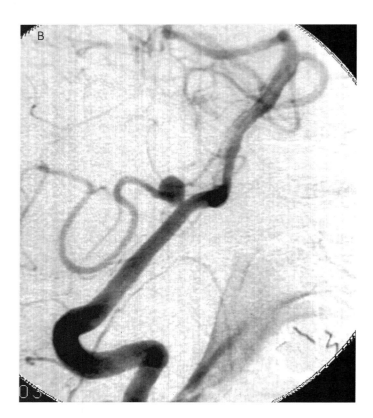

Radiologic Findings

An axial T2-WI (Fig. A) demonstrates a rounded hypointense mass in the left cerebellomedullary angle (*arrowhead*), at the level of the expected origin of the left posterior inferior cerebellar artery (PICA). A lateral view from a cerebral angiogram obtained during selective injection of the left vertebral artery (Fig. B) demonstrates a rounded, contrast-filled mass at the level of the origin of the left PICA.

Diagnosis

Aneurysm of the PICA leading to glossopharyngeal neuralgia (GPN)

Differential Diagnosis

None: This is a pathognomonic appearance.

Discussion

GPN is a rare syndrome that leads to pain in the distribution of the glossopharyngeal nerve. It is far less common than trigeminal neuralgia and has a median age of onset of 64 years. The pain is typically unilateral (75%), lancinating in nature and occurs in the region of the ear, tongue, tonsil, and/or larynx. Attacks tend to be paroxysmal and brief and are often induced by yawning, sneezing, or swallowing. Although symptoms of GPN are usually sensory, disturbances along branches from the carotid sinus may occur, leading to cardiac arrhythmia and syncope. The majority of cases are attributable to vascular compression at the root entry zone of CN IX, and microvascular decompression is highly successful in relieving symptoms of GPN. Vascular loops (usually of the PICA) are often discovered at surgery, although the compression may also be related to an aneurysm or another compressive mass lesion. When the compressed nerves are examined histologically, demyelination, axonal edema, and/or endoneural fibrosis may be seen. Rarely, primary brainstem pathology may lead to GPN, sometimes leading to pain involving multiple anatomic sites in the head and neck and likely due to the fact that multiple cranial nerves contribute to the descending spinal nucleus of the trigeminal nerve. MR may demonstrate brainstem pathology, a compressive lesion, and occasionally the vascular loop itself.

Case 160

Clinical Presentation

A 48-year-old female presents with difficulty swallowing and hoarseness. On examination, she has an absent gag reflex and a vocal cord paralysis.

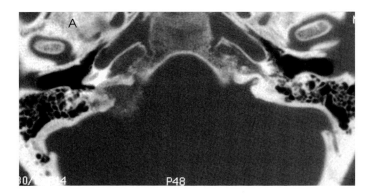

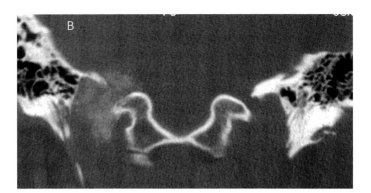

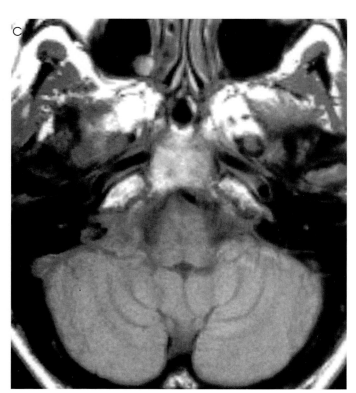

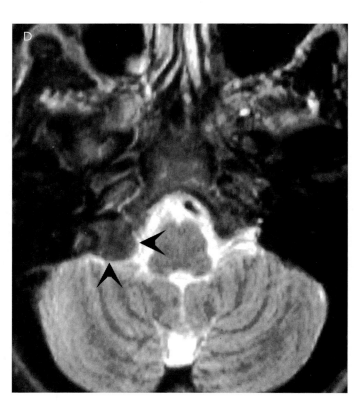

Radiologic Findings

An axial image from a skull base CT scan photographed in bone window (Fig. A) demonstrates irregular calcification at the level of the right cerebellomedullary angle. A coronal image from the same CT scan (Fig. B) demonstrates a calcified mass extending from the right cerebellomedullary angle into the superior aspect of the right jugular foramen. An axial T1-WI from an MR examination (Fig. C) demonstrates an intermediate-signal intensity mass extending toward the right jugular foramen. On an axial T2-WI (Fig. D), the mass is hypointense to brain parenchyma (*arrowheads*).

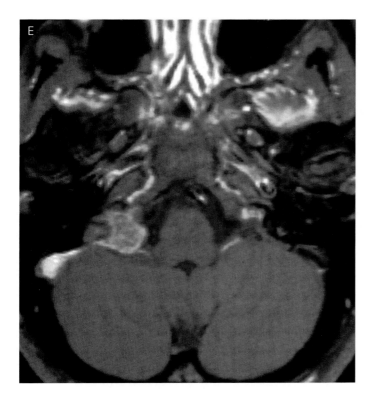

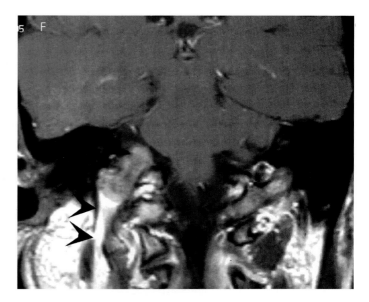

Post-gadolinium, axial (Fig. E) and coronal (Fig. F) T1-WIs with fat saturation demonstrate moderate, homogeneous enhancement of the soft tissue mass that extends from the right cerebellomedullary angle into the superior aspect of the jugular foramen. Note the normal jugular vein inferior to the mass (*arrowheads*, Fig. F).

Diagnosis

Meningioma of the jugular foramen

Differential Diagnosis

- Schwannoma (not generally calcified, often more round, may have areas of cyst formation and hemorrhage when large)
- Paraganglioma (not typically calcified, often contains visible flow voids when larger than 2 cm)
- Metastasis (irregular bone destruction, not typically calcified, may see multiple masses)

Discussion

The jugular foramen is a relatively uncommon location for meningioma. These patients generally present with headache and lower cranial nerve deficits such as hoarseness and dysphagia. In some cases, patients may present with a neck mass when the tumor has descended through the jugular foramen and grown considerably in the neck. Meningiomas are composed of neoplastic meningothelial cells and are well-demarcated but unencapsulated tumors. On CT, these lesions are often calcified. On MR, meningiomas are typically smoothly marginated lesions with a broad dural base. They are isointense to gray matter on T1- and T2-WIs and enhance intensely with gadolinium. At angiography, most jugular foramen meningiomas show only minimal vascularity, unlike the prominent and prolonged vascular blush that is characteristic of supratentorial meningiomas. The treatment of choice is surgical removal, usually by a combined neurosurgical–neurotologic team. Radiation therapy is useful for subtotally resected or recurrent lesions.

Case 161

Clinical Presentation

A 75-year-old woman who has noted progressive headache and gait difficulty over the past year presents with choking episodes. Examination shows loss of the gag reflex.

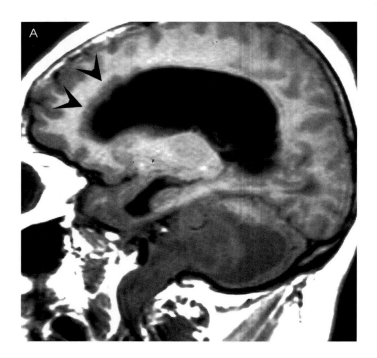

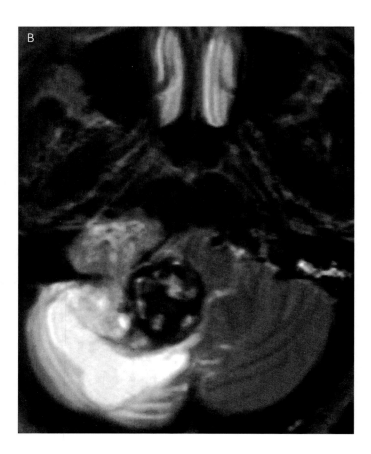

Radiologic Findings

A sagittal T1-WI (Fig. A) demonstrates a mixed cystic and solid posterior fossa mass that extends through a widened jugular foramen into the upper carotid space. Note the massive dilatation of the lateral ventricle consistent with obstructive hydrocephalus, as well as evidence for transependymal flow of CSF in the periventricular white matter (*arrowheads*). An axial T2-WI (Fig. B) demonstrates that the mass is very heterogeneous. Anteromedially, it is quite hypointense, consistent with areas of hemorrhage. Anterolaterally, it is mildly hyperintense to brain parenchyma, and a large component is noted extending into the right jugular foramen. Posteriorly, an area of very bright signal is consistent with a large cyst.

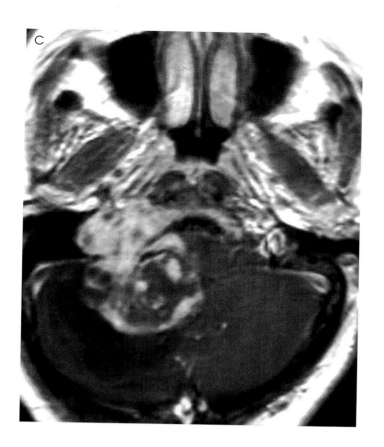

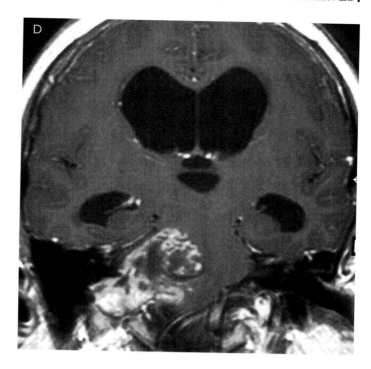

Post-gadolinium, an axial T1-WI (Fig. C) demonstrates moderately homogeneous enhancement of the jugular foramen component of the mass, heterogeneous enhancement of the cerebellomedullary component of the mass, and non-enhancement of the posterior cyst. A coronal post-gadolinium T1-WI (Fig. D) also demonstrates the heterogeneously enhancing extra-axial mass compressing and distorting the right cerebellopontine and cerebellomedullary angles, and extending into the right jugular foramen. The coronal image also demonstrates marked obstructive hydrocephalus, with enlargement of the lateral ventricles and third ventricle.

Diagnosis

Schwannoma of CN IX

Differential Diagnosis

- Meningioma (intermediate-signal intensity on T2-WI, typically a broad dural base, may see a "dural tail")
- Paraganglioma (often irregularly marginated, may see prominent flow voids if larger than 2 cm, may be multiple)
- Giant aneurysm (variable signal intensity, often multiple layers of thrombus of varying ages, extension through jugular foramen would be very unusual)
- Chondrosarcoma (center of lesion usually in a bony or cartilaginous structure, typically strikingly hyperintense on T2-WI unless calcified)

Discussion

Schwannomas may arise from any cranial or spinal nerve, as well as from smaller unnamed nerves. These tumors are typically smoothly marginated, round or ovoid, encapsulated tumors composed of spindle-shaped neoplastic Schwann cells. When arising in the region of the jugular foramen, it is often difficult to determine the nerve of origin preoperatively and even intraoperatively. Presenting symptoms are usually related to lower cranial nerve deficits, but patients may be asymptomatic or have only nonspecific symptoms such as headache. Glossopharyngeal schwannomas are rare, with only 30 or so cases reported. On CT, schwannomas cause smooth enlargement of the jugular foramen and may dumbbell into the posterior fossa or into the infratemporal fossa. Unlike paragangliomas, they rarely extend into the middle ear. On MR, schwannomas are typically intermediate signal intensity on T1-WIs and hyperintense on T2-WIs, with intense enhancement postgadolinium. Hemorrhage and calcification are relatively uncommon, but as tumors enlarge, cystic degeneration is commonly seen. Angiography can be helpful in some cases as schwannomas are typically avascular or hypovascular lesions, while paragangliomas are hypervascular.

Suggested Readings

Caldemeyer KS, Mathews VP, Azzarelli B, Smith RR. The jugular foramen: a review of anatomy, masses, and imaging characteristics. *Radiographics* 17:1123–1139, 1997. (Case 161)

Olds MJ, Woods CI, Winfield JA. Microvascular decompression in glossopharyngeal neuralgia. *Am J Otol* 16:326–330, 1995. (Case 159)

Tekkok IH, Ozcan OE, Turan E, Onol B. Jugular foramen meningioma. *J Neurosurg Sci* 41:283–292, 1997. (Case 160)

Cranial Nerve X

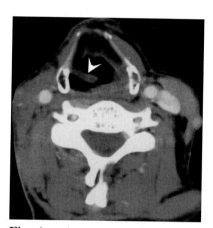

Fig. A. A contrast-enhanced CT of the neck in a patient who has previously undergone a right neck dissection and now presents with hoarseness demonstrates a patulous right pyriform sinus (P) and antero-medial deviation of the right aryepiglottic fold (*arrow*).

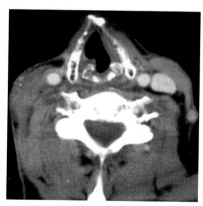

Fig. B. A more inferior image from the same patient as in Figure A demonstrates medial rotation of the right arytenoid, medial deviation of the right true vocal cord, and dilatation of the right laryngeal ventricle. In this patient, recurrent squamous cell carcinoma with involvement of lymph nodes in the right tracheoesophageal groove (*not shown*) led to dysfunction of the right recurrent laryngeal nerve, and paralysis of the right true vocal cord.

Function

The tenth cranial nerve (CN X), also known as the vagus nerve, has both motor and sensory functions, and an extensive distribution. The branchial motor component innervates the striated muscles of the pharynx, tongue, and larynx, with the exception of the stylopharyngeus (CN IX) and the tensor veli palatini (V3). The visceral motor component innervates the smooth muscle and glands of the pharynx and larynx, as well as the thoracic and abdominal viscera. The visceral sensory component receives input from the larynx, trachea, and thoracic and abdominal viscera, as well as from stretch receptors in the walls of the aortic arch and chemoreceptors in the aortic bodies adjacent to the aortic arch. The general sensory component receives input from the pharynx, part of the external surface of the tympanic membrane, and from the skin at the back of the ear and in the external acoustic meatus.

Anatomy

Like CN IX, the functions of CN X are mediated by a group of nuclei within the brainstem. Important nuclei include the nucleus solitarius, the nucleus ambiguus, the spinal nucleus of CN V, and the dorsal vagal (motor) nucleus. Also, like CN IX, CN X emerges from the brainstem as a series of rootlets that exit below the fibers of CN IX. The rootlets converge to form a trunk that traverses the pars vascularis of the jugular foramen. Two sensory ganglia (superior or jugular, and inferior or nodosum) are located within the jugular fossa. Within the jugular foramen, the auricular nerve (nerve of Arnold) emerges from the superior ganglion of the vagus nerve. This branch innervates part of the skin of the external ear, the external ear canal, and the inferior portion of the external surface of the tympanic membrane. Below the jugular foramen, CN X travels in the carotid sheath between the internal jugular vein and the internal carotid artery. Important branches in the neck include the pharyngeal, superior laryngeal, right recurrent laryngeal, and cardiac branches. The right recurrent laryngeal nerve hooks under the right subclavian artery before ascending in the tracheoesophageal groove to the larynx. The left recurrent laryngeal nerve branches off the main trunk of the vagus nerve in the chest, hooks posteriorly under the aortic arch, traverses the aortopulmonic (AP) window, then ascends through the superior mediastinum and along the left tracheoesophageal groove to reach the larynx. The recurrent nerves supply the intrinsic muscles of the larynx except the cricothyroid (which is supplied by the external laryngeal branch of the superior laryngeal nerve).

Pathology

A lesion of CN X results in hoarseness due to dysfunction of the intrinsic laryngeal musculature with resultant paresis or paralysis of the true vocal cord (Figs. A and B) and difficulty swallowing due to the inability to elevate the soft palate. The presence or absence of associated cranial nerve palsies is helpful in localizing pathology. If CNs IX, XI, and/or XII are also affected, pathology is most likely at the level of the brainstem, jugular foramen, or upper carotid sheath (*i.e.*, above the hyoid bone). If CN X is affected in isolation, the lesion may be located from the lower carotid sheath to the AP window (*i.e.*, below the hyoid bone). CN X may be affected along with other cranial nerves by a mass lesion of the jugular foramen or upper carotid sheath such as a schwannoma or paraganglioma. Metastatic disease to the skull base or the structures of the carotid sheath may also result in multiple lower cranial nerve palsies (Figs. C and D). CN X may be affected in isolation if it is injured during surgery (carotid endarterectomy or thyroidectomy), if it is compressed or invaded in the tracheoesophageal groove by tracheal or esophageal masses, or if it is impinged upon in the AP window by an aortic aneurysm or enlarged lymph nodes.

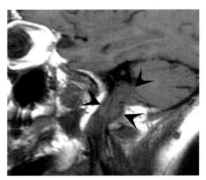

Fig. C. A 56-year-old man with a history of previously treated squamous cell carcinoma of the tongue presents with hoarseness and skull base pain. A sagittal T1-WI demonstrates a soft tissue mass involving the upper carotid sheath, extending through the jugular foramen, and into the posterior fossa (*arrowheads*). On examination, he had an absent gag reflex and weakness of shoulder shrug.

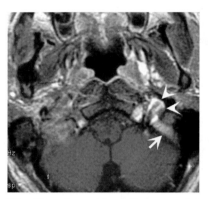

Fig. D. A post-gadolinium axial T1-WI with fat saturation (same patient as in Fig. C) demonstrates moderate homogeneous enhancement of the soft tissue mass which fills the right jugular foramen. Note the normal jugular bulb (*arrowheads*) and sigmoid sinus (*arrow*) on the contralateral side. Biopsy confirmed recurrent squamous cell carcinoma involving the structures of the carotid sheath with intravascular and intracranial extension.

Case 162

Clinical Presentation

A 56-year-old woman presents with acute onset of hoarseness and ataxia.

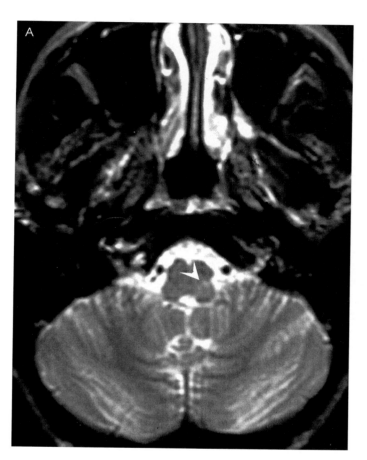

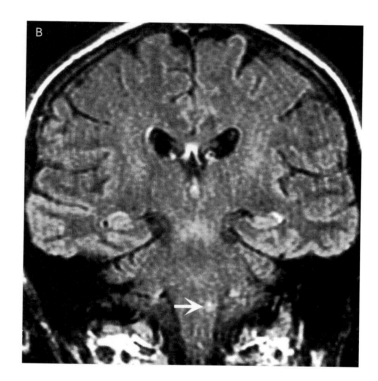

Radiologic Findings

An axial T2-WI (Fig. A) demonstrates a subtle region of T2 prolongation in the left dorsolateral medulla (*arrowhead*). A coronal fluid-attenuated inversion recovery (FLAIR) image (Fig. B) confirms the focal area of T2 prolongation in the left dorsolateral medulla (*arrow*). The skull base and neck were imaged to assess for possible vertebral artery dissection.

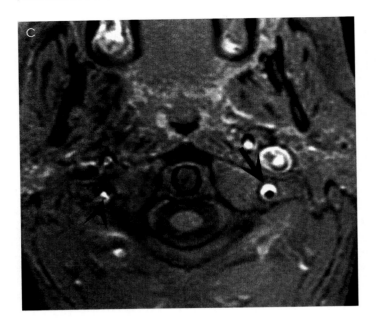

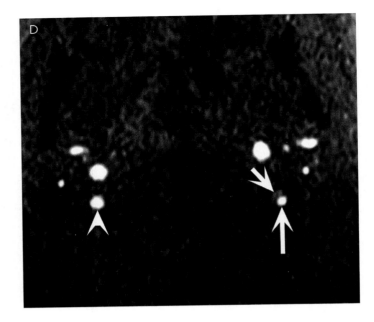

An axial T1-WI with fat saturation (Fig. C) demonstrates a hyperintense crescent (*arrow*) consistent with subintimal methemoglobin around the periphery of the left vertebral artery. High signal within the lumen of the right vertebral artery (*arrowhead*), as well as in the internal carotid arteries, is related to the use of flow compensation. An axial partition image from the corresponding MR angiogram (Fig. D) demonstrates flow-related enhancement within the reduced lumen of the left vertebral artery (*long white arrow*). The methemoglobin crescent is seen faintly "shining through" on this image (*short white arrow*). The lumen of the right vertebral artery (*arrowhead*) is seen to be normal. Evidence of a left true vocal cord paralysis was also noted on the examination of the neck (*not shown*).

Diagnosis

Lateral medullary infarction due to left vertebral artery dissection

Differential Diagnosis

- Brainstem tumor (symptoms usually gradual in onset, mass effect, expansion)
- Brainstem encephalitis (uncommon, more diffuse signal abnormality not confined to a vascular territory)

Discussion

Lateral medullary infarction, also known as Wallenberg's syndrome, may have a variable clinical presentation depending on the extent of the anatomic lesion. Symptoms and signs of Wallenberg's syndrome include pain, numbness, and/or decreased sensation over the ipsilateral half of the face due to involvement of the descending tract and spinal nucleus of CN V; ataxia of limbs due to involvement of spinocerebellar and olivocerebellar fibers; vertigo, nausea and vomiting, nystagmus, and/or diplopia due to involvement of the vestibular nuclei; Horner's syndrome due to involvement of the descending sympathetic tracts; dysphagia, hoarseness, vocal cord paralysis, and/or decreased gag reflex due to involvement of the nuclei of CNs IX and X; and impaired pain and temperature sense over the contralateral half of the body due to involvement of the spinothalamic tracts. Lateral medullary infarction is usually due to occlusion of the vertebral artery or the posterior inferior cerebellar artery (PICA), often in the context of a vertebral artery dissection. Vertebral artery stenosis may also result in lateral medullary infarction, usually due to emboli to the PICA. In a series of 34 patients with lateral medullary infarction, cerebral angiography demonstrated isolated PICA disease in 24%, isolated vertebral artery disease in 38%, involvement of both the vertebral artery and PICA in 26%, and normal results in 12%. Isolated PICA disease tends to cause small, thin lesions in the lateral caudal and/or dorsolateral middle-rostral portion of the medulla. Vertebral artery stenosis or occlusion tends to produce a medium-sized, diagonal band-shaped lesion that leads to the classic lateral medullary syndrome with a crossed sensory pattern. In this case, only a tiny focal lesion was identified, which resulted in a tenth cranial nerve palsy and ataxia.

Case 163

Clinical Presentation

A 67-year-old woman presents with several months of pulsatile tinnitus, as well as increasing hoarseness and difficulty swallowing.

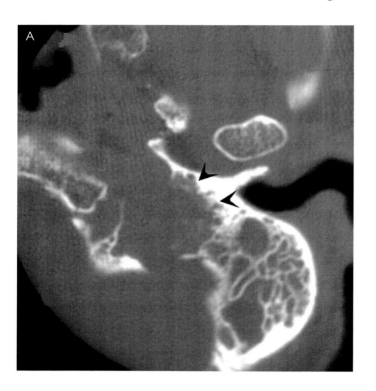

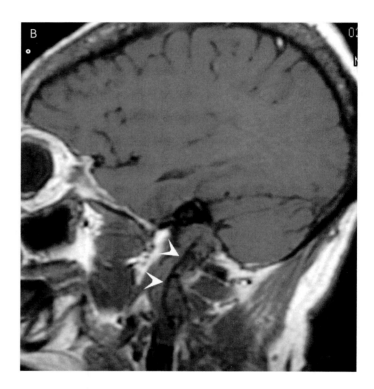

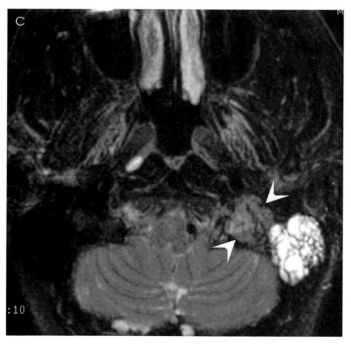

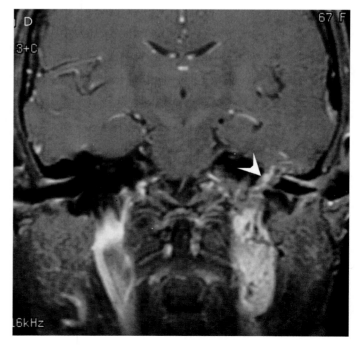

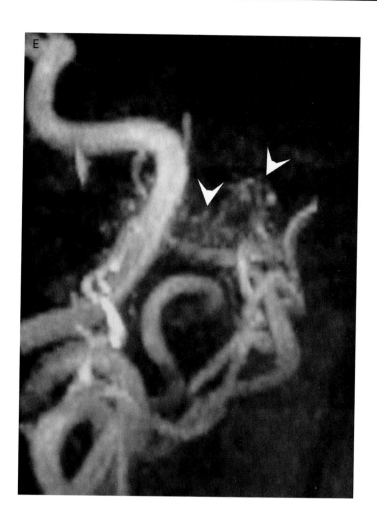

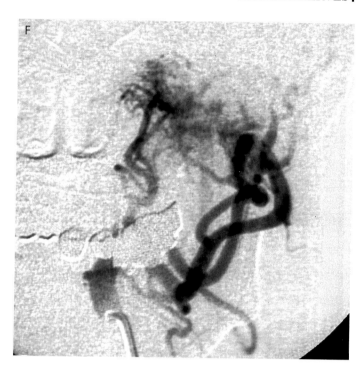

Radiologic Findings

An axial image from a CT scan photographed in bone window (Fig. A) demonstrates irregular enlargement of the left jugular foramen. The lateral margin of the foramen shows irregular erosive changes (*arrowheads*). A sagittal T1-WI from an MR examination (Fig. B) demonstrates a soft tissue mass within the jugular foramen extending inferiorly into the carotid space of the upper neck. Prominent flow voids are identified within the mass (*arrowheads*). An axial fast spin-echo T2-WI with fat saturation (Fig. C) demonstrates an isointense soft tissue mass centered within the left jugular foramen (*arrowheads*) and containing flow voids. Note the high-signal intensity of fluid within adjacent mastoid air cells, likely secondary to eustachian tube compression. A coronal post-gadolinium T1-WI with fat saturation (Fig. D) demonstrates intense enhancement of the soft tissue mass. A superior component of the mass extends into the middle ear (*arrowhead*). A maximum intensity projection image from an MR angiogram (MRA) (Fig. E) demonstrates flow-related enhancement within tumor vessels (*arrowheads*). An AP projection from a conventional arteriogram obtained during selective injection of the left external carotid artery (Fig. F) demonstrates a hypervascular mass supplied by enlarged ascending pharyngeal, occipital, and posterior auricular arteries.

Diagnosis

Glomus jugulare tumor

Differential Diagnosis

- Schwannoma (smooth bone erosion or remodeling on CT, does not show large flow voids or hypervascularity)
- Meningioma (often causes a hyperostotic reaction, has a broad dural base, large flow voids are not usually seen)
- Metastasis (may be hypervascular, typically more infiltrative and destructive)

Discussion

Glomus tumors, also called paragangliomas or chemodectomas, are slow-growing neoplasms arising from glomus bodies. Glomus bodies consist of nonchromaffin cells derived from the neural crest and are normal components of the diffuse neuroendocrine system. Their function is often obscure, but they likely function as chemoreceptors. In the head and neck, favored locations for glomus tumors include the tympanic plexus in the middle ear cavity (glomus tympanicum), the dome of the jugular bulb (glomus jugulare), the nodose ganglion of the vagus nerve (glomus vagale), and the carotid body near the carotid bifurcation (carotid body tumor). Vagal paragangliomas are the least common, representing approximately 5% of head and neck paragangliomas. Because of the proximity of the hypotympanum to the jugular fossa, many tumors will involve both of these locations.

In the temporal bone, glomus bodies accompany the tympanic nerve (nerve of Jacobson, a branch of CN IX) and the auricular branch of the vagus nerve (nerve of Arnold). In the jugular foramen, glomus tumors arise from glomus bodies in the adventitia of the jugular bulb. Depending on their location, lesions may present with symptoms of pulsatile tinnitus or hearing loss, or with symptoms due to mass effect on lower cranial nerves. These tumors may be multiple and/or familial, and they rarely metastasize. (Malignant degeneration occurs in 4% of cases.) On CT, they typically result in irregular permeative destruction of bone. On MR, they are often irregularly marginated tumors that are intermediate-signal intensity on T1-WIs, iso- to mildly hyperintense on T2-WIs, and enhance intensely post-gadolinium. Tumors larger than 2 cm may show prominent intralesional flow voids, which is a helpful feature in the differential diagnosis. In some cases, these tumoral flow voids may be visualized with MRA. Conventional angiography, which is often useful for preoperative embolization, demonstrates a hypervascular mass that is usually supplied by branches of the external carotid artery.

Suggested Readings

Kim JS, Lee JH, Choi CG. Patterns of lateral medullary infarction: vascular lesion-magnetic resonance imaging correlation of 34 cases. *Stroke* 29:645–652, 1998. (Case 162)

Vogl TJ, Juergens M, Balzer JO, et al. Glomus tumors of the skull base: combined use of MR angiography and spin-echo imaging. *Radiology* 192:103–110, 1994. (Case 163)

Cranial Nerve XI

Function

The eleventh cranial nerve (CN XI), also known as the spinal accessory nerve, is a purely motor nerve that innervates the sternocleidomastoid (SCM) and trapezius muscles.

Anatomy

The spinal accessory nucleus is located in the lateral part of the anterior gray column of the spinal cord from the C1 to C5 or C6 levels. It receives input from higher cortical areas via the posterior limb of the internal capsule and the lateral corticospinal tracts. These descending fibers synapse in the accessory nucleus, and the postsynaptic fibers emerge from the lateral aspect of the spinal cord. These rootlets coalesce, ascend intracranially through the foramen magnum, and then exit the cranium via the pars vascularis of the jugular foramen. CN XI travels briefly in the upper carotid sheath, then exits the sheath to descend along the SCM muscle. The nerve penetrates and innervates the SCM and trapezius muscles.

Pathology

A lesion of CN XI results in loss of action of the SCM and trapezius muscles. Trapezius dysfunction results in downward and lateral rotation of the scapula and weakness of shoulder shrug. SCM dysfunction results in difficulty rotating the head to the contralateral side. The most common cause of an isolated lesion of CN XI is prior neck dissection. CN XI may be affected in combination with CNs IX and X by lesions of the jugular foramen or upper carotid sheath.

Case 164

Clinical Presentation

A 55-year-old man with a history of prior neck dissection complains of difficulty lifting his right arm.

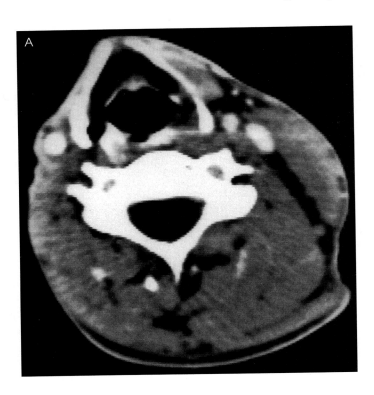

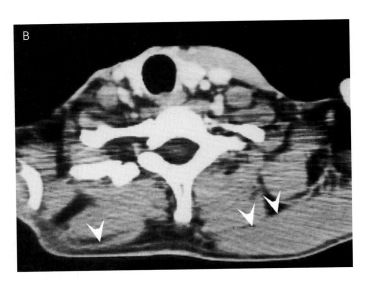

Radiologic Findings

An axial image from a contrast-enhanced CT scan (Fig. A) demonstrates changes due to prior right neck dissection, with absence of the right jugular vein and right sternocleidomastoid muscle. A more inferior image (Fig. B) demonstrates marked atrophy of the right trapezius muscle (*arrowhead*) as compared with the normal left side (*arrowheads*). (*Case courtesy of H. Ric Harnsberger, M.D., Salt Lake City, UT.*)

Diagnosis

Iatrogenic injury to CN XI

Differential Diagnosis

- Recurrent tumor with involvement of CN XI (may see a mass, abnormal lymph nodes, or other evidence of recurrent disease)
- Other traumatic injuries to CN XI (clinical history essential)

Discussion

Iatrogenic injury to the spinal accessory nerve usually occurs secondary to neck dissection or lymph node biopsy in the posterior cervical triangle. In some cases, the nerve must be sacrificed as part of a planned radical neck dissection. Injury to CN XI is often not recognized immediately or is incorrectly diagnosed. Reasons for this delay include partial preservation of trapezius muscle function due to variable innervation, which can lead to variable levels of disability, as well as the fact that there may be compensation for trapezius muscle function (especially shoulder shrug) by the levator scapulae. On imaging, atrophy of the trapezius and/or sternocleidomastoid muscles will be observed depending on the level of the injury. In some cases, a "pseudomass" representing compensatory hypertrophy of the levator scapulae may be seen. In general, nerve exploration should be considered when the patient's clinical exam does not improve within 3 months of injury. However, nerve repair may be beneficial in reducing pain and improving shoulder abduction even as long as 12 months after injury.

Case 165

Clinical Presentation

A patient with neurofibromatosis type 2 (NF2) presents for routine imaging.

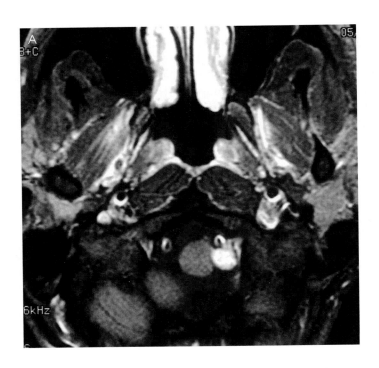

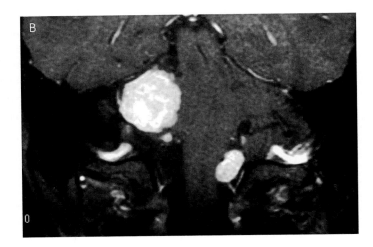

Radiologic Findings

An axial post-gadolinium T1-WI with fat saturation (Fig. A) demonstrates a smooth, round, homogeneously enhancing soft tissue mass lateral to the medulla and posterior to the left vertebral artery. On a coronal post-gadolinium T1-WI with fat saturation (Fig. B), the mass is clearly extra-axial and located at the level of the foramen magnum. In addition, note that the patient has a right cerebellopontine angle mass, representing a known vestibular schwannoma.

Diagnosis

Schwannoma of CN XI

Differential Diagnosis

- Meningioma (broad dural base, may be calcified)
- Paraganglioma (not a typical location, usually more irregularly marginated)

Discussion

Cranial nerve schwannomas are relatively common lesions, but schwannoma involving cranial nerve XI is uncommon. These lesions may arise anywhere along the course of CN XI, including the upper cervical spinal canal, the foramen magnum, the jugular foramen, and the upper neck. In patients without NF2, these lesions are most often seen in the third to sixth decades of life and are slightly more common in females. Symptoms are variable as these lesions may be asymptomatic, may result in compromise of only the nerve of origin, or may affect multiple lower cranial nerves and result in the classic jugular foramen syndrome (loss of taste in the posterior third of the tongue, vocal cord paralysis, dysphagia, and weakness of the sternocleidomastoid and trapezius muscles). The imaging appearance of these lesions is similar to schwannomas elsewhere, with lesions being smoothly marginated, round or ovoid, moderately enhancing, and often containing a cystic component as they enlarge.

Suggested Readings

Matz PG, Barbaro NM. Diagnosis and treatment of iatrogenic spinal accessory nerve injury. *Am Surg* 62:682–685, 1996. (Case 164)

Ortiz O, Reed L. Spinal accessory nerve schwannoma involving the jugular foramen. *AJNR* 16:986–989, 1995. (Case 165)

Cranial Nerve XII

Function

The twelfth cranial nerve (CN XII), or hypoglossal nerve, is a purely motor nerve that supplies all the intrinsic and extrinsic muscles of the tongue except the palatoglossus (which is supplied by CN X).

Anatomy

The hypoglossal nucleus is located in the paramedian dorsal medulla and forms the hypoglossal eminence in the floor of the fourth ventricle. The rootlets of CN XII emerge in the ventrolateral sulcus of the medulla, between the olive and the pyramid. The nerve traverses the subarachnoid space and enters the hypoglossal canal of the occipital bone, which is located at the anterior margin of the occipital condyles. Below the skull base, the nerve travels briefly in the carotid sheath, medial to CNs IX, X, and XI. Once CN XII is below the skull base, it is joined by additional fibers from the nodose ganglion of the vagus nerve, postganglionic sympathetic fibers from the superior cervical ganglion of the sympathetic trunk, and fibers from the first cervical segment of the spinal cord. CN XII exits the carotid sheath, loops anteriorly above the greater cornua of the hyoid bone, passes above the free posterior edge of the mylohyoid muscle, and divides in the floor of mouth to supply the tongue musculature. The C1 fibers follow CN XII until it crosses the internal carotid artery, at which point they separate from the main trunk and course inferiorly as the descending hypoglossal ramus, which, with additional contributions from C2 and C3, innervates the strap muscles.

Fig. A. An axial image from a CECT in an 83-year-old patient with longstanding palsies of cranial nerves X and XII demonstrates a densely enhancing mass adjacent to the left carotid artery (*arrow*), just below the level of the jugular foramen. A patent jugular vein is not observed at this level. The patient has a history of multiple paragangliomas, and this lesion is presumed to represent a glomus jugulare tumor.

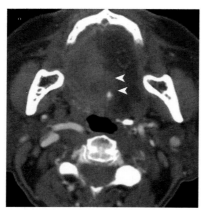

Fig. B. An image through the tongue in the same patient demonstrates marked fatty replacement in the left hemitongue. Note that the midline lingual septum is deviated to the left (*arrowheads*), and the ptotic tongue is flopping posteriorly. While a ptotic tongue can be mistaken for a mass lesion before fatty atrophy occurs, the septum would never be displaced toward the side of a mass.

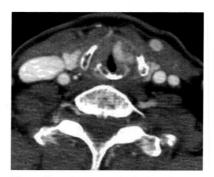

Fig. C. A more inferior image through the larynx (same patient as Figs. A and B) shows high density material within the left vocal cord. The patient had previously undergone Teflon injection into the cord to compensate for her left vocal cord paralysis related to CN X dysfunction.

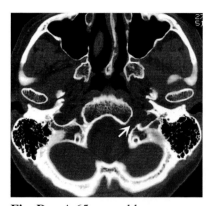

Fig. D. A 65-year-old woman noticed slowly progressive displacement and loss of bulk of the left side of her tongue. An axial CT image photographed in bone window demonstrates smooth widening of the left hypoglossal canal (*arrow*) as compared with the right side.

Pathology

Damage to the upper motor neurons that supply the tongue results in fasciculation of the tongue without atrophy, and the tongue deviates to the side opposite the lesion. Damage to the lower motor neurons results in flaccid paralysis and atrophy, and the tongue deviates to the side of the lesion. Common pathologies affecting CN XII include invasion by tumors of the oral cavity, radiation injury, and compression in the hypoglossal canal by lesions of the skull base. CN XII may also be affected by lesions of the carotid sheath, often in combination with other lower cranial nerves (Figs. A through C). Schwannomas of CN XII may occur but are rare lesions (Figs. D through F). If the strap muscles as well as the tongue are involved, then pathology is infranuclear and distal to the point at which the C1 fibers join CN XII.

Suggested Readings

Hermans R, Fossion E, Sciot R, Baert AL. Hypoglossal schwannoma. *Ann Otol Rhinol Laryngol* 104:490–492, 1995.

Thompson EO, Smoker WRK. Hypoglossal nerve palsy: a segmental approach. *Radiographics* 14:939–958, 1994.

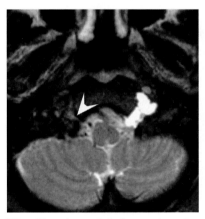

Fig. E. An axial fast spin-echo T2-WI shows a smoothly marginated, slightly lobulated, hyperintense mass filling the mildly expanded left hypoglossal canal. The normal right hypoglossal canal is shown for comparison (*arrowhead*).

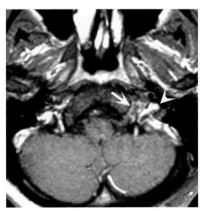

Fig. F. An axial post-gadolinium T1-WI with fat saturation demonstrates moderate, slightly heterogeneous enhancement of the soft tissue mass (*arrow*). Note that the mass is clearly located anteromedial to the jugular foramen, the position of which is indicated by the left jugular bulb (*arrowhead*). A schwannoma was confirmed at surgical biopsy.

Case 166

Clinical Presentation

A 45-year-old woman previously treated for adenoid cystic carcinoma of the nasopharynx complains of skull base pain. On examination, deviation of her tongue to the left upon protrusion is noted.

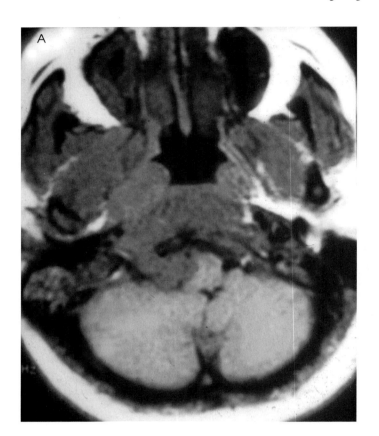
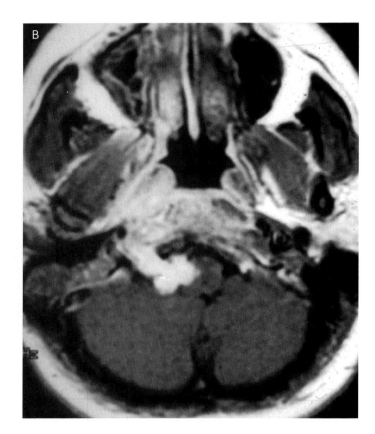

Radiologic Findings

An axial T1-WI (Fig. A) demonstrates an intermediate signal intensity soft tissue mass spreading submucosally in the nasopharynx, encroaching on the parapharyngeal fat, and extending intracranially through a widened hypoglossal canal. A component of the mass is present in the right cerebellomedullary angle and is compressing the right lateral aspect of the medulla. Proteinaceous fluid is present within the right mastoid air cells, presumably related to dysfunction of the eustachian tube. A post-gadolinium T1-WI (Fig. B) demonstrates intense enhancement of the abnormal soft tissue in the posterior fossa, hypoglossal canal, and infiltrating the prevertebral muscles and submucosal nasopharynx.

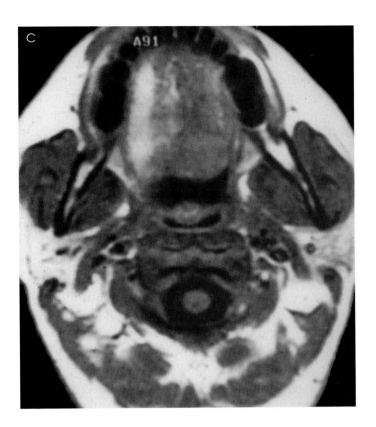 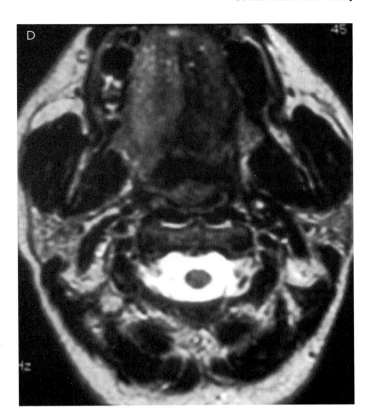

More inferiorly, an axial T1-WI (Fig. C) demonstrates high signal within the right lateral tongue, consistent with fatty atrophy. High signal within the right lateral tongue is seen on an axial T2-WI as well (Fig. D).

Diagnosis

Submucosal recurrence of nasopharyngeal adenoid cystic carcinoma with spread to the hypoglossal canal

Differential Diagnosis

- Hypoglossal schwannoma (encapsulated, well-circumscribed, does not result in skull base pain)
- Nasopharyngeal carcinoma (may be indistinguishable radiographically, requires tissue diagnosis)

Discussion

Neoplastic processes may lead to twelfth nerve palsy via several mechanisms. Primary tumors of the tongue and floor of mouth, and any tumor that accesses the carotid sheath, may spread along CN XII to the level of the hypoglossal canal and may extend intracranially. Alternatively, spread of tumor to retropharyngeal nodes may lead to extracapsular invasion and extension of tumor directly to the occipital bone, with direct involvement of the hypoglossal canal. Finally, hematogenous metastases to the occiput may lead to encroachment on the hypoglossal canal and twelfth nerve palsy. Adenoid cystic carcinoma is a tumor of minor and major salivary glands that often invades the cranial base and intracranial cavity via local and perineural spread. It tends to be locally invasive and slow growing, but has a tendency toward frequent local recurrence and late distant metastasis. When the skull base is involved, patients may complain of headache, neck pain, or progressive occipital pain. Multiple lower cranial neuropathies may be present as well, depending on the extent of the lesion. When CN XII is involved, the affected side of the tongue may initially appear larger than the normal side because of edema. Ptosis of the hemitongue may give a false impression of a tongue base mass. Over weeks to months, hemiatrophy and deviation of the tongue on protrusion become evident. On MR, replacement of normal fatty marrow in the occipital bone may be seen, as well as abnormal soft tissue in and around the hypoglossal canal. Within the ipsilateral tongue, fatty replacement, increased T2 signal, and gadolinium enhancement may become evident.

Case 167

Clinical Presentation

A 45-year-old man with a history of ethmoid sinus surgery presents with headache, low grade fevers, and multiple cranial nerve palsies including right CN IX, X, and XII palsies. CSF examination was unremarkable.

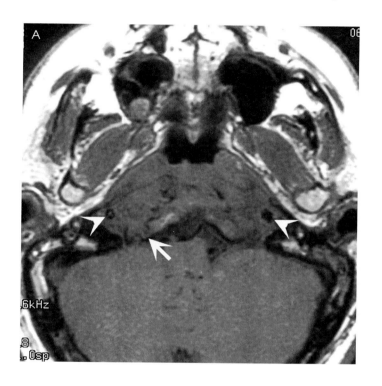

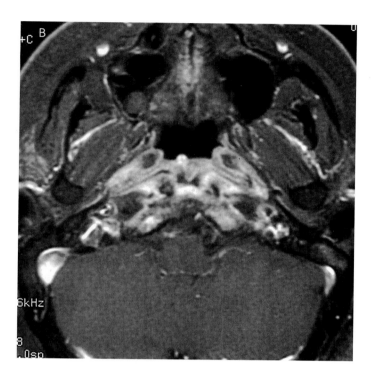

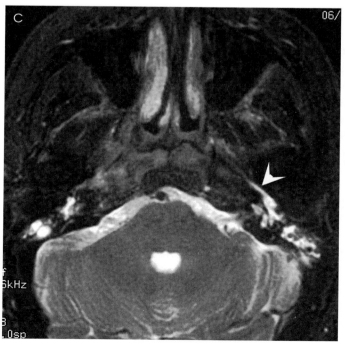

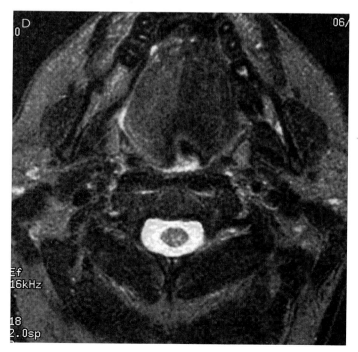

Radiologic Findings

An axial T1-WI (Fig. A) demonstrates abnormal soft tissue isointense to muscle infiltrating submucosally within the nasopharyngeal tissues, extending posteriorly to surround the carotid arteries (*arrowheads*), replacing the normal high-signal intensity fatty marrow within the clivus, and extending to the right hypoglossal canal (*arrow*). Following administration of gadolinium, an axial T1-WI with fat saturation (Fig. B) demonstrates moderately intense enhancement of the infiltrative soft tissue. An axial fast spin-echo T2-WI with fat saturation (Fig. C) demonstrates mildly increased signal within the infiltrated soft tissue as compared with muscle. In addition, there is fluid in the mastoid air cells and middle ear cavities bilaterally. On the left, fluid can be seen extending along the eustachian tube (*arrowhead*). A more inferior fast spin-echo T2-WI with fat saturation (Fig. D) demonstrates mild T2 prolongation within the right tongue, consistent with early denervation changes.

Diagnosis

Skull base osteomyelitis secondary to *Eikenella corrodens* sinusitis

Differential Diagnosis

- Nasopharyngeal carcinoma (typically has a mucosal component, usually asymmetric)
- Lymphoma (often submucosal, infiltrative; could be indistinguishable on imaging, but clinical history helpful)
- Metastatic disease (usually in context of known primary malignancy; may be infiltrative but often more masslike)

Discussion

Osteomyelitis of the skull base (OSB) is a relatively rare but potentially fatal condition. It is typically secondary to infection originating in the external auditory canal, often termed necrotizing or malignant external otitis. Patients who are diabetic or immune compromised are at particularly high risk, and in these patients, *Pseudomonas aeruginosa* is the usual pathogen. However, trauma, surgery, and paranasal sinus infection may also lead to OSB, and in these cases, the pathogens are more variable. *Eikenella corrodens* is increasingly recognized as an important pathogen in sinonasal infections. *Eikenella* is found most often as part of a mixed infection, but independently it is capable of causing serious infections in both normal and immune compromised hosts.

When skull base osteomyelitis is suspected, CT may show bone erosion due to the infectious process, but it may miss early lesions and has little role in monitoring disease progression. CT is helpful in defining sinus and skull base fractures in the setting of trauma. MR is very useful in demonstrating early loss of normal bone marrow signal, infiltration of tissue planes, and abnormal soft tissue edema and enhancement. Nuclear medicine studies may be used to demonstrate disease extent and also to follow response to therapy, particularly when combined technetium[99m]-MDP and gallium[67] scans are performed. Involvement of the jugular bulb may lead to venous sinus thrombosis, and extension to the contralateral side may produce bilateral cranial nerve palsies. Cavernous sinus thrombosis may also complicate skull base osteomyelitis. Treatment includes at least 6 weeks of antibiotics, with surgical intervention reserved for acquiring specimens for culture and for effective debridement of soft tissue.

Suggested Readings

Gormley WB, Sekhar LN, Wright DC, et al. Management and long-term outcome of adenoid cystic carcinoma with intracranial extension: a neurosurgical perspective. *Neurosurgery* 38:1105–1113, 1996. (Case 166)

Malone DG, O'Boynick PL, Ziegler DK, Batnitzky S, Hubble JP, Holladay FP. Osteomyelitis of the skull base. *Neurosurgery* 30:426–431, 1992. (Case 167)

Index

Abscess
    brain, 153–156
    brainstem, 576–578
    fungal, 172–175
Acidopathy, organic, 370–373
Acquired immunodeficiency syndrome. *See* AIDS
Acute disseminated encephalomyelitis, 339–342,
    563–564
ADEM. *See* Acute disseminated encephalomyelitis
Adenoid cystic carcinoma, nasopharyngeal, 620–622
Adrenoleukodystrophy, x-linked, 354–357
Agenesis, corpus callosum, 471–473
AIDS
    congenital, 146–148
    cryptococcosis, 187–190
    cytomegalovirus, 191–193
    HIV encephalitis, 176–178
    lymphoma, 32–35
    neurosyphilis, 194–197
    progressive multifocal leukoencephalopathy, 179–182
    toxoplasmosis, 183–186
ALD. *See* Adrenoleukodystrophy
ALS. *See* Amyotrophic lateral sclerosis
Amyloid angiopathy
    cerebral, primary, 419–421
Amyotrophic lateral sclerosis, 397–400
Anemia, sickle cell, 325–328
Aneurysm
    cranial nerve III dysfunction, 549–551
    giant, 239–242
    saccular, 235–238, 549–551
    vein of Galen, 320–324
Angiitis, central nervous system, 294–297
Anosmia, post-traumatic, 531
Anoxic injury, 268–271, 310–314
Apoplexy, pituitary, 52–54
Arachnoid cyst, 78–81
Arterial infarction, 247–251, 252–255, 256–259
Arteriovenous fistula, dural, 286–289, 290–293
Arteriovenous malformation, 277–281
Arteritis, Takayasu, 302–305
Aspergillosis, central nervous system, 172–175
Astrocytoma
    cerebellar, 91–94
    chiasmal, 542–543
    low-grade, 3–5
    pontine, 101–103
    tectal, 98–100
AVM. *See* Arteriovenous malformation
Axonal injury, diffuse, 431–434

Bacterial meningitis
    group B streptococcus, 139–142
    Haemophilus influenzae, 143–145
    pneumococcal, 223–226
Band heterotopia, 512–514
Basal ganglia disorders, 401–415
Basilar artery, thromboembolic occlusion, 256–259
Bell's palsy, 583–584
Bourneville's disease. *See* Tuberous sclerosis
Brainstem
    abscess, 576–578
    infarction, 554–555
    pontine glioma, 101–103
    tectal glioma, 98–100

Capillary telangiectasia, 275
Carbon monoxide, effects of, 351–353,
Carcinomatous meningitis, 220–222
Carotid cavernous fistula, 286–289
Carotid dissection, 260–263
Cavernous hemangioma, cavernous sinus, 548
Cavernous malformation, 272–276, 539
CCF. *See* Carotid cavernous fistula
Cephalocele, occipital, 484–486
Cerebellar astrocytoma, 91–94
Cerebellar degeneration, 416–418
Cerebellar infarction, 256–258
Cerebellitis, acute, 149–152
Cerebellopontine angle
    acoustic neuroma, 111–114
    epidermoid, 118–120
    glioblastoma, 121–123
    lipoma, 124–126
    meningioma, 115–117
Cerebral amyloid angiopathy, primary, 419–421
Cerebral edema, post-ictal, reversible, 347–350
Cerebritis, secondary to systemic lupus erythematosus,
    377–380
Chiari I malformation, 489–491
Chiari II malformation, 492–494
Chiasmal glioma, 542–543
Choroid plexus papilloma, 75–77
Cholesterol granuloma, 575
CJD. *See* Creutzfeldt-Jakob disease
CMV. *See* Cytomegalovirus
Coccidioides immitis, meningitis secondary to, 227–229
Colloid cyst, 85–87
Congenital malformations/syndromes, supratentorial,
    469–486
Corpus callosum, agenesis, 471–473
Cortical dysplasia, transmantle, 525–527

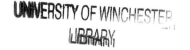

CPM. *See* Myelinolysis, central pontine
Cranial nerves, 529–625
    cranial nerve I, 531–537
    cranial nerve II, 538–546
    cranial nerve III, 547–555
    cranial nerve IV, 556–560
    cranial nerve V, 561–573
    cranial nerve VI, 574–580
    cranial nerve VII, 581–591
    cranial nerve VIII, 592–596
    cranial nerve IX, 597–604
    cranial nerve X, 605–612
    cranial nerve XI, 613–617
    cranial nerve XII, 618–625
Craniopharyngioma, 58–61
Creutzfeldt-Jakob disease, 401–403
Cryptococcosis, 187–190
Cysticercosis, 161–164
Cytomegalovirus
    congenital, 129–131
    ventriculoencephalitis, 191–193

Dandy-Walker malformation, 495–498
DAVF. *See* Arteriovenous fistula, dural
Dermoid cyst, 82–84
Diffuse axonal injury, 431–434
DNET. *See* Dysembryoplastic neuroepithelial tumor
Duane's syndrome, 579–580
Dura, diseases of, 203–219
Dural enhancement, diffuse, 216–219
Dural sinus thrombosis, 329–332
Dysembryoplastic neuroepithelial tumor, 26–28

Empyema
    epidural, 198–201
    subdural, 198–201
Encephalitis
    cytomegalovirus, 191–193
    herpes, type I, 157–160
        type II, 135–138
    HIV, 176–178
Encephalomalacia, post-traumatic, 531
Encephalomyelitis, acute disseminated, 339–342, 563–564
Ependymoma
    infratentorial, 108–110
    supratentorial, 23–25
Epidermoid, 118–120
Epidural hematoma, 425–427
Esthesioneuroblastoma, 532–534

Facial nerve, 581–591
Fibromuscular dysplasia, 298–301
FMD. *See* Fibromuscular dysplasia
Fungal meningitis, 187–190, 227–229

Ganglioglioma, 13–15
GBM. *See* Glioblastoma multiforme

Germinoma, 46–48, 62–64
Glioblastoma multiforme, 121–123
Glioma
    brainstem, 98–100, 101–103
    chiasmal, 542–543
    multicentric, 16–18
    pontine, 101–103
    tectal, 98–100
Gliomatosis, cerebri, 16–18
Gliosarcoma, 6–9
Glomus jugulare tumor, 610–612, 618
Glossopharyngeal neuralgia, 598–599
Glutaric aciduria type II, 370–373

Haemophilus influenzae meningitis, 143–145
Hallervorden-Spatz disease, 404–407
Hamartoma, tuber cinereum, 39–41
Hemangioblastoma, 95–97, 457–460
Hemangioma
    cavernous, cavernous sinus, 548
    facial canal, 587–588
Hematoma
    epidural, 425–427
    parenchymal, 277–281
    subdural, 428–430
Hemifacial spasm, from vascular compression, 585–586
Hemimegalencephaly, 505–507
Hemorrhage
    hypertensive, 264–267
    intraventricular, saccular aneurysm, 235–238
    putaminal, 264–267
    subarachnoid
        aneurysmal, 235–238
        perimesencephalic nonaneurysmal, 243–246
Herniation, tonsillar, 216–219, 489–491
Herpes encephalitis, 135–138, 157–160
Herpetic neuritis, 565–567
Heterotopia
    band, 512–514
    nodular, subependymal, 508–511
Hippocampal sclerosis, 390–393
Histiocytosis, Langerhans' cell, 381–385
HIV
    congenital infection, 146–148
    encephalitis, 176–178
Holoprosencephaly, 474–477
Human immunodeficiency virus. *See* HIV
Huntington's disease, 412–415
Hydranencephaly, 481–484
Hypertension
    intracranial, 216–219
    putaminal hemorrhage, secondary to, 264–267
Hypertensive hemorrhage, 264–267
Hypoperfusion, global, watershed infarction, 252–255
Hypotension, intracranial, spontaneous, 216–219
Hypoxic-ischemic injury, 268–271, 310–314

Infarction, 157–160
  arterial, 247–251, 256–258
  basal ganglia, causes of, 194–197
  bithalamic, basilar artery thromboembolic occlusion,
      256–258
  brainstem, 554–555
  cerebellar, basilar artery thromboembolic occlusion,
      256–258
  embolic, 247–251
  lateral medullary, 607–609
  occipital lobe, 544–546
  venous, 329–332
  watershed, 252–255
Infection, 127–201
Inflammatory/idiopathic disorders, noninfectious, 375–393
Infratentorial malformations, congenital, 487–501
Infratentorial neoplasm, 89–126
Intracranial hypotension, spontaneous, 216–219

Jugular foramen
  meningioma of, 600–601
  paraganglioma, 610–612, 618
  schwannoma, 602–604
Juvenile pilocytic astrocytoma, 91–94

Kallmann's syndrome, 531
Krabbe's disease, 362–365

Labyrinthitis, viral, 594
Langerhans' cell histiocytosis, 381–385
Lateral sclerosis, amyotrophic, 397–400
LCH. See Langerhans' cell histiocytosis
Leigh disease, 358–361
Leptomeningeal process, 220–232
Leukoencephalopathy
  posterior, 347–350
  toxic, 351–353
Leukomalacia, periventricular, 306–309
Lhermitte-Duclos disease, 499–501
Lipoma, 124–126
Lissencephaly, 515–517
Lupus, erythematosus, cerebritis and, 377–380
Lyme disease, 169–171
Lymphoma
  AIDS-related primary, 32–35
  primary, 29–31

Macroadenoma, pituitary, 52–54
Malformations
  congenital, infratentorial, 487–501
  congenital, supratentorial, 471–486
  cortical development, 503–527
Medulloblastoma, 104–107
Melanosis, neurocutaneous, 465–467
Meningioma
  benign, 205–208
  cerebellopontine angle, 115–117

intraventricular, 68–70
jugular foramen, 600–601
neurofibromatosis type II, 499–452
Meningitis
  bacterial, 223–226
    neonatal, 139–142
  carcinomatous, 220–222
  Coccidioides immitis, 227–229
  cryptococcal, with gelatinous pseudocysts, 187–190
  fungal, 227–229
  Haemophilus influenzae, 143–145
  pneumococcal, 223–226
  tuberculous, 165–168
Meningoencephalitis, herpes, neonatal, 135–138
Metastasis, 19–22
Microadenoma, pituitary, 49–51
Mitochondrial disorder, 358–361
Moyamoya disease, 315–319
MS. See Multiple sclerosis
Multiple acyl-CoA dehydrogenase deficiency, 370–373
Multiple sclerosis, 335–338
Mycotic aneurysm, with rupture, 237
Myelinolysis
  central pontine, 343–346

Nasopharyngeal adenoid cystic carcinoma, 620–622
Neonatal bacterial meningitis, 139–142
Neonatal herpes meningoencephalitis, 135–138
Neonatal hypoxic-ischemic injury, 311–314
Neuralgia, glossopharyngeal, 598–599
Neuritis
  Bell's palsy, 583–584
  herpetic, 565–567
  optic, 540–541
Neuroblastoma, olfactory, 532–534
Neurocutaneous melanosis, 465–467
Neurocysticercosis, 161–164
Neurocytoma, 65–67
Neurodegenerative/basal ganglia disorders, 395–421
Neuroectodermal tumor, primitive, 104–107
  supratentorial, 36–38
Neuroepithelial tumor, dysembryoplastic, 26–28
Neurofibromatosis
  type I, 445–448
  type II, 449–452
Neurosarcoidosis, 213–215, 535–537
Neurosyphilis, 194–197

Occipital cephalocele, 484–486
Occipital lobe infarction, 544–546
Olfactory neuroblastoma, 532–534
Olfactory neurosarcoidosis, 535–537
Oligodendroglioma, 10–12
Olivopontocerebellar atrophy, 416–418
OPCA. See Olivopontocerebellar atrophy
Optic nerve
  glioma, 542–543

neuritis, 540–541
septo-optic dysplasia, 478–480
Organic acidopathy, 370–373
Osmotic myelinolysis, 343–346
Osteomyelitis, skull base, 623–625

Papilloma, choroid plexus, 75–77
Parenchymal contusion, traumatic, 435–437
Parenchymal hematoma, 264–267
cavernous malformation, cerebellar peduncle, 272–276
Pelizaeus-Merzbacher disease, 366–369
Perineural disease
cranial nerve V, 571–573
cranial nerve VII, 589–591
Periventricular leukomalacia, 306–309
Phakomatoses, 443–468
Pilocytic astrocytoma, juvenile, 91–94
Pineoblastoma, 42–45
Pituitary cyst, 55–57
Pituitary macroadenoma, 52–54
Pituitary microadenoma, 49–51
Pneumococcal meningitis, 223–226
Poisoning
carbon monoxide, 404–407
Polymicrogyria, 518–521
Pontine glioma, 101–103
Pontine myelinolysis, 343–346
Post-ictal cerebral edema, reversible, 347–350
Putaminal hemorrhage, secondary to hypertension, 264–267

Radiation injury
cranial nerve III, 552–553
Rathke's cleft cyst, 55–57

Saccular aneurysm, 235–238
SAH. See Subarachnoid hemorrhage
Sarcoidosis, 213–215, 535–537
Schizencephaly, 522–524
Schwannoma
cranial nerve V, 568–570
cranial nerve VIII, 111–114, 593–594, 595–596
cranial nerve IX, 602–604
cranial nerve XI, 616–617
cranial nerve XII, 619
Sclerosis, medial temporal, 390–393
tuberous, 453–456
Septo-optic dysplasia, 478–480
Sickle cell disease, 325–328
Siderosis, superficial, 230–232
Skull base osteomyelitis, 623–625
SLE. See Systemic lupus erythematosus
Spasm, hemifacial, 585–586
Sturge-Weber syndrome, 461–464
Subarachnoid hemorrhage
aneurysmal, 235–238
perimesencephalic nonaneurysmal, 243–246

Subdural effusion, 143–145
Subdural empyema, 198–201
Subdural hematoma, 428–430
secondary to metastases, 209–212
secondary to non-accidental trauma, 438–441
Subependymal nodular heterotopia, 508–511
Subependymoma, 71–74
Supratentorial congenital malformations/syndromes, 469–486
Supratentorial neoplasm, 1–88
Systemic lupus erythematosus, 377–380

Takayasu arteritis, 302–305
Telangiectasia, capillary, 275
Thromboembolic occlusion, basilar artery, 256–258
Thrombosis, transverse sinus, 329–332
Tolosa-Hunt syndrome, 558
Toxins, exposure to, 351–353. See also Poisoning
Toxoplasmosis
AIDS-related, 183–186
congenital, 132–134
Transverse sinus thrombosis, 329–332
Trauma, 423–441
non-accidental, 438–441
Tuber cinereum, hamartoma of, 39–41
Tuberculosis, 165–168
Tuberous sclerosis, 453–456

Vascular compression, hemifacial spasm from, 585–586
Vascular malformation, 272–276, 277–281, 282–285,
286–289, 290–293
Vasculitis, 294–297, 302–305
Vein of Galen, aneurysmal malformation, 320–324
Venous infarction, 329–332
Venous malformation, 282–285
and cavernous malformation, 272–276
Venous sinus thrombosis, 329–332
Ventriculitis
bacterial, 154
cytomegalovirus, 191–193
Vertebral artery dissection, 260–263
lateral medullary infarction, 607–609
Vestibular schwannoma, 111–114, 593–594, 595–596
neurofibromatosis, type II with, 449–452
Viral encephalitis
cytomegalovirus, 129–131, 191–193
herpes simplex type I, 157–160
herpes simplex type II, 135–138
human immunodeficiency virus, 176–178
von Hippel-Lindau disease, 457–460

Watershed infarction, 252–255
Wernicke's encephalopathy, 386–389
White matter diseases, 333–373
Wilson's disease, 408–411

X-linked adrenoleukodystrophy, 354–357